Interdisciplinary Cancer Research

Volume 2

The "Interdisciplinary Cancer Research" series publishes comprehensive volumes on different cancers and presents the most updated and peer-reviewed articles on human cancers. Over the past decade, increased cancer research has greatly improved our understanding of the nature of cancerous cells which has led to the development of more effective therapeutic strategies to treat cancers. This translational series is of special value to researchers and practitioners working on cell biology, immunology, hematology, biochemistry, genetics, oncology and related fields.

Nima Rezaei
Editor

Cancer Treatment: An Interdisciplinary Approach

Springer

Editor
Nima Rezaei
Department of Clinical Immunology
Karolinska Institutet
Stockholm, Sweden

Cancer Immunology Project (CIP)
Universal Scientific Education and
Research Network (USERN)
Stockholm, Sweden

ISSN 2731-4561 ISSN 2731-457X (electronic)
Interdisciplinary Cancer Research
ISBN 978-3-031-43982-7 ISBN 978-3-031-43983-4 (eBook)
https://doi.org/10.1007/978-3-031-43983-4

This Springer imprint is published by the registered company Springer Nature Switzerland AG
The registered company address is: Gewerbestrasse 11, 6330 Cham, Switzerland

Paper in this product is recyclable.

Preface

Cancer treatment is a challenging issue, while the treatment modalities have extended from traditional surgery, chemotherapy, and radiation therapy to new therapeutic approaches, including targeted therapy, immunotherapy, stem cell transplantation, and hormone therapy. Therefore, an interdisciplinary approach is needed to find a better therapeutic protocol in order to increase the prognosis and quality of life of patients with cancer.

The Interdisciplinary Cancer Research series publishes comprehensive volumes on different cancers. It plans to present the most updated and peer-reviewed interdisciplinary chapters on cancers. This interdisciplinary book series is of special value to researchers and practitioners working on cell biology, immunology, hematology, biochemistry, genetics, oncology, and related fields. This is the main concept of Cancer Immunology Project (CIP) and Network of Immunity in Infection, Malignancy and Autoimmunity (NIIMA), which are two active interest groups of the Universal Scientific Education and Research Network (USERN).

The second volume of the book, entitled *Cancer Treatment: An Interdisciplinary Approach*, starts with an introduction on cancer, as a complex problem, requiring interdisciplinary research. Tumor immunology and immunotherapy are discussed in general in Chap. 2. New approaches targeting immuno-oncology and tumor microenvironment, tumor infiltrating lymphocytes, and CAR-T Cell therapy are discussed in Chaps. 2, 3, 4 and 5, while a complication of such novel treatment, such as immune checkpoint inhibitors, is presented in Chap. 6. Cancer stem cell as a target for immunotherapy and immunological properties of stem cell grafts are the subjects of Chaps. 7 and 8. Chapter 9 presents a general overview of recent development of quinoline derivatives as anticancer agents. Immunotherapy in certain conditions like COVID-19 and autoimmune diseases are explained in Chaps. 10 and 11. After discussion on effects of radiation on wound healing and cancer in Chap. 12, hyperbaric oxygen therapy is explained in Chap. 13. Interventional oncology techniques, future perspectives of phytochemicals, and integrated palliative cancer care are the main discussion of Chaps. 14, 15 and 16.

I hope that this interdisciplinary book will be comprehensible, cogent, and of special value for researchers and clinicians who wish to extend their knowledge on cancer treatment.

Stockholm, Sweden — Nima Rezaei

Contents

Cancer: A Complex Problem Requiring Interdisciplinary Research 1
Niloufar Yazdanpanah, Filip Dochy, Gary L. Darmstadt, Godefridus J. Peters, Abraham Tsitlakidis, Elias C. Aifantis, Artemi Cerda, Elisabetta Comini, Serge Brand, Manoj Gupta, Bruce D. Cheson, Sabu Thomas, Michael Tanzer, Ralf Weiskirchen, Federico Bella, Seyed-Mohammad Fereshtehnejad, Konstantina Nikita, Imran Ali, Koichi Kato, Alessandro Poggi, Ernest Chua Kian Jon, Idupulapati M. Rao, Xiaoming Tao, Ji-Huan He, Lingamallu Jagan Mohan Rao, Alexander Leemans, Alessio Pomponio, Alfredo Martínez Hernandez, Hamid Ahmadieh, Mohammad Ali Sahraian, Roya Kelishadi, Visith Thongboonkerd, Seema Bahinipati, Masakazu Toi, Matthias von Herrath, Frank Sellke, Steven Sherwood, George Perry, Juan J. Nieto, Sudhir Gupta, Tommaso Dorigo, Bahram Mobasher, Hans D. Ochs, and Nima Rezaei

Tumor Immunology and Immunotherapy 47
Thi Kim Anh Nguyen, Huu-Thinh Nguyen, and Sao-Mai Dam

New Approaches Targeting Immuno-oncology and Tumor Microenvironment 63
Di Zhu and Fenglian He

Tumor-infiltrating Lymphocytes as Markers of the Antitumor Therapy Efficacy: Myth or Reality? 91
Mikhail V. Kiselevskiy, Tatiana N. Zabotina, Elena V. Artamonova, A. N. Kozlov, Igor V. Samoylenko, Zaira G. Kadagidze, and Irina Zh. Shubina

Recent Innovative Approaches to Intensify the Efficacy and Safety of CAR-T Cell Therapy in Cancers 117
Safa Tahmasebi, Elnaz Khosh, Samaneh Rostami, and Nima Rezaei

An Updated Focus on Immune Checkpoint Inhibitors and Tubulointerstitial Nephritis 157
Daniela Picciotto, Carlo Genova, Francesca Costigliolo, Annarita Bottini, Giacomo Garibotto, Francesca Viazzi, and Pasquale Esposito

Cancer Stem Cell as a Target for Immunotherapeutic Approach 185
Kimia Kazemzadeh and Nima Rezaei

Immunological Properties of Manipulated Hematopoietic Stem Cell Grafts 199
Tahereh Rostami, Saeed Mohammadi, and Azadeh Kiumarsi

Recent Development of Quinoline Derivatives as Anticancer Agents: 2015–2022 217
Komalpreet Kaur, Nitish Kumar, Jatinder Vir Singh, Preet Mohinder Singh Bedi, and Harbinder Singh

Antitumor Immunotherapy: Effect of COVID-19 in Cancer Patients . . . 251
Irina Zh. Shubina, Irina O. Chikileva, and Nikolay Yu. Sokolov

The Use of Immunotherapy in Cancer Patients with Autoimmune Diseases 267
Chung-Shien Lee and Nagashree Seetharamu

The Effects of Low-Dose Non-ionizing and Ionizing Radiation on Wound Healing and Cancer 287
Raahilah Zahir Essa, Ming Tsuey Chew, David A. Bradley, Suat-Cheng Peh, and Sin-Yeang Teow

How Is Cancer Under the Sea? Hyperbaric Oxygen Therapy in Cancer 323
Amene Saghazadeh and Nima Rezaei

Interventional Oncology Techniques: A Primer for Non-users 343
Dimitrios K. Filippiadis, Evgenia Efthymiou, Athanasios Gianakis, George Charalampopoulos, and Stavros Spiliopoulos

Future Perspectives of Phytochemicals in Cancer Therapy 383
Bakiye Goker Bagca and Cigir Biray Avci

Integrated Palliative Cancer Care: From an Interdisciplinary Perspective 399
Amene Saghazadeh and Nima Rezaei

Correction to: Cancer: A Complex Problem Requiring Interdisciplinary Research 423
Niloufar Yazdanpanah, Filip Dochy, Gary L. Darmstadt, Godefridus J. Peters, Abraham Tsitlakidis, Elias C. Aifantis, Artemi Cerda, Elisabetta Comini, Serge Brand, Manoj Gupta, Bruce D. Cheson, Sabu Thomas, Michael Tanzer, Ralf Weiskirchen, Federico Bella, Seyed-Mohammad Fereshtehnejad, Konstantina Nikita, Imran Ali, Koichi Kato, Alessandro Poggi, Ernest Chua Kian Jon, Idupulapati M. Rao, Xiaoming Tao, Ji-Huan He, Lingamallu Jagan Mohan Rao, Alexander Leemans, Alessio Pomponio, Alfredo Martínez Hernandez, Hamid Ahmadieh, Mohammad Ali Sahraian, Roya Kelishadi, Visith Thongboonkerd, Seema Bahinipati, Masakazu Toi, Matthias von Herrath, Frank Sellke, Steven Sherwood, George Perry, Juan J. Nieto, Sudhir Gupta, Tommaso Dorigo, Bahram Mobasher, Hans D. Ochs, and Nima Rezaei

Index 425

About the Editor

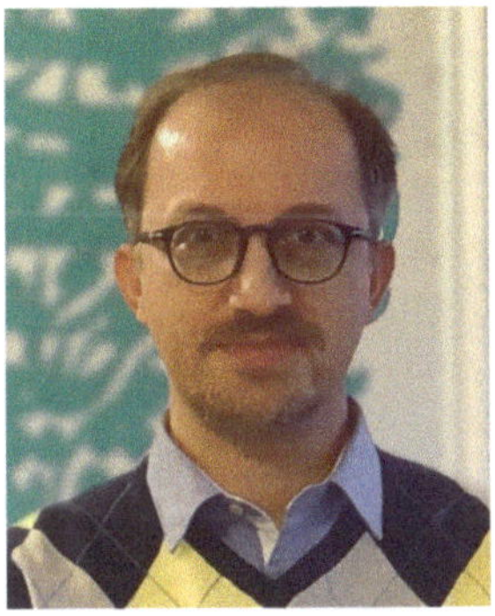

Nima Rezaei, MD, PhD Professor Nima Rezaei gained his medical degree (MD) from Tehran University of Medical Sciences and subsequently obtained an MSc in Molecular and Genetic Medicine and a PhD in Clinical Immunology and Human Genetics from the University of Sheffield, UK. He also spent a short-term fellowship of Pediatric Clinical Immunology and Bone Marrow Transplantation in the Newcastle General Hospital. Professor Rezaei is now the Full Professor of Immunology and Vice Dean of Research and Technologies, School of Medicine, Tehran University of Medical Sciences, and the co-founder and Head of the Research Center for Immunodeficiencies. He is also the Founder of Universal Scientific Education and Research Network (USERN). Prof. Rezaei has already been the Director of more than 100 research projects and has designed and participated in several international collaborative projects. Prof. Rezaei is the editor, editorial assistant, or editorial board member of more than 40 international journals. He has edited more than 50 international books, has presented more than 500 lectures/posters in congresses/meetings, and has published more than 1200 scientific papers in the international journals.

Cancer: A Complex Problem Requiring Interdisciplinary Research

Niloufar Yazdanpanah, Filip Dochy, Gary L. Darmstadt, Godefridus J. Peters, Abraham Tsitlakidis, Elias C. Aifantis, Artemi Cerda, Elisabetta Comini, Serge Brand, Manoj Gupta, Bruce D. Cheson, Sabu Thomas, Michael Tanzer, Ralf Weiskirchen, Federico Bella, Seyed-Mohammad Fereshtehnejad, Konstantina Nikita, Imran Ali, Koichi Kato, Alessandro Poggi, Ernest Chua Kian Jon, Idupulapati M. Rao, Xiaoming Tao, Ji-Huan He, Lingamallu Jagan Mohan Rao, Alexander Leemans, Alessio Pomponio, Alfredo Martínez Hernandez, Hamid Ahmadieh, Mohammad Ali Sahraian, Roya Kelishadi, Visith Thongboonkerd, Seema Bahinipati, Masakazu Toi, Matthias von Herrath, Frank Sellke, Steven Sherwood, George Perry, Juan J. Nieto, Sudhir Gupta, Tommaso Dorigo, Bahram Mobasher, Hans D. Ochs, and Nima Rezaei

Abstract

During decades of cancer research, different disciplines have made important contributions to the development of our knowledge about cancer. Identification of complex problems not being solved using a single discipline has directed scientists toward interdisciplinary approaches. Cancer is a complex problem that, regardless of great advances in different scientific fields, remains to be properly addressed. Early diagnosis, personalized treatment, minimum treatment side effects, optimal treatment outcomes, and effective preventive measures can be achievable by

The original version of this chapter was revised. The affiliation "Universal Scientific Education and Research Network (USERN); the World, Tehran, Iran" was corrected as "Universal Scientific Education and Research Network (USERN), https://usern.tums.ac.ir/" for all authors who were affiliated to it. A correction to this chapter can be found at https://doi.org/10.1007/16833_2023_173.

N. Yazdanpanah · N. Rezaei (✉)
Universal Scientific Education and Research Network (USERN), https://usern.tums.ac.ir/

School of Medicine, Tehran University of Medical Sciences, Tehran, Iran
e-mail: rezaei_nima@yahoo.com; rezaei_nima@tums.ac.ir

Interdisciplinary Cancer Research, https://doi.org/10.1007/16833_2022_116
Published online: 10 February 2023

adopting interdisciplinary approaches in cancer research. This chapter is an interdisciplinary collaboration of scientists from different fields of science, in which the contribution of different disciplines to cancer research is reviewed. In addition, the framework of cancer research in 2050 is depicted as a guide for future research.

Keywords

Cancer · Complex problem · Diagnosis · Interdisciplinary · Research · Transdisciplinary · Treatment

---

F. Dochy
Universal Scientific Education and Research Network (USERN), https://usern.tums.ac.ir/

High Impact Learning Academy, Learning and Development Department, Brussels, Belgium

G. L. Darmstadt
Universal Scientific Education and Research Network (USERN), https://usern.tums.ac.ir/

Department of Pediatrics, Stanford University School of Medicine, Stanford, CA, USA

G. J. Peters
Universal Scientific Education and Research Network (USERN), https://usern.tums.ac.ir/

Laboratory Medical Oncology, Amsterdam University Medical Centers, Location VUMC, Amsterdam, the Netherlands

Department of Biochemistry, Medical University of Gdańsk, Gdańsk, Poland

A. Tsitlakidis
Universal Scientific Education and Research Network (USERN), https://usern.tums.ac.ir/

Aristotle University of Thessaloniki, Thessaloniki, Greece

Department of Neurosurgery, KAT Attica General Hospital, Kifisia, Greece

E. C. Aifantis
Universal Scientific Education and Research Network (USERN), https://usern.tums.ac.ir/

Aristotle University of Thessaloniki, Thessaloniki, Greece

Emeritus, Michigan Technological University, Houghton, MI, USA

Mercator Fellow Friedrich-Alexander University, Erlangen-Nürnberg, Fürth, Germany

A. Cerda
Universal Scientific Education and Research Network (USERN), https://usern.tums.ac.ir/

Soil Erosion and Degradation Research Group, Department of Geography, Valencia University, Blasco Ibàñez, Valencia, Spain

E. Comini
Universal Scientific Education and Research Network (USERN), https://usern.tums.ac.ir/

SENSOR Laboratory, University of Brescia, Brescia, Italy

S. Brand
Universal Scientific Education and Research Network (USERN), https://usern.tums.ac.ir/

University of Basel, Psychiatric Hospital (UPK), Basel, Switzerland

1 Cancer: A Complex Problem

Cancer describes a wide spectrum of malignant conditions, as a result of molecular defects and genetic alterations, which, when not properly treated, progress into a life-threatening disease. Cancer has always been a complicated problem and one of the main causes of death in developed countries, challenging the most advanced treatments. Current treatment options include surgery (in cases of resectable tumors or for palliative purposes), chemotherapy, radiotherapy, and, most recently, targeted agents, immunotherapy, and other novel methods of treatment, of which some are based on targeting the DNA in cancer cells, impairing cell proliferation and

M. Gupta
Universal Scientific Education and Research Network (USERN), https://usern.tums.ac.ir/

Department of Mechanical Engineering, National University of Singapore, Singapore, Singapore

B. D. Cheson
Universal Scientific Education and Research Network (USERN), https://usern.tums.ac.ir/

Lymphoma Research Foundation, New York, NY, USA

S. Thomas
Universal Scientific Education and Research Network (USERN), https://usern.tums.ac.ir/

School of Energy Materials, Mahatma Gandhi University, Kottayam, Kerala, India

M. Tanzer
Universal Scientific Education and Research Network (USERN), https://usern.tums.ac.ir/

McGill University Hospital Centre, Montreal, Quebec, Canada

R. Weiskirchen
Universal Scientific Education and Research Network (USERN), https://usern.tums.ac.ir/

RWTH University Hospital Aachen, Institute of Molecular Pathobiochemistry, Experimental Gene Therapy and Clinical Chemistry (IFMPEGKC), Aachen, Germany

F. Bella
Universal Scientific Education and Research Network (USERN), https://usern.tums.ac.ir/

Department of Applied Science and Technology, Politecnico di Torino, Corso Duca degli Abruzzi, Turin, Italy

S.-M. Fereshtehnejad
Universal Scientific Education and Research Network (USERN), https://usern.tums.ac.ir/

Division of Neurology, Faculty of Medicine, University of Ottawa, Ottawa, ON, Canada

Division of Clinical Geriatrics, NVS Department, Karolinska Institutet, Stockholm, Sweden

K. Nikita
Universal Scientific Education and Research Network (USERN), https://usern.tums.ac.ir/

School of Electrical and Computer Engineering, National Technical University of Athens, Athens, Greece

I. Ali
Universal Scientific Education and Research Network (USERN), https://usern.tums.ac.ir/

Department of Chemistry, Jamia Millia Islamia (Central University), New Delhi, India

metabolism or inducing cell death. Novel cytotoxic agents are commonly designed to target essential steps in cellular proliferation (Bailly 2014). Nevertheless, this selectivity does not always meet the expectations, since the targeted pathways are often involved in the function of normal cells. This (partial) lack of selectivity can result in various adverse effects that in some cases cause serious disabilities for the patient. In addition, treatment with cytotoxic agents can lead to the development of resistant cancerous cells. More recently, radiotherapy and, especially, cytotoxic

K. Kato
Universal Scientific Education and Research Network (USERN), https://usern.tums.ac.ir/

Exploratory Research Center on Life and Living Systems (ExCELLS) and Institute for Molecular Science (IMS), National Institutes of Natural Sciences, Okazaki, Aichi, Japan

A. Poggi
Universal Scientific Education and Research Network (USERN), https://usern.tums.ac.ir/

Molecular Oncology and Angiogenesis Unit, IRCCS Ospedale Policlinico San Martino, Genoa, Italy

E. C. K. Jon
Universal Scientific Education and Research Network (USERN), https://usern.tums.ac.ir/

Department of Mechanical Engineering, National University of Singapore, Singapore, Singapore

I. M. Rao
Universal Scientific Education and Research Network (USERN), https://usern.tums.ac.ir/

Alliance of Bioversity International and International Center for Tropical Agriculture, Cali, Colombia

International Centre of Insect Physiology and Ecology (ICIPE), Nairobi, Kenya

X. Tao
Universal Scientific Education and Research Network (USERN), https://usern.tums.ac.ir/

Research Center of Intelligent Wearable Systems, The Hong Kong Polytechnic University, Hong Kong, China

J.-H. He
Universal Scientific Education and Research Network (USERN), https://usern.tums.ac.ir/

School of Science, Xi'an University of Architecture & Technology, Xi'an, People's Republic of China

L. J. M. Rao
Universal Scientific Education and Research Network (USERN), https://usern.tums.ac.ir/

Spices and Flavor Science Department, CSIR-Central Food Technological Research Institute, Mysore, India

A. Leemans
Universal Scientific Education and Research Network (USERN), https://usern.tums.ac.ir/

Image Sciences Institute, University Medical Center Utrecht, Utrecht, the Netherlands

A. Pomponio
Universal Scientific Education and Research Network (USERN), https://usern.tums.ac.ir/

Dipartimento di Meccanica, Matematica e Management, Politecnico di Bari, Bari, Italy

chemotherapy have been replaced by agents that target the cell surface (e.g., monoclonal antibodies), the intracellular pathways (e.g., protein kinase inhibitors), and the tumor microenvironment (e.g., immunomodulatory agents and checkpoint inhibitors). In addition, newer immunotherapies have emerged, such as bispecific antibodies and cellular therapies, including chimeric antigen receptor (CAR) T-cell.

Importantly, the side effects of some therapies can be so severe that they significantly reduce the quality of life of the patient. It is astonishing that despite rapid

A. M. Hernandez
Universal Scientific Education and Research Network (USERN), https://usern.tums.ac.ir/

Center for Nutrition Research, University of Navarra, Navarra, Spain

H. Ahmadieh
Universal Scientific Education and Research Network (USERN), https://usern.tums.ac.ir/

Ophthalmic Research Center, Research Institute for Ophthalmology and Vision Science, Shahid Beheshti University of Medical Sciences, Tehran, Iran

M. A. Sahraian
Universal Scientific Education and Research Network (USERN), https://usern.tums.ac.ir/

Multiple Sclerosis Research Center, Neuroscience Institute, Tehran University of Medical Sciences, Tehran, Iran

R. Kelishadi
Universal Scientific Education and Research Network (USERN), https://usern.tums.ac.ir/

Department of Pediatrics, Child Growth and Development Research Center, Research Institute for Primordial Prevention of Non-Communicable Disease, Isfahan University of Medical Sciences, Isfahan, Iran

V. Thongboonkerd
Universal Scientific Education and Research Network (USERN), https://usern.tums.ac.ir/

Medical Proteomics Unit, Office for Research and Development, Faculty of Medicine Siriraj Hospital, Mahidol University, Bangkok, Thailand

S. Bahinipati
Universal Scientific Education and Research Network (USERN), https://usern.tums.ac.ir/

Indian Institute of Technology Bhubaneswar, Satya Nagar, Bhubaneswar, Odisha, India

M. Toi
Universal Scientific Education and Research Network (USERN), https://usern.tums.ac.ir/

Department of Breast Surgery, Kyoto University Graduate School of Medicine, Kyoto, Japan

M. von Herrath
Universal Scientific Education and Research Network (USERN), https://usern.tums.ac.ir/

Center for Autoimmunity and Inflammation, La Jolla Institute for Immunology, La Jolla, CA, USA

F. Sellke
Universal Scientific Education and Research Network (USERN), https://usern.tums.ac.ir/

Warren Alpert Medical School, Brown University, Providence, RI, USA

Division of Cardiothoracic Surgery, Rhode Island Hospital, Providence, RI, USA

progress in medical sciences over the last decades, a less toxic and more specific alternative therapy has not yet been developed.

Cancer is characterized by structural and behavioral alterations of cells and impaired interactions with the microenvironment in the context of genetic and epigenetic instabilities that are integrated into a set of environmental factors. Accordingly, the definition of cancer is quite complex, as it originates from a variety of disciplinary points of views. Perhaps cancer could be better described as a disturbance in cell biology that shows certain traits (Hanahan and Weinberg 2000, 2011; Hanahan 2022). Modern biology has improved our understanding of cell biology, cellular features, the molecular level understanding of living things, and interactions with the environment. These novel ideas have resulted in the creation of new medical specialties and subspecialties. Genetic studies not only address cell formation but also more broadly focus on the function of the entire genome. Mathematical, physical, and computational studies have attempted to model cancer as a complex system to facilitate cancer studies and to predict cancer behavior. The environmental science, in close collaboration with medical, biological, and chemical sciences, targets the risk factors and helps prevention of cancer. Thus, a multidisciplinary approach involving chemical, medical, biological, and formal sciences (which the latter include computer sciences, mathematics, statistics, artificial intelligence, etc.) is in a position to open new windows toward understanding and combating cancer by developing new strategies of treatments.

S. Sherwood
Universal Scientific Education and Research Network (USERN), https://usern.tums.ac.ir/

Climate Change Research Centre, UNSW Sydney, Kensington, NSW, Australia

G. Perry
Department of Neuroscience, Developmental and Regenerative Biology, University of Texas at San Antonio, San Antonio, TX, USA

J. J. Nieto
Universal Scientific Education and Research Network (USERN), https://usern.tums.ac.ir/

CITMAga, University of Santiago de Compostela, A Coruña, Spain

S. Gupta
Universal Scientific Education and Research Network (USERN), https://usern.tums.ac.ir/

Division of Basic and Clinical Immunology, Medical Sciences C, University of California, Irvine, CA, USA

T. Dorigo
Universal Scientific Education and Research Network (USERN), https://usern.tums.ac.ir/

Istituto Nazionale di Fisica Nucleare (INFN), Via Francesco Marzolo, Sezione di Padova, Italy

B. Mobasher
Universal Scientific Education and Research Network (USERN), https://usern.tums.ac.ir/

Department of Physics & Astronomy, University of California, Riverside, CA, USA

H. D. Ochs
Universal Scientific Education and Research Network (USERN), https://usern.tums.ac.ir/

Department of Pediatrics, Seattle Children's Research Institute, University of Washington School of Medicine, Seattle, WA, USA

While medical treatment is expected to play a leading role in combatting cancer and improving the quality of life of patients, psychological and social factors, such as mental health and family support, and art and music therapy also play a role in easing the pain and promoting optimal management of cancer patients (Yazdanpanah et al. 2022).

In this chapter, we undertake a comprehensive overview of integrated and multidisciplinary science-based development of a multidimensional approach to cancer. The aim is to develop new strategies for cancer research and treatment that will cover the next three decades, using input from different disciplines suggested by experts and top scientists in different fields of science.

2 An Interdisciplinary Approach Toward Understanding Cancer

2.1 Biological, Chemical, and Environmental Sciences in Cancer Research

Studying the underlying mechanisms of carcinogenesis, cancer progression, behavior of cancer cells, cancer metabolism, and genetics is the fundamental of cancer research. While this approach is taken by the biological sciences, different scientific entities have entered the field to accelerate the progress through interdisciplinary and transdisciplinary collaborations.

Cell biology provides the framework on which cancers emerge and progress. It is generally accepted that most, if not all, types of cancer share some unifying capabilities: to sustain growth signals, to evade the suppression of proliferation, to circumvent immune responses, to remove inherent limits in genome replication, to invade tissues and metastasize, to access or even to induce the formation of blood vessels (angiogenesis), to resist apoptosis, and to dysregulate the metabolism of the cell. Moreover, some general characteristics that enable carcinogenesis have been proposed: the instability of the genome through accumulating mutations, the presence of inflammation, the reprogramming of the cell through epigenetic alterations, and the role of various microorganisms (Hanahan and Weinberg 2000, 2011; Hanahan 2022). Attempts to overcome the complexity of cancer by conceptualizing the different forms of cancer along the same traits have extensively assisted researchers in understanding the mechanisms of cancer progression and defining new targets for cancer treatment. These new insights led the way for the development of more selective, targeted, and effective drugs, diagnostic modalities, and surgical tools. Another contribution of biological sciences to cancer research is the focus on cell surface properties and cellular interactions with the microenvironment and intracellular signaling. Cancer cells' surface properties play an important role in the biologic activity of cancer; like the lotus effect (Li et al. 2021), an unsmooth surface makes the cancer cell more active to obtain its nutritional requirement from its environment.

Chemotherapy, a principal component of cancer treatment, is primarily defined as the administration of chemical substances targeting essential mechanisms required for cancer progression or providing palliative effects, in order to ameliorate/treat and, potentially, cure the disease. Sustainable energy homeostasis, provision of balanced nutrient dense pathogen-free food and a safe source of water, and exploring various biochemical pathways of carcinogenesis are the focus of chemical sciences in the field of oncology, aiming to reduce the risk of cancer development and progression. The interest in proteomics and in the study of the overall protein content of the cell originated from the collaboration of scientists combining chemistry and cancer research. This contribution is not surprising since chemistry has traditionally played a pivotal role in drug discovery. Hence, cancer research has deep roots in chemistry and chemical sciences.

The biosensors are innovative tools with various benefits in drug discovery, biomedicine, food industry, and diagnostic tool design. A biosensor combines a biological sensing element with a physiochemical detector (transducer). These devices assess biochemical reactions by producing signals according to the concentration of a specific analyte (Rasooly and Jacobson 2006). Biosensors have drawn considerable interest from clinicians since they are cost-effective, rapid, easy to use, and independent of the operator's skill. In addition, the sample preparation is performed within the biosensor system, and the system has the power of multi-analyte testing. Collectively, biosensors, as the products of chemical and physical science studies, have emerged as promising devices for the early diagnosis of cancer (Tothill 2009). A major challenge for sensor systems designed for cancer diagnosis is the ability to reveal the relevant biomarkers better than the traditional analytical systems. In this field, not only biosensor but also chemical sensor technologies have been proposed and evaluated for clinical applications. To address the specific requirements for this complex analysis, recent efforts have been directed to develop sensor arrays and other new solutions (e.g., lab-on-a-chip), in which sampling, preparation, high-throughput analysis, and reporting are integrated. The ability of parallelization, miniaturization, and a high degree of automation are the focus of new developments and will be supported by nanotechnology approaches.

In addition to biomarker identification in body tissues and fluidics, another interesting possibility is the detection of cancer markers in exhaled breath or skin odor. Generally, there is more than one single marker in the PPB (parts per billion) range associated with the presence of disease. The distinction in the case of lung cancer was achieved by a combination of 22 volatile organic compounds (Phillips et al. 1999). Chemical sensors and machine learning techniques were used to develop a breath test for lung cancer (Huang et al. 2018). The diagnostic accuracy was assessed using the pathological reports as the reference standard. The combination of the sensor array technique and machine learning was able to detect lung cancer with high accuracy.

Finding the volatile compound biomarkers and the correlation with diseases is extremely important as it will be an easy and fast screening tool for cancer monitoring. Finally, chemical sensor research is pivotal to obtain the desired information in real time. Reliable and fast diagnostic systems will allow the detection of cancer at an early stage; this in turn will lead to more favorable prognosis and responsiveness to therapy.

The recognition and extraction of natural therapeutic compounds from plants, attributed to different branches of chemical sciences, have substantially improved cancer treatment research. For instance, curcumin, resveratrol, paclitaxel, kaempferol, vincristine, and silymarin are extracted from natural compounds, and several of these compounds have proven to be effective in different cancer types, while, for some of compounds, the efficacy in patients still has to be demonstrated (Prasad et al. 2016; Colone et al. 2020).

For the last two decades, ionic liquids (ILs) have been designed as "green" solvents and have been used extensively in various applications including drug delivery and drug formulation. ILs have unusual physicochemical properties including excellent thermal and chemical stability, negligible vapor pressure, low flammability, nonvolatility, high ionic conductivity, recyclability, and broad solvation abilities with organic and inorganic compounds. These extraordinary properties have rendered ILs very useful in biomedical applications (biocatalysis, separation of compounds, energy storage, conversion, etc.) as well as in pharmaceutical applications as a potential component of drug formulations (Chowdhury et al. 2018; Albadawi et al. 2021). In addition, natural deep eutectic solvents (NADES) are highly biocompatible materials designed to serve as carrier molecules that transport drugs to a specific site without any or with minimal side effects; it is a nontoxic solvent prepared by secondary metabolites and does not affect the drug release mechanism. Secondary metabolites such as phenolics, terpenoids, flavonoids, and other natural compounds are crucial for medicinal applications (Pereira et al. 2019; Sun et al. 2020). Compared to organic solvents, the use of NADES has gained attention in the synthesis of carrier systems.

In 1889, Stephen Paget put forward the "seed and soil" hypothesis, which was inspired by the agricultural experience of providing optimal conditions for a seed to grow (Paget 1989). In this theory, Paget tried to rationalize the predilection of tumor metastasis to invade specific body sites. This approach recognizes the importance of the optimal interaction of migrating cancer cells with the surrounding microenvironment of the target destination. In line with this, anticancer therapeutic agents are designed to target the cells, such as some cytotoxic agents, or are aimed at the microenvironment, such as inhibitors of angiogenesis. This approach targets specifically the two principal components of metastasis, according to the "seed and soil" theory. Although initially controversial, there is now consensus in regards to the "anatomical-mechanical" hypothesis (Langley and Fidler 2011), and the "seed and soil" hypothesis is expected to generate interdisciplinary studies that will result in new initiatives using these complex systems. Seed and soil are the cornerstones for the identification of future food systems that are linked to nutrition and health conditions of cancer patients.

The role of environmental sciences in cancer research is not limited to determining environmental risk factors and provides relevant recommendations for cancer prevention. Water sanitation, soil properties, air pollution, and sun radiation are some of the topics discussed by environmental scientists in close collaboration with chemical and, to some extents, biological scientists. One of the most remarkable purposes of environmental sciences is to understand the environment itself and the stress humans place on it that could result in the emergence of factors affecting the incidence of cancer. In addition, the field could work with health scientists to better understand environmental variations in cancer rates. Air pollution and ultraviolet radiation are frequently associated with lung and skin cancer, respectively (Vineis et al. 2007; Narayanan et al. 2010; Josyula et al. 2015). Ultraviolet radiation levels vary significantly with climate, seasonal changes, location, the ozone layer, and air pollution (Barnard and Wenny 2010; Bais et al. 2015; Rafieepour et al. 2015), resulting in different incident rates of some specific cancers in different geographical locations. Detecting risk factors that are more problematic in specific locations could help in developing preventive measures for inhabitants, starting early during childhood to prevent cancer initiation and progression.

Cancer disease and soil properties have been discussed since the 1950s. The pioneer observations of Griffith and Davies (1954) uncovered key information to understand that the health of the soil is related to the health of the planet Earth and of humans. Man et al. (2013) and Davie-Martin et al. (2017) found that soils contaminated with polycyclic aromatic hydrocarbon increase the risk of cancer. Soil is an organized body with different minerals and organic matters, and its composition can induce various rates of cancer. McKinley et al. (2013) researched how some trace elements resulted in an increase in cancer cases. Apart from polycyclic aromatic hydrocarbons, which are recognized as a principal cause of cancer in different regions of the world such as China (Yun et al. 2017), Iran (Mohit et al. 2019), and Nigeria (Inam et al. 2016; Enuneku et al. 2021), there are additional substances in soil that have clearly an impact on the incidence of cancer. Semnani et al. (2010) discovered that selenium in soil contributes to the development of esophageal cancer, and Lee et al. (2016) also found similar results when soil was polluted with nickel. Mohajer et al. observed (Mohajer et al. 2013) that lead and cadmium in soil was associated with increased prevalence of gastrointestinal cancer in the Isfahan region of Iran. Su et al. (2010) reported that nickel and arsenic increased the incidence of oral cancers in Taiwan. Samaila et al. (2022) demonstrated that heavy metals induce higher cancer indexes, and Tang et al. (2014), in a study of Chinese females, found that breast cancer was related to the dietary intake of residual DDT from soil used by agriculture. Most of the research has been performed in soil polluted as a consequence of human activities, but some others found that there are natural elements that can cause cancer. Njinga and Tshivhase (2016) reported that the natural gamma radioactivity found in soil contaminated by the Tudor Shaft mine in South Africa induced higher cancer risk. Granero and Domingo (2002) recognized that increased levels of metals present in soils of Alcalá de Henares in Spain were associated with human health risks, as did Nde et al. (2021) in South Africa, in the upper Crocodile River catchment, and Ibikunle et al. (2018) in Southwestern Nigeria blamed natural radionuclides.

Certain plants have traditionally been seen as a solution to cancer (Cragg and Newman 2005; Desai et al. 2008; Tariq et al. 2017; Buyel 2018). Fauna has also been considered as a source of possible solutions (Wali et al. 2019), although some types of meat, particularly processed meat, might be a cause of cancers (Taylor et al. 2007; Rohrmann et al. 2013; Turner and Lloyd 2017). The consumption of fruits and vegetables, on the contrary, is recognized as a preventive factor against cancer (Terry et al. 2001; Chan et al. 2009). Race and ethnicity play a role, but geography has been shown to be a key issue to understand the cancer distribution. Sariego (2009) observed geographical patterns of breast cancer in the USA, Tan et al. (2016) researched cancer genomics and evaluated the role of ethnicity and geography, and Hongo et al. (2009) explored the incidence of esophageal cancer and found differences between the Orient and the Occident. In addition, Grossi et al. (2003) comprehensively reviewed the control geography exerts on cancer.

Water is another key element in nature that can contribute to understanding the distribution of cancer. Different elements were found in drinking water to increase the risk of cancer. Ferreccio et al. (2000) found that lung cancer and arsenic concentrations in drinking water in Chile were relevant to understand local cancer distribution. Page et al. (1976) found drinking water from the Mississippi River related to cancer mortality in Louisiana, which was attributed to the presence of organic chemicals or some unknown carcinogens in the water. Zhitkovich (2011) pointed out that chromium was the key agent to understand the positive relationship between drinking water and cancer. Hopenhayn-Rich et al. 1998) point out that mortality from lung and kidney cancer was associated with arsenic in the drinking water of Cordoba in Argentina. In addition, McGeehin et al. 1993) demonstrated a correlation between bladder cancer and water disinfection methods.

Some types of cancer are attributed to endemic infections in particular regions of the globe. *Schistosoma haematobium* and *Opisthorchis viverrini* cause chronic parasitic infections that are associated with an increased risk of bladder cancer and cholangiocarcinoma, respectively (Khurana et al. 2005). Some bacterial infections increase the susceptibility to some types of cancer, for example, chronic infection with *Helicobacter pylori* has been associated with gastric cancer, while *Salmonella* spp. with gallbladder carcinoma and colon carcinoma (de Martel et al. 2012; Plummer et al. 2016; van Elsland and Neefjes 2018). In addition, fungal infections can lead to malignancy; liver cancer following infection with *Aspergillus flavus* is an example (van Elsland and Neefjes 2018). Strategies to provide healthy food and safe water supply and improved sanitation facilities potentially reduce the risk of malignancies by decreasing the incidence of infections.

Finally, the overuse of pesticides in agriculture and healthcare is associated with different malignancies, including leukemia, lymphoma, neuroblastoma, gastric cancer, prostate cancer, lung cancer, and colorectal cancer (Bassil et al. 2007; Sabarwal et al. 2018). Investigating the proper amount of a given pesticide and maintaining acceptable safety for human beings and efficiency of the chemical compound and avoiding the induction of resistance to the pesticide are areas covered by environmental sciences in collaboration with biological, chemical, and medical sciences.

2.2 Physics in Cancer Research

The area of cancer research has witnessed the impact of physical sciences on cancer evolution, attitudes, and potential treatments. A pioneering use of physics in understanding biological phenomena is the random mutation hypothesis, leading to bacteriophage resistance, developed in 1943 by Max Delbrück and Salvador Luria (Luria and Delbrück 1943). This hypothesis developed into a model, which is currently used to evaluate whether cancers become resistant to chemotherapy. Meanwhile, the role of physical sciences in cancer treatment is undeniable. Chemotherapy and radiotherapy, two fundamental components of cancer treatment, are linked to physical studies. In addition, physics and mathematics contribute to the design and development of treatment facilities, as well as their application algorithms. Recent developments in personalized cancer medicine are attributed to high-throughput sequencing methods, which are the result of tight collaboration between physical and medical sciences.

Principles derived from studies based on physics have disentangled some features of cancer and displayed them in simplified models. Notable examples of such features are cancer mechanobiology, evolutionary traits of cancer, and information coding and transfer (Michor et al. 2011; Wirtz et al. 2011). Moreover, development of visualization and computational simulation methods has considerably supported cancer research. Photodynamic therapy (PDT), which is the application of light-activated therapeutic agents, was firstly developed with the aim of targeting localized solid tumors. However, PDT is currently used for a number of cancers, central serous chorioretinopathy (CSCR), dermatological diseases, and localized antibiotic resistant infections (Wilson and Patterson 2008). The application of PDT and nuclear medicine for cancer treatment and diagnosis originates from physical studies, which revealed promising insights for the clinical management of cancer (Amaldi 2005; Wilson and Patterson 2008).

Physical scientists are experts of complex systems incorporating unexpected behaviors/events following the interaction of numerous different small components. These systems represent remarkable local variations. Indeed, cancer appropriately fits these criteria. Therefore, adopting an interdisciplinary approach of physical, mathematical, and medical sciences in exploring and confronting cancer might simplify the complexity of cancer and provide a practical set of information, tools, and technologies.

Materials Science and Nanobiotechnology

The understanding and use of relevant materials in cancer management is at a relatively early stage in spite of years of active research worldwide. The interaction of materials, organic and inorganic, with cancer cells is an explored but relatively less well-understood area where much insight needs to be further developed. In particular, the development of nanotechnology, including nanomaterials, for diagnosis, treatment, and prevention of cancer has shown tremendous promises. The main potentials of nanotechnology include, but are not limited to, the following (McNamara and Tofail 2017; Sahoo et al. 2020; Das et al. 2021):

- Ability of nanodevices to interact with biomolecules to assist in cancer detection and treatment development
- Use of nanodevices in early detection of cancer
- Monitoring cancer progression/regression
- Ability of tuning nanoparticles for cancer treatment in targeted fashion
- Cancer therapy using nanoparticles-based drugs

Nanobiotechnology is the integration of chemical, physical, and biological sciences that holds great promises in the diagnosis, drug design, drug delivery, and treatment of different complex diseases, including cancer. The introduction of nanomaterials, nanocarriers, and nanoparticles has the potential to overcome some challenges of drug delivery, such as the optimal pharmacokinetics of therapeutic agents. Nanocarriers may ensure an ideal half-life of drugs in the human body, may avoid probable toxicities, and improve penetration through biological barriers, leading to new opportunities for drug delivery systems (Mitchell et al. 2021). Nevertheless, potential challenges exist concerning the proper application and safety of these materials (De Jong and Borm 2008). A close collaboration of biologists, chemists, material engineers, and medical specialists is required to overcome the existing challenges.

The fractal geometry of cancer cells is one of the key factors for the success of therapeutic regimens (He 2008). Nanotechnological tools are now available to make cancer cells inactive. In brief, due to the high surface energy of cancer cells, nanoparticles can be absorbed onto the cancer cell surface, inhibiting nutrition, thus rendering it metabolically inactive.

Soft and condensed matter physics have emerged as a rapidly growing field in medical research with a wide spectrum of applications. For instance, physical studies on condensed matters have resulted in nuclear magnetic resonance technology that has initiated the development of magnetic resonance imaging (MRI), in DNA manipulation via latex beads and optical traps for treatment purposes, and to advanced drug delivery to the nuclei of cancer cells using star-shaped gold nanoparticles (Jurgons et al. 2006; Naffar-Abu-Amara et al. 2008). An example for soft matter physics is its usefulness in studying the mechanical traits of cancer cell cytoskeleton to figure out how the cytoskeleton self-organizes and rapidly switches through the dynamic instabilities of polymers to induce polarization in the cancer cells (Gonzalez-Rodriguez et al. 2012; Tsukanov and Psakhie 2016).

Wearable technology is an emerging technology that has changed the way of life. Nanotechnology has greatly contributed to advances in wearable technology. In addition to their traditional features, wearable systems have high levels of intelligence. They can effectively see; feel; listen; talk; learn new things; memorize information; display pictures; communicate with others via electronic media, mobile telephones or the Internet; lift weight; and even provide their own power. Development of intelligent wearable technology offers ample opportunities in cancer research (Iqbal et al. 2016).

Flexible, especially fibrous structured, comfortable intelligent wearable systems have been regarded as the major direction of wearable technology development, representing a hot interdisciplinary research field. Most successful examples are intelligent wearable electronic devices for continuous monitoring of physical, physiological, and mental health conditions, communicating with medical professionals, and assisting in establishing a diagnosis and administering drugs. Another group includes assistive wearable systems for advising, healing, mobility enhancing, pain managing, and communicating, as well as mental/physical stress reducing during preventive, restorative, supportive, and palliative phases of patients undergoing cancer treatment (Iqbal et al. 2016; Godfrey et al. 2018).

Mechanics

Biomechanics is the interdisciplinary scientific field that applies the principles of mechanics, i.e., the study of the deformation and translocation of materials on the structure and function of biological systems (Hatze 1974). It involves the study of mechanical processes in a wide spectrum of biological structures, from macromolecules and cells to tissues and multicellular organisms. Specifically, mechanomics (i.e., the study of the interaction between biological and biomechanical processes (Wang et al. 2014)) has attracted the attention of cancer research (Suresh 2007), as the mechanical interactions between the extracellular matrix (ECM) and cancer cells are associated with cell aggressiveness and proliferation (Mouw et al. 2014), cytoskeleton remodeling (Yim et al. 2010), and ECM reorganization (Levental et al. 2009), resulting in the progression of the disease.

As an example, mechanomics has been studied in gliomas, a group of brain tumors. The influence of ECM stiffness on glioma cell aggressiveness has been explored using cell cultures in biomimetic scaffolds simulating the ECM of the brain. This has provided evidence for the influence of the mechanical properties of the ECM on the motility of glioma cells. For instance, on two-dimensional substrates, stiffer scaffolds were associated with more aggressive glioma cells (Thomas and DiMilla 2000; Ulrich et al. 2009), an indication of the role of a stiff substrate on the cell surface in cell engagement and cell motility. On the other hand, three-dimensional substrates with stiffer scaffolds were associated with less aggressive glioma cells (Ananthanarayanan et al. 2011), an indication that the dense extracellular matrix inhibits cell migration (Mair et al. 2018). In order to overcome such hurdles, glioma cells resort to the overproduction of matrix metalloproteinases (Nakada et al. 2001; Rao 2003), enzymes that disintegrate the normal ECM, and induce the turnover and secretion of collagen, fibronectin, tenascin-C, vitronectin (Deryugina and Bourdon 1996), hyaluronic acid (Delpech et al. 1993), and laminin (Tysnes et al. 1999). Consequently, the ECM provides glioma cells both with mechanical stimuli and with a substrate for their adhesion and facilitation of their migration. Likewise, glioma cells remodel the normal brain ECM to their benefit. As a result, structural deregulation occurs, influencing the mechanical properties of the tissue and disturbing mechanical homeostasis of the microenvironment.

Mechanomics and biomechanics offer an emerging perspective on cancer pathophysiology. Along with the well-studied biological hallmarks, a set of physical traits of cancer has been recognized, namely, abnormalities in terms of solid stress, interstitial fluid pressure, cell and tissue stiffness, and disruption of tissue architecture (Nia et al. 2020). Together with other interdisciplinary research approaches in cancer research, it appears that mechanomics will further enrich our knowledge regarding oncogenesis, neoplastic infiltration, and cancer progression. Specifically, mechanomics is expected to contribute to models of oncogenesis and progression of these malignancies (Bondiau et al. 2008; Mierke 2014) to the evolution of the population of cancer cells (Aifantis 2016) and the role of mechanics at the cellular and tissue level. Moreover, cancer mechanobiology provides a novel point of view on the biology of tumors and the development of tools with clinical oncological applications. An important contribution of the study of cancer mechanics could be the accumulation and interpretation of experimental data, necessary to develop and validate models for real-time imaging studies (Liu et al. 2014). Such models are required to achieve accurate surgical navigation systems. Moreover, cancer biomechanics could facilitate the development of haptic devices for robotic applications in support of oncological surgery (Tegin and Wikander 2005; Uribe et al. 2009; Marcus et al. 2014).

2.3 Mathematics in Cancer Research

Cancer prevention, diagnosis, treatment, management, and prognosis have significantly evolved during recent decades. As a result of mathematical modeling of different cancer cell features, our understanding of tumor behavior has grown tremendously. Mathematical models are classified in two main groups, descriptive and mechanistic. Descriptive models focus on dynamics of cancer cell populations, whereas mechanistic models attempt to uncover underlying mechanisms of tumor progression (Araujo and McElwain 2004; Kozusko and Bourdeau 2007). The history of the mathematical modeling of cancer dates back to 1954, when Armitage and Doll introduced the multistage theory of cancer development (Armitage and Doll 1954). This first model of carcinogenesis was derived from interpreting cancer mortality statistics. In 1972, Greenspan proposed the first spatiotemporal model of avascular tumor growth (Greenspan 1972), which was developed to a biomechanical model in 1976 (Greenspan 1976). Subsequently, angiogenesis, as an inseparable phenomenon of carcinogenesis, was first modeled in 1985 by Balding and McElwain (1985).

Tabassum et al. (2019) provide a comprehensive review on the most important deterministic and stochastic models of cancer growth process. The deterministic models have been widely applied to predict cancer cell growth and the rate of change in the volume of the tumor with respect to the changes in time. Stochastic models, instead, are suitable to analyze tumor growth and development by considering the uncontrolled factors of cellular metabolism, energy requirements, hormonal oscillations, respiration, and individual characteristics such as body mass index, genes, smoking, and stress impact.

Besides exploration of underlying mechanisms driving tumor formation and progression, mathematical modeling is beneficial in optimizing cancer treatment approaches (e.g., radiation) and novel drug development. The linear-quadratic law that associates the quantity of remaining cancer cells after radiation with the dose of ionizing radiation was used by Wheldon et al. to combine the exponential growth rate of cancer cells and the linear-quadratic law, estimating the proper number of radiation sessions and intervals, as well as the suitable dosage of radiation to obtain the maximum desirable elimination of cancer cells, while protecting healthy tissues (Wheldon et al. 1977). Other mathematical models are powerful tools to evaluate the outcome of treatment by analyzing the medical records of cancer patients. Alfonso et al. developed a mathematical model of interactions between a tumor and the immune system, to assess the efficacy of radiotherapy after surgical resection of the tumor. They reported that the application of radiation before surgery augmented the antitumor immune response in a group of patients, improving the survival rate (López Alfonso et al. 2019). West et al. applied a mathematical model to data collected from a group of breast cancer patients, known as the game theory model, which has become a branch of mathematics with extensive application in data science, image processing, etc. Based on this model, they proposed a prognostic index and put forward a combination therapy regimen for breast cancer to achieve the lowest risk of metastasis and the least tumor burden (West et al. 2019).

Designing and developing mathematical models to illustrate cancer growth and behavior requires validation, in order to properly demonstrate a biological effect. These models undergo validation through in vitro cell culture studies and in vivo animal studies. In addition, observational studies on human subjects, such as imaging data of cancer patients, contributed to this process (Almeida et al. 2018).

Mathematical models are integral contributors to the development of precision medicine. Several challenges remain to be addressed when entering the characteristics of each individual cancer patient into a therapeutic plan that must be properly tailored to the patient. This requirement is the result of genetic differences and the unique pharmacokinetic details of a given patient that may result in different responses to treatment, different propensity to recurrence and resistance, and different rates of tumor growth and proliferation. Mathematical models can determine the dynamics of a specific patient's disease status by analyzing data already collected from the patient (imaging data, pathological and laboratory data, genetic studies, response to prior treatment regimens, etc.) (Colijn et al. 2017). Mathematical models aim to translate fundamental traits of a system, such as the genetic profile and radiosensitivity of the tumor (Dionysiou et al. 2004) to accurately summarize its expected behaviors in mathematical equations. Hence, a prototype of the system could be designed in silico for further studies (Stamatakos et al. 2002; McKenna et al. 2018). Mathematical studies and in silico facilities potentially accelerate preclinical studies and require lower costs compared to in vitro and in vivo studies. As another example of mathematical modeling, cancer cell metabolism and population evolution can be mathematically predicted using the two-scale fractal theory (Li and He 2019; Anjum et al. 2021). In addition, cancer cell orientation can be explained by the geometrical potential theory (Fan et al. 2019).

One application of mathematical modeling is to use the available data taken from cancer patients to develop a predictive model for tumor growth pattern and pace. This is supervised by modeling, and then, by using the model as it is trained, one could use it to predict tumor growth. This involves regression and classification techniques in data science, which is a very new and innovative approach just being explored. Thus, progress in mathematical modeling will make it a promising tool to translate novel discoveries into clinical settings (Debbouche et al. 2021; Sweilam et al. 2021).

Regardless of vast efforts in cancer research during the last decades, our capabilities to predict and treat cancer have remained inadequate. The complex interconnections of many factors, including different growth, proliferation, and apoptosis rates in addition to the tumor microenvironment-related factors such as inflammatory mediators and ECM components, have eluded a full picture of cancer formation and progression. Mathematical models are tools for in-depth study and prediction of cancer cell behavior. This prediction is based on the successful modeling of cancer metabolism, cell growth, and drug discovery using different mathematical tools to shape the future of cancer diagnosis, treatment, and prognosis (Quaranta et al. 2005; Wang and Deisboeck 2014; Medina 2018; Tabassum et al. 2019).

2.4 Artificial Intelligence in Cancer Research

The term "artificial intelligence" (AI) was introduced in 1956 by John McCarthy (McCarthy et al. 2006). Since then, the role of AI has become prominent in different fields of research, and cancer research is not an exception. AI has already entered the healthcare system as a physicians' assistant to facilitate and accelerate the process of medical decision-making. AI ability of accumulating and processing an immense amount of data in the shortest time makes it a potentially powerful tool in medicine. Establishing the diagnosis, determining the best available treatment for a given case, predicting of prognosis, and establishing a noninvasive prolonged follow-up are some of the promising applications of AI in various medical settings. Considering the AI's notable power in regards to image analysis, medical imaging, radiology, and pathology, it is clear that AI has already affected the field (Radiology ESo 2019). In line with this, FDA-approved Al-based devices in oncology are related predominantly to radiology. Establishing a correct diagnosis can be aided by AI, particularly in visually oriented specialties such as dermatology and gastroenterology. For instance, by adopting a deep convolutional neural network (DCNN) model and training it with 129,450 pathological images, Esteva et al. showed that their trained AI system distinguished different skin malignancies (keratinocyte carcinoma and malignant melanoma) with an acceptable accuracy compared to a dermatologist's visual inspection (Esteva et al. 2017). The IBM intelligence platform, the supercomputer Watson, contributed to the development of a network for advanced investigations in cancer, in which 13 different types of cancer were analyzed. As proof of principle, Somashekhar et al., by conducting a double-blinded validation study, demonstrated that IBM Watson could serve as a reliable assistant in cancer diagnosis (Somashekhar et al. 2017). Finally, Bejnordi et al. reported a remarkable AI capability to diagnose lymph node metastasis in pathological samples from breast cancer patients (Ehteshami Bejnordi et al. 2017). AI is also being evaluated as a tool for the interpretation of positron-emission tomography (PET) scanning (Zaharchuk and Davidzon 2021).

AI has shown promising results in different aspects of cancer research and treatment. For instance, the detection of preneoplastic manifestations, leading to early diagnosis or prevention of cancer development, is one of many benefits expected from AI. After assisting with the early diagnosis, AI will be instrumental, in the future, to determine optimal treatment, including identifying the surgical resection site, optimizing the administered dosage of treatment modalities according to the patients' individual characteristics, and arranging for longitudinal follow-up of individual patients. In addition, predicting the risk and pattern of tumor progression and behavior (metastasis, recurrence, and treatment resistance) will be an important issue expected to be addressed by AI (Huang et al. 2020; Kumar et al. 2022). Beyond clinical applications, AI has provided promising results in cancer research, including drug development, an expensive and time-consuming process that may take as long as 15 years. AI has prominently accelerated this process by introducing large-scale high-throughput screening methods, which predict drug behavior and drug-target interactions. Computational drug repurposing, having recently gained considerable attention, is a method of identifying new indications for drugs already approved for another indication. AI-based systems target the assessment of the efficacy of drug regimens and individual patients' sensitivity to anticancer agents used for different types of cancer, including gastric cancer and ovarian cancer (Hossain et al. 2019; Taninaga et al. 2019; Casimiro-Soriguer et al. 2022). For example, Lind et al. put forward a model to predict the state of drug activity based on the mutated genome of cancer cells (Lind and Anderson 2019). Based on these observations, the role of AI in cancer drug discovery and its contribution to the development of novel treatment strategies for cancer are undeniable. For instance, in regards to adoptive T cell therapy and cancer vaccination, AI is expected to predict the immunogenicity of neo-antigens (Bulik-Sullivan et al. 2019; Jabbari and Rezaei 2019).

Despite the great promises that AI holds for the future of oncology, several challenges remain to be addressed. As examples, discrepancies among the results reported by different imaging and laboratory facilities may stem from variations in the experience of the operators, from differences in devices provided by individual manufacturers, and from proprietary protocols that may lead to different outcome results. As a result, the considerable amount of divergent data used to train AI algorithms has resulted in reduced accuracy of predictions and outputs (Stacke et al. 2021). Furthermore, the application of predictive tools in the clinical setting affects the distribution of medical data among patients; therefore, constantly updated data are needed to train AI systems. This is known as "dataset shift," which is a challenge in working with AI systems (Davis et al. 2019). Accidentally fitting confounders are another challenge in this context; they are defined as accidental signals that are present in a group of input data and lead the AI system to erroneous interpretations of the data (Winkler et al. 2019). Insufficient data input from minority populations may render the model to become biased toward the majority of the population; therefore, predictions and diagnoses concerning the minority populations are missing, and the model cannot be generalized to different populations. The lack of external validation cohorts is another challenge in the extended application and acceptance of AI systems in medical settings. In addition, there are moral and ethical issues that were raised after the introduction of AI tools as well as potential biases in interpreting AI generated data, which remain to be addressed. Nevertheless, AI has the potential to eliminate medical errors despite all these challenges (Basu et al. 2020; Arnold 2021). Recent studies and developments in domain adaptation and robustness to confounders may improve these aspects related to AI. A different challenge concerns moral and ethical issues, which have been raised in connection with the introduction of AI tools, as well as potential biases in interpreting data by using AI, which remain to be addressed (Basu et al. 2020, Arnold 2021).

AI itself is the outcome of substantial interdisciplinary collaboration between computer science, mathematics, linguistics, neurophysiology, and psychology. AI provides a repertoire of data and reflects the experiences of experts beyond the geographical and chronological borders, which potentially facilitate and optimize disease interpretation.

2.5 Medical Sciences in Cancer Research

Multiple biological therapies such as cell cycle and gene repair inhibitors, growth pathway inhibitors, and angiogenesis inhibitors are in clinical use and have changed clinical outcome. Endocrine therapies are used for hormone-dependent cancers, estrogen-dependent breast cancers, and androgen-dependent prostate cancers, resulting in significant improvement of the mortality rates. Treatments can be classified into cancer cell-targeted therapies, immune system activation therapies, and microenvironment or systemic environment-modulation therapies. Recent studies have shown that the physiological condition of the tumor microenvironment, such as hypoxia and poor nutrition, is crucial because the resulting stress, induced by cancer cell progression, contributes to the generation of further genetic mutations, to the downregulation of immune surveillance mechanisms, and to the development of treatment resistance.

Targeting Cancer: Surgery, Radiotherapy, and Chemotherapy

Performing surgery to remove tumors, which was practiced by ancient Greek and Roman physicians, is considered the first step in the evolution of cancer treatment. In the middle of the nineteenth century, the discovery of general anesthesia has notably improved the effectiveness and feasibility of surgical treatments (Wyld et al. 2015). However, surgery was not useful in non-focused or nonsolid cancers. In 1896, about

1 year after the discovery of X-ray, it was noticed that some types of radiations, including the X-rays, are effective against tumors. The researchers did not know the mechanism of action, but they hypothesized that the radiation disrupts the DNA, and as tumor cells proliferate faster, they are more prone to radiation-induced damage. Later in the 1940s, the first steps toward chemotherapy were made. After World War I, soldiers who were exposed to nitrogen mustard gas were diagnosed with impaired function and number of lymphocytes. Therefore, it was hypothesized that nitrogen mustard might treat leukemia (Singh et al. 2018). Research on nitrogen mustard-based alkylating agents has resulted in the designation of a wide spectrum of anticancer medications. The introduction of radiotherapy and chemotherapy has saved many patient lives, but many challenges remained to be addressed. The most considerable improvement in treatment outcomes was achieved when combining surgery and drugs – adjuvant therapy in patient's treatment plan. In some cases, radiotherapy can be included in the treatment process as well. Combining different approaches in the patient's treatment plan is considered a successful multidisciplinary attempt. Both radiotherapy and chemotherapy have been improved remarkably during years of research.

There are some pitfalls and challenges in chemotherapy-based treatments, for instance, intra-tumor and inter-tumor heterogeneity, nonspecific drug distribution that leads to poor drug bioavailability and presence of adverse effects, poor estimation of real-time therapeutic effects that result in drug overuse, resistance to chemotherapeutic agents, and unwanted immune reactions against exogenous carriers (Burrell et al. 2013; Holohan et al. 2013; Qin et al. 2017). Application of smart nanomedicines in targeted drug delivery systems has addressed some of the challenges; they facilitate the selective uptake of the drug by tumor cells, thus enhancing treatment efficacy and lowering the rate of systemic adverse effects (Qin et al. 2018; Abadi et al. 2021). Although chemotherapy has advanced remarkably, some challenges remain to be tackled.

Radiotherapy has considerably progressed, and specific methods were developed for different cancer types; the most common advanced therapies are image-guided radiotherapy and intensity-modulated radiotherapy. Nevertheless, important adverse effects still challenge the patient's treatment process. Following radiotherapy, some patients face structural aberrations in chromosomes and copy number alterations, which can lead to different complications (Grade et al. 2015). In addition, due to advances in cancer treatment and the consequent increase in survival rates, radiation-induced secondary malignant neoplasms have become a significant problem in long-term cancer survivors (Tubiana 2009; De Gonzalez et al. 2011). It is suggested that radiotherapy-related adverse effects would be resolved, to desirable extents, by using radiosensitizers and radioprotectors (Mohan et al. 2019). Advances in radiotherapy and development of methods to overcome these limitations are great examples of interdisciplinary collaboration in cancer research.

Targeting the Tumor Cells Specifically: Immunology and Immunotherapy
Immunology has become an indispensable discipline of cancer research. As the first defense against cancer, the immune system witnesses all stages of tumor initiation and progression and learns how to combat it in unique ways. Therefore, modulation, reprogramming, and augmentation of the immune system are expected to play a beneficial role in combating malignancies. Hence, the concept of cancer immunotherapy was introduced as a promising strategy to fight cancer.

The first documentation of using the immune system to fight tumors has been found in anecdotal reports from ancient Egypt, stating that tumors disappeared spontaneously after contracting a disease associated with high fever (Dobosz and Dzieciątkowski 2019). The initial attempt to induce immune system modulation was performed by Fehleisen and Busch in 1868 (Oiseth and Aziz 2017); they observed the considerable resolution of a tumor after an inducing erysipelas infection in a cancer patient. Later in 1891, William Coley, who has been called the father of immunotherapy, investigated the benefits of immune system modulation in the combat against bone cancer (Coley 1991; McCarthy 2006). Cancer immunotherapy has evolved in some main directions, namely, immune checkpoint inhibitors, monoclonal antibodies, adoptive cell therapies, cancer vaccines, immune system modulators, and oncolytic virus therapy. Efficiency in generating long-term remission (by inducing immune memory) improved specific toxicity and selectivity in targeting cancer cells, and optimization of the cancer treatment strategies is an advantage of immunotherapy in comparison with conventional chemotherapy regimens. Immunotherapy may be the most promising strategy resulting from carefully designed immunological studies in cancer research.

However, the interactions between malignant cells and the immune system are complicated. How tumors can escape immunosurveillance and why some immunotherapy methods have not demonstrated the expected efficacy are questions that could be answered by the elucidation of the complex interactions between the immune system and tumor cells. Currently, prevention of resistance to immunotherapy and reduction of the side effects (particularly the risk of autoimmune disorders) are challenges faced by the field of cancer immunotherapy. These are being met by designing prediction methods to calculate the response to immunotherapy and to follow the patients' prognosis and to investigate the pathways used by some malignancies to evade the treatment (Kroschinsky et al. 2017; Sharma et al. 2017; Hiam-Galvez et al. 2021). Advances in the development of drugs that target intracellular pathways such as Bruton tyrosine kinase, phosphoinositide 3-kinase (PI3K), and bcl-2 pathways have considerably changed the treatment outcome in cancer patients (Liu et al. 2009; Deng et al. 2017); it could be considered as great interdisciplinary collaboration of scientists in chemical, biological, and medical sciences.

Supportive Care: Nutrition and Rehabilitation
Epidemiological studies that investigate the incidence of different types of cancer that occur in migrants will elucidate the role of environmental factors in the

propensity to develop cancer (Menck et al. 1975; Stanford et al. 1995). Diet and nutrition are two important environmental factors that are altered during migration. The association between nutrition and the risk of cancer has also been demonstrated in animal studies (Sapienza and Issa 2016). The effect of diet in cancer initiation and progression has been attributed to the link between nutrition and epigenetic alterations (Sapienza and Issa 2016).

It is estimated that 30–40% of cancer cases could be prevented by controlling weight gain and preventing obesity (Research WCRF 2007). Proper eating behavior, healthy diet, and physical activity contribute to the prevention of obesity and its complications, including cancer. In addition, the alteration of the gut microbiota by probiotic products is a newly suggested beneficial method for decreasing the risk of cancer (Schwabe and Jobin 2013). It should be noted that probiotics and symbiotics (synergistic combination of probiotics and prebiotics) have also shown promising results in cancer prevention research (Raman et al. 2013). Moreover, the recommendation of a healthy diet according to the type of disease and the administered treatments helps the patient to pass the recovery period with fewer complications and may accelerate the treatment process (Ravasco 2019).

Previously, a reduction method to study the effect of nutrition was dominant among scientists, who evaluated the effects of a specific nutrient on the entire biological system. Due to advances in genomic techniques, scientists are focusing their efforts to study the interactions between individual molecules of a nutrient and an entire biological system, which is considered a more holistic method (Go et al. 2001).

Advances in nutrition research have revealed that different dietary patterns are associated with a spectrum of risk for chronic diseases, mainly cardiovascular diseases and cancers. Mediterranean diet recommends higher consumption of fruits, vegetables, olive oil, nuts, as well as fish and poultry instead of large amounts of red meat. This diet is rich in polyphenolic flavonoids, carotenoids, antioxidants, a variety of vitamins and minerals, omega-3 fatty acids, and different amino acids (essential and nonessential), which all have a low dietary inflammatory index, making the Mediterranean diet to be known as an anti-inflammatory diet (Griffiths et al. 2016). Bodén et al. conducted a prospective cohort study, which yielded results indicative of statistically significant associations between a healthier diet rich in anti-inflammatory agents and a lower risk of cancer, particularly lung and gastric cancers; their results were more consistent in men (Bodén et al. 2019). Wang et al. reported that an anti-inflammatory post-diagnosis diet could decrease the risk of breast cancer as well as reducing all-causes mortality rate among breast cancer survivors (Wang et al. 2020). On the other hand, advances in the food industry, the use of different food preservatives, and new methods to prolong the expiration date of food products require the attention of medical research. However, the impact of chemical preservatives and ultra-processed foods on human health remains challenging. Fiolet et al. have studied 104980 participants from the French NutriNet-Santé cohort. They demonstrated that a 10% increase in the consumption of ultra-processed foods correlated with a >10% increase in the risk of overall and breast cancer (Fiolet et al. 2018). Lin et al. reported that more salt-processed foods in the daily diet is associated with higher risk for gastric cancer (Lin et al. 2014). Taken together, nutritional interventions and the correction of unhealthy dietary habits could be helpful in cancer prevention and, in some cases, could lead to more effective cancer treatment results by reducing negative treatment outcomes and lower the mortality rate.

Gut microbiota acts as a double-edge sword in human health and disease. Gut microbiota produce bio substances and metabolites that protect the homeostasis of the immune system and the gut (e.g., LPS, pyridoxine, MPL, ferrichrome, etc.) (Vivarelli et al. 2019). On the other side, some subpopulations grow and propagate better during pathological processes and release high levels of toxins and harmful substances, provoking inflammation and predisposing the host to tumorigenesis (e.g., colibactin, CagA, FadA, VirA, MP toxin, AvrA, superoxide, etc.) (Vivarelli et al. 2019). Probiotics, a select population of the gut microbiota, are potent in maintaining the homeostasis of the intestinal environment. Major research interests have focused on the effect of probiotics to combat dysbiosis in cancer patients who underwent chemo- and radiotherapy (Mego et al. 2013; Redman et al. 2014). Moreover, microbiota is being evaluated for their potential to enhance the efficacy of immunotherapy (Matson et al. 2018; Routy et al. 2018).

Cancer rehabilitation is perceived as a form of medical care that aims to reduce the treatment and disease side effects and improve the quality of life of the patients. It also aims to support patients in coping with both disease and treatment and to help survivors to continue their normal life. Cancer rehabilitation is categorized into four main fields, namely, preventive, restorative, supportive, and palliative (Chowdhury et al. 2020). Preventive rehabilitation starts after the diagnosis is made and before the start of treatment. It evaluates the physical and psychological status of patients and the possible complications of the treatment and tries to prevent further impairment after the treatment course. Restorative rehabilitation starts with the initiation of treatment and continues beyond the treatment period. It aims to keep the patients at the physical and psychological status they had before the disease started or to return the patient to that status, in case the patient deteriorated during treatment. Supportive rehabilitation considers cancer as a chronic condition, helps the patient cope with the sequelae of cancer, and prevents possible future disabilities. Palliative treatment supports patients at the final stages of the disease and attempts to provide physical, psychological, emotional, social, and palliative support. With regard to the support provided during different types of rehabilitation programs, interdisciplinary collaboration between different medical and psychological specialties is required (Chowdhury et al. 2020; Stout et al. 2021).

Self-Care: Thermal Therapy

Self-care includes maintaining an optimistic mood with the help of hydrotherapy and thermal therapy. Hydrotherapy consists of drinking as much water as possible to ensure the normal cells have enough water for normal metabolism (Reger et al. 2022), whereas thermal therapy aims to ensure that the affected part or the whole body reaches a higher temperature to render the normal cells metabolically more active (Glazer and Curley 2011; Li 2020; Abadeer and Murphy 2021). Thermal therapy, also called hyperthermia, has been shown to increase the efficacy of several chemotherapeutic agents. HIPEC (hyperthermic intraperitoneal chemotherapy) in combination with cytoreductive surgery has led to prolonged survival (and even cures) of patients with intraperitoneal metastases (Glazer and Curley 2011; Abadeer and Murphy 2021).

2.6 Social Sciences in Cancer Research

Neuroscience and Behavior

Cancer neuroscience is a burgeoning field in cancer research, mainly devoted to the cancer-related cognitive impairment and the complex mutual connection between the nervous system and cancer.

Formerly known as chemofog or chemo-brain, cancer-related cognitive deficits were recognized during or after the completion of chemotherapy through either subjective or objective reports (Avan et al. 2015; Horowitz et al. 2018). Cognitive deficits are characterized by impaired concentration, losing the ability of multitasking, and experiencing problematic short-term memory (Horowitz et al. 2018; Monje et al. 2020). In addition, peripheral neuropathies, including sensory and motor deficits and pain, have been reported as post chemotherapy effects (Monje et al. 2020). The summation of these cognitive problems considerably diminishes the quality of life of the patient, prevents the patient from getting back to work and premorbid life, compromises the patient's independence, and reduces the patient's compliance with medication, possibly resulting in adverse effects and further complications. It should also be noted that tumors in the brain such as glioblastoma multiforme and metastases from other tumors (e.g., from lung tumors) will affect neurological processes. Cognitive problems are frequently the first indication for the presence of a malignancy in the brain.

An emerging subfield of cancer neuroscience is the recognition of various types of paraneoplastic syndromes involving the central and peripheral nervous systems. Timely recognition of these syndromes leads not only to a more efficient treatment of the neurologic symptoms but also to earlier diagnosis of a potentially hidden cancer. Paraneoplastic neurologic syndromes are a heterogeneous group of neurologic disorders in most cases caused by immunologic reactions to an underlying malignancy in the absence of metastases or side effects of cancer treatment (Dalmau et al. 1999). These syndromes may affect any part of the nervous system, from the cerebral cortex to neuromuscular junction and muscle. The best-known paraneoplastic neurological syndromes include cerebellar degeneration, limbic encephalitis, encephalomyelitis, opsoclonus-myoclonus syndrome, Lambert-Eaton myasthenic syndrome, stiff person syndrome, and rare types of peripheral neuropathy. A growing number of antineuronal antibodies have been discovered in relation to various types of underlying malignancies, contributing to our knowledge of this interesting intersection between cancer and neuroscience.

Studying the bidirectional interaction of cancer and the nervous system opens up new chapters in cancer neuroscience. Recent recognition of both systemic and microenvironmental effects of the nervous system on tumors has brought to light clues to understand mechanisms of cancer initiation and progression (Venkatesh et al. 2015, 2019; Venkataramani et al. 2019). Under certain conditions, neuronal processes and glial cells release growth factors and neurotransmitters for neural growth in normal circumstances; it has been proposed that malignant cell growth and progression are facilitated by these factors when penetrating the malignant tissue (Arranz et al. 2014; Zahalka and Frenette 2020). In addition, nervous circuits modulate the immune responses and, therefore, may aid tumor growth (Saloman et al. 2020). On the other side, malignancies affect the activities of the nervous system by interfering with its remodeling and normal function (Hayakawa et al. 2017; Borniger et al. 2018; Yu et al. 2020). Furthermore, chronic pain syndrome, which is reported in some cancer patients, is attributed to the perineural invasion of cancer cells (Bapat et al. 2011). Considering these points, enhanced efforts should be directed to the field of cancer neuroscience to allow translation of these new insights into clinical practice.

Psychology

Stress is an inevitable factor in daily life, known to be associated with a systemic inflammatory state (Slavich and Irwin 2014; Sin et al. 2015), which highlights the role of mind-body connection. Chronic stress stimulates the hypothalamus-pituitary-adrenal axis (HPA), activates the sympathetic nervous system (SNS), and disrupts the immune system balance, together mediating an inflammatory environment in the human body. Overproduction of stress hormones by the HPA axis and the SNS induces DNA damage, enhances P53 degradation, and triggers different pro-tumor pathways. In addition, stress hormone-mediated inflammation and immunosuppression impede immune cells to properly fight and inhibit cancer cells (Dai et al. 2020; Eckerling et al. 2021). Furthermore, stress hormones directly promote cancer progression, invasion, and metastasis by interacting with the cancer cells and non-cancer cells within the tumor microenvironment (Dai et al. 2020, Eckerling et al. 2021). Hence, stress is an important environmental factor predisposing individuals to cancer formation and progression. In addition, a direct effect of stress on cancer treatment outcomes and prognosis has been established. Chida et al. demonstrated that stress-related psychosocial factors are significantly associated with an increased risk of cancer with poor prognosis in healthy individuals and a higher mortality rate in cancer patients (Chida et al. 2008). Patients with no or poor psychological support may experience a prolonged uncontrolled stress period, which potentially results in an inflammatory state facilitating cancer progression (Lutgendorf and Sood 2011). Meanwhile, uncontrolled stress may lead to depression, conceivably exacerbating the inflammatory state and cancer progression (Krishnadas and Cavanagh 2012). Depressive behavior could be followed by lack of compliance with treatment. Considering all these factors, the release and the accumulation of pro-inflammatory mediators and the inflammatory state could be the major cause linking stressors, depression, cognitive impairment, and cancer exacerbation (Reich 2008; Lutgendorf and Sood 2011; Krishnadas and Cavanagh 2012). Hence, psychological support is an essential element in the care of cancer patients from the initial point of establishing the diagnosis through the period of treatment and recovery. Psychological support has to consider the personality traits, the attachment style, and the coping mechanisms of the patient, as well as the quality of the support by family members and friends (Saita et al. 2015); therefore, interdisciplinary and transdisciplinary approaches are needed to design the best support strategy according to patient characteristics, cancer type and stage, and treatment strategy and duration. More recently, mindfulness-based stress reduction (MBSR) interventions proved to favorably impact cancer- and cancer treatment-related symptoms such as anxiety and depression (Pedro et al. 2021; Lin et al. 2022; Yang et al. 2022). Furthermore, there is growing evidence that physical activity and regular exercise have the power to favorably impact the symptoms of depression and anxiety among a broad range of cancer survivors (see (Cordier et al. 2019) for a more comprehensive overview). More specifically, when compared to strength training, endurance training, along with psychological counseling, has a favorable impact on depression, quality of life, and sleep disturbances among patients with high grade glioma (WHO grade III and IV) (Eisenhut et al. 2022).

Lastly, the psychological health of the cancer caregivers should not be neglected. A considerable number of caregivers develop depressive symptoms and sleep disturbances while caring for their family members with cancer (Baider and Surbone 2014). Hence, providing proper support for the caregivers is a priority, considering that the mental health of cancer patients is closely linked to the caregivers' duty and vice versa.

While there is growing evidence that individuals reporting higher scores for stress and lower scores for social support appear to be at increased risk to report cancer-related illnesses, such observations by no means imply linear, causal, and unidirectional associations. And this is for the following three reasons: First, if true, this would dramatically increase further stress to the individual in terms of guilt feelings, of being a burden to the society, in general, and to close family members, in specific. Second, if true, this would dramatically increase the feeling of thwarted belongingness to the individual, though research on suicidal behavior clearly indicates that the lack of belongingness is associated with higher risks of suicidal ideation (Van Orden et al. 2010). Third, from a methodological and psychological perspective, it is also conceivable that higher perceived stress is a sign of preclinical emergence of cancer.

3 Framework and Perspective of Cancer Research in 2050

New cancer cases are increasing rapidly, and it is predicted that the incidence will increase from 18.1 million per year (which is calculated as the current incidence rate) to 29.5 million by 2040 globally (Baumann et al. 2020). By 2050, the world will witness an even greater number. Weir et al. (Weir et al. 2021) estimated that, in the USA, the yearly cancer patients will upsurge from 1,534,500 in 2015 to 2,286,300 in

2050, with the major percentage growth among adults aged ≥75 years. The most prevalent cancers will be colorectal, lung, and prostate cancers in men, as well as breast cancer in women.

Besides genetic factors, the estimated increase in future cancer cases is attributed to some environmental risk factors, including global climate change associated with higher levels of UV irradiation, extended pollution with microplastics, and unabated contamination of drinking water with harmful germs, pathogenic metals, and other pollutants. Moreover, unbalanced diets enriched in fat and lacking fiber and essential minerals combined with misguided lifestyles avoiding regular physical activity will provoke cancer in many organs and reduce the life expectancy.

On the other hand, advances in medical sciences and the molecular understanding of these diseases will give rise to new forms of therapy. At the same time, the general availability of novel diagnostic methods, such as whole genome sequencing and novel digital technologies, combined with well-designed regular preventive health checkups will provide the tools to identify patients at risk and to recognize the early onset of a cancerous disease. Consequently, tumorigenic lesions can be detected and tackled much earlier than today and, in some cases, even before the disease develops. Furthermore, single step detection of specific cancer types using body fluids has been hypothesized to optimize the diagnostic process. Currently, cancer detection tests are available, but patients are subjected to multiple expensive time-consuming procedures before establishing a diagnosis. However, there are large differences between countries, not only between so-called well-developed and underdeveloped countries but also within these subcategories. This is often due to lack of proper access to healthcare even in well-developed countries. Therefore, in the next decades, diagnostic tools are expected to be developed with the aim of reducing medical expenses, decreasing patient's exposure to different – sometimes unnecessary – diagnostic tests, and achieving early diagnosis.

It is conceivable that the exact identification of the culture conditions necessary for the generation of ex vivo organoids from different patient-derived cancers will be an additional model (although some scientists consider organoids as a substitute) to assess the efficiency of some novel drugs and the ability of the autologous immune system to elicit an antitumor immune response (Dijkstra et al. 2018; Bar-Ephraim et al. 2020). Indeed, the generation of patient-derived organoids has already provided relevant insight into the mechanisms of tumor cell growth and antitumor immunity (Rodrigues et al. 2021). This approach, known as the 3D in vitro model, will reduce the need for experimental animals (Morton et al. 2016; Hahn et al. 2021; Rodrigues et al. 2021). In addition, it is evident that in murine models, tumors are generated in a very short time compared to the situation in humans (Morton et al. 2016; Hahn et al. 2021). Furthermore, immune cell subpopulations and lymphocyte receptors or ligands on murine tumor target cells can differ from the human counterpart (Poggi et al. 2021). In the future, the characterization of chemically defined culture media free of animal or tumor cell-derived growth factors together with tissue matrix isolated from tumors will allow the generation and banking of a representing list of tumor-derived organoids to be used as platforms to identify the right drug, among the plethora of medications already on the market, to which tumor cells of a given patient are sensitive (Reidy et al. 2021). Nevertheless, the implementation of animal models will better characterize and eventually modulate the mechanisms of differentiation of immune cells (Martinov et al. 2021). Together, these platforms will be suitable to identify novel drugs, to study the mechanisms of drug resistance, and to characterize the immune response by patient-derived lymphocytes (Martinov et al. 2021; Reidy et al. 2021). On the other side, the problem with organoids is that they often contain undefined growth media influencing (usually decreasing) the efficacy of anticancer drugs. Moreover, organoids usually do not metabolize drugs similar to an intact organism, often essential for their efficacy. Considering the challenges and limitations, some scientists suggested that organoids could function as an additional platform to select a proper treatment, next to other methods such as gene expression, monitoring protein levels, mutation analysis, and genetic polymorphisms.

One major path into the future of oncology may be through "genome reconstitution" with tandem aligned sequence targeted integrated reagent (TASTIeR) – the successor of clustered regularly interspaced short palindromic repeats (CRISPR). With these novel techniques, the outcomes of cancers could become mostly predictable by 2050. In-depth use of genomics and proteomics, serial biomarker monitoring, and the wealth of open-source information collected from previous patients with similar cancers could continue to facilitate the utilization of early, accurate, and highly effective therapies, turning cancer into a curable disease or one that is chronic and less likely to limit overall survival.

In order to cure cancer, a better understanding of its biology is essential. To accomplish this goal, mathematical and physical models of normal and cancerous cells will be helpful. Using the laws of physics and biological phenomena, individual cells can be modeled and the generated data used to determine the boundary conditions on the cells. However, the body contains billions of cells, and understanding how a cancer cell develops and divides requires sophisticated methods. The interaction of cells with other parts of the body can be modeled using extensive simulations by introducing environmental, psychological, hereditary, and nutritional factors and their effect on converting a healthy cell to a cancerous one. Such models need powerful computers to explain the development of cancer. Moreover, using available and newly generated data, it will be possible to develop data science and machine learning techniques to explore the main parameters that drive tumor formation and growth, as well as the interaction of cancerous cells with other parts of one's body.

Artificial intelligence is expected to play an increasing role in the prevention, diagnosis, and treatment of cancer. While the emphasis in the past has been given in assistance for establishing a diagnosis, with expert systems such as Watson (Somashekhar et al. 2017), in the future we expect that the considerable evolution that AI tools have undergone in recent years will offer application to a much broader set of clinical tasks. The area of domain adaptation will allow algorithms to abstract away from the specific boundaries of datasets and problem-specific parameters, both in unsupervised and adaptive and active learning. The new challenge will be to focus research on the problem of developing and creating the right interfaces for "semi-general" AI tools to be successfully applied to the specific issues arising in medical oncology. It should be expected that by 2050, AI-assisted diagnosis will completely outperform the diagnostic capabilities of today and that targeted drugs will be routinely designed starting with the molecular shape they need to have to perform their task most effectively. Artificial intelligence will be crucial for redesigning investigation and research methodologies in various scientific sectors. In addition to AI's role in cancer research addressed in this chapter, further challenges will concern efforts to integrate different disciplines (medicine, chemistry, biology, and engineering) on a single AI platform. In fact, if the activity is now aimed at implementing AI approaches in single fields or precise applications, the challenge for future cancer treatment will involve the design of a holistic system managed predominantly by AI. With the computing power currently under development and with the growth of a generation of researchers that will be adequately trained on AI topics, this goal will be challenging but feasible between now and 2050.

Mathematical modeling of cancer will help to gain insight into the mechanisms of tumor growth and to implement new treatments (Debbouche et al. 2021). In combination with physical models and artificial intelligence, it will be possible to develop personalized protocols. To study the evolution of a particular cancer, predictive digital twins will be developed (Hernandez-Boussard et al. 2021) in order to interact with the patient in real time and take adequate measures with the help of artificial intelligence. The development of digital twins for cancer patients can play a pivotal role toward optimizing personalized cancer care (Hernandez-Boussard et al. 2021). Cancer patient digital twins (CPDTs) are in silico representations of cancer patients that can dynamically integrate real-time multiscale and multimodal data, leverage advanced computing to train predictive models, and conduct virtual experiments to make treatment predictions and individualized healthcare decisions for cancer patients. By using data from a variety of scales (including both individual- and population-level data), periods (varying from nanoseconds to decades), and modalities (proteomes, clinical features, imaging data, and data from clinical trials and population studies), CPDTs have the potential to revolutionize predictive oncology. Clinicians can use CPDTs to perform virtual experiments, by simulating the patient's disease progression as a result of different treatments. Real-time observational data reflecting changes across timescales from the molecular level to the population level will be used to train CPDTs in a continuous learning loop and predict future states, as the patient's disease state evolves. In this way, CPDTs improve predictive accuracy by accounting for measurement uncertainty, missing data, and limited mechanistic understanding. In the future, a systematic real-world deployment of CPDTs will allow for large cohorts of CPDTs to be employed in in silico clinical trials and population studies. Another potential benefit of CPDTs is that they will provide policymakers with insights into the efficiency of various cancer therapies and serve as a valuable tool toward guiding investment and resource allocation and dynamically shaping healthcare system response to public health issues. Despite the rapid advancement of critical technology and data supporting CPDTs, a number of challenges have to be addressed in order to unleash the potential of CPDTs to advance predictive oncology. CPDT modeling must be scalable and trustworthy, while data must be representative and unbiased. To this end, the development of CPDTs requires the adoption of common rules that regulate the system's reliability, as well as the generation, collection, integration, harmonization, and protection of data. The FAIR (findability, accessibility, interoperability, and reusability) data collecting principles, simple software development best practices, standardized training and validation methods, and regulatory standards for data governance and usage are all examples of standardized rules. The full integration of CPDTs into medical workflows also necessitates the training of clinical staff in advanced technologies, as well as the development of user-friendly CPDT interfaces.

Concerning cancer treatment, there might be enormous progress on two main fronts, based on the cancer knowledge development during previous decades, although the relevant science could be unpredictable. First, the progress in understanding the biologic pathways that are instrumental of subcategories of cancer entities will lead to the development of cancer type (and subtypes within a cancer) specific therapies that only affect the cancerous cells present in a given patient, allowing "cancer type-specific" drugs to be designed. These drugs will only affect cancer cells and not normal cells, avoiding completely the adverse events from chemotherapy or irradiation. Immune checkpoint inhibitors (PD-1, PD-L1, CTLA-4, etc.) are extensively being used but are still limited to certain (sub)types of cancer, are not effective for many patients, and produce serious side effects. However, it is expected that the field will rapidly progress to find a "silver bullet" for each category of cancer. Second, understanding the immunologic makeup of the cancer cells, which is specific for the cancer and not present in the patient's normal tissue, will allow safe and effective immunotherapy that eventually will eliminate any trace of the tumor. Such strategies with CAR T cells (for the treatment of ALL) and monoclonal antibodies (for the treatment of B cell lymphoma) have already been designed. This approach requires a normal immune system and a possible strategy of immunizing the patient with tumor antigens that are specific for a given malignancy.

As we better understand the biology and immunology of cancer, adaptive strategies can be developed. Evaluation of patients prior to therapy with next generation sequencing, evaluation of circulating tumor-derived DNA, and characterizing molecular and genetic signatures will allow for individualized therapies so that patients will not be exposed to treatments with a low likelihood of benefit but can be directed toward those with a greater likelihood of success. Cancer research is going to be directed primarily to be patient-specific. Future research will focus on genetic changes that are unique for a given individual to enable patient-specific care. AI will be used to analyze the pathology, genetic mutations, previous treatments and responses, and other previous clinical information to design the best patient-specific treatment plan. Moreover, the interaction between the microbiome and the patient's treatment response and complications will become increasingly important for developing patient-specific treatment plans. There will be further improvements in immunotherapy and nonsurgical treatment of some tumors. Cancer will become a chronic disease for many patients, being suppressed, rather than cured. Surgery and radiation (e.g., three- and four-dimensional radiation and proton therapy) will become less invasive and more precise, resulting in less morbidity.

Moreover, it is expected that organ transplantation and regenerative medicine will progress, and cyborg technology, which replaces body functions with artificial organs, will spread in a more sophisticated form in medical engineering. This will naturally require the mobilization of interdisciplinary knowledge and technologies. Meanwhile, advances in cryonics technology may benefit cancer research in some aspects.

Finally, extensive scientific developments, particularly affecting chronic diseases such as cancer, will have a major impact on humanity's view of life and death; so, it goes without saying that the development of such technologies must be based on the maturing of bioethics and humanist consciousness around the world.

As to the role of psychology, psychotherapy, and exercise science, in basic research relating to cancer, there is no connection with molecular biology, genetics, or further physiological, endocrinological, or immunological processes. The emphasis is rather on active psychological factors to prevent the emergence of cancer and on the psychological treatment of cancer survivors and their family members. More specifically, key question will be, though not limited to, the following:

1. Which lifestyle factors in terms of nutrition, environmental quality and exposure, regular physical activity, and quality of social networks and interactions do decrease the risk of the emergence of any kind of cancer?
2. Which are the active psychological agents inherent in social interactions and physical activity interventions that might decrease the risk of the emergence of cancer?
3. Which psychological and psychotherapeutic interventions contribute to a reduction of psychological symptoms caused by chemotherapy and radiotherapy among cancer survivors?
4. Which interventions confer to the decrease of psychological burden among family members caring for their family member of cancer survivors?
5. If a cancer survivor reports chronic impairments as affecting their psychological, physical, economical, and social independence, which psychological, psychosocial, and family-centered interventions are needed to keep their current situation stable or to even improve their situation?
6. Which professionals should care for cancer survivors, and which role will have (neuro-) surgeons, psychologists, supportive staff members, and social workers, in guaranteeing an optimal and maximal support for cancer survivors?
7. Considering the point of view mentioned in number 6, what is the minimum number and minimum requirement of team members of a department of oncology?

Overall, while the current state of support of cancer survivors is characterized by modestly interconnected experts in different fields of psychology, social counseling, oncology, and surgery, a more thoroughly organized teamwork is needed to optimize and maximize the treatment and follow-up of cancer survivors.

As illustrated and argued in this chapter, many different fields of research have already contributed to the current progress in cancer treatment. With the growing number of inter-field connections, a multidisciplinary framework is needed to further improve cancer research in the future. Currently, some types of cancer have a considerably high success rate of treatment with a positive outcome. Nevertheless, solving complex problems such as those caused by cancer is not easy and sometimes takes decades. This raises the question whether and how science can become more effective.

One could argue that perhaps some scientists are doing research without a visible impact on the society since "academic freedom" encourages a too diffuse choice of what to investigate. One could argue that more targeted research programs that would lead to have assigned more research investigating key problems in society such as cancer, climate change, energy production, high impact learning, and the like could perhaps be more efficient. However, unexpected results from "high risk research" may catapult a field into new directions. In addition, it is widely accepted that the consequences of research in the long-term can be hardly predicted, with numerous examples from the fields of physics, chemistry, technology, biology, mathematics, sociology, and philosophy. Therefore, at no time should the academic freedom that allows scientists to pursue their interests be restrained.

Reality has shown that in many fields of research, scientists direct their investigations either at receiving funding or, even more likely, at the probability to publish articles in highly ranked journals. With such actions, the majority of scientists aim to boost their own academic career. On top of that, at least in some fields of science, publishing articles becomes easier when "you learn to dance in your own circle," meaning that you stay within your own discipline where the peers that review your manuscripts understand the same scientific jargon. Of course, this is contradictory to any form of interdisciplinary collaboration, which, as we have outlined here, is indispensable to fully solve complex problems such as cancer.

There is not much doubt that complex problem solving, as we showed for cancer research, can be accelerated through a higher level and intensity of interdisciplinary collaboration. With this crucial axiom in mind, the relevant question to consider is how do we bring disciplines together to share their data, methods, and know-how and further to cocreate new approaches, tools, and methods to solve the many complex problem?

Some strategic lines are proposed for higher efficiency in scientific research:

- Redesign funding of research programs in a way that scientists gain advantages when committing to programs that are interdisciplinary in nature.
- Redesign careers of scientists in such a way that interdisciplinary research is higher valued and rated than monodisciplinary research and focuses on interdisciplinary collaboration and high quality work.
- Visible contributions (spin-off) to real problem solving in practice (for organizations, business, and industry) should be endorsed; however, one should bear in mind that the value of a substantial corpus of research is not immediately recognized.

For cancer research, specific aims would be a higher degree of collaboration between researchers, a visible increase of interdisciplinary research, and a much stronger emphasis and policy for "knowledge sharing" between disciplines (think of supporting conferences that are not discipline based but rather problem based).

4 Conclusion

In the next decades, cancer is expected to become more of a chronic disease, and the quality of life will be recognized as a more important topic for further research avenues. The evolution of cancer research during the next decades seems to follow a convergent and multidisciplinary path. The recognition of more emergent aspects of the problem is expected, and the integration of results from multiple study fields will enhance our understanding of cancer causes, progression, and consequences for all parties involved. Detailed modeling of individual and multicell organs is needed to understand the biology of cancer and its development. The number of independent parameters in such models is enormous, and one needs to use dimensional reduction approach. We need codes to incorporate the chemistry of drugs and their interaction with healthy and cancerous cells. This is an enormous undertaking and involves extensive data-driven attempts to model individual and systems of cells and their interactions with one another.

Diagnostic and therapeutic approaches to cancer will be revolutionized in next decades. Diagnoses will involve cellular, molecular, and genetic approaches. Treatments will be designed and personalized based upon molecular and genetic profiles. Indeed, these objectives will be facilitated by the availability of readily accessible methods to quantify and analyze circulating tumor DNA. Genomic sequencing tools, mutation prediction tools, and real targeted therapy would be the routine approach to treat various cancers by immune checkpoint inhibitors, CAR T cell therapy, cell cycle checkpoints, signaling pathways, targeted chemotherapy (e.g., using nano-delivery tools), targeted radiation, gene therapy, and gene editing. However, due to the complex heterogeneous genetic etiology of cancer, designing effective gene therapy strategies would be a challenge for the drug design process and therefore will be mainly based on genomic and predominantly molecular structural analysis to enhance the efficacy of the treatment. Given the global rise in cancer incidence and its harmful effects at individual and public health levels, taking preventive measures should be underscored. Establishment of a healthy lifestyle from early life as well as lifestyle modifications in later years should be emphasized for cancer prevention. In addition, reducing the exposure to environmental chemicals might be effective in preventing epigenetic alterations and other carcinogenic effects of environmental pollutants.

In conclusion, based on the discussions provided here, in 2050, we can anticipate remarkable advances in precision medicine that incorporates genomics, comorbidities, competing health risk scores, microbiome studies, etc. to design the best-tailored treatment plan for each individual cancer patient. In addition, predictive biomarkers of therapeutic response will be developed to evaluate the treatment outcomes and predict the disease response in time, to optimize the treatment period. Systems biology and integrative omics will contribute to increasing our understanding of the complexity of cancer pathophysiology. Besides the development of advanced treatment strategies, cancer research will address mechanisms of resistance in details to design strategies to prevent and combat cancer resistance to treatment. Furthermore, artificial intelligence, data science, and advanced technologies will be successfully integrated into cancer research.

Acknowledgment We appreciate the invaluable contribution of USERN Advisory Board members by commenting on this manuscript to improve it.

Conflict of Interest The authors declare no conflict of interest.

References

Abadeer NS, Murphy CJ (2021) Recent progress in cancer thermal therapy using gold nanoparticles. In: Nanomaterials neoplasms. Jenny Stanford Publishing, pp 143–217

Abadi B, Yazdanpanah N, Nokhodchi A, Rezaei N (2021) Smart biomaterials to enhance the efficiency of immunotherapy in glioblastoma: state of the art and future perspectives. Adv Drug Deliv Rev 179:114035

Aifantis EC (2016) Internal length gradient (ILG) material mechanics across scales and disciplines. Adv Appl Mech 49:1–110

Albadawi H, Zhang Z, Altun I, Hu J, Jamal L, Ibsen KN, Tanner EE, Mitragotri S, Oklu R (2021) Percutaneous liquid ablation agent for tumor treatment and drug delivery. Sci Transl Med 13:eabe3889

Almeida L, Chisholm RH, Clairambault J, Lorenzi T, Lorz A, Pouchol C, Trélat E (2018) Why is evolution important in cancer and what mathematics should be used to treat cancer? Focus on drug resistance. In: Mondaini RP (ed) Trends in biomathematics: modeling, optimization and computational problems: selected works from the BIOMAT consortium lectures, Moscow 2017. Springer International Publishing, Cham, pp 107–120

Amaldi U (2005) Nuclear physics applications in diagnostics and cancer therapy. Nucl Phys A 751:409–428

Ananthanarayanan B, Kim Y, Kumar S (2011) Elucidating the mechanobiology of malignant brain tumors using a brain matrix-mimetic hyaluronic acid hydrogel platform. J Biomater Dent 32:7913–7923

Anjum N, He C-H, He J-H (2021) Two-scale fractal theory for the population dynamics. Fractals 29:2150182

Araujo RP, McElwain DLS (2004) A history of the study of solid tumour growth: the contribution of mathematical modelling. Bull Math Biol 66:1039

Armitage P, Doll R (1954) The age distribution of cancer and a multi-stage theory of carcinogenesis. Br J Cancer 8:1–12

Arnold MH (2021) Teasing out artificial intelligence in medicine: an ethical critique of artificial intelligence and machine learning in medicine. J Bioeth Inq 18:121–139

Arranz L, Sánchez-Aguilera A, Martín-Pérez D, Isern J, Langa X, Tzankov A, Lundberg P, Muntión S, Tzeng Y-S, Lai D-M, Schwaller J, Skoda RC, Méndez-Ferrer S (2014) Neuropathy of haematopoietic stem cell niche is essential for myeloproliferative neoplasms. Nature 512:78–81

Avan A, Postma TJ, Ceresa C, Avan A, Cavaletti G, Giovannetti E, Peters GJ (2015) Platinum-induced neurotoxicity and preventive strategies: past, present, and future. Oncologist 20:411–432
Baider L, Surbone A (2014) Universality of aging: family caregivers for elderly cancer patients. Front Psychol 5:744
Bailly C (2014) Cell-targeted cytotoxics: a new generation of cytotoxic agents for cancer treatment. Phytochem Rev 13:171–181
Bais AF, McKenzie RL, Bernhard G, Aucamp PJ, Ilyas M, Madronich S, Tourpali K (2015) Ozone depletion and climate change: impacts on UV radiation. Photochem Photobiol Sci 14:19–52
Balding D, McElwain DL (1985) A mathematical model of tumour-induced capillary growth. J Theor Biol 114:53–73
Bapat AA, Hostetter G, Von Hoff DD, Han H (2011) Perineural invasion and associated pain in pancreatic cancer. Nat Rev Cancer 11:695–707
Bar-Ephraim YE, Kretzschmar K, Clevers H (2020) Organoids in immunological research. Nat Rev Immunol 20:279–293
Barnard WF, Wenny BN (2010) Ultraviolet radiation and its interaction with air pollution. In: UV radiation in global climate change. Springer, pp 291–330
Bassil KL, Vakil C, Sanborn M, Cole DC, Kaur JS, Kerr KJ (2007) Cancer health effects of pesticides: systematic review. Can Fam Physician 53:1704–1711
Basu K, Sinha R, Ong A, Basu T (2020) Artificial intelligence: how is it changing medical sciences and its future? Indian J Dermatol 65:365–370
Baumann M, Ebert N, Kurth I, Bacchus C, Overgaard J (2020) What will radiation oncology look like in 2050? A look at a changing professional landscape in Europe and beyond. Mol Oncol 14: 1577–1585
Bodén S, Myte R, Wennberg M, Harlid S, Johansson I, Shivappa N, Hébert JR, Van Guelpen B, Nilsson LM (2019) The inflammatory potential of diet in determining cancer risk; a prospective investigation of two dietary pattern scores. PLoS One 14:e0214551
Bondiau P-Y, Clatz O, Sermesant M, Marcy P-Y, Delingette H, Frenay M, Ayache N (2008) Biocomputing: numerical simulation of glioblastoma growth using diffusion tensor imaging. Phys Med Biol 53:879
Borniger JC, Walker Ii WH, Surbhi EKM, Zhang N, Zalenski AA, Muscarella SL, Fitzgerald JA, Smith AN, Braam CJ, TinKai T, Magalang UJ, Lustberg MB, Nelson RJ, DeVries AC (2018) A role for Hypocretin/orexin in metabolic and sleep abnormalities in a mouse model of non-metastatic breast cancer. Cell Metab 28:118–129.e115
Bulik-Sullivan B, Busby J, Palmer CD, Davis MJ, Murphy T, Clark A, Busby M, Duke F, Yang A, Young L, Ojo NC, Caldwell K, Abhyankar J, Boucher T, Hart MG, Makarov V, De Montpreville VT, Mercier O, Chan TA, Scagliotti G, Bironzo P, Novello S, Karachaliou N, Rosell R, Anderson I, Gabrail N, Hrom J, Limvarapuss C, Choquette K, Spira A, Rousseau R, Voong C, Rizvi NA, Fadel E, Frattini M, Jooss K, Skoberne M, Francis J, Yelensky R (2019) Deep learning using tumor HLA peptide mass spectrometry datasets improves neoantigen identification. Nat Biotechnol 37:55–63
Burrell RA, McGranahan N, Bartek J, Swanton C (2013) The causes and consequences of genetic heterogeneity in cancer evolution. Nature 501:338–345
Buyel JF (2018) Plants as sources of natural and recombinant anti-cancer agents. Biotechnol Adv 36:506–520
Casimiro-Soriguer CS, Loucera C, Peña-Chilet M, Dopazo J (2022) Towards a metagenomics machine learning interpretable model for understanding the transition from adenoma to colorectal cancer. Sci Rep 12:1–14
Chan R, Lok K, Woo J (2009) Prostate cancer and vegetable consumption. Mol Nutr Food Res 53: 201–216
Chida Y, Hamer M, Wardle J, Steptoe A (2008) Do stress-related psychosocial factors contribute to cancer incidence and survival? Nat Clin Pract Oncol 5:466–475

Chowdhury MR, Moshikur RM, Wakabayashi R, Tahara Y, Kamiya N, Moniruzzaman M, Goto M (2018) Ionic-liquid-based paclitaxel preparation: a new potential formulation for cancer treatment. Mol Pharm 15:2484–2488

Chowdhury RA, Brennan FP, Gardiner MD (2020) Cancer rehabilitation and palliative care-exploring the synergies. J Pain Symptom Manag 60:1239–1252

Coley WB (1991) The treatment of malignant tumors by repeated inoculations of erysipelas. With a report of ten original cases. 1893. Clin Orthop Relat Res 262:3–11

Colijn C, Jones N, Johnston IG, Yaliraki S, Barahona M (2017) Toward precision healthcare: context and mathematical challenges. Front Physiol 8:136

Colone M, Calcabrini A, Stringaro A (2020) Drug delivery Systems of Natural Products in oncology. Molecules 25:4560

Cordier D, Gerber M, Brand S (2019) Effects of two types of exercise training on psychological Well-being, sleep, quality of life and physical fitness in patients with high-grade glioma (WHO III and IV): study protocol for a randomized controlled trial. Cancer Commun (Lond) 39:46

Cragg GM, Newman DJ (2005) Plants as a source of anti-cancer agents. J Ethnopharmacol 100:72–79

Dai S, Mo Y, Wang Y, Xiang B, Liao Q, Zhou M, Li X, Li Y, Xiong W, Li G (2020) Chronic stress promotes cancer development. Front Oncol 10:1492

Dalmau J, Gultekin HS, Posner JB (1999) Paraneoplastic neurologic syndromes: pathogenesis and physiopathology. Brain Pathol 9:275–284

Das S, Bhardwaj A, Pandey LM (2021) Functionalized biogenic nanoparticles for use in emerging biomedical applications: a review. Curr Nanomater 6:119–139

Davie-Martin CL, Stratton KG, Teeguarden JG, Waters KM, Simonich SLM (2017) Implications of bioremediation of polycyclic aromatic hydrocarbon-contaminated soils for human health and cancer risk. Environ Sci Technol 51:9458–9468

Davis SE, Greevy RA Jr, Fonnesbeck C, Lasko TA, Walsh CG, Matheny ME (2019) A nonparametric updating method to correct clinical prediction model drift. J Am Med Inform Assoc 26: 1448–1457

De Gonzalez AB, Curtis RE, Kry SF, Gilbert E, Lamart S, Berg CD, Stovall M, Ron E (2011) Proportion of second cancers attributable to radiotherapy treatment in adults: a cohort study in the US SEER cancer registries. Lancet Oncol 12:353–360

De Jong WH, Borm PJ (2008) Drug delivery and nanoparticles: applications and hazards. Int J Nanomedicine 3:133–149

de Martel C, Ferlay J, Franceschi S, Vignat J, Bray F, Forman D, Plummer M (2012) Global burden of cancers attributable to infections in 2008: a review and synthetic analysis. Lancet Oncol 13: 607–615

Debbouche A, Nieto JJ, Torres DFM (2021) Focus point: cancer and HIV/AIDS dynamics—from optimality to modelling. Eur Phys J Plus 136:165. Springer

Delpech B, Maingonnat C, Girard N, Chauzy C, Olivier A, Maunoury R, Tayot J, Creissard P (1993) Hyaluronan and hyaluronectin in the extracellular matrix of human brain tumour stroma. Eur J Cancer 29:1012–1017

Deng J, Isik E, Fernandes SM, Brown JR, Letai A, Davids MS (2017) Bruton's tyrosine kinase inhibition increases BCL-2 dependence and enhances sensitivity to venetoclax in chronic lymphocytic leukemia. Leukemia 31:2075–2084

Deryugina EI, Bourdon MA (1996) Tenascin mediates human glioma cell migration and modulates cell migration on fibronectin. J Cell Sci 109:643–652

Desai AG, Qazi GN, Ganju RK, El-Tamer M, Singh J, Saxena AK, Bedi YS, Taneja SC, Bhat HK (2008) Medicinal plants and cancer chemoprevention. Curr Drug Metab 9:581–591

Dijkstra KK, Cattaneo CM, Weeber F, Chalabi M, van de Haar J, Fanchi LF, Slagter M, van der Velden DL, Kaing S, Kelderman S (2018) Generation of tumor-reactive T cells by co-culture of peripheral blood lymphocytes and tumor organoids. Cell 174:1586–1598.e1512

Dionysiou DD, Stamatakos GS, Uzunoglu NK, Nikita KS, Marioli A (2004) A four-dimensional simulation model of tumour response to radiotherapy in vivo: parametric validation considering radiosensitivity, genetic profile and fractionation. J Theor Biol 230:1–20
Dobosz P, Dzieciątkowski T (2019) The intriguing history of cancer immunotherapy. Front Immunol 10:2965
Eckerling A, Ricon-Becker I, Sorski L, Sandbank E, Ben-Eliyahu S (2021) Stress and cancer: mechanisms, significance and future directions. Nat Rev Cancer 21:767–785
Ehteshami Bejnordi B, Veta M, Johannes van Diest P, van Ginneken B, Karssemeijer N, Litjens G, van der Laak JAWM, and the CAMELYON16 Consortium (2017) Diagnostic assessment of deep learning algorithms for detection of lymph node metastases in women with breast cancer. JAMA 318:2199–2210
Eisenhut L, Sadeghi-Bahmani D, Gerber M, Saemann A, Staub L, Brand S, Cordier D (2022) Effects of two types of exercise training on psychological well-being, sleep and physical fitness in patients with high-grade glioma (WHO III and IV). J Psychiatr Res 151:354–364
Enuneku A, Ogbeide O, Okpara B, Kubeyinje BF, Job O, Asemota CO, Imoobe T, Ezemonye LI (2021) Ingestion and dermal cancer risk via exposure to polycyclic aromatic hydrocarbon–contaminated soils in an oil-producing community, Niger Delta, Nigeria. Environ Toxicol Chem 40:261–271
Esteva A, Kuprel B, Novoa RA, Ko J, Swetter SM, Blau HM, Thrun S (2017) Dermatologist-level classification of skin cancer with deep neural networks. Nature 542:115–118
Fan J, Zhang Y, Liu Y, Wang Y, Cao F, Yang Q, Tian F (2019) Explanation of the cell orientation in a nanofiber membrane by the geometric potential theory. Results Phys 15:102537
Ferreccio C, González C, Milosavjlevic V, Marshall G, Sancha AM, Smith AH (2000) Lung cancer and arsenic concentrations in drinking water in Chile. Epidemiology 11:673–679
Fiolet T, Srour B, Sellem L, Kesse-Guyot E, Allès B, Méjean C, Deschasaux M, Fassier P, Latino-Martel P, Beslay M (2018) Consumption of ultra-processed foods and cancer risk: results from NutriNet-Santé prospective cohort. BMJ 360:k322
Glazer ES, Curley SA (2011) The ongoing history of thermal therapy for cancer. Surg Oncol Clin 20:229–235
Go VLW, Wong DA, Butrum R (2001) Diet, nutrition and cancer prevention: where are we going from here? J Nutr 131:3121S–3126S
Godfrey A, Hetherington V, Shum H, Bonato P, Lovell NH, Stuart S (2018) From A to Z: wearable technology explained. Maturitas 113:40–47
Gonzalez-Rodriguez D, Guevorkian K, Douezan S, Brochard-Wyart F (2012) Soft matter models of developing tissues and tumors. Science 338:910–917
Grade M, Difilippantonio MJ, Camps J (2015) Patterns of chromosomal aberrations in solid tumors. Recent Results Cancer Res 200:115–142
Granero S, Domingo JL (2002) Levels of metals in soils of Alcalá de Henares, Spain: human health risks. Environ Int 28:159–164
Greenspan HP (1972) Models for the growth of a solid tumor by diffusion. Stud Appl Math 51:317–340
Greenspan HP (1976) On the growth and stability of cell cultures and solid tumors. J Theor Biol 56:229–242
Griffith GW, Davies RI (1954) Cancer and soils in the county of Anglesey. A revised method of comparison. Br J Cancer 8:594–598
Griffiths K, Aggarwal BB, Singh RB, Buttar HS, Wilson D, De Meester F (2016) Food antioxidants and their anti-inflammatory properties: a potential role in cardiovascular diseases and cancer prevention. Diseases 4:28
Grossi F, Belvedere O, Rosso R (2003) Geography of clinical cancer research publications from 1995 to 1999. Eur J Cancer 39:106–111
Hahn WC, Bader JS, Braun TP, Califano A, Clemons PA, Druker BJ, Ewald AJ, Fu H, Jagu S, Kemp CJ (2021) An expanded universe of cancer targets. Cell 184:1142–1155
Hanahan D (2022) Hallmarks of cancer: new dimensions. Cancer Discov 12:31–46

Hanahan D, Weinberg RA (2000) The hallmarks of cancer. Cell 100:57–70
Hanahan D, Weinberg RA (2011) Hallmarks of cancer: the next generation. Cell 144:646–674
Hatze H (1974) The meaning of the term "biomechanics". J Biomech 7:189–190
Hayakawa Y, Sakitani K, Konishi M, Asfaha S, Niikura R, Tomita H, Renz BW, Tailor Y, Macchini M, Middelhoff M (2017) Nerve growth factor promotes gastric tumorigenesis through aberrant cholinergic signaling. Cancer Cell 31:21–34
He J-H (2008) Fatalness of virus depends upon its cell fractal geometry. Chaos Solitons Fractals 38:1390–1393
Hernandez-Boussard T, Macklin P, Greenspan EJ, Gryshuk AL, Stahlberg E, Syeda-Mahmood T, Shmulevich I (2021) Digital twins for predictive oncology will be a paradigm shift for precision cancer care. Nat Med 27:2065–2066
Hiam-Galvez KJ, Allen BM, Spitzer MH (2021) Systemic immunity in cancer. Nat Rev Cancer 21:345–359
Holohan C, Van Schaeybroeck S, Longley DB, Johnston PG (2013) Cancer drug resistance: an evolving paradigm. Nat Rev Cancer 13:714–726
Hongo M, Nagasaki Y, Shoji T (2009) Epidemiology of esophageal cancer: orient to occident. Effects of chronology, geography and ethnicity. J Gastroenterol Hepatol 24:729–735
Hopenhayn-Rich C, Biggs ML, Smith AH (1998) Lung and kidney cancer mortality associated with arsenic in drinking water in Córdoba, Argentina. Int J Epidemiol 27:561–569
Horowitz TS, Suls J, Treviño M (2018) A call for a neuroscience approach to cancer-related cognitive impairment. Trends Neurosci 41:493–496
Hossain MA, Saiful Islam SM, Quinn JMW, Huq F, Moni MA (2019) Machine learning and bioinformatics models to identify gene expression patterns of ovarian cancer associated with disease progression and mortality. J Biomed Inform 100:103313
Huang C-H, Zeng C, Wang Y-C, Peng H-Y, Lin C-S, Chang C-J, Yang H-Y (2018) A study of diagnostic accuracy using a chemical sensor Array and a machine learning technique to detect lung cancer. Sensors (Basel, Switzerland) 18:2845
Huang S, Yang J, Fong S, Zhao Q (2020) Artificial intelligence in cancer diagnosis and prognosis: opportunities and challenges. Cancer Lett 471:61–71
Ibikunle S, Arogunjo A, Ajayi OJ (2018) Characterization of radiation dose and excess lifetime cancer risk due to natural radionuclides in soils from some cities in Southwestern Nigeria. J Forensic Sci Crim Invest 10:555793
Inam E, Ibanga F, Essien J (2016) Bioaccumulation and cancer risk of polycyclic aromatic hydrocarbons in leafy vegetables grown in soils within automobile repair complex and environ in Uyo, Nigeria. Environ Monit Assess 188:1–9
Iqbal MH, Aydin A, Brunckhorst O, Dasgupta P, Ahmed K (2016) A review of wearable technology in medicine. J R Soc Med 109:372–380
Jabbari P, Rezaei N (2019) Artificial intelligence and immunotherapy. Expert Rev Clin Immunol 15:689–691
Josyula S, Lin J, Xue X, Rothman N, Lan Q, Rohan TE, Hosgood HD (2015) Household air pollution and cancers other than lung: a meta-analysis. Environ Health 14:24
Jurgons R, Seliger C, Hilpert A, Trahms L, Odenbach S, Alexiou CJ (2006) Drug loaded magnetic nanoparticles for cancer therapy. J Phys Condens Matter 18:S2893
Khurana S, Dubey ML, Malla N (2005) Association of parasitic infections and cancers. Indian J Med Microbiol 23:74–79
Kozusko F, Bourdeau M (2007) A unified model of sigmoid tumour growth based on cell proliferation and quiescence. Cell Prolif 40:824–834
Krishnadas R, Cavanagh J (2012) Depression: an inflammatory illness? J Neurol Neurosurg Psychiatry 83:495
Kroschinsky F, Stölzel F, von Bonin S, Beutel G, Kochanek M, Kiehl M, Schellongowski P (2017) New drugs, new toxicities: severe side effects of modern targeted and immunotherapy of cancer and their management. Crit Care 21:1–11

Kumar Y, Gupta S, Singla R, Hu Y-C (2022) A systematic review of artificial intelligence techniques in cancer prediction and diagnosis. Arch Comput Methods Eng 29:2043–2070

Langley RR, Fidler IJ (2011) The seed and soil hypothesis revisited–the role of tumor-stroma interactions in metastasis to different organs. Int J Cancer 128:2527–2535

Lee C-P, Lee Y-H, Lian I-B, Su C-C (2016) Increased prevalence of Esophageal cancer in areas with high levels of nickel in farm soils. J Cancer 7:1724–1730

Levental KR, Yu H, Kass L, Lakins JN, Egeblad M, Erler JT, Fong SF, Csiszar K, Giaccia A, Weninger W (2009) Matrix crosslinking forces tumor progression by enhancing integrin signaling. J Cell 139:891–906

Li L-J (2020) Thermal therapy for eye diseases. Therm Sci 24:2319–2324

Li X-X, He J-H (2019) Along the evolution process kleiber's 3/4 law makes way for rubner's surface law: a fractal approach. Fractals 27:1950015

Li X-X, Tian D, He J-H (2021) High energy surface as a receptor in electrospinning: a good switch for hydrophobicity to hydrophilicity. Therm Sci 25:2205–2212

Lin S-H, Li Y-H, Leung K, Huang C-Y, Wang X-R (2014) Salt processed food and gastric cancer in a Chinese population. Asian Pac J Cancer Prev 15:5293–5298

Lin LY, Lin LH, Tzeng GL, Huang YH, Tai JF, Chen YL, Wu CJ, Chen PH, Lin PC, Hung PL (2022) Effects of mindfulness-based therapy for cancer patients: a systematic review and meta-analysis. J Clin Psychol Med Settings 29:432–445

Lind AP, Anderson PC (2019) Predicting drug activity against cancer cells by random forest models based on minimal genomic information and chemical properties. PLoS One 14:e0219774

Liu P, Cheng H, Roberts TM, Zhao JJ (2009) Targeting the phosphoinositide 3-kinase pathway in cancer. Nat Rev Drug Discov 8:627–644

Liu Y, Yao C, Drakopoulos F, Wu J, Zhou L, Chrisochoides N (2014) A nonrigid registration method for correcting brain deformation induced by tumor resection. Med Phys 41:101710

López Alfonso JC, Poleszczuk J, Walker R, Kim S, Pilon-Thomas S, Conejo-Garcia JJ, Soliman H, Czerniecki B, Harrison LB, Enderling H (2019) Immunologic consequences of sequencing cancer radiotherapy and surgery. JCO Clin Cancer Inform 3:1–16

Luria SE, Delbrück M (1943) Mutations of bacteria from virus sensitivity to virus resistance. Genetics 28:491

Lutgendorf SK, Sood AK (2011) Biobehavioral factors and cancer progression: physiological pathways and mechanisms. Psychosom Med 73:724–730

Mair DB, Ames HM, Li R (2018) Mechanisms of invasion and motility of high-grade gliomas in the brain. J Mol Biol Cell 29:2509–2515

Man YB, Kang Y, Wang HS, Lau W, Li H, Sun XL, Giesy JP, Chow KL, Wong MH (2013) Cancer risk assessments of Hong Kong soils contaminated by polycyclic aromatic hydrocarbons. J Hazard Mater 261:770–776

Marcus HJ, Zareinia K, Gan LS, Yang FW, Lama S, Yang GZ, Sutherland GR (2014) Forces exerted during microneurosurgery: a cadaver study. Int J Med Robot Comput Assist Surg 10:251–256

Martinov T, McKenna KM, Tan WH, Collins EJ, Kehret AR, Linton JD, Olsen TM, Shobaki N, Rongvaux A (2021) Building the next generation of humanized hemato-lymphoid system mice. Front Immunol 12:346

Matson V, Fessler J, Bao R, Chongsuwat T, Zha Y, Alegre M-L, Luke JJ, Gajewski TF (2018) The commensal microbiome is associated with anti–PD-1 efficacy in metastatic melanoma patients. Science 359:104–108

McCarthy EF (2006) The toxins of William B. Coley and the treatment of bone and soft-tissue sarcomas. Iowa Orthop J 26:154–158

McCarthy J, Minsky ML, Rochester N, Shannon CE (2006) A proposal for the Dartmouth summer research project on artificial intelligence, august 31, 1955. AI Mag 27:12–12

McGeehin MA, Reif JS, Becher JC, Mangione EJ (1993) Case-control study of bladder cancer and water disinfection methods in Colorado. Am J Epidemiol 138:492–501

McKenna MT, Weis JA, Brock A, Quaranta V, Yankeelov TE (2018) Precision medicine with imprecise therapy: computational Modeling for chemotherapy in breast cancer. Transl Oncol 11:732–742
McKinley JM, Ofterdinger U, Young M, Barsby A, Gavin A (2013) Investigating local relationships between trace elements in soils and cancer data. Spatial Stat 5:25–41
McNamara K, Tofail SAM (2017) Nanoparticles in biomedical applications. Adv Phys X 2:54–88
Medina MA (2018) Mathematical modeling of cancer metabolism. Crit Rev Oncol Hematol 124:37–40
Mego M, Holec V, Drgona L, Hainova K, Ciernikova S, Zajac V (2013) Probiotic bacteria in cancer patients undergoing chemotherapy and radiation therapy. Complement Ther Med 21:712–723
Menck HR, Henderson BE, Pike MC, Mack T, Martin SP, SooHoo J (1975) Cancer incidence in the Mexican-American. J Natl Cancer Inst 55:531–536
Michor F, Liphardt J, Ferrari M, Widom J (2011) What does physics have to do with cancer? Nat Rev Cancer 11:657–670
Mierke CT (2014) The fundamental role of mechanical properties in the progression of cancer disease and inflammation. Rep Prog Phys 77:076602
Mitchell MJ, Billingsley MM, Haley RM, Wechsler ME, Peppas NA, Langer R (2021) Engineering precision nanoparticles for drug delivery. Nat Rev Drug Discov 20:101–124
Mohajer R, Salehi MH, Mohammadi J, Emami MH, Azarm T (2013) The status of lead and cadmium in soils of high prevalenct gastrointestinal cancer region of Isfahan. J Res Med Sci 18:210
Mohan G, Ayisha Hamna TP, Jijo AJ, Saradha Devi KM, Narayanasamy A, Vellingiri B (2019) Recent advances in radiotherapy and its associated side effects in cancer—a review. The Journal of Basic Applied Zoology 80:1–10
Mohit A, Keshavarzi B, Moore F (2019) Polycyclic aromatic hydrocarbons (PAHs) in urban soils of Ahvaz metropolis; contamination, composition, distribution, potential sources, and cancer risk. Hum Ecol Risk Assess 25:935–948
Monje M, Borniger JC, D'Silva NJ, Deneen B, Dirks PB, Fattahi F, Frenette PS, Garzia L, Gutmann DH, Hanahan D, Hervey-Jumper SL, Hondermarck H, Hurov JB, Kepecs A, Knox SM, Lloyd AC, Magnon C, Saloman JL, Segal RA, Sloan EK, Sun X, Taylor MD, Tracey KJ, Trotman LC, Tuveson DA, Wang TC, White RA, Winkler F (2020) Roadmap for the emerging field of cancer neuroscience. Cell 181:219–222
Morton JJ, Bird G, Refaeli Y, Jimeno A (2016) Humanized mouse xenograft models: narrowing the tumor–microenvironment gap. Cancer Res 76:6153–6158
Mouw JK, Yui Y, Damiano L, Bainer RO, Lakins JN, Acerbi I, Ou G, Wijekoon AC, Levental KR, Gilbert PM (2014) Tissue mechanics modulate microRNA-dependent PTEN expression to regulate malignant progression. J Nat Med 20:360–367
Naffar-Abu-Amara S, Shay T, Galun M, Cohen N, Isakoff SJ, Kam Z, Geiger B (2008) Identification of novel pro-migratory, cancer-associated genes using quantitative, microscopy-based screening. PLoS One 3:e1457
Nakada M, Kita D, Futami K, Yamashita J, Fujimoto N, Sato H, Okada Y (2001) Roles of membrane type 1 matrix metalloproteinase and tissue inhibitor of metalloproteinases 2 in invasion and dissemination of human malignant glioma. J Neurosurg 94:464–473
Narayanan DL, Saladi RN, Fox JL (2010) Review: ultraviolet radiation and skin cancer. Int J Dermatol 49:978–986
Nde SC, Mathuthu M, Massoukou RYM, Bett SK, Richard G, Oluwadamilare OP (2021) Modelling the dynamics of the cancer risk due to potentially toxic elements in agricultural soils, in the upper Crocodile River catchment, north-West province, South Africa. Ecotoxicol Environ Saf 211:111961
Nia HT, Munn LL, Jain RK (2020) Physical traits of cancer. Science 370:eaaz0868
Njinga RL, Tshivhase VM (2016) Lifetime cancer risk due to gamma radioactivity in soils from Tudor shaft mine environs, South Africa. J Radiat Res Appl Sci 9:310–315

Oiseth SJ, Aziz MS (2017) Cancer immunotherapy: a brief review of the history, possibilities, and challenges ahead. J Cancer Metastasis Treat 3:250–261

Page T, Harris RH, Epstein SS (1976) Drinking water and cancer mortality in Louisiana. Science 193:55–57

Paget S (1989) The distribution of secondary growths in cancer of the breast. 1889. Cancer Metastasis Rev 8:98–101

Pedro J, Monteiro-Reis S, Carvalho-Maia C, Henrique R, Jerónimo C, Silva ER (2021) Evidence of psychological and biological effects of structured mindfulness-based interventions for cancer patients and survivors: a meta-review. Psychooncology 30:1836–1848

Pereira CV, Silva JM, Rodrigues L, Reis RL, Paiva A, Duarte ARC, Matias A (2019) Unveil the anticancer potential of limomene based therapeutic deep eutectic solvents. Sci Rep 9:1–11

Phillips M, Gleeson K, Hughes JM, Greenberg J, Cataneo RN, Baker L, McVay WP (1999) Volatile organic compounds in breath as markers of lung cancer: a cross-sectional study. Lancet 353: 1930–1933

Plummer M, de Martel C, Vignat J, Ferlay J, Bray F, Franceschi S (2016) Global burden of cancers attributable to infections in 2012: a synthetic analysis. Lancet Glob Health 4:e609–e616

Poggi A, Villa F, Fernadez JLC, Costa D, Zocchi MR, Benelli R (2021) Three-dimensional culture models to study innate anti-tumor immune response: advantages and disadvantages. Cancers (Basel) 13:3417

Prasad NR, Muthusamy G, Shanmugam M, Ambudkar SV (2016) South Asian medicinal compounds as modulators of resistance to chemotherapy and radiotherapy. Cancers (Basel) 8:32

Qin S-Y, Zhang A-Q, Cheng S-X, Rong L, Zhang X-Z (2017) Drug self-delivery systems for cancer therapy. Biomaterials 112:234–247

Qin SY, Zhang AQ, Zhang XZ (2018) Recent advances in targeted tumor chemotherapy based on smart nanomedicines. Small 14:1802417

Quaranta V, Weaver AM, Cummings PT, Anderson AR (2005) Mathematical modeling of cancer: the future of prognosis and treatment. Clin Chim Acta 357:173–179

Radiology ESo (2019) What the radiologist should know about artificial intelligence–an ESR white paper. Insights Imaging 10:1–8

Rafieepour A, Ghamari F, Mohammadbeigi A, Asghari M (2015) Seasonal variation in exposure level of types a and B ultraviolet radiation: an environmental skin carcinogen. Ann Med Health Sci Res 5:129–133

Raman M, Ambalam P, Kondepudi KK, Pithva S, Kothari C, Patel AT, Purama RK, Dave JM, Vyas BR (2013) Potential of probiotics, prebiotics and synbiotics for management of colorectal cancer. Gut Microbes 4:181–192

Rao JS (2003) Molecular mechanisms of glioma invasiveness: the role of proteases. J Nat Rev Cancer 3:489–501

Rasooly A, Jacobson J (2006) Development of biosensors for cancer clinical testing. Biosens Bioelectron 21:1851–1858

Ravasco P (2019) Nutrition in cancer patients. J Clin Med 8:1211

Redman M, Ward E, Phillips R (2014) The efficacy and safety of probiotics in people with cancer: a systematic review. Ann Oncol 25:1919–1929

Reger M, Kutschan S, Freuding M, Schmidt T, Josfeld L, Huebner J (2022) Water therapies (hydrotherapy, balneotherapy or aqua therapy) for patients with cancer: a systematic review. J Cancer Res Clin Oncol 148:1–21

Reich M (2008) Depression and cancer: recent data on clinical issues, research challenges and treatment approaches. Curr Opin Oncol 20:353–359

Reidy E, Leonard NA, Treacy O, Ryan AE (2021) A 3D view of colorectal cancer models in predicting therapeutic responses and resistance. Cancers 13:227

Research WCRF (2007) Food, nutrition, physical activity, and the prevention of cancer: a global perspective. American Institute for Cancer Research, Washington, DC

Rodrigues J, Heinrich MA, Teixeira LM, Prakash J (2021) 3D in vitro model (R) evolution: unveiling tumor–stroma interactions. Trends Cancer 7:249–264

Rohrmann S, Overvad K, Bueno-de-Mesquita HB, Jakobsen MU, Egeberg R, Tjønneland A, Nailler L, Boutron-Ruault MC, Clavel-Chapelon F, Krogh V, Palli D, Panico S, Tumino R, Ricceri F, Bergmann MM, Boeing H, Li K, Kaaks R, Khaw KT, Wareham NJ, Crowe FL, Key TJ, Naska A, Trichopoulou A, Trichopoulos D, Leenders M, Peeters PH, Engeset D, Parr CL, Skeie G, Jakszyn P, Sánchez MJ, Huerta JM, Redondo ML, Barricarte A, Amiano P, Drake I, Sonestedt E, Hallmans G, Johansson I, Fedirko V, Romieux I, Ferrari P, Norat T, Vergnaud AC, Riboli E, Linseisen J (2013) Meat consumption and mortality–results from the European Prospective Investigation into Cancer and Nutrition. BMC Med 11:63

Routy B, Le Chatelier E, Derosa L, Duong CP, Alou MT, Daillère R, Fluckiger A, Messaoudene M, Rauber C, Roberti MP (2018) Gut microbiome influences efficacy of PD-1–based immunotherapy against epithelial tumors. Science 359:91–97

Sabarwal A, Kumar K, Singh RP (2018) Hazardous effects of chemical pesticides on human health–cancer and other associated disorders. Environ Toxicol Pharmacol 63:103–114

Sahoo BM, Kumar BVVR, Patra CN, Panda JR, Mohanta BC, Palei NN (2020) Nanotechnology: a novel approach for drug development in health care system. Curr Nanomater 5:12–25

Saita E, Acquati C, Kayser K (2015) Coping with early stage breast cancer: examining the influence of personality traits and interpersonal closeness. Front Psychol 6:88

Saloman JL, Cohen JA, Kaplan DH (2020) Intimate neuro-immune interactions: breaking barriers between systems to make meaningful progress. Curr Opin Neurobiol 62:60–67

Samaila B, Maidamma B, Usman B, Jega AI, Alhaji SA (2022) Assessment of hazard index and incremental life cancer risk associated with heavy metals in the soils. Sci Prog Res 2. https://doi.org/10.52152/spr/2022.155

Sapienza C, Issa J-P (2016) Diet, nutrition, and cancer epigenetics. Annu Rev Nutr 36:665–681

Sariego J (2009) Patterns of breast cancer presentation in the United States: does geography matter? Am Surg 75:545–549; discussion 549–550

Schwabe RF, Jobin C (2013) The microbiome and cancer. Nat Rev Cancer 13:800–812

Semnani S, Roshandel G, Zendehbad A, Keshtkar A, Rahimzadeh H, Abdolahi N, Besharat S, Moradi A, Mirkarimi H, Hasheminasab SJ (2010) Soils selenium level and esophageal cancer: an ecological study in a high risk area for esophageal cancer. J Trace Elem Med Biol 24:174–177

Sharma P, Hu-Lieskovan S, Wargo JA, Ribas A (2017) Primary, adaptive, and acquired resistance to cancer immunotherapy. Cell 168:707–723

Sin NL, Graham-Engeland JE, Ong AD, Almeida DM (2015) Affective reactivity to daily stressors is associated with elevated inflammation. Health Psychol 34:1154

Singh RK, Kumar S, Prasad D, Bhardwaj T (2018) Therapeutic journey of nitrogen mustard as alkylating anticancer agents: historic to future perspectives. Eur J Med Chem 151:401–433

Slavich GM, Irwin MR (2014) From stress to inflammation and major depressive disorder: a social signal transduction theory of depression. Psychol Bull 140:774

Somashekhar SP, Kumarc R, Rauthan A, Arun KR, Patil P, Ramya YE (2017) Abstract S6-07: double blinded validation study to assess performance of IBM artificial intelligence platform, Watson for oncology in comparison with Manipal multidisciplinary tumour board – first study of 638 breast cancer cases. Cancer Res 77:S6–S07

Stacke K, Eilertsen G, Unger J, Lundstrom C (2021) Measuring domain shift for deep learning in histopathology. IEEE J Biomed Health Inform 25:325–336

Stamatakos GS, Dionysiou DD, Zacharaki EI, Mouravliansky NA, Nikita KS, Uzunoglu NK (2002) In silico radiation oncology: combining novel simulation algorithms with current visualization techniques. Proc IEEE 90:1764–1777

Stanford JL, Herrinton LJ, Schwartz SM, Weiss NS (1995) Breast cancer incidence in Asian migrants to the United States and their descendants. Epidemiology 6:181–183

Stout NL, Santa Mina D, Lyons KD, Robb K, Silver JK (2021) A systematic review of rehabilitation and exercise recommendations in oncology guidelines. CA Cancer J Clin 71:149–175

Su C-C, Lin Y-Y, Chang T-K, Chiang C-T, Chung J-A, Hsu Y-Y, Lian I-B (2010) Incidence of oral cancer in relation to nickel and arsenic concentrations in farm soils of patients' residential areas in Taiwan. BMC Public Health 10:1–10

Sun X, Pradeepkumar P, Rajendran NK, Shakila H, Houreld NN, Al Farraj DA, Elnahas YM, Elumalai N, Rajan M (2020) Natural deep eutectic solvent supported targeted solid–liquid polymer carrier for breast cancer therapy. RSC Adv 10:36989–37004

Suresh S (2007) Biomechanics and biophysics of cancer cells. J Acta Biomater 3:413–438

Sweilam N, Al-Mekhlafi S, Albalawi A, Machado JT (2021) Optimal control of variable-order fractional model for delay cancer treatments. Appl Math Model 89:1557–1574

Tabassum S, Rosli NB, Mazalan MSAB (2019) Mathematical modeling of cancer growth process: a review. J Phys Conf Ser 1366:article id. 012018, IOP Publishing

Tan DS, Mok TS, Rebbeck TR (2016) Cancer genomics: diversity and disparity across ethnicity and geography. J Clin Oncol 34:91–101

Tang M, Zhao M, Shanshan Z, Chen K, Zhang C, Liu W (2014) Assessing the underlying breast cancer risk of Chinese females contributed by dietary intake of residual DDT from agricultural soils. Environ Int 73:208–215

Taninaga J, Nishiyama Y, Fujibayashi K, Gunji T, Sasabe N, Iijima K, Naito T (2019) Prediction of future gastric cancer risk using a machine learning algorithm and comprehensive medical check-up data: a case-control study. Sci Rep 9:12384

Tariq A, Sadia S, Pan K, Ullah I, Mussarat S, Sun F, Abiodun OO, Batbaatar A, Li Z, Song D (2017) A systematic review on ethnomedicines of anti-cancer plants. Phytother Res 31:202–264

Taylor EF, Burley VJ, Greenwood DC, Cade JE (2007) Meat consumption and risk of breast cancer in the UK Women's cohort study. Br J Cancer 96:1139–1146

Tegin J, Wikander J (2005) Tactile sensing in intelligent robotic manipulation–a review. Ind Robot Int J. https://doi.org/10.1108/01439910510573318

Terry P, Terry JB, Wolk A (2001) Fruit and vegetable consumption in the prevention of cancer: an update. J Intern Med 250:280–290

Thomas T, DiMilla P (2000) Spreading and motility of human glioblastoma cells on sheets of silicone rubber depend on substratum compliance. J Med Biol Eng Comput 38:360–370

Tothill IE (2009) Biosensors for cancer markers diagnosis. Semin Cell Dev Biol 20:55–62

Tsukanov A, Psakhie S (2016) Adhesion effects within the hard matter–soft matter interface: molecular dynamics. Facta Univ Ser Mech Eng 14:269–280

Tubiana M (2009) Can we reduce the incidence of second primary malignancies occurring after radiotherapy? A critical review. Radiother Oncol 91:4–15

Turner ND, Lloyd SK (2017) Association between red meat consumption and colon cancer: a systematic review of experimental results. Exp Biol Med (Maywood) 242:813–839

Tysnes BB, Mahesparan R, Thorsen F, Haugland HK, Porwol T, Enger PØ, Lund-Johansen M, Bjerkvig R (1999) Laminin expression by glial fibrillary acidic protein positive cells in human gliomas. Int J Dev Neurosci 17:531–539

Ulrich TA, de Juan Pardo EM, Kumar S (2009) The mechanical rigidity of the extracellular matrix regulates the structure, motility, and proliferation of glioma cells. J Cancer Res 69:4167–4174

Uribe DO, Stroop R, Wallaschek J (2009) Piezoelectric self-sensing system for tactile intraoperative brain tumor delineation in neurosurgery. In: 2009 annual international conference of the IEEE engineering in medicine and biology society. IEEE

van Elsland D, Neefjes J (2018) Bacterial infections and cancer. EMBO Rep 19:e46632

Van Orden KA, Witte TK, Cukrowicz KC, Braithwaite SR, Selby EA, Joiner TE Jr (2010) The interpersonal theory of suicide. Psychol Rev 117:575

Venkataramani V, Tanev DI, Strahle C, Studier-Fischer A, Fankhauser L, Kessler T, Körber C, Kardorff M, Ratliff M, Xie R, Horstmann H, Messer M, Paik SP, Knabbe J, Sahm F, Kurz FT, Acikgöz AA, Herrmannsdörfer F, Agarwal A, Bergles DE, Chalmers A, Miletic H, Turcan S, Mawrin C, Hänggi D, Liu H-K, Wick W, Winkler F, Kuner T (2019) Glutamatergic synaptic input to glioma cells drives brain tumour progression. Nature 573:532–538

Venkatesh HS, Johung TB, Caretti V, Noll A, Tang Y, Nagaraja S, Gibson EM, Mount CW, Polepalli J, Mitra SS (2015) Neuronal activity promotes glioma growth through neuroligin-3 secretion. Cell 161:803–816

Venkatesh HS, Morishita W, Geraghty AC, Silverbush D, Gillespie SM, Arzt M, Tam LT, Espenel C, Ponnuswami A, Ni L, Woo PJ, Taylor KR, Agarwal A, Regev A, Brang D, Vogel H, Hervey-Jumper S, Bergles DE, Suvà ML, Malenka RC, Monje M (2019) Electrical and synaptic integration of glioma into neural circuits. Nature 573:539–545

Vineis P, Hoek G, Krzyzanowski M, Vigna-Taglianti F, Veglia F, Airoldi L, Overvad K, Raaschou-Nielsen O, Clavel-Chapelon F, Linseisen J, Boeing H, Trichopoulou A, Palli D, Krogh V, Tumino R, Panico S, Bueno-De-Mesquita HB, Peeters PH, Lund EE, Agudo A, Martinez C, Dorronsoro M, Barricarte A, Cirera L, Quiros JR, Berglund G, Manjer J, Forsberg B, Day NE, Key TJ, Kaaks R, Saracci R, Riboli E (2007) Lung cancers attributable to environmental tobacco smoke and air pollution in non-smokers in different European countries: a prospective study. Environ Health 6:7

Vivarelli S, Salemi R, Candido S, Falzone L, Santagati M, Stefani S, Torino F, Banna GL, Tonini G, Libra M (2019) Gut microbiota and cancer: from pathogenesis to therapy. Cancers 11:38

Wali AF, Majid S, Rasool S, Shehada SB, Abdulkareem SK, Firdous A, Beigh S, Shakeel S, Mushtaq S, Akbar I, Madhkali H, Rehman MU (2019) Natural products against cancer: review on phytochemicals from marine sources in preventing cancer. Saudi Pharm J 27:767–777

Wang Z, Deisboeck TS (2014) Mathematical modeling in cancer drug discovery. Drug Discov Today 19:145–150

Wang J, Lü D, Mao D, Long M (2014) Mechanomics: an emerging field between biology and biomechanics. Protein Cell 5:518–531

Wang K, Sun J-Z, Wu Q-X, Li Z-Y, Li D-X, Xiong Y-F, Zhong G-C, Shi Y, Li Q, Zheng J, Shivappa N, Hébert JR, Foukakis T, Zhang X, Li H-Y, Xiang T-X, Ren G-S (2020) Long-term anti-inflammatory diet in relation to improved breast cancer prognosis: a prospective cohort study. npj Breast Cancer 6:36

Weir HK, Thompson TD, Stewart SL, White MC (2021) Peer reviewed: cancer incidence projections in the United States between 2015 and 2050. Prev Chronic Dis 18:E59

West J, Robertson-Tessi M, Luddy K, Park DS, Williamson DFK, Harmon C, Khong HT, Brown J, Anderson ARA (2019) The immune checkpoint kick start: optimization of Neoadjuvant combination therapy using game theory. JCO Clin Cancer Inform 3:1–12

Wheldon TE, Kirk J, Orr JS (1977) Optimal radiotherapy of tumour cells following exponential-quadratic survival curves and exponential repopulation kinetics. Br J Radiol 50:681–682

Wilson BC, Patterson MS (2008) The physics, biophysics and technology of photodynamic therapy. Phys Med Biol 53:R61–R109

Winkler JK, Fink C, Toberer F, Enk A, Deinlein T, Hofmann-Wellenhof R, Thomas L, Lallas A, Blum A, Stolz W, Haenssle HA (2019) Association between surgical skin markings in Dermoscopic images and diagnostic performance of a deep learning convolutional neural network for melanoma recognition. JAMA Dermatol 155:1135–1141

Wirtz D, Konstantopoulos K, Searson PC (2011) The physics of cancer: the role of physical interactions and mechanical forces in metastasis. Nat Rev Cancer 11:512–522

Wyld L, Audisio RA, Poston GJ (2015) The evolution of cancer surgery and future perspectives. Nat Rev Clin Oncol 12:115–124

Yang X, Huang L, Li C, Ji N, Zhu H (2022) The effectiveness of mindfulness-based stress reduction intervention on alleviating anxiety and depression in postoperative patients with cervical cancer: a protocol for systematic review and meta-analysis. Medicine (Baltimore) 101:e28706

Yazdanpanah N, Mojtabavi H, Ziaei H, Pirkoohi ZR, Rayzan E, Rezaei N (2022) The clinical benefits of art therapy: definition, history, and outcomes with a focus on music therapy. Springer, Multidisciplinarity and Interdisciplinarity in Health, pp 457–482

Yim EK, Darling EM, Kulangara K, Guilak F, Leong KW (2010) Nanotopography-induced changes in focal adhesions, cytoskeletal organization, and mechanical properties of human mesenchymal stem cells. J Biomater Dent 31:1299–1306

Yu K, Lin C-CJ, Hatcher A, Lozzi B, Kong K, Huang-Hobbs E, Cheng Y-T, Beechar VB, Zhu W, Zhang Y, Chen F, Mills GB, Mohila CA, Creighton CJ, Noebels JL, Scott KL, Deneen B (2020) PIK3CA variants selectively initiate brain hyperactivity during gliomagenesis. Nature 578:166–171

Yun Y, Gao R, Yue H, Liu X, Li G, Sang N (2017) Polycyclic aromatic hydrocarbon (PAH)-containing soils from coal gangue stacking areas contribute to epithelial to mesenchymal transition (EMT) modulation on cancer cell metastasis. Sci Total Environ 580:632–640

Zahalka AH, Frenette PS (2020) Nerves in cancer. Nat Rev Cancer 20:143–157

Zaharchuk G, Davidzon G (2021) Artificial intelligence for optimization and interpretation of PET/CT and PET/MR images. Semin Nucl Med 51:134–142

Zhitkovich A (2011) Chromium in drinking water: sources, metabolism, and cancer risks. Chem Res Toxicol 24:1617–1629

Tumor Immunology and Immunotherapy

Thi Kim Anh Nguyen, Huu-Thinh Nguyen, and Sao-Mai Dam

Abstract

Understanding immune mechanisms in cancer and immunotherapy has made cancer diagnosis and treatment more effective. The immune system can recognize and elicit a response against tumor cells. However, tumor cells also have mechanisms to evade the immune system. This chapter focuses on discussing up-to-date issues related to tumor immunology and immunotherapy, including innate immunity, adaptive immunity, different therapeutic approaches, including dendritic cells, T cells, antibodies, cancer vaccines, checkpoint blockade, and the future trends in clinical trials applying immunotherapy.

Keywords

Antibody · Checkpoint blockade · Dendritic cell · Immunotherapy · T-cell response · Tumor

1 Introduction

Globally, cancer is the second leading cause of death, with nearly ten million deaths in 2020 (Ferlay et al. 2020). Traditional cancer treatments for decades have mainly been surgery, radiation, and chemotherapy, either individually or in combination (Abbas and Rehman 2018). Surgery still has limitations in mortality and

T. K. A. Nguyen · S.-M. Dam (✉)
Institute of Biotechnology and Food Technology, Industrial University of Ho Chi Minh City, Ho Chi Minh City, Vietnam
e-mail: damsaomai@iuh.edu.vn

H.-T. Nguyen
University of Medicine and Pharmacy in Ho Chi Minh City, Ho Chi Minh City, Vietnam

Interdisciplinary Cancer Research, https://doi.org/10.1007/16833_2023_135
Published online: 14 February 2023

complications after treatment (GlobalSurg Collaborative and National Institute for Health Research Global Health Research Unit on Global Surgery 2021). Treatment with surgery and radiation alone is not as effective as using these two therapeutic methods in combination to control cancer. High energy radiation from electron, protons, and number of ions damage genetic material of cancerous cells, consequently, block cell division and prevent them to proliferate (Abbas and Rehman 2018). To date, chemotherapy is considered the most effective and widely used method in the treatment of most types of cancers. Chemotherapy drugs target the tumor cells and produce reactive oxygen species with the majority killing tumor cells by the means of genotoxicity (DeVita and Chu 2008). Chemotherapy, however, damages normal cells leading to different side effects depending on the dose such as fatigue, nausea, hair loss, and vomiting or even death in severe case (Aslam et al. 2014). In addition, drug resistance is the majority limitation of chemotherapy, when cancer cells develop resistance to drug that they initially were susceptible to (Houseman et al. 2014).

Finding new therapy approaches for cancer to reduce side effects caused by conventional therapies have been concerned in many research studies (Pucci et al. 2019). Immunotherapy is a cancer treatment approach that aims to stimulate or restore the immune system of the patient against cancer cells. The immune system with its white blood cells, organs, and tissues of the lymph system helps the body fight infections and other diseases. Immunotherapy is a type of biological therapy that is safe for patient.

In this chapter, a general overview of tumor immunology including innate and adaptive immunity and immunotherapeutic approaches based on dendritic cells, T cells, antibodies, vaccines, and checkpoint blockade has been provided. Immunotherapy strategies among other novel cancer therapies have been considered as potential safe approaches to treat cancer patients.

2 Antitumor Immunity

The physiological role of the adaptive immune system is to prevent the growth of deformed cells or destroy these cells before they become harmful tumors. This phenomenon is called immune screening. There is strong evidence that immune screening has an important role in the development of tumor suppression. Tumors forming in healthy people show that the immunity to the tumor is usually very weak and is easily overwhelmed by the growth rate of the tumor.

3 The Tumor Antigens

Malignant tumors express many different types of molecules that the immune system can recognize as foreign. Antigens are produced by many tumor cells, and some of these antigens are discharged into the bloodstream, while others are retained on the cell surface. An antigen is any molecule that the immune system may recognize.

Antigens can be found in many different forms. If an individual's immune system can react against a tumor, the tumor must express antigens that are considered foreign to that individual's immune system. In experimental tumors produced by carcinogenic chemicals or ultraviolet rays, tumor antigens may be mutant products of common cellular proteins. Any protein can mutate in different tumors; usually, these proteins play no role in tumor formation. Mutations of many of these cellular proteins are less common in spontaneous human tumors than in experimentally induced ones. Some tumor antigens are the product of mutated or translocated oncogenes or tumor suppressor genes, and antigens are implicated in malignant transformation. In some human tumors, antibodies that trigger a purely immune response are proteins that are usually only overexpressed or dysregulated in tumor expression. Typically, these autoantigens do not trigger an immune response, but their aberrant expression is sufficient to trigger these responses. For example, proteins expressed only in embryonic tissue may not be induced to tolerate in adults. In tumors caused by oncogenic viruses, tumor antigens are usually viral products.

Antigens have been found in almost all of human cancer types, including Burkitt lymphoma, neuroblastoma, melanoma, osteoblastoma, renal carcinoma, breast cancer, prostate cancer, lung cancer, and colon cancer. An essential role of the immune system is to detect these cancer antigens to target and kill cancer cells. However, despite the foreign structure, the immune response to cancer antigens is highly variable and is often insufficient to suppress tumor growth.

The antigens known as tumor-associated antigens (TAAs) are particular to tumor cells. Tumor-specific antigens (TSAs) are unique to tumor cells. TSAs and TAAs are frequently found to be components of intracellular molecules expressed on the cell surface as a component of the major histocompatibility complex.

Proposed mechanisms for the origin of cancer antigens include the following:

- The emergence of new genetic information from viruses (e.g., the E6 and E7 proteins of the human papillomavirus in cervical cancer).
- Changes in oncogenes or tumor suppressor genes by the action of carcinogens lead to the formation of new cancer antigens (new protein sequences or accumulations of proteins that are generally not expressed or expressed at deficient levels, such as ras or p53), by directly generating new protein sequences or by stimulating the accumulation of these proteins.
- Some mutations of many genes are not directly related to tumor suppressor genes or oncogenes but can cause the appearance of new tumor-specific antigens on the cell surface.
- Abnormally high levels of proteins are generally expressed at significantly lower levels (e.g., prostate-specific antigens, melanoma-associated antigens) or only during embryonic development (embryonic cancer antigen).
- Regular antigen expression is masked by cell membranes due to impaired membrane homeostasis in tumor cells.
- The release of antigens is usually trapped in cells or organelles when tumor cells die.

Cancer antigens recognized by T cells can be mutated forms of normal self-proteins, oncogene, or tumor suppressor gene products, overexpressed or abnormal self-proteins, or effects of cancer-causing viruses. Tumor antigens can be recognized by TCD4 (lymphocyte T CD4) cells, but the role of TCD4 in antitumor immunity is poorly understood.

4 Immune Mechanism of Tumor Elimination

The primary immunological mechanism of tumor elimination is the destruction of tumor cells by tumor antigen-specific cytotoxic T lymphocyte (CTL). Most tumor antigens that trigger the immune response are proteins synthesized intracellularly and presented as peptide-MHCI (major histocompatibility complex class I) complexes. Thus, these antigens are recognized by MHCI-restricted CTL/CD8+ cells, whose function is to destroy the cells that produce this antigen. The role of CTL in tumor suppression has been established in animal models, where tumor transplantation can be eliminated by the transfer of antitumor CD8+ T cells into tumor-bearing animals.

The antitumor-responsive CTL is usually induced by the recognition of antigens on the host APC, which captures tumor cells or tumor antigens and presents these antigens to T cells. Tumors can be formed from any normal nucleated cells. These cells can present peptides on MHC I (since all nucleated cells express the MHC I molecule). Still, usually, the tumor does not represent either the excitatory co-receptor or major histocompatibility complex class II (MHCII). However, we do know that the activation of naive $CD8^+$ T cells to proliferate and differentiate into CTL-specific cells requires not only antigen recognition (MHC I-binding peptide) but also co-receptors stimulation and/or help from MHC II-restricted $CD4^+$ T cells. Tumor cells are captured by host APCs (dendritic cells), and tumor antigens are processed and presented on both MHC I and MHC II so that tumor antigens can be recognized by $CD8^+$ and $CD4^+$ T cells. At the same time, professional APCs express stimulated co-receptors that provide a second signal for T-cell activation. This process is called cross-presentation because one cell type (APC) presents antigens from another cell (tumor) and activates T cells specific to this second cell. This cross-presentation concept has been applied to the development of vaccines against tumors. Once CD8+ T cells differentiate into CTLs, they can kill tumor cells that express the respective antigens without the need for co-stimulatory receptors or help from T cells. Thus, CTL can be induced by cross-presenting tumor antigens by host APC cells, but CTL is a practical response factor to the tumor itself. Some other mechanisms may play a role in tumor elimination, such as the antitumor response of $CD4^+$ T and antibodies, which have also been detected in these patients. Still, the evidence is inconclusive on the role of these responses against tumors. Experimental results have shown that activated NKs and macrophages can also kill tumors in vitro, but the protective role of these mechanisms in tumor carriers is unclear.

5 Immune Escape from Tumors

Immune responses are often unsuccessful in controlling tumor growth because these responses are ineffective or because tumors have evolved to escape the immune system. The immune system must be effective against malignancies since the immune responses must destroy all tumor cells while the tumor grows rapidly. Often the growth rate surpasses the defenses of the immune system. Immune responses are often weak because many tumor antigens are immunogenic, perhaps because they are just slightly different from autologous antigens. Growing tumors also form immune-escape mechanisms. Some tumors stop expressing antigens that are targets of the immune response. These tumors are called antigen-loss variants. If this antigen loss is not related to the malignancy of the tumor, which variant will continue to grow and metastasize? Other tumors cease to express MHC I and do not present antigens for CD8+ T. Because NK recognizes MHC I-deficient cells, they can kill tumor cells that do not have MHC I. Other tumors can produce transforming growth factor β (TGF-β) molecules that suppress the immune response.

The immune response to foreign antigens includes humoral and cellular mechanisms.

Most humoral immune responses (e.g., antibodies) cannot prevent tumor growth. However, effector cells, such as T lymphocytes, macrophages, and natural killer cells, are relatively effective at killing tumor cells. This effector cell activity is enhanced by the presence of cancer-specific antigens (TSA) or tumor-associated antigens (TAA) on their surface (these cells are referred to as tumor-associated antigen-presenting cells) and is supported by cytokines (such as interleukins or interferons). However, despite the activity of effector cells, the body's immune responses may fail to control tumor appearance and growth.

6 Cellular Immunity

T lymphocytes are the primary cells responsible for detecting and destroying tumor cells. T lymphocytes perform immunosurveillance, then proliferate and destroy the newly transformed tumor cells after recognizing TAA. The response of T-lymphocytes to the tumor is regulated by other immune cells; some cells require the presence of humoral antibodies directed against tumor cells (antibody-dependent cytotoxicity) to initiate interactions that lead to tumor cell death. In contrast, suppressor T lymphocytes suppress the immune response against the tumor.

Cytotoxic T lymphocytes, often known as CTLs, are responsible for lysing target cells after recognizing antigens on those cells. These antigens could be cell surface proteins, or intracellular proteins (like TAAs) expressed on the cell surface along with MHC class I molecules. Tumor-specific cytotoxic T cells have been found in the following tumor types:

- Neuroblastoma
- Melanoma

- Sarcomas
- Colon cancer
- Lung carcinoma
- Breast carcinoma breast cancer
- Cervical carcinoma
- Endometrial cancer
- Ovarian cancer
- Testicular cancer
- Nasopharyngeal carcinoma
- Renal carcinoma

Natural killer (NK) cells are another subpopulation of effector cells with tumor cell-killing potential. In contrast to CTLs, NK cells do not have receptors to recognize antigens but still recognize virus-infected normal cells or tumor cells. Their tumor-killing activity is naturally named because these responses are independent of a specific antigen. The mechanism by which NK cells differentiate between normal and abnormal cells is still being studied. Evidence shows that molecules of class I MHC are present on the surface of normal cells, where they inhibit NK cells and prevent cell lysis. Thus, a specific decrease in MHC class I expression in tumor cells may induce NK cell activation and, ultimately, cell lysis.

Macrophages can kill tumor cells when activated by combining with starting factors, including lymphokines (soluble factors produced by T lymphocytes) and interferons. The tumor-killing ability of macrophages is inferior to that of T-lymphocyte-mediated cytotoxicity. Under certain circumstances, macrophages may present TAA to T-lymphocytes. And stimulate an antitumor-specific immune response. There are at least two groups of tumor-associated macrophages (TAMs), including activated macrophages (TAM-1 or M1) and alternatively activated macrophages (TAM-2 or M2). M1 cells facilitate the destruction of tumors by T lymphocytes, while M2 cells enhance tumor immune tolerance.

M1 and M2 are still considered to be cell types that persist in succession until they fully differentiate (polarize) into M1 and M2 cells. This differentiation can change over time and depends on the state and type of cancer cells and the treatment (Zhou et al. 2020). M1 and M2 are only two broad descriptions of the polarization state of macrophages that have a wide range of subpopulations (Murray 2017). There are many TAMs in tumor tissues of CD169+ macrophages and TCR+ macrophages, two types of macrophage subpopulations (Chávez-Galán et al. 2015).

Dendritic cells are antigen-presenting cells found in immune barriers (e.g., skin, lymph nodes). They play a central role in the initiation of an antitumor-specific immune response. These cells capture tumor-associated proteins, process them, and present TAA to T lymphocytes to stimulate a CTL immune response against the tumor. Several classes of dendritic cells may mediate tumor promotion or inhibition.

Lymphokines are produced by stimulating the growth of immune cells or increasing other immune cells' activity. These lymphokines include interleukin-2 (IL-2), the T-lymphocyte growth factor, and interferons. IL-12 is produced by dendritic cells and activates explicitly CTLs, thereby enhancing the antitumor immune response.

Regulatory T lymphocytes, typically present in the body, aid in preventing autoimmune reactions. They are produced during the active phase of the immune response to pathogens and limit an overly aggressive immune response that can harm the body. The accumulation of these cells in cancer suppresses the immune response against the tumor. The immune system's regulatory T (Treg) cells play crucial functions in preserving self-tolerance. Treg cells are an immunosuppressive subset of $CD4^+$ T cells distinguished by the presence of the master transcription factor forkhead box protein P3 (FOXP3). Treg cells can suppress antitumor immunity, thus impeding protective immune surveillance of tumors and impeding effective antitumor immune responses in tumor-bearing hosts, thereby promoting tumor growth and progression (Togashi et al. 2019). Tregs are present in solid tumors and promote immunosuppression by several mechanisms, including the secretion of immunosuppressive cytokines, competition for the activation of cytokines with effector cells, and direct contact with invading effector cells (Budhu et al. 2017; Togashi et al. 2019).

Immature bone marrow cells and the precursors of mature bone marrow cells are examples of bone marrow-derived suppressor cells. Cancer, inflammation, and infections all cause an increase in the number of these cells in the body. These cells have solid immunosuppressive capacity. There are two recognized cell populations: granulosa cells and mono lineage cells. Bone marrow-derived suppressor cells can accumulate in large numbers in cancers and have a poor prognosis in many cancers.

7 Humoral Immunity

In contrast to CTL immunity, antibodies do not play an essential role in protecting the body against tumor growth. Most antibodies cannot recognize TAAs. However, experimentally, antibodies in the serum have been shown to react with cancer cells in many types of cancer, such as:

- Burkitt lymphoma
- Melanoma
- Osteosarcoma
- Neuroblastoma
- Lung carcinoma
- Breast carcinoma breast cancer
- Carcinoma of the gastrointestinal tract

Antibodies cause cytotoxicity by a natural resistance to surface antigens of cancer cells. These antibodies may induce antitumor responses through complement fixation or serve as a guide for tumor-killing activity via CTLs (antibody-dependent cellular). Another group of humoral antibodies, called booster antibodies (blocking antibodies), can stimulate rather than inhibit tumor growth. The mechanisms and relative importance of immune enhancement are still not fully understood.

Although many tumors are eliminated by the immune system (and therefore never detected), many others continue to grow despite TAA expression. Multiple mechanisms have been proposed to explain the inadequate immune response to TAA, including:

- TAA-specific immune tolerance involves antigen-presenting cells and suppressor T lymphocytes, possibly secondary to antigen exposure during the fetal stage.
- Suppression of the immune response to physicochemical or viral agents (e.g., HIV-induced T-helper lymphocyte destruction).
- Suppression of the immune response due to cytotoxic drugs or radiation.
- Immunosuppression by the tumor itself by complex and nonspecific mechanisms can cause many consequences such as impaired T-lymphocyte, B-lymphocyte, and antigen-presenting cell function, decreased production of IL-2, increasing circulating soluble IL-2 receptors (binding and inactivating IL-2).
- Presence and activity of differentiated TAM-2 (M2) cells increase tumor tolerance.

8 Immunotherapy

Immunotherapy employs compounds produced by the body or in a laboratory to stimulate the immune system and assist the body in locating and eliminating cancer cells. Different types of cancers can be treated by immunotherapy. Other types of immunotherapies include checkpoint inhibitors, cellular therapy, vaccine, tumor microenvironment, oncolytic virus therapy, and biomarkers.

9 Checkpoint Inhibitor

Immune checkpoints are regular and considered regulators of the immune system. Their role is to prevent the immune system from attacking cells indiscriminately. Immune checkpoints are involved when proteins on the surface of T cells recognize and bind to partner proteins on other cells, such as tumor cells. These proteins are called immune checkpoint proteins. When the checkpoint and partner proteins bind together, they send an "off" signal to the T cells. This can prevent the immune system from attacking cancer.

Immunotherapy drugs called immune checkpoint inhibitors to work by blocking checkpoint proteins from binding to their partner proteins. This prevents the "off" signal from being sent, allowing the T cells to kill the cancer cells. The first immune-checkpoint inhibitor (ICI) to be approved by the U.S. Food and Drug Administration (FDA) was ipilimumab (anti-cytotoxic T lymphocyte antigen 4 (CTLA-4) therapy) in 2011 after it was found to increase overall survival in patients with advanced melanoma (Schadendorf et al. 2015). CTLA-4 blocks checkpoint protein. Since then, several inhibitors have been approved with the incorporation of blocking programmed cell death protein 1 (PD1)/PD-Ligand 1 (PD-L1) pathway (Vaddepally et al. 2020). Immune-checkpoint inhibitors (ICIs) have provided a paradigm shift in cancer treatment. Most immunological checkpoint molecules are expressed in T_{reg} cells. However, the effects of ICIs on T_{reg} cells and the contributions of these cells to treatment responses are unknown. Notably, research suggests that ICIs that target programmed cell death 1 (PD-1) could boost the immunosuppressive function of T_{reg} cells, but CTLA-4 inhibitors could deplete these cells (Togashi et al. 2019).

Immune checkpoint inhibitors have been given the go-ahead to treat certain patients suffering from a wide range of cancers, including breast cancer, bladder cancer, cervical cancer, colon cancer, head and neck cancer, Hodgkin lymphoma, liver cancer, lung cancer, renal cell carcinoma, and others.

10 Cellular Therapies

Cellular immunotherapy is adoptive cell therapy. Cells isolated from the host immune system or genetically engineered immune cells are used to eliminate cancer. T cells can bind antigens on the surface of cancer cells and kill them. Cellular therapy takes advantage of T cells and can be developed in different ways, including tumor infiltrating lymphocyte (TIL) therapy, engineered T-cell receptor (TCR) therapy, chimeric antigen receptor (CAR) T-cell therapy, and natural killer (NK) cell therapy. TIL and CAR T cell therapy are major T cell transfer therapy types. Immune cells are collected, cultured in the laboratory, and transfer back to the host in a vein using a needle.

TIL therapy uses tumor-infiltrating lymphocytes from a patient's tumor. Lymphocytes are then tested to find out the ones that recognize tumor cells. Selected lymphocytes are treated with substances to stimulate them to grow to a considerable number quickly. T-cell transfer therapy was initially investigated for the treatment of metastatic melanoma because melanomas frequently produce a robust immune response and are often rich in TILs. Some people with melanoma were treated rather effectively with TIL. In addition, TIL therapy has produced promising findings in other cancers, such as cervical squamous cell carcinoma and cholangiocarcinoma.

CAR T-cell therapy is similar to TIL therapy, but T cells are modified in the laboratory to make a type of protein known as CAR before being cultured and given back to patients. CARs are meant to help T cells adhere to particular proteins on the surface of cancer cells, enhancing their potential to attack cancer cells. CARs can bind to cancer cells even if their antigen is not presented on the cell surface via MHC, rendering more cancer cells vulnerable to attacks. However, CAR T cells can only naturally recognize antigens expressed on the cell surface. FDA approved the first CAR T cells therapy to treat certain types of large B-cell lymphoma in adults in 2017. To present, FDA approved six CAR T-cell therapies for blood cancers.

- Axicabtagene ciloleucel (Yescarta®): a CD19-targeting CAR T cell immunotherapy; approved for subsets of patients with lymphoma
- Brexucabtagene autoleucel (Tecartus™): a CD19-targeting CAR T cell immunotherapy; approved for subsets of patients with leukemia and lymphoma

- Ciltacabtagene autoleucel (Carvykti™): a BCMA-targeting CAR T cell immunotherapy; approved for subsets of patients with advanced multiple myelom
- Idecabtagene vicleucel (Abecma™): a BCMA-targeting CAR T cell immunotherapy; approved for subsets of patients with advanced multiple myeloma
- Lisocabtagene maraleucel (Breyanzi®): a CD19-targeting CAR T Cell immunotherapy; approved for subsets of patients with lymphoma
- Tisagenlecleucel (Kymriah®): a CD19-targeting CAR T cell immunotherapy; approved for subsets of patients with leukemia and lymphoma

Cytokine release syndrome is a potentially life-threatening adverse event that may be brought on by CAR T-cell treatment. This condition is brought on when the T cells that were put into the body, or other immune cells that were responding to the incoming T cells, release a significant amount of cytokines into the bloodstream. Fever, nausea, headache, rash, rapid heartbeat, low blood pressure, and difficulty in breathing are only some symptoms that might result from a sudden spike in their levels.

In addition, although CAR T cells are programmed to recognize proteins unique to cancer cells, they are nevertheless capable of recognizing healthy cells on occasion. This can result in various adverse outcomes, including organ harm, depending on which normal cells are targeted.

Up to now, CAR-T has been the best-known cellular therapy. It is shown to be hugely effective against that cancer the CAR can be reengineered to target. There are limited subsets of cancers; this type treats mostly blood-borne cancers of therapy. Lymphocytic leukemia patients treated with CAR T therapy were effectively recovered (Miliotou and Papadopoulou 2018; Singh et al. 2016). CAR T-cell therapy has also been studied to treat solid tumors, including breast and brain cancers, but limited results were observed (Lin et al. 2022; Wang and Zhou 2017).

Several genes can be inserted into a T cell, which may lead to CARs with multiple protein targets, which is the advantage of therapy. Ongoing research suggests CAR may also be possible to edit the T cell so that it has built-in defenses against the tumor microenvironment. CAR-T is also being tested in combination with checkpoint inhibitors and other immunotherapies.

11 Vaccines

The primary strategy for anticancer immunotherapies is to deliver cancer-specific mechanisms (antibodies and T cells) to patients, proactively immunizing patients with their tumor cells and stimulating their immune response.

Treatments of cancer, especially metastatic cancer, with chemotherapy and radiation methods strongly affect normal non-tumor tissues. Therefore, particular immune responses should be expected to eliminate the tumor without affecting the patient. Immunotherapy remains a significant target for oncology immunologists, and numerous therapeutic approaches have been tested, and some are used in treatment.

Passive vaccination was one of the earliest used immunotherapies. Immune-specific cells are taken from the patient, processed, and then introduced into the cancer patients. Monoclonal antibodies against tumor antigens bound to toxins have been tested for various tumors. This antibody binds to the tumor and activates host-specific mechanisms such as phagocytosis, complement, or delivery of toxins to tumor cells. An antibody of this type, which is an antibody against the product of the HER2/neu cancer gene that is often overexpressed in breast cancer, is currently approved for use in breast cancer patients. CD20-specific antibodies, expressed on B cells, are used to treat B-cell cancers and are often combined with chemotherapy. Since CD20 is not defined in hematopoietic stem cells, normal B cells will be regenerated after the treatment has ended. T cells can be isolated from the patient's blood or tumor-infiltrating cells, multiplied by growth factors, and injected back into the patient. These T cells are thought to contain tumor-specific CTLs, which will find and destroy tumors. This is called adaptive cellular immunotherapy and is being tested for many metastatic cancers, but results vary by patient and tumor type.

Some vaccines against viruses are also vaccines against cancer caused by viruses, such as hepatitis B and human papillomavirus vaccines. These are preventive vaccines. A therapeutic cancer vaccine would be used to treat cancer after it has already occurred. There are two major types of therapeutic vaccines, including autologous and allogeneic vaccines.

Autologous cancer vaccines are produced from their immune system cells or cancer cells. Cells from patients' tumors are collected and treated to make them become a target for the immune system. Subsequently, treated cells are injected into the patient. The immune cells will recognize and destroy them; simultaneously, they do the same to other cancer cells in the body. The memory cells will act and eliminate cancer cells if they return. The aim is to treat cancer in the body or prevent a tumor from returning after more conventional cancer treatments, such as surgery, radiation, or chemotherapy, have removed most or all of it. Using an individual's immune cells to develop autologous cancer vaccines is an alternative method. The U.S. Food and Drug Administration has approved an autologous vaccine manufactured from immune cells. Sipuleucel-t (Provenge®) is an autologous immune cell prostate cancer vaccination. In clinical trials, it has been found to prolong the lives of men with treatment-resistant metastatic prostate cancer.

Several allogeneic cancer cell vaccines have been evaluated, such as those for pancreatic cancer, melanoma (skin cancer), leukemia, non-small cell lung cancer, and prostate cancer. Allogeneic cancer vaccines are appealing because they are less costly to develop and produce than autologous vaccines. However, none is effective enough to be licensed yet. Several allogeneic immune cell vaccines have been tested in early stages (Avigan et al. 2007; de Gruijl et al. 2008).

12 The Tumor Microenvironment and Other Targets

The tumor microenvironment is a barrier to effector immune cells. Tumors create a microenvironment that inhibits T cells by enzymes and immunosuppressants. That environment surrounds the proteins expressed on the cell surface of the tumor.

Several checkpoint inhibitors are known. However, there are about 50 potential targets to hit in this environment. In the case of agonists, which stimulate (rather than inhibit) immune cells are also studied. Several targets, such as CD-27, CD40, GITR, ICO, and others, have been reviewed. So do the cytokines. IL-2 and IL-15 are considered candidates for cancer immunotherapy (Fehniger et al. 2002).

Furthermore, the role of other immune cells in T-cell capture and activation and how they may contribute to the control of immunosuppressive factors in the tumor microenvironment is concerned. Unregulated cancer cell growth can lead to intrinsic immunosuppressive features of the tumor, such as hypoxic regions, and high lactate levels can inhibit effector T cell function (Fischer et al. 2007). Most immune suppression is due to normal immune regulatory cells and molecules within the tumor that inhibit T-cell priming or suppress cytotoxic T-cell function (Vander Heiden et al. 2009; Zhang and Ertl 2016).

The microenvironment, which generates cytokines, recruits macrophages to the tumor site. As proposed in previous studies, the recruitment and differentiation progress are related to local anoxia, inflammation, and high levels of lactic acid. The CC chemokines, such as CCL2, CCL11, CCL16, and CCL21, which are critical determinants of macrophage infiltration and angiogenesis, have been shown to function in the cancer of breast, lung, esophagus, ovary, and cervix, and CCL2 primarily contributes to the recruitment of macrophages (Qiu et al. 2018; Santoni et al. 2014). CCL2 (also known as monocyte chemotactic protein-1, MCP-1) is available on activated macrophages, monocytes, and dendritic cells. Notably, the interaction between resident macrophages and newly recruited macrophages is bidirectional since resident TAMs can recruit macrophages to worsen tumor metastasis. As a peritoneal function of TAMs, CCL2 is considered a good target site to protect tissue not harmed by TAMs (Tang and Tsai 2012).

13 Oncolytic Virus Therapy

Oncolytic viruses (OV) have expressed excellent benefits in cancer treatment because it mediates antitumor effects in several ways. Viruses can infect cancer cells, especially normal cells, to produce tumor-associated antigens to trigger a "danger signal" that generates a tumor microenvironment that is less immunogenic and serves as transporters for the expression of inflammatory and immunomodulatory cytokines (Santos Apolonio et al. 2021). Genetically modified herpes virus called talimogene laherparepvec, which FDA approves, was first used as OV for melanoma treatment. Melanoma cells are infected with a genetically modified virus, and the melanoma is reprogrammed to create immune-stimulating proteins. Cancer-infecting viruses also increase in time for melanoma cells to break out, producing many tumor antigens that signal the immune system to coordinate the fighting.

Afterward, clinical trials investigate several OVs as a potential cancer treatment (Fu et al. 2019). Furthermore, OV can stimulate the immune system against tumor cells, influencing the development of an antitumor response (Desjardins et al. 2016). The clinical use of OV is seen as an alternative to modulating the tumor environment from an immune desert state due to the evasion mechanism that contributes to tumor progression to a form that is suppressed inflammation, where the immune system can destroy abnormal cells (Rosewell Shaw and Suzuki 2018). Furthermore, viruses have different mechanisms that expose infected cells to cell lysis, contributing to tumor cell death and increasing the effectiveness of immunotherapy (Lawler et al. 2017). Oncolytic viruses can turn tumors that the body's immune system does not appear to detect into immunogenic material. Modulating the tumor microenvironment with oncolytic viruses allows T-cell therapies to work in solid tumors.

Several oncolytic viruses, including adenoviruses, herpes viruses, measles viruses, coxsackie viruses, polioviruses, reoviruses, poxviruses, and Newcastle disease viruses, are currently undergoing preclinical and clinical development for use in cancer therapy (Kaufman et al. 2015). Adenovirus has been considered a potential antitumor candidate with minimum toxicity (Hemminki and Hemminki 2016). Insertion of therapeutic transgenes into the adenovirus genome enhances the efficacy of immunotherapy. A commonly used modification is adding granulocyte-macrophage cytokine gene transfer factor (GMCSF) to the adenovirus genome. Viral replication produces multiple GMCSF products, leading to the recruitment and maturation of dendritic cells (DCs). The decomposition process releases subsequent priming of T cells with tumor-associated antigens (Cerullo et al. 2010). CGTG-102 (also named ONCOS-102) is an oncolytic adenovirus expressing GMCSF. Patients' data reported increases in T cells' peripheral levels against tumor-associated antigens (Kanerva et al. 2013). These findings show that dendritic cell priming in humans is predicted by the established mechanism of action of GMCSF (Simmons et al. 2007). The increased CD8+ T-cell infiltration found in tumor biopsies after treatment of advanced cancer patients with ONCOS-102 emphasizes the immunological potency of this approach (Ranki et al. 2016).

Antibodies can also be inserted as transgenes to enhance the efficacy of oncolytic virotherapy. For example, anti-CTLA4, a checkpoint inhibitor, has been successfully inserted into an oncolytic adenovirus platform. Experiments carried out in mouse models, and ex vivo cultures of cancer patients' peripheral blood mononuclear cells (PBMCs) revealed that the antitumor activity of T cells increased (Dias et al. 2012).

14 Biomarkers

Immune checkpoint inhibitors (ICIs) have changed the treatment circumstances for advanced malignancies. However, response rates remain widely variable. Therefore, high sensitivity and specificity biomarkers are needed to identify patients most likely to elicit a sustained response. Since tumor cells have antigens that are different from themselves, patients with solid and hematologic cancers have the potential to respond to ICI predicted. However, intrinsic features of the tumor, tumor microenvironment (TME), and deficiency of the patient's innate and adaptive immune responses may settle an effective antitumor immune response and influence the host's response to ICI. The development of standardization and predictive biomarkers is essential in treating cancers. Researchers have been focused on biomarkers to find out those can predict response to ICI. The investigation of predictive biomarkers of ICIs' efficacy revealed a complex interaction between the regulation of the immune system network and tumors, reflecting more comprehensively the complexity and diversity of the effects of immunotherapy on tumors and even the whole body (Bai et al. 2020). Biomarkers may be detected and measured in the tumor tissue and the peripheral blood (Sankar et al. 2022). Currently, the FDA approves several tissue biomarkers for the solid tumor, such as PD-L1, tumor mutational burden (TMB), and microsatellite instability (MSI). In addition, other biomarkers can be used, such as exploratory tissue biomarkers like tumor gene expression profiling (GEP), multiplex immunohistochemistry (IHC), immunofluorescence (IF), tumor-infiltrating lymphocytes (TILs), Immunocore, T-cell receptor (TCR) diversity, and the microbiome, as well as cellular and soluble peripheral blood biomarkers (Sankar et al. 2022).

15 Conclusion

Recently, cancer immunotherapy based on tumor immunology has been widely covered in research and clinical application. Immune checkpoint inhibitors are drugs that can block checkpoint proteins to bind to their partner proteins, allowing immune system to attack cancer. TIL and CAR T are adopted cells that can eliminate cancer. Vaccination and monoclonal antibodies against tumor antigens have been applied in various tumor treatments. Several oncolytic viruses are currently undergoing preclinical and clinical development for use in cancer therapy since they can generate tumor microenvironment. Cytokines generated by microenvironment recruit macrophages to the tumor site play important role in treatment of many types of cancers. Furthermore, the standardization and predictive biomarkers development are needed in treating cancers.

Immunotherapy strategies are biological treatment approaches that reduce the side effect of the conventional cancer treatment methods.

References

Abbas Z, Rehman S (2018) An overview of cancer treatment modalities. Neoplasma 1:139–157. https://doi.org/10.5772/intechopen.76558

Aslam MS, Naveed S, Ahmed A, Abbas Z, Gull I, Athar MA (2014) Side effects of chemotherapy in cancer patients and evaluation on patients opinion about starvation based differential chemotherapy. J Cancer Ther 5(8):817. https://doi.org/10.4236/jct.2014.58089

Avigan DE, Vasir B, George DJ, Oh WK, Atkins MB, McDermott DF, Kantoff PW, Figlin RA, Vasconcelles MJ, Xu Y, Kufe D, Bukowski RM (2007) Phase I/II study of vaccination with electrofused allogeneic dendritic cells/autologous tumor-derived cells in patients with stage IV renal cell carcinoma. J Immunother 30:749–761. https://doi.org/10.1097/CJI.0b013e3180de4ce8

Bai R, Lv Z, Xu D, Cui J (2020) Predictive biomarkers for cancer immunotherapy with immune checkpoint inhibitors biomark. Res 8:34. https://doi.org/10.1186/s40364-020-00209-0

Budhu S, Schaer DA, Li Y, Toledo-Crow R, Panageas K, Yang X, Zhong H, Houghton AN, Silverstein SC, Merghoub T, Wolchok JD (2017) Blockade of surface-bound TGF-β on regulatory T cells abrogates suppression of effector T cell function in the tumor microenvironment. Sci Signal 10. https://doi.org/10.1126/scisignal.aak9702

Cerullo V, Pesonen S, Diaconu I et al (2010) Oncolytic adenovirus coding for granulocyte macrophage colony-stimulating factor induces antitumoral immunity in cancer patients. Cancer Res 70:4297–4309. https://doi.org/10.1158/0008-5472.CAN-09-3567

Chávez-Galán L, Olleros ML, Vesin D, Garcia I (2015) Much more than M1 and M2 macrophages, there are also CD169+ and TCR+ macrophages. Front Immunol 6:1–15. https://doi.org/10.3389/fimmu.2015.00263

de Gruijl TD, van den Eertwegh AJM, Pinedo HM, Scheper RJ (2008) Whole-cell cancer vaccination: from autologous to allogeneic tumor- and dendritic cell-based vaccines. Cancer Immunol Immunother 57:1569–1577. https://doi.org/10.1007/s00262-008-0536-z

Desjardins A, Vlahovic G, Friedman HS (2016) Vaccine therapy, oncolytic viruses, and gliomas. Oncology (Williston Park) 30:211–218

DeVita VT, Chu E (2008) A history of cancer chemotherapy. Cancer Res 68(21):8643–8653. https://doi.org/10.1158/0008-5472.CAN-07-6611

Dias JD, Hemminki O, Diaconu I, Hirvinen M, Bonetti A, Guse K, Escutenaire S, Kanerva A, Pesonen S, Löskog A, Cerullo V, Hemminki A (2012) Targeted cancer immunotherapy with oncolytic adenovirus coding for a fully human monoclonal antibody specific for CTLA-4. Gene Ther 19:988–998. https://doi.org/10.1038/gt.2011.176

Fehniger TA, Cooper MA, Caligiuri MA (2002) Interleukin-2 and interleukin-15: immunotherapy for cancer. Cytokine Growth Factor Rev 13:169–183. https://doi.org/10.1016/s1359-6101(01)00021-1

Ferlay J, Ervik M, Lam F, Colombet M, Mery L, Piñeros M et al (2020) Global cancer observatory: cancer today. International Agency for Research on Cancer, Lyon. https://gco.iarc.fr/today

Fischer K, Hoffmann P, Voelkl S et al (2007) Inhibitory effect of tumor cell-derived lactic acid on human T cells. Blood 109:3812–3819. https://doi.org/10.1182/blood-2006-07-035972

Fu L-Q, Wang S-B, Cai M-H, Wang X-J, Chen J-Y, Tong X-M, Chen X-Y, Mou X-Z (2019) Recent advances in oncolytic virus-based cancer therapy. Virus Res 270:197675. https://doi.org/10.1016/j.virusres.2019.197675

GlobalSurg Collaborative and National Institute for Health Research Global Health Research Unit on Global Surgery (2021) Global variation in postoperative mortality and complications after cancer surgery: a multicentre, prospective cohort study in 82 countries. Lancet 397:387–397. https://doi.org/10.1016/S0140-6736(21)00001-5

Hemminki O, Hemminki A (2016) A century of oncolysis evolves into oncolytic immunotherapy. Onco Targets Ther 5:e1074377. https://doi.org/10.1080/2162402X.2015.1074377

Housman G, Byler S, Heerboth S, Lapinska K, Longacre M (2014) Drug resistance in cancer: an overview. Cancers 6(3):1769–1792. https://doi.org/10.3390/cancers6031769

Kanerva A, Nokisalmi P, Diaconu I et al (2013) Antiviral and antitumor T-cell immunity in patients treated with GM-CSF-coding oncolytic adenovirus. Clin Cancer Res an Off J Am Assoc Cancer Res 19:2734–2744. https://doi.org/10.1158/1078-0432.CCR-12-2546

Kaufman HL, Kohlhapp FJ, Zloza A (2015) Oncolytic viruses: a new class of immunotherapy drugs. Nat Rev Drug Discov 14:642–662. https://doi.org/10.1038/nrd4663

Lawler SE, Speranza M-C, Cho C-F, Chiocca EA (2017) Oncolytic viruses in cancer treatment: a review. JAMA Oncol 3:841–849. https://doi.org/10.1001/jamaoncol.2016.2064

Lin YJ, Mashouf LA, Lim M (2022) CAR T cell therapy in primary brain tumors: current investigations and the future front. Immunol 13:1–12. https://doi.org/10.3389/fimmu.2022.817296

Miliotou AN, Papadopoulou LC (2018) CAR T-cell therapy: a new era in cancer immunotherapy. Curr Pharm Biotechnol 19:5–18. https://doi.org/10.2174/1389201019666180418095526

Murray PJ (2017) Macrophage polarization. Annu Rev Physiol 79:541–566. https://doi.org/10.1146/annurev-physiol-022516-034339

Pucci C, Martinelli C, Ciofani (2019) Innovative approaches for cancer treatment: current perspectives and new challenges. Ecancermedicalscience 13:961. https://doi.org/10.3332/ecancer.2019.961

Qiu S-Q, Waaijer SJH, Zwager MC, de Vries EGE, van der Vegt B, Schröder CP (2018) Tumor-associated macrophages in breast cancer: innocent bystander or important player? Cancer Treat Rev 70:178–189. https://doi.org/10.1016/j.ctrv.2018.08.010

Ranki T, Pesonen S, Hemminki A et al (2016) Phase I study with ONCOS-102 for the treatment of solid tumors – an evaluation of clinical response and exploratory analyses of immune markers. J Immunother Cancer 4:17. https://doi.org/10.1186/s40425-016-0121-5

Rosewell Shaw A, Suzuki M (2018) Oncolytic viruses partner with T-cell therapy for solid tumor treatment. Front Immunol 9:2103. https://doi.org/10.3389/fimmu.2018.02103

Sankar K, Ye JC, Li Z, Zheng L, Song W, Hu-Lieskovan S (2022) The role of biomarkers in personalized immunotherapy. Biomark Res 10:32. https://doi.org/10.1186/s40364-022-00378-0

Santoni M, Bracarda S, Nabissi M, Massari F, Conti A, Bria E, Tortora G, Santoni G, Cascinu S (2014) CXC and CC chemokines as angiogenic modulators in nonhaematological tumors. Biomed Res Int 2014:768758. https://doi.org/10.1155/2014/768758

Santos Apolonio J, de Souza L, Gonçalves V, Cordeiro Santos ML et al (2021) Oncolytic virus therapy in cancer: a current review. World J Virol 10:229–255. https://doi.org/10.5501/wjv.v10.i5.229

Schadendorf D, Hodi FS, Robert C, Weber JS, Margolin K, Hamid O, Patt D, Chen T-T, Berman DM, Wolchok JD (2015) Pooled analysis of long-term survival data from phase II and phase III trials of ipilimumab in unresectable or metastatic melanoma. J Clin Oncol Off J Am Soc Clin Oncol 33:1889–1894. https://doi.org/10.1200/JCO.2014.56.2736

Simmons AD, Li B, Gonzalez-Edick M, Lin C, Moskalenko M, Du T, Creson J, VanRoey MJ, Jooss K (2007) GM-CSF-secreting cancer immunotherapies: preclinical analysis of the mechanism of action. Cancer Immunol Immunother 56:1653–1665. https://doi.org/10.1007/s00262-007-0315-2

Singh N, Frey NV, Grupp SA, Maude SL (2016) CAR T cell therapy in acute lymphoblastic leukemia and potential for chronic lymphocytic leukemia. Curr Treat Options in Oncol 17:28. https://doi.org/10.1007/s11864-016-0406-4

Tang C-H, Tsai C-C (2012) CCL2 increases MMP-9 expression and cell motility in human chondrosarcoma cells via the Ras/Raf/MEK/ERK/NF-κB signaling pathway. Biochem Pharmacol 83:335–344. https://doi.org/10.1016/j.bcp.2011.11.013

Togashi Y, Shitara K, Nishikawa H (2019) Regulatory T cells in cancer immunosuppression—implications for anticancer therapy. Nat Rev Clin Oncol 16:356–371. https://doi.org/10.1038/s41571-019-0175-7

Vaddepally RK, Kharel P, Pandey R, Garje R, Chandra AB (2020) Review of indications of FDA-approved immune checkpoint inhibitors per NCCN guidelines with the level of evidence. Cancers (Basel) 12. https://doi.org/10.3390/cancers12030738

Vander Heiden MG, Cantley LC, Thompson CB (2009) Understanding the Warburg effect: the metabolic requirements of cell proliferation. Science 324:1029–1033. https://doi.org/10.1126/science.1160809

Wang J, Zhou P (2017) New approaches in CAR-T cell immunotherapy for breast cancer. Adv Exp Med Biol 1026:371–381. https://doi.org/10.1007/978-981-10-6020-5_17

Zhang Y, Ertl HCJ (2016) Starved and asphyxiated: how can CD8(+) T cells within a tumor microenvironment prevent tumor progression. Front Immunol 7:32. https://doi.org/10.3389/fimmu.2016.00032

Zhou J, Tang Z, Gao S, Li C, Feng Y, Zhou X (2020) Tumor-associated macrophages: recent insights and therapies. Front Oncol 10:1–13. https://doi.org/10.3389/fonc.2020.00188

New Approaches Targeting Immuno-oncology and Tumor Microenvironment

Di Zhu and Fenglian He

Abstract

Immune checkpoint blockade therapy is now a key tool in the war against cancer. Antibody medications, such as anti-PD-1 and anti-PD-L1, have several clear benefits, including broad applicability across cancer types and long-lasting clinical response. The overall response rates, especially for tumors with a modest mutational burden, are still unsatisfactory. In addition to traditional checkpoint blocking, novel therapeutic approaches targeting these pathways have recently surfaced and have been studied in preclinical models, opening up new possibilities for the development of the next generation of immunotherapies such as inhibitory checkpoints such as TIM-3, LAG-3, TIGHT, VISTA and BILA, and costimulatory checkpoint agonists such as CD28, OX40, CD137, IOS, GITA and CD27. Targeting immunosuppressive cells and antitumor by combining targeted drugs with PD-1/PD-L1 antibodies may also improve clinical outcomes and overcome immune resistance.

Keywords

Immune checkpoint · Immune resistance · Immuno-oncology · Immunotherapy · Tumor microenvironment

D. Zhu (✉)
Department of Pharmacology, School of Basic Medical Sciences, Fudan University, Shanghai, China
e-mail: zhudi@fudan.edu.cn

F. He
Department of Pharmacology, School of Pharmacy, Fudan University, Shanghai, China

Interdisciplinary Cancer Research, https://doi.org/10.1007/16833_2022_89
Published online: 23 December 2022

Abbreviations

ACC	antibody-dependent cellular cytotoxicity
BELA	B and T lymphocytes attenuator
CEACAM-1	carcinoembryonic antigen cell adhesion molecule-1
cGAMP	cyclin GMP-AMP
cGAS	cyclic GMP-AMP synthase
CTLA-4	cytotoxic T lymphocyte antigen 4
DAMP	damage-associated molecular patterns
FGL1	fibrinogen-like protein 1
Gal-3	galectin-3
Gal-9	galectin-9
GITR	glucocorticoid-induced tumor necrosis factor receptor
HAVCR2	hepatitis A virus cellular receptor 2
HMGB1	high mobility group box 1
HSV-gD	herpes simplex virus glycoprotein D
HVEM	herpesvirus entry mediator
ICIs	immune checkpoint inhibitors
ICOS	inducible T-cell costimulatory
IMCs	immature myeloid cells
iNOS	inducible nitric oxide synthase
LAG-3	lymphocyte activation gene-3
LTα	lymphotoxin-α
MDSCs	myeloid-derived suppressor cells
MHC II	major histocompatibility complex II
MMR	deficient mismatch repair
MSI-H	microsatellite instability-high
MSI-L	microsatellite instability-low
MSS	microsatellite stability
NK cells	natural killer cells
NO	nitric oxide
PAMPs	pathogen-associated molecular patterns
PD-1	programmed cell death protein 1
PSGL-1	P-selectin glycoprotein ligand-1
PVR	poliovirus receptor
SIRPα	signal regulatory protein-α
STING	stimulator of interferon genes
TAB08	theralizumab
TAM	tumor-associated macrophages
TIM-3	T-cell immunoglobulin mucin-3
TLRs	toll-like receptors
Treg	regulatory T cells

VISTA	V-domain immunoglobulin suppressor of T-cell activation
VSIG-3	V-Set and immunoglobulin domain containing protein 3

1 Introduction

In 2020, there will be about 19.3 million new cancer cases and about ten million cancer deaths worldwide (Sung et al. 2021). Immune checkpoints are key molecules that regulate T-cell activation signals in immune responses (Zhao and Subramanian 2017). There are two types of immune checkpoints: one is the costimulatory checkpoint, which inhibits the activation of immune cells, such as programmed cell death protein 1 (PD-1), cytotoxic T-lymphocyte-associated protein 4 (CTLA-4), T-cell immunoglobulin mucin-3 (TIM-3), lymphocyte activation gene-3 (LAG-3), V-domain immunoglobulin suppressor of T-cell activation (VISTA), TIM domain (T-cell immunoglobulin and TIM domain, TIGHT), and B and T lymphocytes attenuator (BELA); the second is the co-inhibitory checkpoint, which stimulates the activation of immune cells, such as CD28, OX40, CD137, inducible T-cell costimulatory molecules (ICOS), glucocorticoid-induced tumor necrosis factor receptor (GITA), and CD27 (Galon and Bruni 2019; Choi et al. 2020). In recent years, significant progress has been made in tumor immunotherapy research, especially immune checkpoint inhibitors (ICIs) represented by PD-1/PD-L1 and CTLA-4 antibodies, including pembrolizumab, nivolumab, atezolizumab, toripalimab, and several PD-1/PD-L1 antibodies and CTLA-4 antibodies, including ipilimumab, have been approved for marketing (Bagchi et al. 2021). Currently, ICIs are the first-line immunotherapy for melanoma, NSCLC, liver cancer, and colorectal cancer, and widely prolong the survival of cancer patients. Although recent clinical data has shown that patients with solid tumors having high microsatellite instability (Microsatellite Instability-High, MSI-H) or mismatch repair deficiency (Deficient Mismatch Repair, MMR) show good clinical efficacy, but the most patients with solid tumors having microsatellite stability (MSS) or low-grade microsatellite instability (Microsatellite Instability-Low, MSI-L) barely benefit from immunotherapy (Cui 2021). In particular, some tumor patients are prone to developing drug resistance soon after they respond (Morad et al. 2021). Therefore, how to improve the efficacy of ISIs and overcome drug resistance is the focus of current clinical and basic research fields. Numerous studies have shown that the combination of ICIs with chemotherapy, radiotherapy, and other immunotherapies (including tumor vaccines, CAR-T therapy, and oncolytic viruses) can increase the efficacy. In addition, new-generation ICIs such as TIM-3, LAG-3, TIGHT, VISTA, and BILA, costimulatory checkpoint agonists such as CD28, OX40, CD137, IOS, GITA, and CD27, drugs targeting immunosuppressive cells and antitumor combining targeted drugs with PD-1/PD-L1 antibodies may also improve clinical outcomes and overcome immune resistance (Choi et al. 2020; Archilla-Ortega et al. 2022).

2 Co-suppression Checkpoint

2.1 PD-1

PD-1, also known as CD279, belongs to the co-suppressive immune checkpoint and is expressed by activated T cells, B cells, natural killer cells (NK cells), and myeloid cells. In particular, in the tumor environment or chronic infection, T cells are continuously stimulated by antigens, and T cells become exhausted T cells, which will continue to highly express PD-1 (Kallies et al. 2020). Currently, known PD-1 ligands include PD-L1 (CD274) and PD-L2 (CD273). PD-L1 is expressed on a variety of immune cells, including T cells, B cells, macrophages, and DCs. In addition, epithelial, stromal, and endothelial cells, especially various types of tumor cells, also express PD-L1. PD-L2 is mainly expressed by immune cells such as DCs, macrophages, and B cells. Normally, PD-1 binds to its ligands PD-L1/PD-L2, inhibits T-cell activation and cytokine production, and protects the body from attack by the autoimmune system. In the tumor microenvironment, PD-1 on activated T cells binds to PD-L1 expressed on tumor cells, inhibiting T-cell activation, blocking the body's immune recognition and attack, and promoting tumor immune escape. Therefore, blocking the interaction between PD-1 and PD-L1 can enhance the activity of T cells. At present, several PD-1-targeted ICIs represented by pembrolizumab, nivolumab, and toripalimab have been approved for first-line treatment of cancers such as melanoma, NSCLC, and colorectal cancer (Majidpoor and Mortezaee 2021). Similar to PD-1, the PD-L1 target can also block the immunosuppression mediated by the binding of PD-L1 of tumor cells to PD-1 on the surface of T cells, and re-stimulate T cells to recognize and kill tumor cells. At present, ICIs of PD-L1 targets represented by durvalumab, atezolizumab, and avelumab have also been approved for the immunotherapy of bladder cancer, NSCLC, and urothelial cancer (Banchereau et al. 2021). Currently, PD-1/PD-L1-targeted ICIs have shown significant antitumor activity in a variety of tumor types, and have gradually become "broad-spectrum" antitumor drugs (Yap et al. 2021). However, PD-1/PD-L1 inhibitors are only effective in a minority of patients and are prone to drug resistance. At the same time, due to blocking the negative immune regulation mechanism of the body, the immune status of the body is changed, resulting in some adverse reactions related to immunotoxicity. Therefore, how to improve the response rate of PD-1/PD-L1 inhibitors, improve drug resistance, and reduce adverse reactions is the focus of current immunotherapy. At present, the combination of PD-1/PD-L1 inhibitor monotherapy and other antitumor drugs, PD-1/PD-L1 inhibitor monotherapy and other antitumor target bispecific antibodies and PD-1/PD – "second-generation" PD-1/PD-L1 inhibitors represented by bispecific antibodies against L1 targets and other checkpoints have become a research hotspot in this field, and it is expected that these combination therapies can improve the limitations of current tumor immunotherapy.

2.2 CTLA-4

CTLA-4, also known as CD152, is a transmembrane protein receptor that belongs to the co-suppressive immune checkpoint. CTLA-4 is mainly expressed in activated T cells, especially constitutively expressed in regulatory T cells (Treg). CTLA-4 is highly homologous to the T-cell costimulatory molecule CD28, and both molecules share the same ligands CD80 and CD86 on the surface of antigen-presenting cells. CD28 is a costimulatory checkpoint, responsible for T cells transmitting activation signals and promoting T-cell activation and proliferation; CTLA-4 is a co-inhibitory checkpoint. Activated T cells upregulate their cell surface CTLA-4 expression, responsible for the transmission of inhibitory signals, and inhibit T-cell activation. In particular, CTLA-4 has a higher affinity for CD80/CD86 than CD28, and can competitively block the activation of CD28 on T cells. Therefore, blocking the interaction between CTLA-4 and CD80/CD86 can enhance T-cell activation. Currently, Ipilimumab, a monoclonal antibody targeting CTLA-4, has been approved for the immunotherapy of melanoma and advanced renal cell carcinoma (Larkin et al. 2019). With the deepening of research, it has been found that ipilimumab can inhibit tumor growth by selectively removing Treg cells in the tumor microenvironment. This new mechanism believes that Treg cells in tumors highly express CTLA-4, and CTLA-4 antibody may selectively remove these Treg cells through antibody Fc receptor-mediated antibody-dependent cellular cytotoxicity (ACC). The immunosuppressive effect of Treg cells, and then an antitumor effect (Liu and Zheng 2020; Zhang et al. 2021a). At present, whether the antitumor effect of CTLA-4 antibody depends on the blockade of immune checkpoints or the clearance of tumor Treg cells, or the combined effect of the two, is still some controversy. In addition, although Ipilimumab has been approved for marketing as early as 2011, the development of inhibitors of CTLA-4 targets has been slow. At the same time, studies have found that the side effects of inhibitors of CTLA-4 targets are significantly higher than those of inhibitors of PD-1/PD-L1 targets (Lam and Goldszmid 2021). However, although the response rate of ipilimumab mAb is not as good as that of PD-1/PD-L1 mAb, ipilimumab combined with PD-1/PD-L1 mAb is used in the treatment of advanced melanoma, metastatic NSCLC without EGFR or ALL genomic tumor aberrations, hepatocellular carcinoma, MSI-H/mMR metastatic colorectal cancer, renal cell carcinoma and malignant pleural mesothelioma have high response rates and have been approved for clinical trials in the past (Olson et al. 2021; Paz-Ares et al. 2022; Llovet et al. 2022; Korman et al. 2022). At the same time, studies have shown that PD-1/PD-L1 and CTLA-4 dual-target specific antibodies represented by MDG019, AK104, XmAb20717, KN046, MEDI5752, and PSB205 have shown obvious advantages (Lee et al. 2021a; Dovedi et al. 2021). In addition, CTLA-4 antibodies can induce long-term immune memory, and the activation of the immune system lasts for a long time (Pedicord et al. 2011). Therefore, the development of inhibitors of CTLA-4 targets still has great development prospects. How to expand the clinical application of CTLA-4-targeted inhibitors, improve the clinical efficacy, and reduce side effects of CTLA-4 inhibitors is an important direction of CTLA-4-targeted inhibitor research.

2.3 TIM-3

TIM-3, also known as hepatitis A virus cellular receptor 2 (HAVCR2), is a member of the TIM family of immunomodulatory proteins and a co-suppressive immune checkpoint. TIM-3 is expressed in cells such as T cells, Treg cells, DCs, B cells, macrophages, and NK cells. The ligands of TIM-3 include phosphatidylserine (Ptdser), galectin-9 (Gal-9), high mobility group box 1 (HMGB1), and carcinoembryonic antigen cell adhesion molecule-1 (CEACAM-1). In the tumor microenvironment, TIM-3 can promote myeloid-derived suppressor cells (MDSCs) by suppressing T helper cells, inducing CD8+ T-cell exhaustion, promoting Treg cells to become highly immunosuppressive cell subset, and promoting myeloid-derived suppressor cells (MDSCs). Pathways such as amplifying and promoting innate immunosuppression exert immunosuppressive effects (Solinas et al. 2019). In recent years, TIM-3 has received extensive attention as a novel co-inhibitory checkpoint, in the hope that it can improve the response rate of existing immune checkpoint inhibitors and overcome immune resistance (Wolf et al. 2020). At present, no inhibitors targeting TIM-3 have been approved for clinical use. Inhibitors of TIM-3 targets such as TSR-022, LY3321367, MGB453, BGB-A425, IBI104, INCAGN-02390, BMS-986258, and SHR-1702 are undergoing clinical evaluation. However, research data shows that TIM-3 mAb data is not ideal (Hollebecque et al. 2021). However, in mouse models of melanoma, colorectal cancer, and AML, TIM-3 mAb combined with PD-1 mAb is more effective than PD-1 mAb (Acharya et al. 2020; Yi et al. 2022; Rezaei et al. 2021). Currently, bispecific antibodies RO-7121661 and LY3415244 target TIM-3 and PD-1, and clinical trials of TIM-3 monoclonal antibody combined with PD-1/PD-L1 monoclonal antibody are also in progress (Hellmann et al. 2021; Tian and Li 2021). Based on the current research data, targeting TIM-3 has the potential to enhance the efficacy of PD-1/PD-L1 antibodies, which will bring new hope to cancer patients who cannot benefit from PD-1/PD-L1 antibodies. Therefore, inhibitors of TIM-3 targets deserve further investigation.

2.4 LAG-3

LAG-3, also known as CD233, is a type I transmembrane protein and belongs to one of the immunoglobulin superfamilies. Similar to PD-1 and CTLA-4, LAG-3 is a co-suppressive immune checkpoint, which can negatively regulate the activation and proliferation of T cells by directly inhibiting the proliferation and activation of T cells or promoting the suppressive function of Treg cells. LAG-3 is mainly expressed in activated CD4+ T and CD8+ T cells, Treg cells, NK cells, B cells, and DCs (Shi et al. 2021). In the tumor environment or chronic infection, antigens continuously stimulate T cells, and T cells become exhausted T cells, which will continue to express LAG-3 at a high level (Jiang et al. 2020). The ligands of LAG-3 mainly include major histocompatibility complex II (MHC II), galectin-3 (Gal-3), and hepatic sinusoidal endothelial cell lectin (hepatic sinusoidal endothelial cell lectin, LSECtin) and fibrinogen-like protein 1 (FGL1) (Wang et al. 2019). MHC-II is mainly expressed in antigen-presenting cells and is also highly expressed in various types of tumor cells. Gal-3 is mainly expressed in various types of tumor cells as well as stromal cells and CD8+ T cells in the tumor microenvironment. LSECtin and FGL1 are also highly expressed in various types of tumor cells. Therefore, LAG-3 target blockade of LAG-3-mediated immunosuppression enhances T-cell activity and inhibits tumor growth. Currently, no inhibitors targeting LAG-3 have been approved for clinical use. However, in March 2022, the dual immunotherapy Relatlimab (LAG-3 antibody) + Nivolumab (PD-1 antibody) fixed-dose combination Opdualag was approved for the treatment of adults and children (12 years and older) with unresectable or metastatic melanoma) patients (Tawbi et al. 2022). Relatlimab is the first LAG-3 antibody approved by the US FDA. LAG-3 has thus become the third immune checkpoint applied in clinical after PD-1/PD-L1 and CTLA-4. At present, the research of a new generation of ICIs for LAG-3 has received extensive attention. Drugs under development against LAG-3 include LAG-3 monomers (including LAG525, BI754111, MK-4280, TSR-033, Sym022, REGN3767, INCAGN2385-101, and BI754111), bispecific antibodies (PD-1/MGD013 for LAG-3 target, FS118 for PD-L1/LAG-3 target, XmAb22841 for CTLA-4/LAG-3 target, etc.) and IMP321 (Eftilagimod alpha) represented by soluble LAG-3 fusion protein and other three class (Kraman et al. 2020; Ghosh et al. 2019; Catenacci et al. 2021; Maruhashi et al. 2020). Drug research based on the LAG-3 target, especially its combination therapy with PD-1/PD-L1 antibodies, makes LAG-3 a very promising immunotherapy target.

2.5 VISTA

VISTA, a member of the immunoglobulin superfamily and a member of the B7 family of molecules, is a co-inhibitory checkpoint. Unlike other immune checkpoints, VISTA is constitutively expressed on naive T cells. In particular, VISTA expression on T cells is reduced under inflammatory conditions. Therefore, VISTA is a unique inhibitory checkpoint on naive T cells that can effectively inhibit T-cell activation and proliferation (ElTanbouly et al. 2020). V-Set and Immunoglobulin Domain Containing Protein 3 (VSIG-3) is a ligand of VISTA, which is hardly expressed in normal tissues, but highly expressed in the tumor microenvironment. VSIG-3/VISTA signaling-mediated co-inhibitory signaling inhibits T-cell activation. In addition, VISTA binds to P-selectin glycoprotein ligand-1 (PSGL-1) under acidic pH conditions to promote VISTA-mediated immunosuppression. Studies have shown that VISTA inhibition enhances the infiltration, proliferation, and effector functions of T cells in the tumor microenvironment, thereby promoting antitumor immune responses (Johnston et al. 2019). Therefore, VISTA is a valuable new immune checkpoint for tumor immunotherapy. However, no single drug targeting VISTA has been approved for clinical use. Currently, the drugs targeting VISTA targets mainly include monoclonal antibodies represented by JNJ-61610588

(CI-8993) and oral small molecule inhibitor CA-170 that selectively targets PD-L1 and VISTA and are undergoing clinical trials (Musielak et al. 2019). Data show that VISTA-targeted drugs show positive antitumor effects, and blocking VISTA and PD-1/PD-L1 can significantly enhance the antitumor immune response (Yuan et al. 2021). Therefore, immune checkpoint inhibitors targeting VISTA deserve further study.

2.6 TIGIT

TIGIT, a member of the poliovirus receptor (PVR)/Nectin family, belongs to the co-inhibitory checkpoint. TIGIT is expressed in lymphocytes, especially in effector and regulatory CD4+ T cells, effector CD8+ T cells, and NK cells. CD155, also known as PVR, is a high-affinity ligand for TIGIT. CD155 is mainly expressed in DC cells, T cells, B cells, and macrophages, and is also highly expressed in various types of tumor cells. CD155 is highly expressed on the surface of tumor cells, and when combined with TIGIT on the surface of NK and T cells, the killing effect of NK and T cells on tumor cells is inhibited (Freed-Pastor et al. 2021; Ge et al. 2021). Therefore, TIGIT/CD155 signaling may be one of the mechanisms of tumor immune escape. In addition, CD112 and CD113 can also bind to TIGIT, but with weaker affinity than CD155. CD112 is widely expressed on the surface of both hematopoietic cells and non-hematopoietic cells, and is highly expressed in various types of tumor cells, but CD113 is only expressed on the surface of non-hematopoietic cells. Studies have shown that TIGIT can bind to CD155, and CD226 and CD96 can also interact with CD155, but these interactions are weaker than the interaction between TIGIT-CD155. CD226 produces downstream signals that activate immune responses, while TIGIT downstream signals suppress immune responses (Chan et al. 2014; Sun et al. 2019a). TIGIT can compete with CD226 for binding to CD155, thereby attenuating the downstream signaling activity of CD226. TIGIT can inhibit the activation and function of immune cells at multiple steps of the tumor immune cycle and promote immune escape. Therefore, TIGIT can serve as a novel immune checkpoint for tumor therapy. At present, a new generation of immune checkpoint research on TIGIT targets is in full swing. The drugs under development against TIGIT mainly include at least 20 inhibitors including MK-7684, BMS-986207, Tiragolumab, BGB-A1217, and IBI-939 (Harjunpaa and Guillerey 2020; Rotte et al. 2021). In particular, TIGIT mAb combined with PD-1/PD-L1 mAb, PD-1/TIGIT-targeted bispecific antibodies AZD2936 and IBI321, and PD-L1/TIGIT-targeted bispecific antibodies HLX301 and PM1022 and others have gained widespread attention. Data show that the combination of TIGIT mAb and PD-1 mAb is likely to benefit patients who do not respond to existing immune checkpoint inhibitors (American Association for Cancer Research 2020a, 2022; Han et al. 2021). Therefore, despite the complex mechanism of action of TIGIT, inhibitors of TIGIT targets deserve further study (Fig. 1).

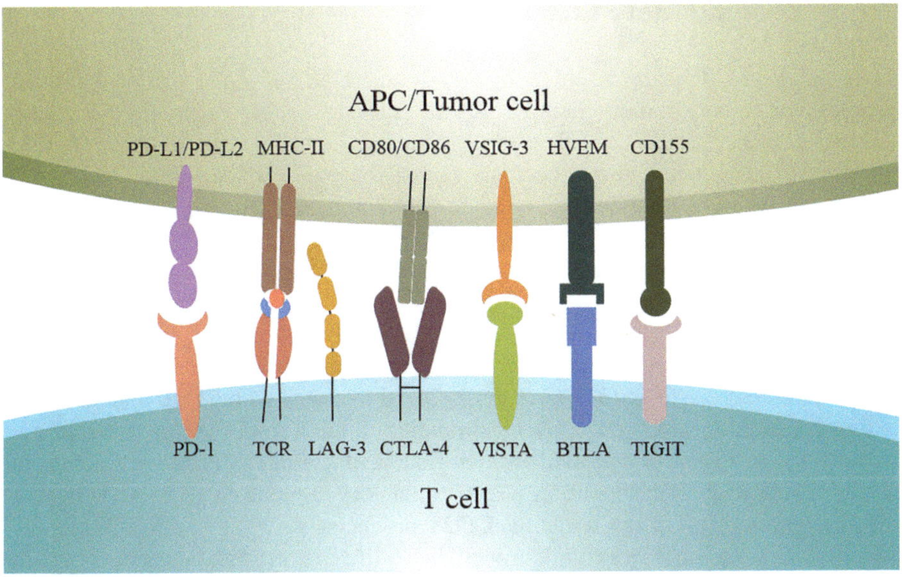

Fig. 1 Current and emerging immune checkpoint receptors and their respective ligands. Various immune checkpoint molecules expressed on T cells were shown with their ligands. Immune checkpoints such as PD-1, CTLA-4, LAG-3, VISTA, TIGIT, and BTLA bound with their respective ligands on APCs and/or tumor cells

2.7 BTLA

BTLA, also known as CD272, is a type I glycosylated transmembrane protein that belongs to a co-inhibitory receptor of the CD28 superfamily. BTLA is expressed in T cells, B cells, macrophages, DCs, and NK cells. Herpesvirus entry mediator (HVEM), also known as tumor necrosis factor receptor superfamily, member 14, TNFRSF14, is a BTLA ligand. HVEM is expressed on T cells, DCs, and various types of tumor cells. In addition, HVEM can also bind to CD160, LIGHT, lymphotoxin-α (LTα), and Herpes simplex virus glycoprotein D (HSV-gD) (Liu et al. 2021). HVEM binds to LIGHT or LTα and is responsible for transmitting costimulatory signals. The binding of HVEM to BTLA or CD160 is responsible for transmitting co-inhibitory signals. HVEM transmits co-inhibitory signals stronger than costimulatory signals. Therefore, binding of BTLA to HVEM inhibits T-cell activity. Especially in the tumor microenvironment, BTLA is upregulated in the later stages of T-cell depletion (Demerle et al. 2021). Tumor cells upregulate HVEM and participate in tumor immune escape through BTLA/HVEM signaling (Lan et al. 2017). Therefore, inhibitors against BTLA targets deserve further research, especially the combination therapy with PD-1/PD-L1 antibodies is a direction worth exploring. At present, clinical trials targeting BTLA targets are mostly in the basic research stage. Only the antitumor BTLA mAb JS004 is in clinical trials. Research on BTLA-targeted drugs is in its infancy, and BTLA is gradually gaining attention as a new immune checkpoint.

3 Costimulatory Checkpoints

In recent years, ICIs represented by PD-1 and CTLA-4 have made significant progress in tumor immunotherapy. At the same time, the activating receptors CD28, OX40, CD137 on T cells, inducible T-cell costimulatory (ICOS), glucocorticoid-induced tumor necrosis factor receptor (GITR), and CD27 have also been extensively studied as targets for immunotherapy.

3.1 CD28

CD28, a member of the B7 receptor family, is a costimulatory molecule constitutively expressed on the surface of T cells. CD28 interacts with CD80 and CD86 on antigen-presenting cells, provides costimulatory signals for T-cell activation, and participates in T-cell activation, proliferation, and cytokine secretion. Therefore, CD28 has attracted much attention as a costimulatory immune checkpoint. However, the development of drugs targeting CD28 has been slow. In 2006, research on costimulatory agonists was undermined by a life-threatening cytokine storm in clinical trials of the CD28 mAb agonist Theralizumab (Stebbings et al. 2009). In 2013, Theralizumab (TAB08) underwent another I clinical trial after a reduced dose with success (Hunig 2016). In 2017, the phase I clinical trial of TAB08 in patients with solid tumors was carried out, which made the CD28 target attract attention again (Mishra et al. 2020). In January 2020, Sanofi published data showing that the CD28/CD3/CD38 trispecific antibody SAR442257 developed by Sanofi can enhance costimulatory signals to promote antitumor immunity, and will advance it to clinical research in May 2020 (Wu et al. 2020). Similarly, in January 2020, Regeneron published experimental data showing that CD28-involved bispecific antibodies enhanced the antitumor effect of CD3-involved bispecific antibodies without significant cytokine storm (Skokos et al. 2020). In June 2020, Regeneron once again published experimental data showing that its new bispecific antibody TSA×CD28 and PD-1 antibody synergistically enhance the efficacy of PD-1 antibody, and impart better reactivity and long-term immune memory, and no obvious toxic effects (Waite et al. 2020). Subsequently, the three bispecific antibodies MUC16×CD28 (REGN5668), PSMA×CD28 (REGN5678), and EGFR×CD28 (REGN7075) developed by it were pushed to the clinical trial stage. In August 2021, Sanofi also advanced its trispecific antibody SAR443216 targeting CD28/CD3/HER2 into clinical research, and published experimental data in March 2022 showing that the CD28/CD3/HER2 trispecific antibody stimulating T-cell activation can effectively mediate tumor regression, providing new hope for the majority of breast cancer patients who do not respond to HER2-based therapy (Seung et al. 2022). In addition, the second-generation CAR-T therapy with CD28 as a costimulatory domain has also received extensive attention in recent years (Guedan et al. 2020). However, CAR-T therapy with CD28 as a costimulatory domain is also controversial due to side effects such as cytokine storm. Therefore, the development of drugs targeting CD28 has a long way to go. However, it is believed that with the continuous deepening of basic research, the development of drugs targeting CD28 will become clearer, bringing new ideas for tumor immunotherapy.

3.2 OX40

OX40, also known as tumor necrosis factor receptor superfamily, member 4, TNFRSF4, is a T-cell costimulatory molecule. OX40 is mainly expressed in activated effector T cells, Treg cells, and NK cells. OX40L is the ligand of OX40 and is mainly expressed in antigen-presenting cells, activated T cells, and NK cells. In the tumor microenvironment, immune activation can lead to the upregulation of OX40 expression, enhance the activation and proliferation of effector T cells, and reduce the suppressive effect of Treg cells, thereby enhancing the antitumor immune response (Alves Costa Silva et al. 2020). The antitumor activity of OX40-targeted agonists has been demonstrated in several preclinical studies (Messenheimer et al. 2017; Ma et al. 2020). Therefore, OX40 is a potentially valuable costimulatory immune checkpoint. Several OX40 agonists are currently in clinical trials, including AGX-051, IBI101, ABBV-368, BGB-A445, and mRNA-2416. However, preliminary clinical data of OX40 agonists represented by BMS-986178 and MOXR0916 show that the antitumor effect of OX40 agonists as a single agent is not ideal (Gutierrez et al. 2021; Cebada et al. 2021). Combination therapy with OX40 agonists is a direction worth exploring. Currently, the combination therapy of OX40 target agonist and PD-1/PD-L1 monoclonal antibody and CAR-T therapy of OX40 costimulatory domain are undergoing clinical research (Zhang et al. 2021b). In addition, bispecific antibodies that combine PD-L1/OX40 antagonism and agonism, represented by IBI327 and KN052, are also under clinical research (Kvarnhammar et al. 2019; Kuang et al. 2020). Preliminary clinical trial results show that OX40 agonists have great development value, but they are very difficult to develop. Therefore, there is a long way to go to promote the research of OX40 agonists.

3.3 CD137

CD137, also known as 4-1BB or tumor necrosis factor receptor superfamily, member 9, TNFRSF9, is a type II membrane glycoprotein on the cell membrane surface and is a costimulatory immune checkpoint. CD137 is expressed in activated T cells, Treg cells, NK cells, DCs, and macrophages. CD137L is a ligand for CD137, which is mainly expressed on professional antigen -presenting cells such as DCs, macrophages, and B cells. The interaction of CD137 with CD137L expressed by professional antigen-presenting cells provides a costimulatory signal for T-cell activation, and is involved in T-cell activation, proliferation, and cytokine secretion (Etxeberria et al. 2020). CD137 agonists mainly act by inducing T-cell proliferation and cytokine secretion. In addition, CD137 agonists can enhance the ADCC effect of NK cells, as well as promote DC- and macrophage-mediated antitumor immune responses (Cabo et al. 2021; Segal et al. 2018). Therefore, CD137 is a potentially valuable costimulatory immune checkpoint. However, clinical data based on CD137 agonists represented by BMS-663513 and PF-05082566 show that their efficacy is not high and has liver toxicity (Chin et al. 2018). Several other CD137 agonists, including CTX-471, AGEN2373, ATOR-1017, and ADG-106, are currently undergoing clinical studies (Chester et al. 2018). In order to improve the efficacy and reduce the side effects of CD137 agonists, a number of bispecific antibodies targeting CD137 and PD-1/PD-L1 including GEN1046, PRS-344, ES101, and IBI319 have been developed and are also under clinical evaluation (Muik et al. 2022). In addition, second-generation CD19-CAR-T therapies with CD137 as the costimulatory domain, such as Liso-cel, Tisa-cel, and Relma-cel, have been approved for marketing one after another (Ying et al. 2021; Rejeski et al. 2021; Abramson et al. 2020). Therefore, the CD137 target has gained obvious advantages in CAR-T therapy due to its safety and durability, but the development of CD137 agonists still has a long way to go.

3.4 ICOS

ICOS, also known as CD278, is a type I transmembrane glycoprotein, a member of the CD28 family like CTLA-4, and a costimulatory immune checkpoint. ICOS is mainly expressed on activated T cells. ICOS-L is the ligand of ICOS and belongs to the B7 family member. ICOS-L is mainly expressed on antigen-presenting cells such as B cells, macrophages, and DCs. ICOS binds to its ligand ICOS-L, provides costimulatory signals to induce cell activation, proliferation, and differentiation, and regulates multiple T-cell functions. In the tumor microenvironment, ICOS/ ICOS-L costimulatory signaling enhances the antitumor activity of T cells (Amatore et al. 2020; Hanson et al. 2020). Therefore, ICOS is a potentially valuable costimulatory immune checkpoint. At present, no drugs targeting ICOS targets have been approved for marketing, but many drugs targeting ICOS have entered the clinical evaluation stage. However, the clinical data of ICOS agonists represented by Vopratelimab and GSK3359609 show that the single-agent efficacy of ICOS agonists is not ideal (Nooka et al. 2021). Currently, Vopratelimab combined with CTLA-4 antibody Ipilimumab, GSK3359609 combined with PD-1 antibody Pembrolizumab, and PD-1/ICOS bispecific antibody XmAb23104 are being explored as ICOS agonists and combined therapy with other therapies, which are expected to improve the current limitations of ICIs (Penter et al. 2021; Boudjema et al. 2021) (Fig. 2).

3.5 GITR

GITR, also known as tumor necrosis factor receptor superfamily, member 18, TNFRSF18, is a type I transmembrane protein that belongs to the costimulatory immune checkpoint. GITR is highly expressed on activated T cells, especially activated Treg cells. In addition, B cells, macrophages, DCs, and NK cells also

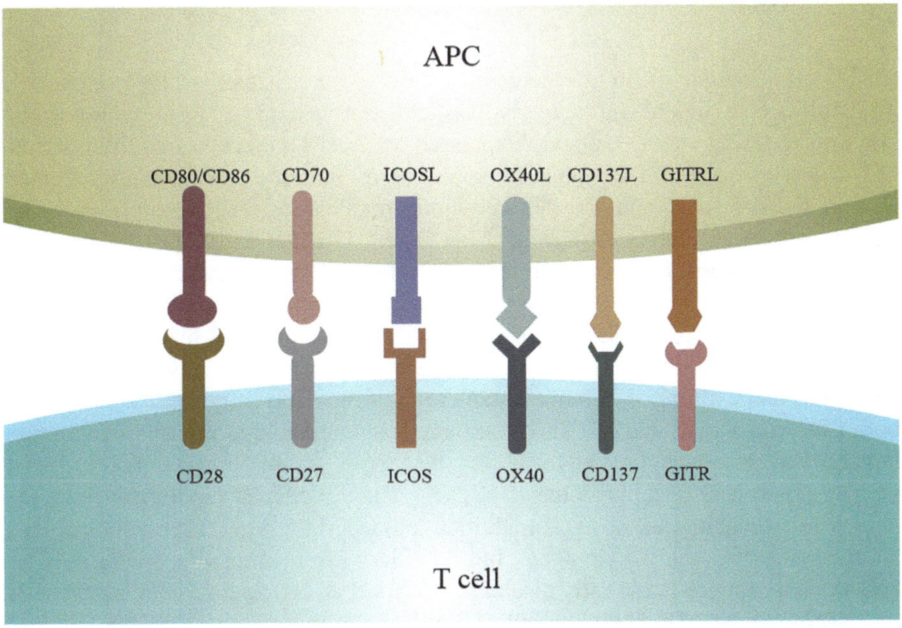

Fig. 2 Current and emerging immune checkpoint receptors and their respective ligands. Various immune checkpoint molecules expressed on T cells were shown with their ligands. Immune checkpoints such as CD28, CD27, ICOS OX40, CD137, and GITR bound with their respective ligands on APCs and/or tumor cells

express GITR. GITRL is a ligand of GITR and is mainly expressed in activated antigen-presenting cells such as macrophages, B cells, and DCs. GITR binds to the ligand GITRL and provides a costimulatory signal to enhance T-cell activation and effector function. Meanwhile, GITR/GITRL signaling can inhibit the activity of Treg cells (Zappasodi et al. 2019; Amoozgar et al. 2021). Therefore, GITR is a potentially valuable costimulatory immune checkpoint that can synergistically enhance antitumor responses with existing PD-1/PD-L1 antibodies. In recent years, research on GITR agonists has gained extensive attention. However, the clinical efficacy of single-agent GITR agonists represented by AMG 228, BMS-986156, and TRX518 is not ideal (Buzzatti et al. 2020). Studies have shown that the safety of BMS-986156 in the treatment of advanced solid tumors is controllable, but the efficacy and safety of BMS-986156 in combination with PD-1 antibody Nivolumab are similar to those of Nivolumab alone (Heinhuis et al. 2020). However, the GITR agonist MK-4166 enhanced the antitumor immune response of the PD-1 antibody Pembrolizumab with less adverse effects (Sun et al. 2021). Currently, other GITR agonists, including ASP-1951, Ragifilimab, and GWN-323, are under clinical research, especially in combination with other immune checkpoints. It is expected that these GITR agonists might have the potential detected with positive signals in clinical trial.

3.6 CD27

CD27, also known as tumor necrosis factor receptor superfamily, member 7, TNFRSF7, is a transmembrane glycoprotein that belongs to the costimulatory checkpoint. CD27 is constitutively expressed on T cells, NK cells, and thymocytes. CD70 is a ligand for CD27, and its expression on immune cells such as activated T cells, B cells, DCs, and NK cells is tightly regulated. CD27 binds to its ligand CD70, and costimulatory signals such as OX40, CD137, and ICOS promote the survival of activated T cells and enhance the effector function and cytokine production of T cells (Gennery 2020). In addition, CD70 is highly expressed in various types of tumor cells. The high expression of CD70 in tumor cells binds to the T-cell receptor CD27, and the inhibition of the effector function of T cells may be one of the mechanisms of tumor immune escape (van de Ven and Borst 2015). Therefore, both CD27 on T cells and CD70 on tumor cells are potential tumor immunotherapy targets. Preclinical studies have shown that PD-1 antibody and CD27 agonist varlilumab synergistically enhance CD8+ T-cell-mediated antitumor immune responses (Buchan et al. 2018). In addition, clinical data show that varlilumab has antitumor activity as a single agent, but its efficacy in combination with the PD-1 antibody Nivolumab is not fully disclosed (Burris et al. 2017). Phase II clinical trials of CD27 agonist MK-5890 and PD-1 antibody Pembrolizumab in NSCLC are ongoing. In addition, preclinical data based on CD27/PD-L1-targeted bispecific antibody CDX-527 showed that its antitumor activity was superior to PD-L1 monoclonal antibody and CD27 agonist monotherapy, and CDX-527 was subsequently pushed to Phase I clinical study (Vitale et al. 2020). At the same time, CD70-targeted inhibitors represented by cusatuzumab, CD70-targeted CAR-T therapy, and CD70-targeted antibody-drug conjugates (ADCs) have all entered the clinical evaluation stage. It is expected that these combination therapies can improve the limitations of current ICIs (American Association for Cancer Research 2020b; Sauer et al. 2021; Phillips et al. 2019).

4 Targeting Immunosuppressive Cells

There are a large number of immunosuppressive cells in the tumor microenvironment. These immunosuppressive cells can inhibit the infiltration and effect of antitumor immune cells, which is one of the important mechanisms of tumor immune escape and immunotherapy resistance (Park et al. 2022). Immunosuppressive cells mainly refer to Treg cells, myeloid-derived suppressor cells (MDSC), and M2 tumor-associated macrophages (TAM). Targeting immunosuppressive cells in the tumor microenvironment and using drugs to block their inhibitory pathways can effectively inhibit the immune escape of tumor cells, enhance the response rate of tumor immunotherapy and improve the drug resistance of tumor immunotherapy.

4.1 Treg Cells

Treg cells mainly refer to CD4+ CD25+ FoxP3+ T cells. The CCR4/CCL17 or CCR4/CCL22 pathway is the main pathway regulating Treg cell chemotaxis. CCL17 or CCL22 secreted by tumor cells, TAMs, and MDSCs recruit CCR4+ Treg cells to the tumor microenvironment (Li et al. 2020a). In the tumor microenvironment, Treg cells promote tumor immune escape mainly by secreting inhibitory cytokines such as IL-10, TGF-β, and IL-35, or by directly contacting antitumor immune cells such as effector T cells or DCs (Scott et al. 2021). Therefore, targeting Treg cells is an important strategy for tumor immunotherapy. In recent years, studies have found that CTLA-4 antibody may play an antitumor effect by removing Treg cells and releasing the immunosuppressive effect of Treg cells (Marangoni et al. 2021). In particular, a preclinical study of the CTLA-4/OX40 dual-target-specific antibody ATOR-1015, which activates effector T cells and clears Treg cells, has shown that it can enhance the antitumor activity of PD-1 antibodies (Kvarnhammar et al. 2019). At present, the ATOR-1015 research has advanced to the clinical trial stage. In addition, Treg cells highly express the costimulatory immune checkpoint GITR, and the binding of GITR to its ligand GITRL can inhibit the activity of Treg cells and promote the activation of effector T cells. However, the current research progress of GITR agonists is slow, and it is expected to be further studied in the future. In addition, Treg cells highly express CD25. Studies have found that Fc-optimized CD25 antibodies can clear Treg cells in the tumor microenvironment and enhance the antitumor response rate of PD-1 antibodies (Arce Vargas et al. 2017). However, the interaction of CD25 antibody with IL-2 simultaneously blocks IL-2 signaling on effector T cells, affecting the survival and effector function of effector T cells. Therefore, CD25 antibodies that suppress Treg cells without suppressing effector T cells require further investigation. Fortunately, a modified CD25 antibody, RO7296682 (RG6292), was reported to be able to clear Treg cells while preserving IL-2 signaling on effector T cells (Solomon et al. 2020). At present, the research of RO7296682 has entered the clinical trial stage. In addition, studies have found that drugs targeting CD25-ADC significantly inhibit tumor growth by removing Treg cells, and at the same time can enhance the antitumor response of PD-1 antibodies (Zammarchi et al. 2020). At present, the research of ADCT-301, a drug targeting CD25-ADC, has been advanced to the clinical trial stage. Therefore, targeting Treg cells, especially their combination therapy with ICIs, will help to improve the limitations of existing tumor immunotherapy and improve immune resistance.

4.2 MDSC

MDSCs are a heterogeneous group of bone marrow-derived cells that can significantly inhibit the function and effect of immune cells. MDSCs are derived from myeloid progenitor cells and immature myeloid cells (IMCs), which are precursors of DCs, macrophages, and granulocytes, and can rapidly differentiate into mature DCs, macrophages, and granulocytes. Soluble and pro-inflammatory factors such as IFN-γ, IL-1β, IL-4, and IL-10 in the tumor environment promote the differentiation of IMCs into MDSCs. In addition, CCL2, CCL12, and CXCL5 secreted by tumor cells can recruit MDSCs to the tumor microenvironment (Li et al. 2020b). MDSCs in the tumor microenvironment can secrete IL-10, TGF-β, inducible nitric oxide synthase (iNOS), nitric oxide (NO), and arginase-1 inhibits the function and effect of immune cells and induces Treg cells to indirectly inhibit antitumor immune responses and promote immune escape (Hegde et al. 2021; Orillion et al. 2017). Therefore, targeting MDSC cells is an important strategy for antitumor immunotherapy. However, targeting MDSC cells is challenging due to the lack of uniform molecular markers. Studies have shown that chemotherapy drugs such as 5-Fluorouracil and Oxaliplatin can enhance the antitumor response of PD-1 antibody and improve drug resistance by reducing the number of MDSCs (Kim et al. 2021). In addition, it was found that the STAT3 inhibitor Galiellalactone inhibited prostate cancer cells from producing MDSC-like monocytes and reduced immunosuppressive and tumorigenic factors (Hellsten et al. 2019). Studies have reported that the receptor tyrosine kinase inhibitor Sunitinib inhibits MDSCs and promotes antitumor responses (Fu et al. 2020). Meanwhile, inhibitors that inhibit the recruitment of MDSCs have also gained widespread attention. Studies have reported that the CXCR2 small molecule inhibitor SX-682 can enhance the antitumor response of adoptively transferred T cells and NK cells by eliminating MDSC tumor infiltration (Greene et al. 2020; Sun et al. 2019b). At present, clinical trials of SX-682 monotherapy and PD-1 antibody Pembrolizumab have been launched. The CXCR2 inhibitor AZD5069 is also in clinical studies. In addition, studies have reported that Entinostat, a class I histone deacetylase inhibitor, can neutralize MDSCs and enhance the antitumor effect of PD-1 antibodies (Orillion et al. 2017). At present, clinical trials of the combination therapy of Entinostat and Pembrolizumab have also been carried out, and it is expected to obtain positive effects.

4.3 TAM

TAMs are macrophages that infiltrate tumors and are one of the most abundant immune cells in the tumor microenvironment. TAM can be divided into M1-type classical macrophages and M2-type activated macrophages. M1-type TAMs exert antitumor effects by promoting Th1-type immune responses and secreting TNF-α, IL-1, IL-6, IL-12, type I IFN, CXCL1–3, CXCL5, and CXCL8–10; M2-type TAMs exert their antitumor effects by Promote Th2-type immune response and secrete IL-10, TGF-β, CCL17, CCL18, CCL22, and CCL24 to play an immunosuppressive effect (Pittet et al. 2022). In particular, M2-type TAMs can also promote angiogenesis by secreting adrenomedullin and VEGF and upregulate PD-L1 expression to promote immune escape (Jayasingam et al. 2019). Adenosine, CCL2, and CXCL12 produced in the tumor microenvironment can recruit TAMs to the tumor microenvironment through the adenosine pathway, the CCL2/CCR2 axis, and CXCL12/CXCR4 (Li et al. 2019). CSF-1R is a cell surface receptor expressed by macrophages and other myeloid cells.

Inflammatory cytokines such as IFN-γ and TNF-α can induce tumor cells to produce CSF-1, which can promote the activation or recruitment of M2-type TAMs to the tumor microenvironment through CSF/CSF-1R signaling (Mily et al. 2020). In addition, tumor cells highly express CD47, which binds to signal regulatory protein-α (SIRPα) on the surface of TAMs, which can initiate inhibitory signaling pathways and lead to tumor immune escape (Logtenberg et al. 2020). Therefore, how to specifically reduce the M2 type becomes the key to targeting TAM. Preclinical studies have shown that blocking CSF/CSF-1R signaling can specifically remove M2-type TAMs and enhance the antitumor effect of ICIs (Ries et al. 2014; Akkari et al. 2020; Magkouta et al. 2021). CSF-1R inhibitors represented by Cabiralizumab, Emactuzumab, and ARRY-382 have entered clinical trials (Johnson et al. 2022; Weiss et al. 2021; Gomez-Roca et al. 2019). Furthermore, blocking the CXCL12/CXCR4 pathway also reduces the infiltration of M2-type TAMs in the tumor microenvironment (Mota et al. 2016; O'Connor and Heikenwalder 2021). At present, the CXCR4 inhibitor represented by LY2510924 and the CXCR4 antibody represented by Ulocuplumab have been advanced to the clinical evaluation stage (O'Hara et al. 2020; Treon et al. 2021). In addition, blocking the CD47/SIRPα inhibitory signal can also promote the phagocytosis of tumor cells by macrophages and enhance the antitumor effect. At present, CD47 antibodies represented by Hu5F9-G4, IBI188, and TJC4, SIRPα-Fc fusion proteins represented by TTI-621 and ALX148, and CD47 bispecific antibodies represented by HX009, IMM0306, and IBI-322 have entered the market clinical evaluation stage (Zhang et al. 2020; Jiang et al. 2021). However, since CD47 is also expressed on cells of the hematopoietic system, the off-target effect of CD47-targeted drugs is significant. In view of the important role of CD47/SIRPα signaling in tumor immune escape, it is possible to develop novel antitumor drugs targeting CD47/SIRPα by further studying the mechanism of CD47/SIRPα signaling and improving primer design. In addition, PI3Kγ is a molecule widely expressed by myeloid cells but not by tumor cells. Studies have shown that blocking PI3Kγ signaling in macrophages can activate immune responses and inhibit tumor growth, while also enhancing sensitivity to antitumor drugs and ICIs (Kaneda et al. 2016; Joshi et al. 2020; Sai et al. 2017). Therefore, antitumor immunity can be promoted by targeting PI3Kγ. At present, PI3Kγ inhibitors represented by IPI-549 have entered the clinical evaluation stage, and positive results are expected.

5 Drugs that Regulate Innate Immunity and Promote Tumor Immune Infiltration

5.1 STING Agonists

Cyclic GMP-AMP synthase (cGAS) is an intracellular DNA sensor that is located in the cytoplasm and can recognize DNA in the cytoplasm and catalyze the synthesis of cyclic guanosine-adenosine from GTP and ATP (cyclin GMP-AMP, cGAMP), cGAMP acts as a second messenger, binds and activates interferon gene stimulator (stimulator of interferon genes, STING), and then activates the downstream TBK1 and transcription factor IRF3, inducing the production of type I interferon. In the tumor microenvironment, the cGAS/STING signaling pathway can activate the killing activity of the immune system against tumors. In DC cells, DNA leaked into the cytoplasm from tumor or genomic instability can be recognized by the STING-mediated cytoplasmic DNA recognition signaling pathway, ultimately leading to the production of type I interferons. On the one hand, type I interferon can promote DC cross-presentation to initiate tumor-specific CD8+ T cells. On the other hand, type I interferon further activates the STING signaling pathway and leads to the production of chemokines, which help recruit CD8+ T cells to the tumor microenvironment to kill tumor cells. Studies have found that one of the mechanisms of action of certain chemotherapy drugs or tumor radiation is by causing DNA damage and ultimately tumor cell death. Leakage of nuclear DNA into the cytoplasm after tumor cell death can cause activation of the STING signaling pathway and further activate the immune response. Therefore, the STING signaling pathway plays an important role in tumor immunity, and STING agonists have become a hot spot in the development of antitumor drugs. Currently, STING agonists represented by IMSA-101, GSK3745417, BMS-986301, and MK-1454 have been clinically studied (Motedayen Aval et al. 2020). Studies have found that STING agonists can promote antigen presentation, enhance CD8+ T-cell activation and tumor infiltration, promote NK activation, and promote the transformation of M2-type TAMs to M1-type (Nakamura et al. 2021; Lam et al. 2021; Lee et al. 2021b). Existing clinical research data have preliminarily verified the feasibility of combining STING agonists with immunotherapy, which is expected to improve the limitations of existing immunotherapy (Shi et al. 2020; Yang et al. 2019).

5.2 TLR Agonists

Toll-like receptors (TLRs) are a class of important protein receptors in innate immunity that can recognize pathogen-associated molecular patterns (PAMPs) and damage-associated molecular patterns (DAMP), which lead to the activation of innate immune cells through a cascade of reactions, which in turn secrete pro-inflammatory cytokines and initiate specific immunity. Therefore, in the tumor microenvironment, TLR agonists can be used to enhance innate immunity, promote DC-mediated antigen presentation, and enhance the antitumor response of CD8+ T cells. In recent years, TLR agonists represented by TLR9 agonists have attracted widespread attention. After TLR9 activation, DCs secrete a large amount of type 1 interferons, activate traditional DCs and T cells, and then reshape the tumor-killing activity of immune cells in the tumor microenvironment. TLR9 agonists represented by CMP-001, SD-101, and AZD1419 have entered the clinical evaluation stage (Ribas et al. 2018). Studies have found that TLR9 agonists can promote the activation and tumor infiltration of DCs, CD8+ T cells, and NK cells, promote the activation of B cells, and enhance the antitumor effect of ICIs (Cohen et al. 2022). Clinical data have shown great potential for a combination strategy of TLR9 agonists with other ICIs (Ribas et al. 2021; Garon et al. 2021).

Acknowledgments We thank Anqi Li for providing suggestions in reference and figure formatting in this chapter.

Conflict of Interest Statement The authors certify that they have no affiliations with or involvement in any organization or entity with any financial interest or nonfinancial interest in the subject matter or materials discussed in this manuscript. The authors declare no competing financial interests.

Funding This work was supported by projects on the Science and Technology Commission of Shanghai (18ZR1403900 and 20430713600) (D. Zhu) and Jinan Science and Technology Bureau, Innovation team for the development and evaluation of new drugs for oncology immunotherapy (2020GXRC041 to DZ).

Compliance with Ethical Standards

Ethical Approval and Consent to Participate This work had the approval from Research and Ethical committee of School of Pharmacy, Fudan University. This work was not performed studies on individuals, so no individual participated in the study. Informed consent was not taken from individuals.

Consent for Publication In this work, we didn't perform study on any individuals and this work doesn't include details, images, or videos relating to any individual person. There are no details on individuals reported within the manuscript.

Data Availability Data repository: https://figshare.com/s/75ed36bdd8506bea8495

References

Abramson JS, Palomba ML, Gordon LI, Lunning MA, Wang M, Arnason J, Mehta A, Purev E, Maloney DG, Andreadis C, Others (2020) Lisocabtagene maraleucel for patients with relapsed or refractory large B-cell lymphomas (TRANSCEND NHL 001): a multicentre seamless design study. Lancet 396:839–852. https://doi.org/10.1016/S0140-6736(20)31366-0

Acharya N, Sabatos-Peyton C, Anderson AC (2020) Tim-3 finds its place in the cancer immunotherapy landscape. J Immunother Cancer 8. https://doi.org/10.1136/jitc-2020-000911

Akkari L, Bowman RL, Tessier J, Klemm F, Handgraaf SM, de Groot M, Quail DF, Tillard L, Gadiot J, Huse JT, Others (2020) Dynamic changes in glioma macrophage populations after radiotherapy reveal CSF-1R inhibition as a strategy to overcome resistance. Sci Transl Med 12. https://doi.org/10.1126/scitranslmed.aaw7843

Alves Costa Silva C, Facchinetti F, Routy B, Derosa L (2020) New pathways in immune stimulation: targeting OX40. ESMO Open 5. https://doi.org/10.1136/esmoopen-2019-000573

Amatore F, Gorvel L, Olive D (2020) Role of Inducible Co-Stimulator (ICOS) in cancer immunotherapy. Expert Opin Biol Ther 20:141–150. https://doi.org/10.1080/14712598.2020.1693540

American Association for Cancer Research (2020a) Tiragolumab impresses in multiple trials. Cancer Discov 10:1086–1087. https://doi.org/10.1158/2159-8290.CD-NB2020-063

American Association for Cancer Research (2020b) The CD70 antibody Cusatuzumab shows promise in acute myeloid leukemia. Cancer Discov 10:1251. https://doi.org/10.1158/2159-8290.CD-RW2020-106

American Association for Cancer Research (2022) An anti-TIGIT antibody with a PD-1 inhibitor shows promise in solid tumors. Cancer Discov 12:14. https://doi.org/10.1158/2159-8290.CD-RW2021-170

Amoozgar Z, Kloepper J, Ren J, Tay RE, Kazer SW, Kiner E, Krishnan S, Posada JM, Ghosh M, Mamessier E, Others (2021) Targeting Treg cells with GITR activation alleviates resistance to immunotherapy in murine glioblastomas. Nat Commun 12:2582. https://doi.org/10.1038/s41467-021-22885-8

Arce Vargas F, Furness AJS, Solomon I, Joshi K, Mekkaoui L, Lesko MH, Miranda Rota E, Dahan R, Georgiou A, Sledzinska A, Others (2017) Fc-optimized anti-CD25 depletes tumor-infiltrating regulatory T cells and synergizes with PD-1 blockade to eradicate established tumors. Immunity 46:577–586. https://doi.org/10.1016/j.immuni.2017.03.013

Archilla-Ortega A, Domuro C, Martin-Liberal J, Munoz P (2022) Blockade of novel immune checkpoints and new therapeutic combinations to boost antitumor immunity. J Exp Clin Cancer Res 41:62. https://doi.org/10.1186/s13046-022-02264-x

Bagchi S, Yuan R, Engleman EG (2021) Immune checkpoint inhibitors for the treatment of cancer: clinical impact and mechanisms of response and resistance. Annu Rev Pathol 16:223–249. https://doi.org/10.1146/annurev-pathol-042020-042741

Banchereau R, Leng N, Zill O, Sokol E, Liu G, Pavlick D, Maund S, Liu LF, Kadel E 3rd, Baldwin N, Others (2021) Molecular determinants of response to PD-L1 blockade across tumor types. Nat Commun 12:3969. https://doi.org/10.1038/s41467-021-24112-w

Boudjema K, Locher C, Sabbagh C, Ortega-Deballon P, Heyd B, Bachellier P, Metairie S, Paye F, Bourlier P, Adam R, Others (2021) Simultaneous versus delayed resection for initially Resectable synchronous colorectal cancer liver metastases: a prospective, open-label, randomized, controlled trial. Ann Surg 273:49–56. https://doi.org/10.1097/SLA.0000000000003848

Buchan SL, Fallatah M, Thirdborough SM, Taraban VY, Rogel A, Thomas LJ, Penfold CA, He LZ, Curran MA, Keler T, Others (2018) PD-1 blockade and CD27 stimulation activate distinct transcriptional programs that synergize for CD8(+) T-cell-driven antitumor immunity. Clin Cancer Res 24:2383–2394. https://doi.org/10.1158/1078-0432.CCR-17-3057

Burris HA, Infante JR, Ansell SM, Nemunaitis JJ, Weiss GR, Villalobos VM, Sikic BI, Taylor MH, Northfelt DW, Carson WE 3rd, Others (2017) Safety and activity of Varlilumab, a novel and first-in-class agonist anti-CD27 antibody, in patients with advanced solid tumors. J Clin Oncol 35:2028–2036. https://doi.org/10.1200/JCO.2016.70.1508

Buzzatti G, Dellepiane C, Del Mastro L (2020) New emerging targets in cancer immunotherapy: the role of GITR. ESMO Open 4:e000738. https://doi.org/10.1136/esmoopen-2020-000738

Cabo M, Santana-Hernandez S, Costa-Garcia M, Rea A, Lozano-Rodriguez R, Ataya M, Balaguer F, Juan M, Ochoa MC, Menendez S, Others (2021) CD137 Costimulation counteracts TGFbeta inhibition of NK-cell antitumor function. Cancer Immunol Res 9:1476–1490. https://doi.org/10.1158/2326-6066.CIR-21-0030

Catenacci DV, Rosales M, Chung HC, Yoon HH, Shen L, Moehler M, Kang YK (2021) MAHOGANY: margetuximab combination in HER2+ unresectable/metastatic gastric/gastroesophageal junction adenocarcinoma. Future Oncol 17:1155–1164. https://doi.org/10.2217/fon-2020-1007

Cebada J, Perez-Santos M, Bandala C, Lara-Padilla E, Herrera-Camacho I, Rosas-Murrieta NH, Millan-Perez Pena L, Monjaraz E, Flores A, Anaya-Ruiz M (2021) OX40 agonists for cancer treatment: a patent review. Expert Opin Ther Pat 31:81–90. https://doi.org/10.1080/13543776.2021.1825688

Chan CJ, Martinet L, Gilfillan S, Souza-Fonseca-Guimaraes F, Chow MT, Town L, Ritchie DS, Colonna M, Andrews DM, Smyth MJ (2014) The receptors CD96 and CD226 oppose each other in the regulation of natural killer cell functions. Nat Immunol 15:431–438. https://doi.org/10.1038/ni.2850

Chester C, Sanmamed MF, Wang J, Melero I (2018) Immunotherapy targeting 4-1BB: mechanistic rationale, clinical results, and future strategies. Blood 131:49–57. https://doi.org/10.1182/blood-2017-06-741041

Chin SM, Kimberlin CR, Roe-Zurz Z, Zhang P, Xu A, Liao-Chan S, Sen D, Nager AR, Oakdale NS, Brown C, Others (2018) Structure of the 4-1BB/4-1BBL complex and distinct binding and functional properties of utomilumab and urelumab. Nat Commun 9:4679. https://doi.org/10.1038/s41467-018-07136-7

Choi Y, Shi Y, Haymaker CL, Naing A, Ciliberto G, Hajjar J (2020) T-cell agonists in cancer immunotherapy. J Immunother Cancer 8. https://doi.org/10.1136/jitc-2020-000966

Cohen EEW, Nabell L, Wong DJ, Day T, Daniels GA, Milhem M, Deva S, Jameson M, Guntinas-Lichius O, Almubarak M, Others (2022) Intralesional SD-101 in combination with Pembrolizumab in anti-PD-1 treatment-naive head and neck squamous cell carcinoma: results from a multicenter, phase II trial. Clin Cancer Res 28:1157–1166. https://doi.org/10.1158/1078-0432.CCR-21-1411

Cui G (2021) The mechanisms leading to distinct responses to PD-1/PD-L1 blockades in colorectal cancers with different MSI statuses. Front Oncol 11:573547. https://doi.org/10.3389/fonc.2021.573547

Demerle C, Gorvel L, Olive D (2021) BTLA-HVEM couple in health and diseases: insights for immunotherapy in lung cancer. Front Oncol 11:682007. https://doi.org/10.3389/fonc.2021.682007

Dovedi SJ, Elder MJ, Yang C, Sitnikova SI, Irving L, Hansen A, Hair J, Jones DC, Hasani S, Wang B, Others (2021) Design and efficacy of a monovalent bispecific PD-1/CTLA4 antibody that enhances CTLA4 blockade on PD-1(+) activated T cells. Cancer Discov 11:1100–1117. https://doi.org/10.1158/2159-8290.CD-20-1445

ElTanbouly MA, Zhao Y, Nowak E, Li J, Schaafsma E, Le Mercier I, Ceeraz S, Lines JL, Peng C, Carriere C, Others (2020) VISTA is a checkpoint regulator for naive T cell quiescence and peripheral tolerance. Science 367. https://doi.org/10.1126/science.aay0524

Etxeberria I, Glez-Vaz J, Teijeira A, Melero I (2020) New emerging targets in cancer immunotherapy: CD137/4-1BB costimulatory axis. ESMO Open 4:e000733. https://doi.org/10.1136/esmoopen-2020-000733

Freed-Pastor WA, Lambert LJ, Ely ZA, Pattada NB, Bhutkar A, Eng G, Mercer KL, Garcia AP, Lin L, Rideout WM 3rd, Others (2021) The CD155/TIGIT axis promotes and maintains immune evasion in neoantigen-expressing pancreatic cancer. Cancer Cell 39:1342–1360 e1314. https://doi.org/10.1016/j.ccell.2021.07.007

Fu SY, Wang CC, Chen FH, Yu CF, Hong JH, Chiang CS (2020) Sunitinib treatment-elicited distinct tumor microenvironment dramatically compensated the reduction of myeloid-derived suppressor cells. In Vivo 34:1141–1152. https://doi.org/10.21873/invivo.11886

Galon J, Bruni D (2019) Approaches to treat immune hot, altered and cold tumours with combination immunotherapies. Nat Rev Drug Discov 18:197–218. https://doi.org/10.1038/s41573-018-0007-y

Garon EB, Spira AI, Johnson M, Bazhenova L, Leach J, Cummings AL, Candia A, Coffman RL, Janatpour MJ, Janssen R, Others (2021) A phase Ib open-label, multicenter study of inhaled DV281, a TLR9 agonist, in combination with Nivolumab in patients with advanced or metastatic non-small cell lung cancer. Clin Cancer Res 27:4566–4573. https://doi.org/10.1158/1078-0432.CCR-21-0263

Ge Z, Peppelenbosch MP, Sprengers D, Kwekkeboom J (2021) TIGIT, the next step towards successful combination immune checkpoint therapy in cancer. Front Immunol 12:699895. https://doi.org/10.3389/fimmu.2021.699895

Gennery AR (2020) CD27-CD70 defects: a wolf in wolf's clothing? Blood 136:2600–2602. https://doi.org/10.1182/blood.2020007763

Ghosh S, Sharma G, Travers J, Kumar S, Choi J, Jun HT, Kehry M, Ramaswamy S, Jenkins D (2019) TSR-033, a novel therapeutic antibody targeting LAG-3, enhances T-cell function and the activity of PD-1 blockade in vitro and in vivo. Mol Cancer Ther 18:632–641. https://doi.org/10.1158/1535-7163.MCT-18-0836

Gomez-Roca CA, Italiano A, Le Tourneau C, Cassier PA, Toulmonde M, D'Angelo SP, Campone M, Weber KL, Loirat D, Cannarile MA, Others (2019) Phase I study of emactuzumab single agent or in combination with paclitaxel in patients with advanced/metastatic solid tumors reveals depletion of immunosuppressive M2-like macrophages. Ann Oncol 30:1381–1392. https://doi.org/10.1093/annonc/mdz163

Greene S, Robbins Y, Mydlarz WK, Huynh AP, Schmitt NC, Friedman J, Horn LA, Palena C, Schlom J, Maeda DY, Others (2020) Inhibition of MDSC trafficking with SX-682, a CXCR1/2 inhibitor, enhances NK-cell immunotherapy in head and neck cancer models. Clin Cancer Res 26:1420–1431. https://doi.org/10.1158/1078-0432.CCR-19-2625

Guedan S, Madar A, Casado-Medrano V, Shaw C, Wing A, Liu F, Young RM, June CH, Posey AD Jr (2020) Single residue in CD28-costimulated CAR-T cells limits long-term persistence and antitumor durability. J Clin Invest 130:3087–3097. https://doi.org/10.1172/JCI133215

Gutierrez M, Moreno V, Heinhuis KM, Olszanski AJ, Spreafico A, Ong M, Chu Q, Carvajal RD, Trigo J, Ochoa de Olza M, Others (2021) OX40 agonist BMS-986178 alone or in combination with Nivolumab and/or Ipilimumab in patients with advanced solid tumors. Clin Cancer Res 27: 460–472. https://doi.org/10.1158/1078-0432.CCR-20-1830

Han D, Xu Y, Zhao X, Mao Y, Kang Q, Wen W, Yu X, Xu L, Liu F, Zhang M, Others (2021) A novel human anti-TIGIT monoclonal antibody with excellent function in eliciting NK cell-mediated antitumor immunity. Biochem Biophys Res Commun 534:134–140. https://doi.org/10.1016/j.bbrc.2020.12.013

Hanson A, Elpek K, Duong E, Shallberg L, Fan M, Johnson C, Wallace M, Mabry GR, Sazinsky S, Pepper L, Others (2020) ICOS agonism by JTX-2011 (vopratelimab) requires initial T cell priming and Fc cross-linking for optimal T cell activation and anti-tumor immunity in preclinical models. PLoS One 15:e0239595. https://doi.org/10.1371/journal.pone.0239595

Harjunpaa H, Guillerey C (2020) TIGIT as an emerging immune checkpoint. Clin Exp Immunol 200:108–119. https://doi.org/10.1111/cei.13407

Hegde S, Leader AM, Merad M (2021) MDSC: markers, development, states, and unaddressed complexity. Immunity 54:875–884. https://doi.org/10.1016/j.immuni.2021.04.004

Heinhuis KM, Carlino M, Joerger M, Di Nicola M, Meniawy T, Rottey S, Moreno V, Gazzah A, Delord JP, Paz-Ares L, Others (2020) Safety, tolerability, and potential clinical activity of a glucocorticoid-induced TNF receptor-related protein agonist alone or in combination with Nivolumab for patients with advanced solid tumors: a phase 1/2a dose-escalation and cohort-expansion clinical trial. JAMA Oncol 6:100–107. https://doi.org/10.1001/jamaoncol.2019.3848

Hellmann MD, Bivi N, Calderon B, Shimizu T, Delafontaine B, Liu ZT, Szpurka AM, Copeland V, Hodi FS, Rottey S, Others (2021) Safety and immunogenicity of LY3415244, a bispecific antibody against TIM-3 and PD-L1, in patients with advanced solid tumors. Clin Cancer Res 27: 2773–2781. https://doi.org/10.1158/1078-0432.CCR-20-3716

Hellsten R, Lilljebjorn L, Johansson M, Leandersson K, Bjartell A (2019) The STAT3 inhibitor galiellalactone inhibits the generation of MDSC-like monocytes by prostate cancer cells and decreases immunosuppressive and tumorigenic factors. Prostate 79:1611–1621. https://doi.org/10.1002/pros.23885

Hollebecque A, Chung HC, de Miguel MJ, Italiano A, Machiels JP, Lin CC, Dhani NC, Peeters M, Moreno V, Su WC, Others (2021) Safety and antitumor activity of alpha-PD-L1 antibody as monotherapy or in combination with alpha-TIM-3 antibody in patients with microsatellite instability-high/mismatch repair-deficient tumors. Clin Cancer Res 27:6393–6404. https://doi.org/10.1158/1078-0432.CCR-21-0261

Hunig T (2016) The rise and fall of the CD28 superagonist TGN1412 and its return as TAB08: a personal account. FEBS J 283:3325–3334. https://doi.org/10.1111/febs.13754

Jayasingam SD, Citartan M, Thang TH, Mat Zin AA, Ang KC, Ch'ng ES (2019) Evaluating the polarization of tumor-associated macrophages into M1 and M2 phenotypes in human cancer tissue: technicalities and challenges in routine clinical practice. Front Oncol 9:1512. https://doi.org/10.3389/fonc.2019.01512

Jiang W, He Y, He W, Wu G, Zhou X, Sheng Q, Zhong W, Lu Y, Ding Y, Lu Q, Others (2020) Exhausted CD8+T cells in the tumor immune microenvironment: new pathways to therapy. Front Immunol 11:622509. https://doi.org/10.3389/fimmu.2020.622509

Jiang Z, Sun H, Yu J, Tian W, Song Y (2021) Targeting CD47 for cancer immunotherapy. J Hematol Oncol 14:180. https://doi.org/10.1186/s13045-021-01197-w

Johnson M, Dudek AZ, Sukari A, Call J, Kunk PR, Lewis K, Gainor JF, Sarantopoulos J, Lee P, Golden A, Others (2022) ARRY-382 in combination with Pembrolizumab in patients with advanced solid tumors: results from a phase 1b/2 study. Clin Cancer Res 28:2517–2526. https://doi.org/10.1158/1078-0432.CCR-21-3009

Johnston RJ, Su LJ, Pinckney J, Critton D, Boyer E, Krishnakumar A, Corbett M, Rankin AL, Dibella R, Campbell L, Others (2019) VISTA is an acidic pH-selective ligand for PSGL-1. Nature 574:565–570. https://doi.org/10.1038/s41586-019-1674-5

Joshi S, Liu KX, Zulcic M, Singh AR, Skola D, Glass CK, Sanders PD, Sharabi AB, Pham TV, Tamayo P, Others (2020) Macrophage Syk-PI3Kgamma inhibits antitumor immunity: SRX3207, a novel dual Syk-PI3K inhibitory Chemotype relieves tumor immunosuppression. Mol Cancer Ther 19:755–764. https://doi.org/10.1158/1535-7163.MCT-19-0947

Kallies A, Zehn D, Utzschneider DT (2020) Precursor exhausted T cells: key to successful immunotherapy? Nat Rev Immunol 20:128–136. https://doi.org/10.1038/s41577-019-0223-7

Kaneda MM, Messer KS, Ralainirina N, Li H, Leem CJ, Gorjestani S, Woo G, Nguyen AV, Figueiredo CC, Foubert P, Others (2016) PI3Kgamma is a molecular switch that controls immune suppression. Nature 539:437–442. https://doi.org/10.1038/nature19834

Kim W, Chu TH, Nienhuser H, Jiang Z, Del Portillo A, Remotti HE, White RA, Hayakawa Y, Tomita H, Fox JG, Others (2021) PD-1 signaling promotes tumor-infiltrating myeloid-derived suppressor cells and gastric tumorigenesis in mice. Gastroenterology 160:781–796. https://doi.org/10.1053/j.gastro.2020.10.036

Korman AJ, Garrett-Thomson SC, Lonberg N (2022) The foundations of immune checkpoint blockade and the ipilimumab approval decennial. Nat Rev Drug Discov 21:509–528. https://doi.org/10.1038/s41573-021-00345-8

Kraman M, Faroudi M, Allen NL, Kmiecik K, Gliddon D, Seal C, Koers A, Wydro MM, Batey S, Winnewisser J, Others (2020) FS118, a bispecific antibody targeting LAG-3 and PD-L1, enhances T-cell activation resulting in potent antitumor activity. Clin Cancer Res 26:3333–3344. https://doi.org/10.1158/1078-0432.CCR-19-3548

Kuang Z, Pu P, Wu M, Wu Z, Wang L, Li Y, Zhang S, Jing H, Wu W, Chen B, Others (2020) A novel bispecific antibody with PD-L1-assisted OX40 activation for cancer treatment. Mol Cancer Ther 19:2564–2574. https://doi.org/10.1158/1535-7163.MCT-20-0226

Kvarnhammar AM, Veitonmaki N, Hagerbrand K, Dahlman A, Smith KE, Fritzell S, von Schantz L, Thagesson M, Werchau D, Smedenfors K, Others (2019) The CTLA-4 x OX40 bispecific antibody ATOR-1015 induces anti-tumor effects through tumor-directed immune activation. J Immunother Cancer 7:103. https://doi.org/10.1186/s40425-019-0570-8

Lam KC, Goldszmid RS (2021) Can gut microbes predict efficacy and toxicity of combined immune checkpoint blockade? Cancer Cell 39:1314–1316. https://doi.org/10.1016/j.ccell.2021.09.013

Lam KC, Araya RE, Huang A, Chen Q, Di Modica M, Rodrigues RR, Lopes A, Johnson SB, Schwarz B, Bohrnsen E, Others (2021) Microbiota triggers STING-type I IFN-dependent monocyte reprogramming of the tumor microenvironment. Cell 184:5338–5356 e5321. https://doi.org/10.1016/j.cell.2021.09.019

Lan X, Li S, Gao H, Nanding A, Quan L, Yang C, Ding S, Xue Y (2017) Increased BTLA and HVEM in gastric cancer are associated with progression and poor prognosis. Onco Targets Ther 10:919–926. https://doi.org/10.2147/OTT.S128825

Larkin J, Chiarion-Sileni V, Gonzalez R, Grob JJ, Rutkowski P, Lao CD, Cowey CL, Schadendorf D, Wagstaff J, Dummer R, Others (2019) Five-year survival with combined Nivolumab and Ipilimumab in advanced melanoma. N Engl J Med 381:1535–1546. https://doi.org/10.1056/NEJMoa1910836

Lee JB, Ha SJ, Kim HR (2021a) Clinical insights into novel immune checkpoint inhibitors. Front Pharmacol 12:681320. https://doi.org/10.3389/fphar.2021.681320

Lee SJ, Yang H, Kim WR, Lee YS, Lee WS, Kong SJ, Lee HJ, Kim JH, Cheon J, Kang B, Others (2021b) STING activation normalizes the intraperitoneal vascular-immune microenvironment and suppresses peritoneal carcinomatosis of colon cancer. J Immunother Cancer 9. https://doi.org/10.1136/jitc-2020-002195

Li X, Liu R, Su X, Pan Y, Han X, Shao C, Shi Y (2019) Harnessing tumor-associated macrophages as aids for cancer immunotherapy. Mol Cancer 18:177. https://doi.org/10.1186/s12943-019-1102-3

Li C, Jiang P, Wei S, Xu X, Wang J (2020a) Regulatory T cells in tumor microenvironment: new mechanisms, potential therapeutic strategies and future prospects. Mol Cancer 19:116. https://doi.org/10.1186/s12943-020-01234-1

Li BH, Garstka MA, Li ZF (2020b) Chemokines and their receptors promoting the recruitment of myeloid-derived suppressor cells into the tumor. Mol Immunol 117:201–215. https://doi.org/10.1016/j.molimm.2019.11.014

Liu Y, Zheng P (2020) Preserving the CTLA-4 checkpoint for safer and more effective cancer immunotherapy. Trends Pharmacol Sci 41:4–12. https://doi.org/10.1016/j.tips.2019.11.003

Liu W, Chou TF, Garrett-Thomson SC, Seo GY, Fedorov E, Ramagopal UA, Bonanno JB, Wang Q, Kim K, Garforth SJ, Others (2021) HVEM structures and mutants reveal distinct functions of binding to LIGHT and BTLA/CD160. J Exp Med 218. https://doi.org/10.1084/jem.20211112

Llovet JM, Castet F, Heikenwalder M, Maini MK, Mazzaferro V, Pinato DJ, Pikarsky E, Zhu AX, Finn RS (2022) Immunotherapies for hepatocellular carcinoma. Nat Rev Clin Oncol 19:151–172. https://doi.org/10.1038/s41571-021-00573-2

Logtenberg MEW, Scheeren FA, Schumacher TN (2020) The CD47-SIRPalpha immune checkpoint. Immunity 52:742–752. https://doi.org/10.1016/j.immuni.2020.04.011

Ma Y, Li J, Wang H, Chiu Y, Kingsley CV, Fry D, Delaney SN, Wei SC, Zhang J, Maitra A, Others (2020) Combination of PD-1 inhibitor and OX40 agonist induces tumor rejection and immune memory in mouse models of pancreatic cancer. Gastroenterology 159:306–319 e312. https://doi.org/10.1053/j.gastro.2020.03.018

Magkouta SF, Vaitsi PC, Pappas AG, Iliopoulou M, Kosti CN, Psarra K, Kalomenidis IT (2021) CSF1/CSF1R Axis blockade limits mesothelioma and enhances efficiency of anti-PDL1 immunotherapy. Cancers (Basel) 13. https://doi.org/10.3390/cancers13112546

Majidpoor J, Mortezaee K (2021) The efficacy of PD-1/PD-L1 blockade in cold cancers and future perspectives. Clin Immunol 226:108707. https://doi.org/10.1016/j.clim.2021.108707

Marangoni F, Zhakyp A, Corsini M, Geels SN, Carrizosa E, Thelen M, Mani V, Prussmann JN, Warner RD, Ozga AJ, Others (2021) Expansion of tumor-associated Treg cells upon disruption of a CTLA-4-dependent feedback loop. Cell 184:3998–4015 e3919. https://doi.org/10.1016/j.cell.2021.05.027

Maruhashi T, Sugiura D, Okazaki IM, Okazaki T (2020) LAG-3: from molecular functions to clinical applications. J Immunother Cancer 8. https://doi.org/10.1136/jitc-2020-001014

Messenheimer DJ, Jensen SM, Afentoulis ME, Wegmann KW, Feng Z, Friedman DJ, Gough MJ, Urba WJ, Fox BA (2017) Timing of PD-1 blockade is critical to effective combination immunotherapy with Anti-OX40. Clin Cancer Res 23:6165–6177. https://doi.org/10.1158/1078-0432.CCR-16-2677

Mily A, Kalsum S, Loreti MG, Rekha RS, Muvva JR, Lourda M, Brighenti S (2020) Polarization of M1 and M2 human monocyte-derived cells and analysis with flow cytometry upon mycobacterium tuberculosis infection. J Vis Exp. https://doi.org/10.3791/61807

Mishra A, Sarangi SC, Reeta K (2020) First-in-human dose: current status review for better future perspectives. Eur J Clin Pharmacol 76:1237–1243. https://doi.org/10.1007/s00228-020-02924-x

Morad G, Helmink BA, Sharma P, Wargo JA (2021) Hallmarks of response, resistance, and toxicity to immune checkpoint blockade. Cell 184:5309–5337. https://doi.org/10.1016/j.cell.2021.09.020

Mota JM, Leite CA, Souza LE, Melo PH, Nascimento DC, de-Deus-Wagatsuma VM, Temporal J, Figueiredo F, Noushmehr H, Alves-Filho JC, Others (2016) Post-sepsis state induces tumor-associated macrophage accumulation through CXCR4/CXCL12 and favors tumor progression in mice. Cancer Immunol Res 4:312–322. https://doi.org/10.1158/2326-6066.CIR-15-0170

Motedayen Aval L, Pease JE, Sharma R, Pinato DJ (2020) Challenges and opportunities in the clinical development of STING agonists for cancer immunotherapy. J Clin Med 9. https://doi.org/10.3390/jcm9103323

Muik A, Altintas I, Gieseke F, Schoedel KB, Burm SM, Toker A, Salcedo TW, Verzijl D, Eisel D, Grunwitz C, Others (2022) An Fc-inert PD-L1x4-1BB bispecific antibody mediates potent anti-tumor immunity in mice by combining checkpoint inhibition and conditional 4-1BB co-stimulation. Onco Targets Ther 11:2030135. https://doi.org/10.1080/2162402X.2022.2030135

Musielak B, Kocik J, Skalniak L, Magiera-Mularz K, Sala D, Czub M, Stec M, Siedlar M, Holak TA, Plewka J (2019) CA-170 – a potent small-molecule PD-L1 inhibitor or not? Molecules 24. https://doi.org/10.3390/molecules24152804

Nakamura T, Sato T, Endo R, Sasaki S, Takahashi N, Sato Y, Hyodo M, Hayakawa Y, Harashima H (2021) STING agonist loaded lipid nanoparticles overcome anti-PD-1 resistance in melanoma lung metastasis via NK cell activation. J Immunother Cancer 9. https://doi.org/10.1136/jitc-2021-002852

Nooka AK, Weisel K, van de Donk NW, Routledge D, Otero PR, Song K, Quach H, Callander N, Minnema MC, Trudel S, Others (2021) Belantamab mafodotin in combination with novel agents in relapsed/refractory multiple myeloma: DREAMM-5 study design. Future Oncol 17: 1987–2003. https://doi.org/10.2217/fon-2020-1269

O'Connor T, Heikenwalder M (2021) CCL2 in the tumor microenvironment. Adv Exp Med Biol 1302:1–14. https://doi.org/10.1007/978-3-030-62658-7_1

O'Hara MH, Messersmith W, Kindler H, Zhang W, Pitou C, Szpurka AM, Wang D, Peng SB, Vangerow B, Khan AA, Others (2020) Safety and pharmacokinetics of CXCR4 peptide antagonist, LY2510924, in combination with Durvalumab in advanced refractory solid tumors. J Pancreat Cancer 6:21–31. https://doi.org/10.1089/pancan.2019.0018

Olson DJ, Eroglu Z, Brockstein B, Poklepovic AS, Bajaj M, Babu S, Hallmeyer S, Velasco M, Lutzky J, Higgs E, Others (2021) Pembrolizumab plus Ipilimumab following anti-PD-1/L1 failure in melanoma. J Clin Oncol 39:2647–2655. https://doi.org/10.1200/JCO.21.00079

Orillion A, Hashimoto A, Damayanti N, Shen L, Adelaiye-Ogala R, Arisa S, Chintala S, Ordentlich P, Kao C, Elzey B, Others (2017) Entinostat neutralizes myeloid-derived suppressor cells and enhances the antitumor effect of PD-1 inhibition in murine models of lung and renal cell carcinoma. Clin Cancer Res 23:5187–5201. https://doi.org/10.1158/1078-0432.CCR-17-0741

Park K, Veena MS, Shin DS (2022) Key players of the immunosuppressive tumor microenvironment and emerging therapeutic strategies. Front Cell Dev Biol 10:830208. https://doi.org/10.3389/fcell.2022.830208

Paz-Ares LG, Ramalingam SS, Ciuleanu TE, Lee JS, Urban L, Caro RB, Park K, Sakai H, Ohe Y, Nishio M, Others (2022) First-line Nivolumab plus Ipilimumab in advanced NSCLC: 4-year outcomes from the randomized, open-label, phase 3 CheckMate 227 part 1 trial. J Thorac Oncol 17:289–308. https://doi.org/10.1016/j.jtho.2021.09.010

Pedicord VA, Montalvo W, Leiner IM, Allison JP (2011) Single dose of anti-CTLA-4 enhances CD8+ T-cell memory formation, function, and maintenance. Proc Natl Acad Sci U S A 108: 266–271. https://doi.org/10.1073/pnas.1016791108

Penter L, Zhang Y, Savell A, Huang T, Cieri N, Thrash EM, Kim-Schulze S, Jhaveri A, Fu J, Ranasinghe S, Others (2021) Molecular and cellular features of CTLA-4 blockade for relapsed myeloid malignancies after transplantation. Blood 137:3212–3217. https://doi.org/10.1182/blood.2021010867

Phillips T, Barr PM, Park SI, Kolibaba K, Caimi PF, Chhabra S, Kingsley EC, Boyd T, Chen R, Carret AS, Others (2019) A phase 1 trial of SGN-CD70A in patients with CD70-positive diffuse large B cell lymphoma and mantle cell lymphoma. Investig New Drugs 37:297–306. https://doi.org/10.1007/s10637-018-0655-0

Pittet MJ, Michielin O, Migliorini D (2022) Clinical relevance of tumour-associated macrophages. Nat Rev Clin Oncol 19:402–421. https://doi.org/10.1038/s41571-022-00620-6

Rejeski K, Perez A, Sesques P, Hoster E, Berger C, Jentzsch L, Mougiakakos D, Frolich L, Ackermann J, Bucklein V, Others (2021) CAR-HEMATOTOX: a model for CAR T-cell-related hematologic toxicity in relapsed/refractory large B-cell lymphoma. Blood 138:2499–2513. https://doi.org/10.1182/blood.2020010543

Rezaei M, Tan J, Zeng C, Li Y, Ganjalikhani-Hakemi M (2021) TIM-3 in Leukemia; immune response and beyond. Front Oncol 11:753677. https://doi.org/10.3389/fonc.2021.753677

Ribas A, Medina T, Kummar S, Amin A, Kalbasi A, Drabick JJ, Barve M, Daniels GA, Wong DJ, Schmidt EV, Others (2018) SD-101 in combination with Pembrolizumab in advanced melanoma: results of a phase Ib, multicenter study. Cancer Discov 8:1250–1257. https://doi.org/10.1158/2159-8290.CD-18-0280

Ribas A, Medina T, Kirkwood JM, Zakharia Y, Gonzalez R, Davar D, Chmielowski B, Campbell KM, Bao R, Kelley H, Others (2021) Overcoming PD-1 blockade resistance with CpG-A Toll-Like eceptor 9 agonist Vidutolimod in patients with metastatic melanoma. Cancer Discov 11: 2998–3007. https://doi.org/10.1158/2159-8290.CD-21-0425

Ries CH, Cannarile MA, Hoves S, Benz J, Wartha K, Runza V, Rey-Giraud F, Pradel LP, Feuerhake F, Klaman I, Others (2014) Targeting tumor-associated macrophages with anti-CSF-1R antibody reveals a strategy for cancer therapy. Cancer Cell 25:846–859. https://doi.org/10.1016/j.ccr.2014.05.016

Rotte A, Sahasranaman S, Budha N (2021) Targeting TIGIT for immunotherapy of cancer: update on clinical development. Biomedicine 9. https://doi.org/10.3390/biomedicines9091277

Sai J, Owens P, Novitskiy SV, Hawkins OE, Vilgelm AE, Yang J, Sobolik T, Lavender N, Johnson AC, McClain C, Others (2017) PI3K inhibition reduces mammary tumor growth and facilitates antitumor immunity and anti-PD1 responses. Clin Cancer Res 23:3371–3384. https://doi.org/10.1158/1078-0432.CCR-16-2142

Sauer T, Parikh K, Sharma S, Omer B, Sedloev D, Chen Q, Angenendt L, Schliemann C, Schmitt M, Muller-Tidow C, Others (2021) CD70-specific CAR T cells have potent activity against acute myeloid leukemia without HSC toxicity. Blood 138:318–330. https://doi.org/10.1182/blood.2020008221

Scott EN, Gocher AM, Workman CJ, Vignali DAA (2021) Regulatory T cells: barriers of immune infiltration into the tumor microenvironment. Front Immunol 12:702726. https://doi.org/10.3389/fimmu.2021.702726

Segal NH, He AR, Doi T, Levy R, Bhatia S, Pishvaian MJ, Cesari R, Chen Y, Davis CB, Huang B, Others (2018) Phase I study of single-agent Utomilumab (PF-05082566), a 4-1BB/CD137 agonist, in patients with advanced cancer. Clin Cancer Res 24:1816–1823. https://doi.org/10.1158/1078-0432.CCR-17-1922

Seung E, Xing Z, Wu L, Rao E, Cortez-Retamozo V, Ospina B, Chen L, Beil C, Song Z, Zhang B, Others (2022) A trispecific antibody targeting HER2 and T cells inhibits breast cancer growth via CD4 cells. Nature 603:328–334. https://doi.org/10.1038/s41586-022-04439-0

Shi Y, Zheng W, Yang K, Harris KG, Ni K, Xue L, Lin W, Chang EB, Weichselbaum RR, Fu YX (2020) Intratumoral accumulation of gut microbiota facilitates CD47-based immunotherapy via STING signaling. J Exp Med 217. https://doi.org/10.1084/jem.20192282

Shi AP, Tang XY, Xiong YL, Zheng KF, Liu YJ, Shi XG, Lv Y, Jiang T, Ma N, Zhao JB (2021) Immune checkpoint LAG3 and its ligand FGL1 in cancer. Front Immunol 12:785091. https://doi.org/10.3389/fimmu.2021.785091

Skokos D, Waite JC, Haber L, Crawford A, Hermann A, Ullman E, Slim R, Godin S, Ajithdoss D, Ye X, Others (2020) A class of costimulatory CD28-bispecific antibodies that enhance the antitumor activity of CD3-bispecific antibodies. Sci Transl Med 12. https://doi.org/10.1126/scitranslmed.aaw7888

Solinas C, De Silva P, Bron D, Willard-Gallo K, Sangiolo D (2019) Significance of TIM3 expression in cancer: from biology to the clinic. Semin Oncol 46:372–379. https://doi.org/10.1053/j.seminoncol.2019.08.005

Solomon I, Amann M, Goubier A, Arce Vargas F, Zervas D, Qing C, Henry JY, Ghorani E, Akarca AU, Marafioti T, Others (2020) CD25-Treg-depleting antibodies preserving IL-2 signaling on effector T cells enhance effector activation and antitumor immunity. Nat Cancer 1:1153–1166. https://doi.org/10.1038/s43018-020-00133-0

Stebbings R, Poole S, Thorpe R (2009) Safety of biologics, lessons learnt from TGN1412. Curr Opin Biotechnol 20:673–677. https://doi.org/10.1016/j.copbio.2009.10.002

Sun H, Huang Q, Huang M, Wen H, Lin R, Zheng M, Qu K, Li K, Wei H, Xiao W, Others (2019a) Human CD96 correlates to natural killer cell exhaustion and predicts the prognosis of human hepatocellular carcinoma. Hepatology 70:168–183. https://doi.org/10.1002/hep.30347

Sun L, Clavijo PE, Robbins Y, Patel P, Friedman J, Greene S, Das R, Silvin C, Van Waes C, Horn LA, Others (2019b) Inhibiting myeloid-derived suppressor cell trafficking enhances T cell immunotherapy. JCI Insight 4. https://doi.org/10.1172/jci.insight.126853

Sun JM, Shen L, Shah MA, Enzinger P, Adenis A, Doi T, Kojima T, Metges JP, Li Z, Kim SB, Others (2021) Pembrolizumab plus chemotherapy versus chemotherapy alone for first-line treatment of advanced oesophageal cancer (KEYNOTE-590): a randomised, placebo-controlled, phase 3 study. Lancet 398:759–771. https://doi.org/10.1016/S0140-6736(21)01234-4

Sung H, Ferlay J, Siegel RL, Laversanne M, Soerjomataram I, Jemal A, Bray F (2021) Global cancer statistics 2020: GLOBOCAN estimates of incidence and mortality worldwide for 36 cancers in 185 countries. CA Cancer J Clin 71:209–249. https://doi.org/10.3322/caac.21660

Tawbi HA, Schadendorf D, Lipson EJ, Ascierto PA, Matamala L, Castillo Gutierrez E, Rutkowski P, Gogas HJ, Lao CD, De Menezes JJ, Others (2022) Relatlimab and Nivolumab versus Nivolumab in untreated advanced melanoma. N Engl J Med 386:24–34. https://doi.org/10.1056/NEJMoa2109970

Tian T, Li Z (2021) Targeting Tim-3 in cancer with resistance to PD-1/PD-L1 blockade. Front Oncol 11:731175. https://doi.org/10.3389/fonc.2021.731175

Treon SP, Meid K, Hunter ZR, Flynn CA, Sarosiek SR, Leventoff CR, White TP, Cao Y, Roccaro AM, Sacco A, Others (2021) Phase 1 study of ibrutinib and the CXCR4 antagonist ulocuplumab in CXCR4-mutated Waldenstrom macroglobulinemia. Blood 138:1535–1539. https://doi.org/10.1182/blood.2021012953

van de Ven K, Borst J (2015) Targeting the T-cell co-stimulatory CD27/CD70 pathway in cancer immunotherapy: rationale and potential. Immunotherapy 7:655–667. https://doi.org/10.2217/imt.15.32

Vitale LA, He LZ, Thomas LJ, Wasiuk A, O'Neill T, Widger J, Crocker A, Mills-Chen L, Forsberg E, Weidlick J, Others (2020) Development of CDX-527: a bispecific antibody combining PD-1 blockade and CD27 costimulation for cancer immunotherapy. Cancer Immunol Immunother 69:2125–2137. https://doi.org/10.1007/s00262-020-02610-y

Waite JC, Wang B, Haber L, Hermann A, Ullman E, Ye X, Dudgeon D, Slim R, Ajithdoss DK, Godin SJ, Others (2020) Tumor-targeted CD28 bispecific antibodies enhance the antitumor efficacy of PD-1 immunotherapy. Sci Transl Med 12. https://doi.org/10.1126/scitranslmed.aba2325

Wang J, Sanmamed MF, Datar I, Su TT, Ji L, Sun J, Chen L, Chen Y, Zhu G, Yin W, Others (2019) Fibrinogen-like protein 1 is a major immune inhibitory ligand of LAG-3. Cell 176:334–347 e312. https://doi.org/10.1016/j.cell.2018.11.010

Weiss SA, Djureinovic D, Jessel S, Krykbaeva I, Zhang L, Jilaveanu L, Ralabate A, Johnson B, Levit NS, Anderson G, Others (2021) A phase I study of APX005M and Cabiralizumab with or without Nivolumab in patients with melanoma, kidney cancer, or non-small cell lung cancer resistant to anti-PD-1/PD-L1. Clin Cancer Res 27:4757–4767. https://doi.org/10.1158/1078-0432.CCR-21-0903

Wolf Y, Anderson AC, Kuchroo VK (2020) TIM3 comes of age as an inhibitory receptor. Nat Rev Immunol 20:173–185. https://doi.org/10.1038/s41577-019-0224-6

Wu L, Seung E, Xu L, Rao E, Lord DM, Wei RR, Cortez-Retamozo V, Ospina B, Posternak V, Ulinski G, Others (2020) Trispecific antibodies enhance the therapeutic efficacy of tumor-directed T cells through T cell receptor co-stimulation. Nat Cancer 1:86–98. https://doi.org/10.1038/s43018-019-0004-z

Yang H, Lee WS, Kong SJ, Kim CG, Kim JH, Chang SK, Kim S, Kim G, Chon HJ, Kim C (2019) STING activation reprograms tumor vasculatures and synergizes with VEGFR2 blockade. J Clin Invest 129:4350–4364. https://doi.org/10.1172/JCI125413

Yap TA, Parkes EE, Peng W, Moyers JT, Curran MA, Tawbi HA (2021) Development of immunotherapy combination strategies in cancer. Cancer Discov 11:1368–1397. https://doi.org/10.1158/2159-8290.CD-20-1209

Yi M, Zheng X, Niu M, Zhu S, Ge H, Wu K (2022) Combination strategies with PD-1/PD-L1 blockade: current advances and future directions. Mol Cancer 21:28. https://doi.org/10.1186/s12943-021-01489-2

Ying Z, Yang H, Guo Y, Li W, Zou D, Zhou D, Wang Z, Zhang M, Wu J, Liu H, Others (2021) Relmacabtagene autoleucel (relma-cel) CD19 CAR-T therapy for adults with heavily pretreated relapsed/refractory large B-cell lymphoma in China. Cancer Med 10:999–1011. https://doi.org/10.1002/cam4.3686

Yuan L, Tatineni J, Mahoney KM, Freeman GJ (2021) VISTA: a mediator of quiescence and a promising target in cancer immunotherapy. Trends Immunol 42:209–227. https://doi.org/10.1016/j.it.2020.12.008

Zammarchi F, Havenith K, Bertelli F, Vijayakrishnan B, Chivers S, van Berkel PH (2020) CD25-targeted antibody-drug conjugate depletes regulatory T cells and eliminates established syngeneic tumors via antitumor immunity. J Immunother Cancer 8. https://doi.org/10.1136/jitc-2020-000860

Zappasodi R, Sirard C, Li Y, Budhu S, Abu-Akeel M, Liu C, Yang X, Zhong H, Newman W, Qi J, Others (2019) Rational design of anti-GITR-based combination immunotherapy. Nat Med 25:759–766. https://doi.org/10.1038/s41591-019-0420-8

Zhang W, Huang Q, Xiao W, Zhao Y, Pi J, Xu H, Zhao H, Xu J, Evans CE, Jin H (2020) Advances in anti-tumor treatments targeting the CD47/SIRPalpha Axis. Front Immunol 11:18. https://doi.org/10.3389/fimmu.2020.00018

Zhang A, Ren Z, Tseng KF, Liu X, Li H, Lu C, Cai Y, Minna JD, Fu YX (2021a) Dual targeting of CTLA-4 and CD47 on T_{reg} cells promotes immunity against solid tumors. Sci Transl Med 13. https://doi.org/10.1126/scitranslmed.abg8693

Zhang H, Li F, Cao J, Wang X, Cheng H, Qi K, Wang G, Xu K, Zheng J, Fu YX, Others (2021b) A chimeric antigen receptor with antigen-independent OX40 signaling mediates potent antitumor activity. Sci Transl Med 13. https://doi.org/10.1126/scitranslmed.aba7308

Zhao X, Subramanian S (2017) Intrinsic resistance of solid tumors to immune checkpoint blockade therapy. Cancer Res 77:817–822. https://doi.org/10.1158/0008-5472.CAN-16-2379

Tumor-infiltrating Lymphocytes as Markers of the Antitumor Therapy Efficacy: Myth or Reality?

Mikhail V. Kiselevskiy, Tatiana N. Zabotina, Elena V. Artamonova, A. N. Kozlov, Igor V. Samoylenko, Zaira G. Kadagidze, and Irina Zh. Shubina

Abstract

Tumor-infiltrating lymphocytes (TIL) are an important prognostic factor of the antitumor therapy effectiveness and the course of the malignant disease. Clinical and epidemiological studies have demonstrated that the presence and quantification of TILs correlates with relapse-free and overall survival. However, other studies report the contrasting data that cannot confirm the prognostic significance of TILs. Such contradictions are primarily associated with various methodological approaches for the evaluation of qualitative and quantitative TIL content. This chapter discusses the results of clinical studies and meta-analyses considering the prognostic value of TILs in different tumor types and presents a comparative analysis of various methods for TIL assessment.

The conventional histological methods with a semi-quantitative assessment of stromal TILs provide an opportunity for splitting patients into groups of high and low TIL levels. This method is largely subjective and depends on the selected fields of vision and the pathologist's experience. In addition, this approach allows only a qualitative or semi-quantitative assessment of infiltrates. Immunohistochemistry provides a more accurate identification of lymphocytes and their subpopulations, though lymphocyte number count is still subjective and laborious. Multiparameter flow cytometry is a promising approach to increase the objectivity and accuracy of TIL assessment with an advantage of quantitative analysis and detection of different lymphocyte subsets.

M. V. Kiselevskiy · T. N. Zabotina · E. V. Artamonova · A. N. Kozlov · I. V. Samoylenko · Z. G. Kadagidze · I. Zh. Shubina (✉)
N.N. Blokhin National Medical Research Center of Oncology, Ministry of Health of Russia, Moscow, Russia
e-mail: irinashubina@mail.ru

Interdisciplinary Cancer Research, https://doi.org/10.1007/16833_2022_59
Published online: 5 October 2022

The TIL numbers, their subsets, and localization in the stroma or parenchyma may have prognostic value in certain tumor types. Histological, immunohistochemical examinations and multiparameter flow cytometry analysis provide relevant data for tumor immunoprofiling.

Keywords

Immunotherapy · Prognostic biomarkers · Tumor-infiltrating lymphocytes

1 Introduction

The immune system plays the central role in the control of malignant neoplasms. Tumor-infiltrating lymphocytes (TILs) are a population of immune cells that have a greater immunological activity against tumor cells compared to circulating lymphocytes. Thus, the tumor lymphocyte infiltration and the content of lymphocyte subpopulations are considered as prognostic biomarkers for a number of malignant neoplasms, including breast cancer, head and neck cancer, melanoma, colorectal cancer, non-small cell lung cancer, malignant pleural mesothelioma, and esophageal cancer. Recently, morphological analysis of tumor-infiltrating lymphocytes has been regarded as an important prognostic marker of the therapy effectiveness and overall survival for cancer patients (Dieci et al. 2018). The data accumulated as a result of clinical studies indicate the prognostic significance of the TIL content for the effectiveness of neoadjuvant and adjuvant chemotherapy (Denkert et al. 2015; Liu et al. 2022; Orhan et al. 2022). These data support the suggestion that clinical response to the antitumor therapy of a number of malignancies depends on the TIL infiltration. Some authors propose to evaluate the TIL content along with the standard histological analysis (Park et al. 2019; Chen et al. 2019). Although TIL evaluation has not been yet included in the standard histopathological study, immunohistochemical (IHC) analysis was used to estimate the TIL infiltration density and specific subsets of lymphocytes. CD3+, CD4+, CD8+, and FOXP3+ TILs are reported to be among the most frequently assessed markers (Idos et al. 2020). Higher numbers of CD3+, CD4+, and CD8+TILs in the tumor microenvironment show an active antitumor immune reaction. In contrast, high levels of FOXP3+TIL were associated with immunosuppressive tumor microenvironment (McCoy et al. 2017). Revealing TIL infiltration, in particular CD8+T cells, in tumor tissue prior to treatment correlates with improved survival of patients with various types of gastrointestinal cancers, including stomach cancer, hepatocellular carcinoma, and pancreatic cancer (Lee et al. 2018; Ding et al. 2018; Orhan et al. 2020).

TILs include T- and B-cells, natural killers that moved from circulation and settled in the stroma or parenchyma of the tumor. The studies have found that CD8+ or CD4+T lymphocytes can recognize tumor antigens or overexpressed tumor-associated antigens and cause tumor regression.

Therefore, the importance of evaluation of immune infiltration in tumors is increasing when optimal biomarkers are needed to select patients with the highest probability of responding to up-to-date chemo- or immunotherapy and prognosis for the course of the disease. However, the accuracy and complexity of the techniques for TIL assessment vary in different research and in different types of tumors. TILs in the tumor and surrounding microenvironment show the current antitumor immune response of the organism. Three main categories of tumor microenvironment (TME) were identified for different types of tumors: immune-desolate ("cold" tumors with lack of lymphocytes), immune-devoid (lymphocytes are found in the peritumoral stroma only), and immune-infiltrated/inflammatory ("hot" tumors) (Chen and Mellman 2017).

The development of prognostic biomarker profiles in oncology requires a careful evaluation of the analytical reliability and clinical value of the tests. The researchers accumulate the data that support the benefit of TIL assessment as a prognostic biomarker in various solid tumors, and, currently, various techniques for TIL evaluation are used along with routine histological methods. Though semi-quantitative tests on the base of standard histological examination were recommended by the International Working Group on Immuno-Oncological Biomarkers for TIL evaluation, they have low accuracy and reproducibility. Immunohistochemical methods are quite labor-consuming and depend on the subjective evaluation determined by the pathologist's qualification, the selected fields for analysis, and the number of serial biopsy sections. The clinical validity of the TIL assessment requires implementation of a standardized and reproducible method. As such method, flow cytometry may complement histological tests and give an accurate quantitative assessment of the lymphocyte numbers and their subpopulations.

TILs may be regarded as potential biomarkers for the prognosis of the course of disease and the treatment effectiveness for cancer. In 1931 McCarfy et al. (1931) suggested that TILs represented manifestation of the immune system antitumor activity. In the late 1990s, a number of studies showed that the infiltration of tumors by immune inflammatory cells corresponded to tumor progression. Later, the dual role of TILs in the tumor microenvironment was demonstrated for cancer progression. TILs may not only suppress tumor growth by destroying transformed cells, or inhibiting their proliferation, but also contribute to the tumor progression by selecting immune-resistant clones or by modulating the microenvironment that promotes tumor growth (Schreiber et al. 2011). TILs are a heterogeneous population consisting mainly of T-lymphocytes and, to a lesser extent, B-lymphocytes and natural killer cells (NKs). The content of TIL subpopulations is essential due to their various physiological and pathological effects in the tumor microenvironment. The progress of immunohistochemistry has led to extensive studies of different TIL subtypes. Thus, CD3, a biomarker of T-lymphocytes, is expressed on almost all T-lymphocytes. Major T-lymphocyte subsets include the following subtypes: CD8+ cytotoxic T-lymphocytes (CTL), CD4+ T-helper lymphocytes (Th), CD45RO+ memory T cells (Tm), and FOXP3+ regulatory cells (T-reg). The correlation between TIL content and clinical outcome has been studied in different neoplasms, such as lung cancer (Al-Shibli et al. 2008), colorectal cancer (Mlecnik et al. 2011), breast cancer (Mahmoud et al. 2011), melanoma (Mackensen et al. 1993), ovarian cancer (Zhang et al. 2003), pancreatic cancer (Fukunaga et al. 2004), etc. Some reports regarded TILs as a more significant prognostic factor for patient survival than the TNM classification. However, the predictive value of TILs in a number of tumor types remains controversial.

Kawai et al. reported that only CD8+T cells infiltrating tumor nests, but not those of the tumor stroma, are associated with longer overall survival (Kawai et al. 2008). Goc et al. showed that both types of CD8+ T cells had prognostic value for patients with lung cancer (Goc et al. 2014). The same contradictory results were obtained for the CD3+T cell predictive role (Kayser et al. 2012). Most comparative studies with CD8+ and CD3+T cells showed the contradictory effects of regulatory Foxp3+T cells for the prognosis of the course of the disease (Suzuki et al. 2013).

2 TILs as Prognostic Markers of the Therapy Effectiveness and the Course of Malignant Disease

The International TILs Working Group (The Working Group) developed a consensus on TIL evaluation (Salgado et al. 2015). The Working Group made recommendations on the standardization of TIL assessment summarized in Table 1.

The TIL content in the stroma is defined as the percentage of stromal TIL. The denominator for determining the percentage of the stromal TILs is the area of stromal tissue (i.e., the area occupied by the inflammatory mononuclear cells across the intratumoral stromal site), but not the number of stromal cells. Most pathologists seldom report the exact TIL numbers; they rather present the approximate data in their everyday practice. The percentage of stromal TILs is a semi-quantitative parameter. For instance, 80% of stromal TILs mean that 80% of the stromal site is occupied by a dense mononuclear infiltrate. Lymphocytes usually do not form dense cell clusters, so the statement of "100% stromal TILs" still has some loose tissue between single lymphocytes. At this stage, no formal recommendations exist regarding a clinically significant threshold of TIL content. The consensus for clinical recommendations suggests that the current methodology is more important than the discussion of thresholds which will be determined after a robust methodology is established. The definition of lymphocyte-predominant breast cancer can be used as a descriptive term for tumors that include "more lymphocytes than tumor cells." However, the threshold ranges from 50% to 60% of stromal lymphocytes.

Table 1 Recommendations for TIL evaluation in breast cancer

TILs should be evaluated within the boundaries of the invasive tumor
TILs should be excluded beyond the tumor border and around DCIS (ductal carcinoma in situ) and normal lobules
TILs should be excluded in tumor zones with artifacts (crushing, necrosis, regressive hyalinization)
All mononuclear cells (including lymphocytes and plasma cells) should be analyzed, but polymorphonuclear leukocytes should be excluded
One section of 4–5 μm is sufficient per patient with magnification ×200–400

3 Methodological Approaches to TIL Evaluation

The magnification of the microscope hardly has any importance, though ×200–400 is usually recommended (10 × 20; 10 × 40). The section thickness is not critical, the standard thickness of 4–5 μm is considered optimal. Most of the existing experiments are based on the analysis of preparations obtained from paraffin blocks, while the evaluation of TILs on cryosections is not well studied and cannot be recommended for routine use. TILs can be evaluated using core biopsies in the neoadjuvant mode, as well as surgical samples in the adjuvant mode. Taking into account the above-mentioned, it is sufficient to analyze one block for a patient for neoadjuvant and adjuvant modes. In some studies the prognostic or predictive values of TILs were evaluated, but additional studies are needed before making recommendations on the standard methodology for assessing TIL after neoadjuvant treatment (Dieci et al. 2014).

Initially, tissue microarrays (TMs) were not recommended for the TIL evaluation because little evidence was reported about the capacity of TMs to assess the potential TIL heterogeneity. However, the recently published results obtained with TMs are consistent with other immunohistochemical methods studying TIL subtypes, but not with hematoxylin-eosin TIL staining (Schalper et al. 2014). Further research should finally define the technical details of the methodology.

The section analysis should include all mononuclear cells, including lymphocytes and plasmocytes, while granulocytes and other polymorphonuclear leukocytes should be excluded from the count. Quantitative count of other mononuclear cells, such as dendritic cells and macrophages, is currently not recommended, although there is increasing evidence that they may have functional potential.

Immunohistochemistry has been used to assess the clinical significance of lymphocyte subtypes such as CD45, CD8, CD3, etc. However, although immunohistochemistry can improve the assessment accuracy, the value of these markers is currently unclear. The TIL Working Group has no recommendations for the use of immunohistochemistry to detect specific subpopulations until additional evidence is available.

PCR diagnostics of TILs may improve the count accuracy of lymphocyte subpopulations achieved by simple morphology. However, the effectiveness of this approach has not been confirmed, yet. Researchers continue developing other methods, such as CyTOF (Bendall et al. 2011), which should gain formal approval.

4 The Concept of Stromal and Intratumoral TILs

Initial studies evaluated stromal and intratumoral lymphocytes separately. Intratumoral TILs (iTIL) are defined as lymphocytes in tumor nests that have direct intercellular contacts with no intermediate stroma and interact directly with tumor cells, whereas stromal TILs (sTILs) are located in the stroma amid tumor cells and have no direct contact with the latter. Since both TIL variants are localized in the tumor tissue, it should be emphasized that both categories represent true TILs. In addition, since TILs can move within the live tumor microenvironment, the difference may be somewhat unnatural, and such definition is associated with the static histological preparations that are used for diagnostic evaluation. The initial hypothesis was that lymphocytes directly interacting with tumor cells may be more relevant and therefore more useful for diagnostic evaluation. Although this hypothesis may still be biologically and/or clinically relevant for diagnostic purposes, recent studies have found that sTILs are a good and more reproducible parameter in hematoxylin-eosin stained slides. The main explanation is that iTILs usually present in smaller numbers, less frequently detected, more heterogeneous, and difficult to observe on hematoxylin-eosin stained slides (i.e., without immunohistochemistry or immunofluorescence).

Counting iTIL does not add to the information received with sTILs, since they usually present in parallel. However, focusing on the stromal component (but not on the tumor as a whole) has a clear advantage, because the density and growth pattern of the carcinoma nests do not affect the TIL count, since sTILs are estimated only in the sites between the carcinoma nests. Nevertheless, recent studies have shown that both stromal and iTILs are factors in predicting the pathomorphological response to neoadjuvant chemotherapy with platinum-based drugs (Vinayak et al. 2014).

On the other hand, some studies found no connection between TILs and improved outcome; moreover, they reported the opposite effect (Mao et al. 2016).

Immunohistochemistry determining intratumoral CD3+ or CD8+TILs can potentially be used to detect sTILs. However, the current recommendations focus on evaluating sTILs as the main parameter. Additional parameters, including TILs in the peri-tumoral area, TILs in the invasive margin, or iTILs may be included in the analysis, though more data should be provided for their potential clinical significance. The TIL calculation technique described by Denkart et al. in 2010 was used in most of the subsequently published studies, thereby sufficient data were provided for the initial stage of designing a unique methodology. Pathologists who used that approach were discussing different aspects of the method since 2010 and slightly changed the original version. The alternative assessment of TILs does not abolish the previously published results based on other methods of TIL evaluation, but provides a basis for future standardization. According to Denkart's recommendations, sTILs should be evaluated as a percentage of stromal areas, while the areas with tumor cells should not be included in the total estimated surface area (Denkert et al. 2010). That is an important notice, otherwise the size of the epithelial cell nests, as well as the pattern of tumor growth, can affect the sTIL assessment. For example, an estimate of 50% sTILs means that 50% of the stromal surface area is occupied by TILs.

5 Clinical Studies of the TIL Prognostic Significance

The retrospective studies initiated by the German Breast Group evaluated the prognostic role of TILs using hematoxylin-eosin stained slides that were prepared as part of translational studies. The number of sTILs was determined in the core-biopsy samples obtained before the start of the neoadjuvant chemotherapy. TILs were evaluated using the guidelines of the International Working Group for TILs (Salgado et al. 2015). Stromal TILs were estimated as the percentage of immune cells in the stroma of the tumor tissue, which were regarded as a mononuclear immunological infiltrate. In addition, three categories of infiltration were determined: low (TILs – 0–10%), intermediate (TILs – 11–59%), and high (TILs – 60–100%). The number of iTILs correlated with the number of stromal TILs, though iTIL concentrations were lower.

6 TILs and Breast Cancer

The most number of clinical studies that evaluated the prognostic significance of TILs were performed in breast cancer (BC). The molecular subtype of this tumor has a great effect on its interaction with the immune system. Triple-negative breast cancer (TNBC) and HER2-positive (HER2+) breast cancer are more often infiltrated by more lymphocytes than hormone (HR)-positive tumors (Denkert et al. 2018). However, all subtypes of breast cancer may present cases with TIL infiltration. Some authors suggested that the grade of TIL infiltration reflects the tumor mutation burden, which is lower in HR-positive tumors (Hammerl et al. 2018). Immune infiltrates in early HER2-positive and triple-negative breast cancers are detected in up to 75% of tumors, and a particularly dense infiltrate and smaller TIL numbers in luminal subtypes are found in up to 20% of tumors.

Morphological evaluation of TILs in breast cancer is widely introduced into clinical practice. The data of several studies show that TIL density is a prognostic factor of response to neoadjuvant chemotherapy and in patients with certain subtypes of breast cancer receiving adjuvant chemotherapy. The response to treatment and the BC outcome correlate with different TIL levels. Therefore, the assessment of TIL density in clinical trials, as well as in routine histopathological practice, may be of ultimate importance (Dieci et al. 2018).

The meta-analysis was based on six clinical trials which involved 9125 patients. Core biopsy for TIL evaluation was performed in 3771 patients with primary breast cancer prior to the start of therapy, 1366 (37%) of them had HER2-negative tumors (HER2–), 906 (25%) had triple-negative tumors, and 1379 (38%) were HER2-positive (HER2+), 1677 (44%) patients had a low TIL content in tumors, 1369 (36%) had an average TIL content, and 725 (19%) patients had high TIL concentrations. The percentage of tumors with high TIL concentrations was registered more often in patients with TNBC, 273 (30%) of 906 patients and in patients with HER2+ BC, 262 (19%) of 1379, than in patients with HER2– tumors, 172 (13%) of 1 366 patients. The increased TIL concentration was a predictor of the response to neoadjuvant chemotherapy: the complete response was achieved in 328 (20%) of 1677 patients with tumors with a low TIL content, in 369 (27%) of 1369 patients with tumors with an intermediate TIL content, and in 317 (44%) of 725 patients with tumors with a high TIL content. The increasing TIL concentrations correlated with the complete response in all subtypes of breast cancer in case if TILs were evaluated as a categorical or continuous parameter. In patients with the luminal

HER2-negative subtype, the complete response was achieved in 45 (6%) of 759 patients with low TIL level, in 48 (11%) of 435 patients with intermediate TILs, and in 49 (28%) of 172 patients with high TIL level. In patients with HER2+ subtype. The complete response was achieved in 194 (32%) of 605 patients with low TILs, in 198 (39%) of 512 patients with intermediate TILs, and in 127 (48%) of 262 with high TILs. The complete response was achieved in 80 (31%) of 260 patients with low TIL levels, 117 (31%) of 373 patients with intermediate TIL levels, and 136 (50%) of 273 patients with high TIL levels. The authors' regression analysis of the tumor lymphocyte infiltration and the complete response in the TNBC, HER2+ breast cancer, and luminal-HER2– breast cancer showed that the association between immunological infiltrates and the response to chemotherapy was similar in the studied categories, and did not depend on the breast cancer subtype (Denkert et al. 2018).

Another study evaluated TILs as a prognostic marker for relapse-free breast cancer and overall survival in 2570 patients in five sets of clinical trials (Von Minckwitz et al. 2014). The average follow-up for overall survival was 62.8 months, and the median follow-up for relapse-free survival was 63.3 months. The data showed that patients with TNBC and high TIL concentrations had significantly longer relapse-free and overall survival than patients with TNBC and low TIL concentrations. High TIL concentrations in patients with HER2+ BC correlated with a longer relapse-free period, compared with patients with HER2+ BC and low TIL concentrations. However, there was no statistically significant difference in overall survival in these two subgroups. In contrast, TIL concentrations in patients with luminal HER2– BC were not significantly associated with relapse-free survival, and low TIL concentrations correlated with longer overall survival than high TIL concentrations. Univariate and multivariate analysis showed that the relationship between TIL concentration and survival was similar in all subtypes of breast cancer. However, when complete response was included in the multivariate analysis, TIL concentrations were no longer significantly associated with relapse-free survival in all patients or with overall survival in patients with TNBC and with HER2+BC. The survival analysis using the Kaplan-Meyer model, which included 986 patients with HER2+BC and 832 patients with luminal HER2– BC, showed that high TIL concentrations were a positive prognostic factor for relapse-free survival in the TNBC and HER2+ subgroup. On the contrary, low TIL concentrations in the luminal HER2– BC subgroup were a positive prognostic factor for relapse-free survival. Overall survival also did not depend on the rate of the tumor lymphocyte infiltration. The complete response in the TNBC and luminal HER2– BC subgroups correlated with good prognosis regardless of the TIL concentrations. Patients with TNBC with no complete response had similar prognosis in all three TIL categories; in contrast, patients with luminal HER2– BC with no complete response had better prognosis with low TIL levels than with high or intermediate TIL concentrations. An additional "post-hoc" analysis of survival based on molecular subtypes and clinical and pathological parameters showed that high TIL concentrations were associated with a longer period of relapse-free and overall survival than low TIL levels in TNBC and HER2+ BC. On the contrary, in patients with luminal HER2– BC the results were ambiguous for both relapse-free and overall survival. Regarding TNBC, the presence of most types of immune cells, including various T-cell subsets, natural killer cells, B cells, monocytes, and dendritic cells, significantly correlated with good prognosis for overall survival. Conversely, in luminal HER2– BC, most T-cell markers were not associated with overall survival; and although dendritic myeloid cells and B cells correlated with a better prognosis, the presence of monocytes or macrophages was associated with poor prognosis for overall survival. Thus, the prognostic significance of TILs may essentially depend on particular TIL subpopulations and, accordingly, the antitumor immune response.

The joint analysis of six randomized trials of neoadjuvant chemotherapy (NACT) in patients with breast cancer found that TIL concentrations in all BC subtypes had a high correlation with complete response to the NACT, but the association of the TIL content and relapse-free and overall survival was different in patients with HER2+ BC or TNBC (positive correlation for both BC subtypes) and luminal HER2– BC (negative correlation).

Regression analysis showed an increase of the odds ratio for complete response with every 10% increase of TIL concentration. The authors of the study (Von Minckwitz et al. 2014) focused on sTILs, because it was the dominating localization in breast cancer. The amount of iTILs correlates with the amount of sTILs, but usually iTILs are found at a much lower density, and therefore are less suitable as a predictive biomarker.

Although the connection of TILs and the response to neoadjuvant chemotherapy was similar in BC subtypes, significant differences of the survival endpoints were noted across the subtypes. Thus, the increased TIL numbers in TNBC and HER2+ BC were associated with a longer relapse-free survival than low TIL numbers; in addition, the increased TILs in TNBC were associated with the increased overall survival. Taking into account the basic parameters, the multivariate analysis showed the significant prognostic role of TILs in these BC subtypes.

TILs in luminal HER2– tumors had no prognostic significance for relapse-free survival. Interestingly, a better prognosis for overall survival was associated with low TIL concentrations in this BC subtype. Thus, the effect of TILs on overall survival had the opposite effect in luminal tumors compared to TNBC and HER2+ BC.

The different effect of TILs on survival in patients with TNBC and luminal BC is unlikely to result from the differences of the response to chemotherapy, since the complete response rates increased with the increase of TIL concentrations in all subtypes.

The differences between luminal tumors and TNBC might be related to different types of infiltrating immune cells. The immune cell subtypes in TNBC associated with improved survival included B cells, T cells, and macrophages. In contrast, the presence of T cells in luminal-HER2– BC was not prognostically significant for survival, and the only cell types associated with an improved prognosis were B cells and myeloid dendritic cells, although macrophages in the tumor were associated with the decreased survival. These findings show differences of the cell subsets and prognostic effect of immune cells in TNBC compared to luminal HER2– BC.

The study report (Iglesia et al. 2016) presented various approaches to the analysis of immune cell phenotypes in malignant tumor datasets. MCP counter is used to make the TIL count automatic, which measures the absolute content of immune cell subtypes, and it can be used to analyze tumors with a low number of immune cells, such as breast cancer. The CIBERSORT method (Gentles et al. 2015) focused on the relative quantification of the immune cell subtypes and was less suitable for tumors with a low TIL content. However, other studies by CIBERSORT identified a number of different subpopulations of immune cells in breast cancer (Bense et al. 2016).

Over the recent decades, the studies have demonstrated the relationship between certain subpopulations of immune cells and clinical response in patients with various solid tumors (Galon et al. 2013). In addition, the data have presented the evidence that adaptive immunity mediated by T- and B-lymphocytes is extensively involved in the tumor growth control (Liu et al. 2014). Seo et al. found that marked tumor infiltration with cytotoxic CD8+T cells in breast cancer patients correlated with overall survival (Seo et al. 2013) and response to chemotherapy (West et al. 2013). The subpopulation of CD4+ regulatory T cells (Treg) was associated with both good response and no response (Gu-Trantien et al. 2013). Another subset of CD4+T cells, Th1 lymphocytes (the main cell source of interferon-γ) were associated with favorable clinical outcomes, whereas Th2 cells were associated with tumor progression (Teschendorff et al. 2010). Follicular CD4+T helpers were positively associated with the outcome of both adjuvant and neoadjuvant therapy (Denkert et al. 2010). Th17 cells producing pro-inflammatory cytokines of the IL-17 family seem to have ambiguous prognostic significance (Qi et al. 2013). The exact role of B cells infiltrating the tumor is still unclear (Mahmoud et al. 2012).

Cytotoxic therapies, such as chemo- and radiation therapy, can sometimes act as triggers of the immune system, initiating an antitumor immune response to a wider range of antigens, which may determine the control over a heterogeneous cell population in primary tumors and emerging metastases (2014). This hypothesis is supported by the studies showing that the rate of lymphocyte infiltration may predict the response to neoadjuvant therapy, relapse-free, and overall survival (Loi et al. 2013).

7 TILs and Lung Cancer

The prognostic value of TILs in lung cancer is still controversial and depends on the cell localization and cell types. A meta-analysis of 29 studies and 8,600 lung cancer (LC) patients confirmed that high TIL density was associated with favorable relapse-free rather than overall survival (Geng et al. 2015). The analysis of the LC patients included subpopulations of sTILs with CD8+, CD3+, CD4+, and FOXP3+T cells and showed better overall survival in patients with high levels of infiltration of both stromal and intratumoral CD8+T cells. At the same time, similar to breast cancer, sTILs had a greater prognostic value. However, the high infiltration density of FOXP3+T cells can be considered a negative prognostic factor. These results were interpreted as follows: different TIL subtypes and their localizations are associated with the outcome of the disease, but the assessment of the TIL population as a whole did not show significant differences in survival. A high infiltration level of CD8+ and CD3+T cells in the tumors of patients with RL is regarded as a positive prognosis, whereas a high density of FOXP3+T cell infiltration can be admitted as a negative prognostic factor (Geng et al. 2015).

A recent retrospective study involving 1,191 patients with resected lung adenocarcinoma and squamous cell carcinoma performed histological evaluation on the basis of the criteria proposed by the International Immuno-Oncology Biomarkers Working Group. The study results revealed no reliable prognostic significance of TILs for the patient outcome (Mlika et al. 2022). Analyzing the prognostic significance of the TIL subset content, the authors showed that high CD8+ expression significantly correlated with an increase in relapse-free survival, while CD4+ expression had no significant correlation with overall and relapse-free survival (Yan and Jiao 2015). More prospective multicenter studies with a large number of samples are necessary to reveal the most appropriate TIL content for RL prognosis outcomes.

8 TILs and Colorectal Cancer

Some studies suggested that TILs such as CD8+ and FoxP3+ T cells may be associated with the prognosis of treatment for colorectal cancer. In particular, TIL connection with the effectiveness of preoperative radiation therapy and survival was studied in 237 patients with locally advanced rectal cancer. The density of TIL (CD8+ and FoxP3+) in the intraepithelial and stromal compartments was evaluated in surgical samples and biopsies. The primary endpoint was to assess the effect of tumor or tumor node lymphocyte infiltration after preoperative radiation therapy on progression-free survival and overall survival. Secondary endpoints were the effect of the radiation therapy dose fractionation scheme on TIL. The single-variate analysis found that a high level of FOXP3+ TIL density after radiation therapy significantly correlated with better progression-free survival ($p = 0.007$). Multivariate analysis showed that a decrease of CD8+/FOXP3+ iTIL ratio after radiation therapy correlated with better relapse-free and overall survival ($p = 0.049$ and $p = 0.024$, respectively). The dose fractioning scheme significantly affected the CD8+/FOXP3+ ratio after treatment. On the base of the obtained data, the authors made a conclusion that patients with a significant decrease of the CD8+/FOXP3+ ratio after radiation therapy had a higher overall survival.

An assessment system Immunoscore was designed to assess the TIL content, and it passed international validation as a prognostic tool for colon cancer (Mlecnik et al. 2020). Immunoscore classifies patients as low, medium, or high, according to the density of CD8+ and CD3+T cells and their number in the center and on the edge of the tumor. The international validation studies of the Immunoscore in colon cancer have shown that this method allows a reliable assessment of recurrence in patients with colon cancer and it was superior to some other commonly assessed parameters, such as histopathological differentiation, microsatellite instability status (MSI), vascular and perineural invasion (Mlecnik et al. 2020).

9 TILs and Ovarian Cancer

So far, numerous data have been accumulated demonstrating that ovarian cancer (OC) is an immunogenic malignancy that can be identified by the immune system. Therefore, over the recent years, numerous studies have been completed to detect and characterize TILS in ovarian cancer (Benedet et al. 2000). A number of papers were published evaluating the prognostic value of TILs for OC outcome. Zhang et al. analyzed 186 tumor samples of patients with advanced OC and found that intratumoral CD3+ TILs corresponded to a better survival (Zhang et al. 2003).

However, Sato et al. failed to record survival benefits in patients with CD3+ TIL. The authors demonstrated that the only subtype associated with favorable prognosis was intraepithelial CD8+ TILs (Sato et al. 2005).

The discrepancy in the results shows that the prognostic value of TIL in OC remains controversial. Li et al. analyzed 21 clinical studies of the TIL prognostic significance involving 2,903 patients with OC (Li et al. 2017). The authors evaluated the prognostic significance of various TIL subtypes. The analysis found that high density of intraepithelial CD3+, CD8+, or CD103+ TILs indicated better survival, but solely FOXP3+ TILs (Treg) and the ratio of CD8+/FOXP3+ or CD8+/CD4+ was not associated with the prognosis.

Evaluation of the prognostic role of FOXP3+TILs in different studies showed ambiguous results. Thus, some studies showed that Treg infiltration was associated with a decrease of overall survival in patients with OC, while other authors did not find such an association (Vermeij et al. 2011) or established a positive effect of Treg infiltration on the survival of patients with OC (Leffers et al. 2009).

These discrepancies can be partly explained by differences in the studied populations, the method of processing, and histological studies of tumor samples. Besides, the choice of different Treg markers in each study may also contribute to the inconsistency of the results. The reason is that FOXP3 expression in Treg cells can be unstable, and lymphocyte differentiation is characterized by a high degree of plasticity (Zhou et al. 2009).

A recent retrospective study involving 119 patients (63 with endometrioid and 56 with clear cell ovarian carcinomas) assessed the association of patient survival with both systemic ratio of neutrophils to lymphocytes or the presence of endometriosis, and CD3+ and CD8+ TILs (Gallego et al. 2022).

The analysis showed that medium and high levels of intraepithelial CD8+ TILs were associated with longer survival in patients with endometrioid ovarian cancer. While intraepithelial CD3+ and CD8+ TILs were established as prognostic biomarkers for better clinical outcome, systemic immune markers had no prognostic significance. The patients with endometrioid clear cell ovarian cancer with moderate to high levels of CD8+ and CD3+ intraepithelial TILs had a higher overall survival. On the contrary, systemic inflammation, evaluated according to the ratio of neutrophils to lymphocytes or endometriosis, had no prognostic significance in these histological subtypes (Gallego et al. 2022).

Thus, TILs have prognostic significance in patients with OC that is determined by the content of various TIL subtypes. It should be noted that more than 1,200 experimental and clinical studies, as well as review articles and comments have been published to date, but the clinical significance of TILs as a prognostic factor has yet to be definitely assessed, and well-planned randomized controlled trials are needed to confirm these findings.

10 TILs for Prognosis of Head and Neck Cancer

The study involving 182 patients with oropharyngeal cancer showed that TILs were a simple and promising prognostic method for patient's survival (Almangush et al. 2022). The analysis of TIL subpopulations demonstrated that high CD3+ TIL level correlated with favorable prognosis for both HPV-negative and HPV-positive head and neck cancer. Such result is consistent with the hypothesis that immune cells in the tumor microenvironment play an important role in clinical outcomes, and this is also consistent with the results in other cancers (Gooden et al. 2011).

The studies of TILs in squamous cell carcinoma of head and neck mainly evaluated the prognostic significance of CD8+ TILs. The authors assumed that CD8+, a marker of cytotoxic T lymphocytes that directly target tumor cells, was a more reliable biomarker than CD3. Indeed, a number of studies that evaluated CD8+ TILs for disease prognosis showed that the best result was achieved in patients with high infiltration of CD8+ T cells in tumors (de Ruiter et al. 2017).

Meta-analysis also showed that high CD4+ TIL concentration was a favorable prognostic biomarker of treatment outcomes in these patients. However, most studies of the prognostic role of CD4+ lymphocytes do not provide a proper analysis of statistical significance. Other studies found that the amount of FOXP3+ TILs could simply reflect the total number of T cells in the tumor epithelium, and the effect of CD8+ T cells exceeded the immunosuppressive effect of Tregs (Park et al. 2019). Therefore, the authors proposed to evaluate not only the Treg content, but also the CD8/FOXP3+ ratio. The high ratio, which reflected the relative depletion of Tregs, was a potential biomarker of a favorable clinical outcome for different tumor types. A study evaluated this ratio in patients with squamous cell carcinoma of head and neck with promising results. Therefore, the authors proposed to evaluate not only the infiltrating Treg content, but also the CD8/FOXP3+ ratio. However, additional studies are needed to confirm the prognostic value of the CD8/FOXP3+ ratio in such patients. Given the ambiguous role of CD4+ lymphocytes in the tumor microenvironment and the small amount of this marker, the prognostic role of CD4 remains doubtful. Unexpectedly, meta-analysis showed that high FOXP3+ lymphocyte tumor infiltration may predict a better clinical outcome in patients with squamous cell carcinoma of head and neck. Some evidence was presented that immunosuppressive T cells in the tumor microenvironment were associated with better clinical outcomes in colorectal cancer and esophageal cancer (Shang et al. 2015). The phenomenon might be explained by the suggestion that Tregs suppress the ongoing ineffective inflammatory response, which is associated with tumor progression and inflammatory cytokines produced by the immune cells such as macrophages and dendritic cells. Meta-analysis confirmed the prognostic role of the infiltration of CD3+T cells and CD8+T cells in squamous cell carcinoma of the head and neck. High rates of CD3+ and CD8+ lymphocytes predicted a better clinical outcome. Nevertheless, in order to include any T-cell subsets as prognostic biomarkers in clinical practice, TILs should be studied by up-to-date methods in homogeneous cohorts with respect to the histological variant of the tumor, stage of the disease, and therapy.

11 TILs in Esophageal Cancer

Although several studies suggested that TILs may be regarded as a potential prognostic biomarker for patients with esophageal cancer, other studies claimed that the prognostic role of TILs remains controversial (Vacchelli et al. 2015). Zhang et al. reported that patients with high levels of CD8+TILs had better overall survival (Zhang et al. 2011), whereas other authors have shown that they CD8+TILs had no prognostic value in many cancer types (Chen et al. 2011; Grabenbauer et al. 2006; Nakano et al. 2001). Noble et al. stated that a high level of FOXP3+TILs was associated with better survival (Noble et al. 2016).

Taking into account these contradictory results, a meta-analysis including 2,909 patients of 22 studies was completed to assess the TIL prognostic role in esophageal cancer. The analysis of the data confirmed that a high level of TILs was associated with better survival, given that each of TIL subsets plays a different role in the development of esophageal cancer. Thus, a high level of CD8+TILs correlated with better survival of patients with esophageal cancer. Some studies showed that a high level of Tregs was an unfavorable prognostic factor in several tumor types (Gao et al. 2007). However, other authors reported that a high level of FOXP3+TILs was associated with better relapse-free, but not with overall survival in patients with esophageal cancer. This evidence results from the suggestion that the FOXP3+TIL immunosuppression represents a negative feedback mechanism where high levels of FOXP3+TILs are often accompanied by high levels of CD8+TILs (Zingg et al. 2010).

The role of CD4+TILs is ambiguous, on the one hand, this subset can induce antitumor activity, but on the other hand, it can promote tumor growth, which is consistent with the ambiguous prognostic significance of CD4+TILs. CD45RO is an important marker of memory T cells. CD45RO+T cells can induce an effective antitumor immune response after repeated stimulation by tumor-associated antigens (Levy et al. 2009). However, CD45RO+TILs were not associated with patient survival, while high levels of CD57+TILs, natural killers, correlated with better survival of patients with esophageal cancer.

12 TILs in Melanoma

The recent data showed a higher content FOXP3+T lymphocytes in the peripheral blood of patients with stage III-IV melanoma compared with healthy donors. The content of FOXP3+T cells in the lymphoid infiltrate of the tumor in patients with melanoma is significantly higher than in the peripheral blood, and peritumoral expression of FOXP3+T lymphocytes is higher than that of intratumoral infiltration (Ahmadzadeh et al. 2008). According to another study, a high level of FOXP3+T lymphocytes in the lymphoid infiltrate of the tumor correlated with low relapse-free and overall survival of patients and was an independent prognostic factor (Gerber et al. 2014). A flow cytometry study showed that an increase of FOXP3+T lymphocytes in the lymphoid infiltrate of melanoma correlated with the disease progression (Fujii et al. 2014). At the same time, Knol et al. found no significant differences in the amount of FOXP3+ T-lymphocytes in patients with and without metastases in the sentinel lymph node (Knol et al. 2011). However, the high content of FOXP3+TILs in melanoma stage III correlated with a decrease in the relapse-free survival, but not with the overall survival of patients. However, Ladányi et al. found no correlation between tumor infiltration by FOXP3+T lymphocytes with melanoma thickness and the survival rate of patients with melanoma (Ladányi et al. 2010).

Thus, the analysis shows that, despite numerous clinical studies of the prognostic significance of TILs in various types of malignant neoplasms, there is still no single point of view on this problem. The most data have been accumulated on the evaluation of TILs as a prognostic factor for overall and relapse-free survival and the effectiveness of neoadjuvant therapy in patients with breast cancer. Although meta-analysis of the reviews showed a high level of correlation between TILs and the survival of BC patients, as well as with the effectiveness of neoadjuvant therapy, these findings were noted just for a few BC types.

Even more contradictions arise when assessing the predictive role of various lymphocyte subpopulations. In particular, some studies showed a positive correlation between the percentage of both cytotoxic CD8+ TILs and suppressor FOXP3+ TILs. Obviously, for this reason, the German Breast Cancer Group recommendations proposed to evaluate the infiltration of tumor lymphocytes using standard histological staining with hematoxylin-eosin without isolation of individual lymphocyte subpopulations. Yet, TILs in other types of malignant tumors have an even more complicated and ambiguous interpretation of their prognostic significance, which seems to be associated with a small number of patients included in the studies.

Along with the predictive role of TILs for chemo- and radiation therapy, these lymphocyte subpopulations can also be prognostic biomarkers for the effectiveness of immunotherapy. In particular, immunotherapies based on pembrolizumab, nivolumab, etc. enhance the antitumor effect of CD8+ TILs. Therefore, the amount and subsets of TILs might serve as a prognostic factor for the disease outcome and these factors should be considered when making a decision about a personalized therapy, including up-to-date immunotherapies.

13 Predictive and Prognostic Biomarkers for the Effectiveness of the Inhibitors of the Immune Checkpoints

Immunotherapy by the immune checkpoint inhibitors (ICI) has started a new era in oncology and significantly improved the effectiveness of antitumor treatment (Larkin et al. 2015). Immune checkpoints belong to a receptor class, including co-stimulating (CD27, CD28, and CD137) and co-inhibiting receptors (CTLA-4, PD-1, BTLA), which regulate T-cell effector functions. The most clinically effective strategies include blockade of the programmed cell death receptor 1 (PD-1) or its ligand PD-L1. Interaction between the PD-1 receptor of cytotoxic T-lymphocytes and PD-L1 on a tumor cell reduces T-cell activity as a result of several mechanisms, including inhibition of T-cell receptor signaling and increased activity of Tregs while reducing the activity of B cells and natural killers (Curran et al. 2010).

Another important immune checkpoint is CTLA-4 that competes for binding B7 co-stimulation molecules to the CD28 co-stimulating receptor reducing T-cell activation (Shi et al. 2016). PD-1 and CTLA-4 blockade restores the antitumor immune response by inducing the expansion of depleted CD8+TILs. In addition, CTLA-4 blockade contributes to the increase of Th1 CD4+T cells and TILs, as well as the development of memory T cells and increased cytolytic activity of CD8+T cells (Hodi et al. 2010).

ICIs have demonstrated the efficacy in different malignant neoplasms such as melanoma, non-small cell lung cancer (NSCLC), renal cancer, squamous cell carcinoma of head and neck, Hodgkin's lymphoma, cancer of the urethra, gastric cancer, cervical cancer, hepatocellular carcinoma, etc. Although various clinical trials showed an objective immune response in most patients, some patients do not respond to ICI therapy as a result of primary or acquired resistance to the treatment (Sharma et al. 2017). The least effective ICI therapy seems anti-CTLA-4 with the clinical response in only 15% of patients (Thorsson et al. 2018). A number of clinical studies registered a much greater clinical effect (up to 40% of patients) with anti-PD1 drugs that presented less side effects. Combined immunotherapy regimens were most effective (in 50% of patients), though showing significant side effects (Larkin et al. 2015). Therefore, it is important to search for predictor markers that potentially determine the patients most sensitive to ICI therapy.

14 Tumor-infiltrating Lymphocytes: Biomarkers of the ICI Effectiveness

Retrospective studies have shown that TILs are associated with increased survival rates in patients with various malignancies, such as colorectal cancer, melanoma, BC, and NSCLC. Most clinical trials of TIL prognostic significance involved patients with breast cancer (Schirosi et al. 2020).

Patients with NSCLC stage III receiving chemo-radiotherapy had a longer relapse-free survival and overall survival rates if a high density of CD8+ TILs were detected in tumor biopsies before treatment. The prognostic significance of

TILs has also been shown in other malignant neoplasms. Presumably, TILs improve tumor recognition and therefore may be regarded as a prognostic biomarker. Alterations of the concentration of the pro-inflammatory factors in the T-cell micro-environment are also associated with the clinical efficacy of the therapy with interleukins and antitumor vaccines (Mansfield et al. 2016). TILs in various malignant neoplasms were investigated as a predictive biomarker for ICI effectiveness (Rizk et al. 2019). The increase of the TIL amount is the main indicator of the immune inflammation and the intensity of immune-mediated elimination of tumor cells.

15 TILs for the Prognosis of the ICI Effectiveness

Clinical studies have shown that prognostic significance in various malignant neoplasms has both the TIL increase and the absolute number of peripheral blood lymphocytes (PBL) and may represent a prognostic biomarker for the ICI effectiveness (Simeone et al. 2014). The role of PBL as a prognostic biomarker was confirmed in patients with metastatic melanoma treated with ipilimumab (IPI). The patients with a 1.35-fold increase of the PBL compared to the baseline in the first two weeks of IPI therapy had significantly higher overall survival. Early increase of the PBL with a subsequent delayed increase of CD4+ and CD8+ T cells characterizes a favorable rearrangement of the immune system and may indicate a clinically significant transition from a nonspecific (innate) to a specific (adaptive) immune response. However, a dynamic assessment of various leukocyte subsets: the number of eosinophils, CD4+ Ki67+ and CD8+ Ki67+ T cells, CD127+low CD25+ FoxP3+ Treg and Lin–CD14–CD16+ HLA-DR+ monocytes in melanoma patients during ICI therapy revealed any association of disease stabilization with these parameters (Martens et al. 2016). Progression-free survival of patients receiving IPI therapy was positively associated with a low serum lactate dehydrogenase (LDH$\leq$ 1.2 times), low absolute number of monocytes (less than 650 cells/ml), low number of myeloid suppressor cells (less than 50 cells/ml), the PBL content was not less than 10.5%, and CD4+ CD25+ FOXP3+ Treg level less than 1.5%. Numerous studies that proved LDH as a prognostic biomarker showed that patients with elevated LDH levels also responded to ICI therapy. J. Manolo et al. found that LDH was a potential prognostic biomarker for overall survival, but not for immunotherapy (Manola et al. 2000). Other biomarkers are also used for monitoring IPI treatment, including Ki 67, a marker for cell proliferation, which expression increased on CD4+ and CD8+ T cells with IPI therapy (Wang et al. 2012). Similar to Ki 67, induced expression of T-cell co-stimulator (ICOS) on CD4+ T cells was also considered as a pharmacodynamic marker for IPI therapy. Patients with enhanced numbers of circulating ICOS+T cells at week 7 of the IPI therapy had better overall survival (Ng Tang et al. 2013).

At present, studying predictive biomarkers of the ICI effectiveness in cancer patients is still an experimental approach, therefore making conclusions about their clinical use seems too early. Nevertheless, several observations are worth mentioning. Thus, the most promising biomarkers for predicting the response to ICI are the subset content of TILs and localization of immune cells, as well as the amount of activated CD8+T lymphocytes. Obviously, the prognostic significance of TILs can be improved by evaluating lymphocyte PD-1 expression, as well as PDL-1 on tumor cells.

16 Methods of TIL Detection

Most of the studies on the prognostic role of TILs used histological or immunohistochemical methods to assess the content and intensity of lymphocytic infiltration of the tumor. Sections of paraffin blocks prepared for TIL counts are preferable, while evaluation of TIL on cryosections has not been thoroughly investigated, yet: therefore, this method has not been recommended for routine practice. Magnification of the microscope does not matter much, though ×200–400 is conventionally applied (eyepiece ×10, lens ×20, ×40). The section thickness is not critical, and the standard thickness of 4–5 μm is optimal. TILs may be evaluated using core biopsies in neoadjuvant modes, as well as surgical material in adjuvant modes. TIL counts of one block for a patient are considered sufficient in both neoadjuvant and adjuvant modes.

In 2012 the International Immuno-Oncology Biomarker Working Group was established in order to standardize the approach to the TIL assessment in breast cancer (Denkert et al. 2016). The Working Group developed and published a guidance for TIL evaluation. At the first stage, hematoxylin-eosin stain was recommended (Salgado et al. 2015). The evaluation should involve all mononuclear cells, including lymphocytes and plasmatic cells, whereas granulocytes and other polymorphonuclear leukocytes should be excluded. The recommendations establish three categories of infiltration: low (TILs – 0–10%), intermediate (TILs – 11–59%), and high (TILs – 60–100%). Quantification of other mononuclear cells, such as dendritic cells and macrophages, is currently not recommended, although there is increasing evidence that they may be functionally important. To estimate the prognostic significance of TIL, single- and multi-factor analysis should be performed. The endpoints include complete response, relapse-free, and overall survival. Clinical significance of lymphocyte subtypes is conventionally assessed by immunohistochemistry. The significance of the most informative biomarkers such as CD45, CD3, CD8, and Foxp3 expressed on lymphoid cells is still unclear, though immunohistochemistry can improve the accuracy of TIL marker assessment.

According to the recommendations of the Working Group, the assessment focuses on stromal TIL (Fig. 1a, b). However, some authors showed the prognostic significance of peritumoral lymphocyte infiltration (Hussein 2006) and both intratumoral and peritumoral TILs could be evaluated.

Although PCR (polymerase chain reaction) is also used for TIL estimation, it is not clear whether the method can improve the accuracy achieved by conventional

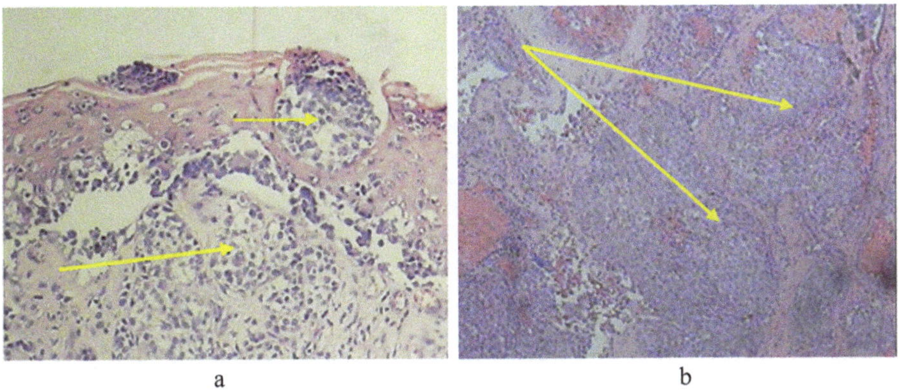

Fig. 1 Immunohistochemical study of TILs: (**a**) melanoma lymphocyte infiltration; (**b**) breast cancer lymphocyte infiltration; hematoxylin-eosin staining; ×500. The arrows show lymphocyte infiltrates

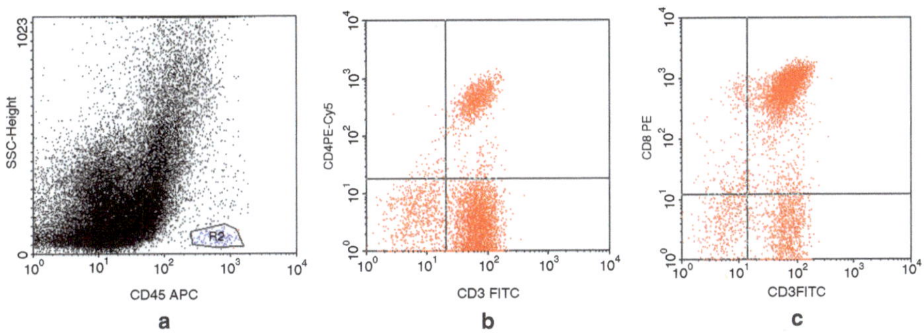

Fig. 2 Flow cytometry analysis of TILs, (**a**) DotPlot with gated CD45+ cell population; (**b**) analysis of CD45+ cell population for CD4+ and CD3+ subsets; (**c**) analysis of CD45+ cell population for CD8+ and CD3+ subsets

immunohistochemistry. Other methods, such as CyTOF (Bendall et al. 2011) seem to have additional potential.

Most studies of TIL content performed immunohistochemical analysis of fixed sections, which provides information only about the rate of infiltration (low/high). Multiparameter flow cytometry allows evaluation of various TIL subpopulations and estimation of the immune response at the tissue level, as well as the assessment of the phenotypic heterogeneity of the immunocompetent cells (Fig. 2a–c).

The number of TIL lymphocytes in the cell suspension samples was comparable when studied by flow cytometry and standard cytological examination (Fig. 3a, b) (Zabotina et al. 2016).

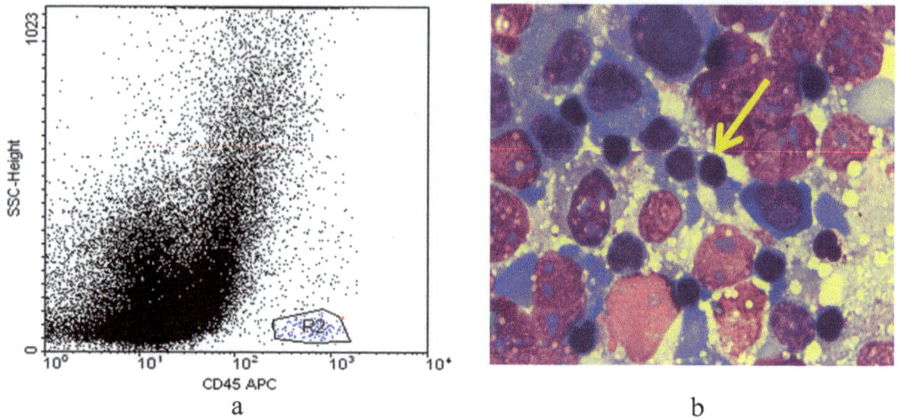

Fig. 3 Comparative analysis of breast cancer core-biopsy samples with TILs after enzyme-based disaggregation: (**a**) flow cytometry analysis of CD45+cells, gate 2; (**b**) cytomorphology, hematoxylin-eosin staining, ×1000, arrow points to a lymphocyte infiltrate

17 Conclusion

The International Immuno-Oncology Biomarker Working Group on Breast Cancer recommended standard histological methods and semi-quantitative calculation of the percentage of stromal TILs, which allows subdivision of patients with tumors of high (>10%) and low (<10%) TIL levels. However, it should be noted that the recommended method is largely subjective and depends on the selected fields of vision and pathologist's experience. Though immunohistochemistry seems a more accurate method for lymphocyte identification and subset evaluation, calculation of the lymphocyte proportions is also semi-quantitative and subjective. Besides, false-positive results may occur, in particular, in case of pigmented melanoma, and the assessment of the TIL subsets appears rather time-consuming.

Multiparameter flow cytometry allows evaluation of a wide range of lymphocyte antigens, including CTLA-4 and PD-1, which may be important for the patient selection for immunotherapy. The TIL number and subsets may have prognostic significance, as well as their localization in the stroma or parenchyma of the tumor, and standard histological examination is recommended to evaluate stromal TILs and peritumoral TILs. Immunohistochemical staining reveals major TIL subsets (CD3, CD16, CD19).

Thus, the review analysis has shown that a more comprehensive information about TIL numbers and various subsets may be obtained by histological and immunohistochemical examination with additional multiparameter flow cytometry analysis.

Disclosure of Interests All authors declare they have no conflict of interest.

Funding This work had no special funding.

References

Ahmadzadeh M, Felipe-Silva A, Heemskerk B et al (2008) FOXP3 expression accurately defines the population of intratumoral regulatory T cells that selectively accumulate in metastatic melanomalesions. Blood 112(13):4953–4960

Almangush A, Jouhi L, Atula T, Haglund C, Mäkitie AA, Hagström J, Leivo I (2022) Tumour-infiltrating lymphocytes in oropharyngeal cancer: a validation study according to the criteria of the international immuno-oncology biomarker working group. Br J Cancer 126(11):1589–1594

Al-Shibli KI, Donnem T, Al-Saad S, Persson M, Bremnes RM, Busund LT (2008) Prognostic effect of epithelial and stromal lymphocyte infiltration in non-small cell lung cancer. Clin Cancer Res 14:5220–5227

Bendall SC, Simonds EF, Qiu P, Amir EAD, Krutzik PO, Finck R et al (2011) Single-cell mass cytometry of differential immune and drug responses across a human hematopoietic continuum. Science 332(6030):687–696

Benedet JL, Bender H, Jones H, Ngan HY, Pecorelli S (2000) FIGO staging classifications and clinical practice guidelines in the management of gynecologic cancers. FIGO committee on gynecologic oncology. Int J Gynaecol Obstet 70:209–262

Bense RD, Sotiriou C, Piccart-Gebhart MJ et al (2016) Relevance of tumor-infiltrating immune cell composition and functionality for disease outcome in breast cancer. J Natl Cancer Inst 109: djw192

Chen DS, Mellman I (2017) Elements of cancer immunity and the cancer-immune set point. Nature 541:321–330

Chen JG, Xia JC, Liang XT, Pan K, Wang W, Lv L, Zhao JJ, Wang QJ, Li YQ, Chen SP, He J, Huang LX, Ke ML, Chen YB, Ma HQ, Zeng ZW, Zhou ZW, Chang AE, Li Q (2011) Intratumoral expression of IL-17 and its prognostic role in gastric adenocarcinoma patients. Int J Biol Sci 7(1):53–60

Chen XY, Yeong J, Thike AA, Bay BH, Tan PH (2019) Prognostic role of immune infiltrates in breast ductal carcinoma in situ. Breast Cancer Res Treat 27. https://doi.org/10.1007/s10549-019-05272-2

Curran MA, Montalvo W, Yagita H, Allison JP (2010) PD-1 and CTLA-4 combination blockade expands infiltrating T cells and reduces regulatory T and myeloid cells within B16 melanoma tumors. Proc Natl Acad Sci U S A 107(9):4275–4280

de Ruiter EJ, Ooft ML, Devriese LA, Willems SM (2017) The prognostic role of tumor infiltrating T-lymphocytes in squamous cell carcinoma of the head and neck: a systematic review and meta-analysis. Oncoimmunology 6(11):e1356148

Denkert C, Loibl S, Noske A et al (2010) Tumor-associated lymphocytes as an independent predictor of response to neoadjuvant chemotherapy in breast cancer. J Clin Oncol 28:105–113

Denkert C, von Minckwitz G, Brase JC, Sinn BV, Gade S, Kronenwett R et al (2015) Tumor-infiltrating lymphocytes and response to neoadjuvant chemotherapy with or without Carboplatin in human epidermal growth factor receptor 2-positive and triple-negative primary breast cancers. J Clin Oncol 33(9):983–991

Denkert C, Wienert S, Poterie A, Loibl S (2016) Standardized evaluation of tumor-infiltrating lymphocytes in breast cancer: results of the ring studies of the international immuno-oncology biomarker working group. Mod Pathol 10:1155–1164

Denkert C, von Minckwitz G, Darb-Esfahani S, Lederer B et al (2018) Tumour-infiltrating lymphocytes and prognosis in different subtypes of breast cancer: a pooled analysis of 3771 patients treated with neoadjuvant therapy. Lancet Oncol 19:40–50

Dieci MV, Criscitiello C, Goubar A et al (2014) Prognostic value of tumor-infiltrating lymphocytes on residual disease after primary chemotherapy for triple-negative breast cancer: a retrospective multicenter study. Ann Oncol 25:611–618

Dieci MV, Radosevic-Robin N, Fineberg S (2018) Update on tumor-infiltrating lymphocytes (TILs) in breast cancer, including recommendations to assess TILs in residual disease after neoadjuvant

therapy and in carcinoma in situ: A report of the international immuno-oncology biomarker working group on breast cancer. Semin Cancer Biol Pt2:16–25
Ding W, Xu X, Qian Y, Xue W, Wang Y, Du J, Jin L, Tan Y (2018) Prognostic value of tumor-infiltrating lymphocytes in hepatocellular carcinoma a meta-analysis. Medicine 97:e13301
Fujii H, Arakawa A, Kitoh A et al (2014) Perturbations of both nonregulatory and regulatory FOXP3+ Tcells in patients with malignant melanoma. J Dermatol 164(5):1052–1560
Fukunaga A, Miyamoto M, Cho Y, Murakami S et al (2004) CD8+ tumor-infiltrating lymphocytes together with CD4+ tumor-infiltrating lymphocytes and dendritic cells improve the prognosis of patients with pancreatic adenocarcinoma. Pancreas 28:e26–e31
Gallego A, Mendiola M, Hernando B, Berjon A, Cadiz A, Chaves-Urbano B, Heredia-Soto V, Spagnolo E, Hernández Gutiérrez A, Hardisson D, Macintyre G, Redondo A, Garçia MJ (2022) Prognostic markers of inflammation in endometrioid and clear cell ovarian cancer. Int J Gynecol Cancer 18:ijgc-2022-003353
Galon J, Angell HK, Bedognetti D et al (2013) The continuum of cancer immunosurveillance: prognostic, predictive, and mechanistic signatures. Immunity 39:11–26
Gao Q, Qiu SJ, Fan J, Zhou J, Wang XY et al (2007) Intratumoral balance of regulatory and cytotoxic T cells is associated with prognosis of hepatocellular carcinoma after resection. J Clin Oncol 25:2586–2593
Geng Y, Shao Y, He W, Hu W, Xu Y, Chen J, Wu C (2015) Prognostic role of tumor-infiltrating lymphocytes in lung cancer: a meta-analysis Jiang. J Cell Physiol Biochem 37(4):1560–1571
Gentles AJ, Newman AM, Liu CL et al (2015) The prognostic landscape of genes and infiltrating immune cells across human cancers. Nat Med 21:938–945
Gerber AL, Münst A, Schlapbach C et al (2014) High expression of FOXP3 in primary melanoma is associated with tumour progression. Br J Dermatol 170(1):103–109
Goc J, Germain C, Vo-Bourgais TK, Lupo A, Klein C et al (2014) Dendritic cells in tumor-associated tertiary lymphoid structures signal a Th1 cytotoxic immune contexture and license the positive prognostic value of infiltrating CD8+ T cells. Cancer Res 74:705–715
Gooden MJ, de Bock GH, Leffers N, Daemen T, Nijman HW (2011) The prognostic influence of tumour-infiltrating lymphocytes in cancer: a systematic review with meta-analysis. Br J Cancer 105(1):93–103
Grabenbauer GG, Lahmer G, Distel L et al (2006) Tumor-infiltrating cytotoxic T cells but not regulatory T cells predict outcome in anal squamous cell carcinoma. Clin Cancer Res 12(11 Pt 1):3355–3360
Gu-Trantien C, Loi S, Garaud S et al (2013) CD4(+) follicular helper T cell infiltration predicts breast cancer survival. J Clin Invest 123:2873–2892
Hammerl D, Smid M, Timmermans AM, Sleijfer S, Martens M, JW, Debets R. (2018) Breast cancer genomics and immuno-oncological markers to guide immune therapies. Semin Cancer Biol 52 (Pt 2):178–188
Hodi FS, O'Day SJ, McDermott DF (2010) Improved survival with ipilimumab in patients with metastatic melanoma. N Engl J Med 363(8):711–772
Hussein MR (2006) Immunohistologicalcharacterisation of tumour infiltrating lymphocytes in melanocytic skin lesions. Fadeletal J Clin Pathol 59(3):316–332
Idos GE, Kwok J, Bonthala N, Kysh L, Gruber SB, Qu C (2020) The prognostic implications of tumor infiltrating lymphocytes in colorectal cancer: a systematic review and meta-analysis. Sci Rep 10:1–14. https://doi.org/10.1038/s41598-020-60255-4
Iglesia MD, Parker JS, Hoadley KA et al (2016) Genomic analysis of immune cell infiltrates across 11 tumor types. J Natl Cancer Inst 108:djw144
Kawai O, Ishii G, Kubota K, Murata Y et al (2008) Predominant infiltration of macrophages and CD8(+) T Cells in cancer nests is a significant predictor of survival in stage IV nonsmall cell lung cancer. Cancer 113:1387–1395
Kayser G, Schulte-Uentrop L, Sienel W, Werner M et al (2012) Stromal CD4/CD25 positive T-cells are a strong and independent prognostic factor in non-small cell lung cancer patients, especially with adenocarcinomas. Lung Cancer 76:445–451

Knol AC, Nguyen JM, Quéreux G et al (2011) Prognostic value of tumor-infiltrating Foxp3+ T-cellsubpopulations in metastatic melanoma. Exp Dermatol 20(5):430–434

Ladányi A, Mohos A, Somlai B et al (2010) FOXP3+ cell density in primary tumor has no prognostic impact in patients with cutaneous malignant melanoma. Pathol Oncol Res 16(3): 303–309

Larkin J, Chiarion-Sileni V, Gonzales R, Grob JJ, Cowey CL, Lao CD, Schadendorf D, Dummer R, Smylie M, Rutkowski P et al (2015) Combined nivolumab and ipilimumab or monotherapy in untreated melanoma. N Engl J Med 373:23–34. https://doi.org/10.1056/NEJMoa1504030

Lee JS, Won HS, Sun DS, Hong JH, Ko YH (2018) Prognostic role of tumor-infiltrating lymphocytes in gastric cancer a systematic review and meta-analysis. Medicine 97:e11769

Leffers N, Gooden MJ, de Jong RA, Hoogeboom BN (2009) Prognostic significance of tumor-infiltrating T-lymphocytes in primary and metastatic lesions of advanced stage ovarian cancer. Cancer Immunol Immunother 58:449–459

Levy Y, Lacabaratz C, Weiss L, Viard JP, Goujard C et al (2009) Enhanced T cell recovery in HIV-1-infected adults through IL-7 treatment. J ClinInvest 119:997–1007

Li J, Wang J, Chen R, Bai Y, Lu X (2017) The prognostic value of tumor-infiltrating T lymphocytes in ovarian cancer. Oncotarget 8(9):15621–15631

Liu S, Foulkes WD, Leung S et al (2014) Prognostic significance of FOXP3+ tumor infiltrating lymphocytes in breast cancer depends on estrogen receptor and human epidermal growth factor receptor-2 expression status and concurrent cytotoxic T-cell infiltration. Breast Cancer Res 16: 432

Liu D, Heij LR, Czigany Z, Dahl E, Lang SA, Ulmer TF, Luedde T, Neumann UP, Bednarsch J (2022) The role of tumor-infiltrating lymphocytes in cholangiocarcinoma. J Exp Clin Cancer Res 41(1):127. https://doi.org/10.1186/s13046-022-02340-2

Loi S, Sirtaine N, Piette F et al (2013) Prognostic and predictive value of tumor-infiltrating lymphocytes in a phase III randomized adjuvant breast cancer trial in node-positive breast cancer comparing the addition of docetaxel to doxorubicin with doxorubicin-based chemotherapy: BIG 02-98. J Clin Oncol 31:860–867

Mackensen A, Ferradini L, Carcelain G, Triebel F, Faure F, Viel S, Hercend T (1993) Evidence for in situ amplification of cytotoxic T-lymphocytes with antitumor activity in a human regressive melanoma. Cancer Res 53:3569–3573

Mahmoud SM, Paish EC, Powe DG, Macmillan RD, Grainge MJ, Lee AH, Ellis IO, Green AR (2011) Tumor-infiltrating CD8+ lymphocytes predict clinical outcome in breast cancer. J Clin Oncol 29:1949–1955

Mahmoud SM, Lee AH, Paish EC et al (2012) The prognostic significance of B lymphocytes in invasive carcinoma of the breast. Breast Cancer Res Treat 132:545–553

Manola J, Atkins M, Ibrahim J, Kirkwood J (2000) Prognostic factors in metastatic melanoma: A pooled analysis of eastern cooperative oncology group trials. J Clin Oncol 18:3782–3793. https://doi.org/10.1200/JCO.2000.18.22.3782

Mansfield AS, Murphy SJ, Peikert T et al (2016) Heterogeneity of programmed cell death ligand 1 expression in multifocal lung cancer. Clin Cancer Res 22:2177–2182

Mao Y, Qu Q, Chen X, Huang O, Wu J, Shen K (2016) The prognostic value of tumor-infiltrating lymphocytes in breast cancer: a systematic review and meta-analysis. PLoS One 11(4): e0152500

Martens A, Wistuba-Hamprecht K, Yuan J, Postow MA, Wong P, Capone M, Madonna G, Khammari A et al (2016) Increases in absolute lymphocytes and circulating CD4+ and CD8+ T cells are associated with positive clinical outcome of melanoma patients treated with Ipilimumab. Clin Cancer Res 22(19):4848–4858

McCarty WC (1931) Principles of prognosis in cancer. JAMA 96:30–33

McCoy MJ, Hemmings C, Anyaegbu CC, Austin SJ, Lee-Pullen TF, Miller TJ, Bulsara MK, Zeps N, Nowak AK, Lake RA et al (2017) Tumour-infiltrating regulatory T Cell density before Neoadjuvant Chemoradiotherapy for rectal cancer does not predict treatment response. Oncotarget 8:19803–19813. https://doi.org/10.18632/oncotarget.15048

Mlecnik B, Tosolini M, Kirilovsky A, Berger A, Bindea G, Meatchi T, Bruneval P, Trajanoski Z, Fridman WH, Pages F, Galon J (2011) Histopathologic-based prognostic factors of colorectal cancers are associated with the state of the local immune reaction. J Clin Oncol 29:610–618

Mlecnik B, Bifulco C, Bindea G, Marliot F, Lugli A, Lee JJ, Zlobec I, Rau TT, Berger MD, Nagtegaal ID et al (2020) Multicenter international society for immunotherapy of cancer study of the consensus Immunoscore for the prediction of survival and response to chemotherapy in stage III colon cancer. J Clin Oncol 38:3638–3651. https://doi.org/10.1200/JCO.19.03205,57

Mlika M, Saidi A, Mejri N, Abdennadher M, Haddouchi C, Labidi S, Khiari H, Boussen H, Hsairi M, Mezni F (2022) Prognostic impact of tumor-infiltrating lymphocytes in non-small cell lung carcinomas. Asian Cardiovasc Thorac Ann 30(2):177–184

Nakano O, Sato M, Naito Y et al (2001) Proliferative activity of intratumoral CD8+ T-lymphocytes as a prognostic factor in human renal cell carcinoma: clinicopathologic demonstration of antitumor immunity. Cancer Res 61(13):5132–5136

Ng Tang D, Shen Y, Sun J, Wen S, Wolchok JD, Yuan J et al (2013) Increased frequency of ICOS +CD4 T cells as a pharmacodynamic biomarker for anti-CTLA-4 therapy. Cancer Immunol Res 1:229–234

Noble F, Mellows T, McCormick Matthews LH, Bateman AC (2016) Tumour infiltrating lymphocytes correlate with improved survival in patients with oesophageal adenocarcinoma. Cancer Immunol Immunother 65:651–662

Orhan A, Vogelsang RP, Andersen MB, Madsen MT, Hölmich ER, Raskov H, Gögenur I (2020) The prognostic value of tumour-infiltrating lymphocytes in pancreatic cancer: a systematic review and meta-analysis. Eur J Cancer 132:71–84. https://doi.org/10.1016/j.ejca.2020.03.013

Orhan A, Khesrawi F, Tvilling Madsen M, Peuliche Vogelsang R, Dohrn N, Kanstrup Fiehn AM, Gögenur I (2022) Tumor-infiltrating lymphocytes as biomarkers of treatment response and long-term survival in patients with rectal cancer: a systematic review and meta-analysis. Cancers (Basel) 14(3):636. https://doi.org/10.3390/cancers14030636

Park JH, Lee HJ, Lee SB, Ahn JH (2019) Intrinsic prognostic impact of tumor-infiltrating lymphocytes in systemically untreated patients with early-stage triple-negative. Breast Cancer Anticancer Res 39(6):3111–3119

Qi W, Huang X, Wang J (2013) Correlation between Th17 cells and tumor microenvironment. Cell Immunol 285:18–22

Rizk EM, Gartrell RD, Barker LW, Esancy CL, Finkel GG, Bordbar DD, Saenger YM (2019) Prognostic and predictive immunohistochemistry-based biomarkers in cancer and immunotherapy. Hematol Oncol Clin North Am 33(2):291–299. https://doi.org/10.1016/j.hoc.2018.12.005

Salgado R, Denkert C, Demaria S et al (2015) The evaluation of tumor-infiltrating lymphocytes (TILs) in breast cancer:recommendations by an International TILs Working Group 2014. Ann Oncol 26:259–271

Sato E, Olson SH, Ahn J, Bundy B, Nishikawa H et al (2005) Intraepithelial CD8+ tumor-infiltrating lymphocytes and a high CD8+/regulatory T cell ratio are associated with favorable prognosis in ovarian cancer. Proc Natl Acad Sci U S A 102:18538–18543

Schalper KA, Velcheti V, Carvajal D et al (2014) In situ tumor PD-L1 mRNA expression is associated with increased TILs and better outcome in breast carcinomas. Clin Cancer Res 20: 2773–2782

Schirosi L, Saponaro C, Giotta F, Popescu O, Pastena MI, Scarpi E, Mangia A (2020) Tumor infiltrating lymphocytes and NHERF1 impact on prognosis of breast cancer. Patients Transl Oncol 13(2):186–192. https://doi.org/10.1016/j.tranon.2019.10.020

Schreiber RD, Old LJ, Smyth MJ (2011) Cancer immunoediting: integrating immunity's roles in cancer suppression and promotion. Science 331:1565–1570

Seo AN, Lee HJ, Kim EJ et al (2013) Tumour-infiltrating CD8+ lymphocytes as an independent predictive factor for pathological complete response to primary systemic therapy in breast cancer. Br J Cancer 109:2705–2713

Shang B, Liu Y, Jiang SJ, Liu Y (2015) Prognostic value of tumor-infiltrating FoxP3+ regulatory T cells in cancers: A systematic review and meta-analysis. Sci Rep 5:1517914

Sharma P, Hu-Lieskovan S, Wargo JA, Ribas A (2017) Primary, adaptive, and acquired resistance to cancer immunotherapy. Cell 168:707–723

Shi LZ, Fu T, Guan B (2016) Interdependent IL-7 and IFN-gamma signalling in T-cell controls tumour eradication by combined alpha-CTLA-4+alpha-PD-1 therapy. Nat Commun 7:12335

Simeone E, Gentilcore G, Giannarelli D, Grimaldi AM, Caraco C, Curvietto M et al (2014) Immunological and biological changes during ipilimumab treatment and their potential correlation with clinical response and survival in patients with advanced melanoma. Cancer Immunol Immunother 63:675–683

Suzuki K, Kadota K, Sima CS, Nitadori J et al (2013) Clinical impact of immune microenvironment in stage I lung adenocarcinoma: tumor interleukin-12 receptor beta2 (IL-12Rbeta2), IL-7R, and stromal FoxP3/CD3 ratio are independent predictors of recurrence. J Clin Oncol 31:490–498

Teschendorff AE, Gomez S, Arenas A et al (2010) Improved prognostic classification of breast cancer defined by antagonistic activation patterns of immune response pathway modules BMC. Cancer 10:604

Thorsson V, Gibbs DL, Brown SD, Wolf D, Bortone DS, Ou Yang TH, Porta-Pardo E, Gao GF, Plaisier CL, Eddy JA et al (2018) The immune landscape of cancer. Immunity 48:812–830

Vacchelli E, Semeraro M, Enot DP, Chaba K (2015) Negative prognostic impact of regulatory T cell infiltration in surgically resected esophageal cancer post-radiochemotherapy. Oncotarget 6: 20840–20850

Vermeij R, de Bock GH, Leffers N, Ten HK (2011) Tumor-infiltrating cytotoxic T lymphocytes as independent prognostic factor in epithelial ovarian cancer with wilms tumor protein 1 overexpression. J Immunother 34:516–523

Vinayak S, Gray RJ, Adams S et al (2014) Association of increased tumor-infiltrating lymphocytes (TILs) with immunomodulatory (IM) triple-negative breast cancer (TNBC) subtype and response to neoadjuvant platinum-based therapy in PrECOG0105. J Clin Oncol 32(5s):1000

Von Minckwitz G, Schneeweiss A, Loibl S et al (2014) Neoadjuvant carboplatin in patients with triple-negative and HER2-positive early breast cancer (GeparSixto; GBG 66): a randomised phase 2 trial. Lancet Oncol 15:747–756

Wang W, Yu D, Sarnaik AA, Yu B, Hall M, Morelli D et al (2012) Biomarkers on melanoma patient T cells associated with Ipilimumab treatment. J Transl Med 10:146

West NR, Kost SE, Martin SD et al (2013) Tumour-infiltrating FOXP3(+) lymphocytes are associated with cytotoxic immune responses and good clinical outcome in oestrogen receptor-negative breast cancer. Br J Cancer 108:155–162

Yan X, Jiao SC (2015) Roles of tumor-infiltrating lymphocytes in non-small cell lung cancer recurrence and metastasis: a meta analysis. Zhongguo Yi Xue Ke Xue Yuan Xue Bao 37(4): 406–414

Zabotina TN, Korotkova OV, Borunova AA (2016) Multiparameter study of the immunophenotype of tumor-infiltrating lymphocytes in cancer patients. Russian Journal of Oncology 21:51–54

Zhang L, Conejo-Garcia JR, Katsaros D, Gimotty PA, Massobrio M, Regnani G, Makrigiannakis A, Gray H, Schlienger K, Liebman MN, Rubin SC, Coukos G (2003) Intratumoral T cells, recurrence, and survival in epithelial ovarian cancer. N Engl J Med 348: 203–213

Zhang G, Liu WL, Zhang L, Wang JY, Kuang MH et al (2011) Involvement of indoleamine 2, 3-dioxygenase in impairing tumor-infiltrating CD8 T-cell functions in esophageal squamous cell carcinoma. Clin Dev Immunol 2011:384726

Zhou L, Chong MM, Littman DR (2009) Plasticity of CD4+ T cell lineage differentiation. Immunity 30:646–655

Zingg U, Montani M, Frey DM, Dirnhofer S, Esterman AJ, Went P, Oertli D (2010) Tumour-infiltrating lymphocytes and survival in patients with adenocarcinoma of the oesophagus. Eur J Surg Oncol 36:670–677

Recent Innovative Approaches to Intensify the Efficacy and Safety of CAR-T Cell Therapy in Cancers

Safa Tahmasebi, Elnaz Khosh, Samaneh Rostami, and Nima Rezaei

Abstract

In recent decades, the advent of chimeric antigen receptor (CAR)-T cell therapy has revolutionized cancer treatment, especially hematological malignancies. Despite the promising results of this therapeutic approach, tumor degradation, and patient improvement, there are some concerns about the efficacy and safety of the widespread use of this treatment in the clinic. Complex and suppressing tumor microenvironment (TME), tumor antigen heterogeneity, the difficulty of cell trafficking, CAR-T cell exhaustion, and reduced cytotoxicity in the tumor site limit the applicability of CAR-T cell therapy and highlight the requiring to improve the performance of this treatment. On the other hand, the life-threatening side effects of CAR-T cell therapy, such as cytokine release syndrome (CRS), on-target/off-tumor toxicity, neurotoxicity, and anaphylaxis, cast doubt on the clinical use of this treatment, cause the need for crucial control of their activity. Accordingly, enhancing the therapeutic potential of CAR-T cells with

S. Tahmasebi
Department of Immunology, School of Medicine, Shahid Beheshti University of Medical Sciences, Tehran, Iran

E. Khosh · S. Rostami
Department of Immunology, School of Medicine, Zanjan University of Medical Sciences, Zanjan, Iran

N. Rezaei (✉)
Research Center for Immunodeficiencies, Children's Medical Center, Tehran University of Medical Sciences, Tehran, Iran

Department of Immunology, School of Medicine, Tehran University of Medical Sciences, Tehran, Iran

Network of Immunity in Infection, Malignancy and Autoimmunity (NIIMA), Universal Scientific Education and Research Network (USERN), Stockholm, Sweden
e-mail: rezaei_nima@tums.ac.ir

Interdisciplinary Cancer Research, https://doi.org/10.1007/16833_2022_64
Published online: 22 November 2022

combination therapies and improving both the efficiency and safety of these cells by equipping them with genetic engineering methods would help to better respond to tumors. Hence, this study aims to comprehensively discuss the challenges and side effects of CAR-T cell therapy and emphasize the types and applications of combination therapies and armored CARs to intensify the efficiency and safety of CAR-T cell therapy in cancer treatment.

Keywords

Cell therapy · Chimeric antigen receptor · Combination therapy · Tumor microenvironment

1 Introduction

Recently, redoubled efforts have been made to find fully effective cancer treatments, but none have yet been introduced. Chemotherapy, radiotherapy, surgery, and other treatments have been used to treat cancers for many years. Immunotherapy against cancer is not a new concept, but it rose to prominence with the development of immune-based therapies such as cytokine therapy, cancer vaccines, checkpoint inhibitors, adoptive cell therapy (ACT), tumor-infiltrating lymphocytes (TILs), monoclonal antibodies (mAbs), bispecific antibodies, and chimeric antigen receptor (CAR)-T cells (Khalil et al. 2015; Oiseth and Aziz 2017). CAR-T cells are genetically engineered T cells with synthetic receptors to improve their efficacy in recognizing a wide range of target antigen epitopes on tumor cells. CAR is a chimeric receptor, which means there is a combination of an antigen-binding domain and T cell signaling domain. In other words, these synthetic receptors recognize antigens in a non-MHC-restricted way using the ability of antibodies as advantage of taking T cell function (Feins et al. 2019). In general, CAR-T cells are called "the living drugs" because their signaling and activity are almost similar to T lymphocytes. So far, successful and promising applications of CAR-T cell therapy in various diseases have been reported, including cancers, allergies, autoimmune diseases, and infections (Esmaeilzadeh et al. 2020; Marofi et al. 2021a, b).

In the last few years, some drugs with the basis of CAR-T cells were developed and received the license by the US Food and Drug Administration (FDA) and the European Commission (EC) to be used in hematological malignancies. Tisagenlecleucel (Kymriah, Novartis) was approved in August 2017 by the FDA to treat acute lymphocytic leukemia (ALL), and in August 2018 the EC licensed the Kymriah for refractory pediatric and young adult patients with B cell ALL (NCT02435849 and NCT05075603) (Bach et al. 2017; Maude et al. 2018). In October 2017, another CAR-T cell, called Axicabtagene ciloleucel (Yescarta, Gilead), got the license to be used in adult patients with relapsed or refractory (R/R) large B cell lymphoma (NCT02348216, NCT04002401, and NCT03391466) (Bouchkouj et al. 2019). In February 2021, the newest CAR-T cell-based drug named lisocabtagene maraleucel (Breyanzi, Celgene) was approved for medical use in the United States to treat adult patients with R/R large B cell lymphoma, including diffuse large B cell lymphoma (DLBCL) not otherwise specified (including DLBCL arising from indolent lymphoma), high-grade B cell lymphoma, primary mediastinal large B cell lymphoma, and follicular lymphoma grade 3B (NCT03744676 and NCT03483103) (Abramson et al. 2020).

Encouragingly, the use of CAR-T cells in the treatment of patients with hematological malignancies has had promising results (Marofi et al. 2021a, b). However, in solid tumors, due to the complex inhibitory tumor microenvironment (TME), antigen heterogeneity, and the difficulty of cell trafficking to the tumor site, CAR-T cell efficiency has faced several challenges (Tahmasebi et al. 2019; Marofi et al. 2021a, b, c). Also, as a significant concern, this strategy has multiple worrying side effects that need to improve the safety of these engineered cells more and more. Up to now, several efforts have been developed to increase the CAR-T cell efficacy clinical responses of cancers to CAR-T cells and limited the side effects of this therapeutic regimen (Elahi et al. 2018; Tahmasebi et al. 2021). Genetically engineering strategies, producing the armored CAR-T cells, and recruiting the other cancer treatment approaches in combination with CAR-T cell therapy are the most valuable solutions developed to intensify the safety and efficacy of CAR-T cells, which have been comprehensively described in the current study.

2 Structure, Generations, and Function of CAR-T Cell

The CAR structure results from binding the different components next to each other. This chimeric receptor consists of three parts: ectodomain, a transmembrane domain, and endodomain (Liu et al. 2017). The antigen recognition domain, so-called single-chain Fragment variant (ScFv), is a part of the ectodomain bound to potential target antigens and directs CAR-T cells to target cells. This domain is composed of variable portions of light (VL) and heavy (VH) chains from a tumor specific monoclonal antibody (Sadelain et al. 2013). The ScFv acts as a signal peptide and can distinguish the amount of ligand and differentiate between tumor cells and normal healthy cells (Chmielewski et al. 2004; Miliotou and Papadopoulou 2018). The next part of the ectodomain is the hinge domain (Spacer), which gives the CAR considerable flexibility and indirectly plays a vital role in recognizing the target epitope by promoting the synapse formation (Guest et al. 2005). The transmembrane domain is an important structural section responsible for keeping the CAR constant on the cell. This part is usually derived from type 1 proteins like CD3-zeta, CD8a, CD28, and even CD4, which each gives different features to CAR-T cells (Bridgeman et al. 2010). CD3ζ, an intracellular signaling domain or endodomain, is the essential part of the receptor. This section is responsible for functional actions of the receptor and initiating a signaling cascade (Tasian and Gardner 2015). CD3ζ is fixed and identical in all generations of CARs. The classification of CAR generations is based on co-stimulatory domains, which have key roles in conveying and sustaining the signaling pathway, differentiation of T cells, metabolic cycles, apoptosis, and activation-induced cell death (AICD) (Weinkove et al. 2019) (Fig. 1).

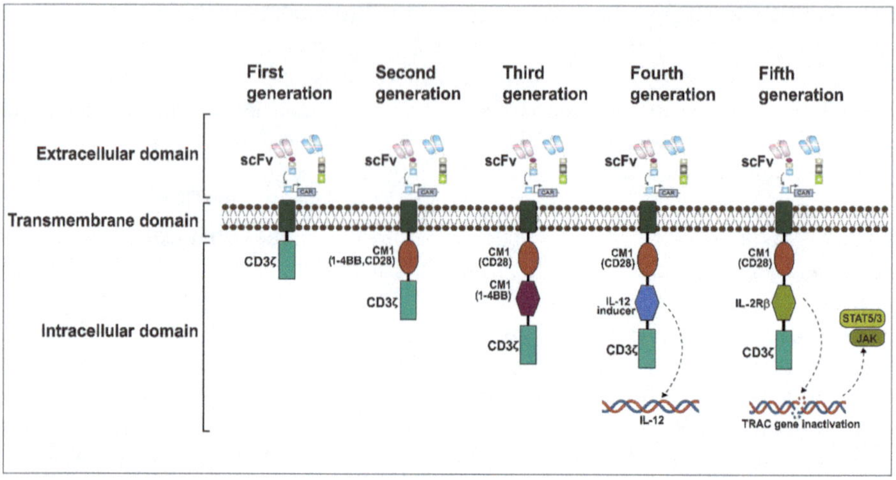

Fig. 1 Chimeric antigen receptor (CAR) generations. All generation of CARs consists of an extracellular antigen-binding domain (ScFv), a transmembrane domain, and intracellular signaling domains which are different in generations. First-generation CARs only contain one intracellular signal domain, CD3ζ. The second-generation CARs consist of a co-stimulatory domain, including 4-1BB (CD137) or CD28, whereas the third-generation CARs have two co-stimulatory domains. The fourth-generation CAR-T cells are also referred to as TRUCKs, can activate the downstream transcription factor, and induce cytokine production such as IL-12. The fifth-generation CAR-T cells use gene editing to inactivate the TRAC gene and contain intracellular domains of cytokine receptors, such as IL-2Rβ chain fragment

The first-generation CARs only include ScFv and CD3ζ, providing primary activating signals (signal 1). Due to a lack of co-stimulatory signals, they cannot induce persistent signals (signal 2). Multiple experiments showed low cytotoxicity, proliferation, and persistence of this generation of CAR to destroy tumor cells (Weinkove et al. 2019). The second-generation CARs include additional co-stimulatory signaling by coupling CD28 or CD137 (4-1BB) with CD3ζ in the signal transduction region, boosting CAR-T cell proliferation, toxicity, and consistent activity while also extending their half-life (van der Stegen et al. 2015). The third-generation CARs have been designed with more than one co-stimulatory domain besides CD3ζ like CD3ζ-CD28-OX40 or CD3ζ-CD28-41BB to enhance CAR efficiency with more outstanding cytokine production and tumor cell killing capacity. Based on some studies, third-generation CARs have better signal strengths, tumor eradication, persistence, and expansion than their second-generation counterparts (Zhong et al. 2010; Ramos et al. 2018). The fourth-generation CARs have also been introduced as T cells redirected for universal cytokine-mediated killing (TRUCKs), created with the additional transgenes of co-stimulatory ligands or pro-inflammatory cytokines such as IL-12 on the base of the second-generation CARs. Compared to the previous three generations, TRUCK cells have more advantages in acting against the immune suppressors in the tumor microenvironment. They, therefore, have a higher potential for tumor cell destruction. The fifth generation of CAR was developed using the structure of the second-generation

CAR, which also has cytokine receptors in the intracellular domain, such as an IL-2Rβ chain segment. (Chmielewski and Abken 2015).

3 CAR-T Cell Challenges

As mentioned earlier, the effectiveness and clinical applications of CAR-T cells are limited due to their many challenges and obstacles, especially in solid tumors. Thereby, manipulating the tumor microenvironment, equipping the CAR-T cells, and using combination therapies can help overcome these limitations (Lanitis et al. 2020; Bansal and Reshef 2021). The most critical restricting barriers include the heterogeneity and the misplaced or excessive expression of tumor antigens, the difficulty of targeting the tumor-specific antigens, resistant tumor stroma, improper CAR-T cell accessing to the target area, and mainly inhibitory and complex tumor microenvironment that suppresses immune responses and reduces CAR-T cell function (Tahmasebi et al. 2019). Resistant tumor stroma [cancer-associated stromal cells (CASCs), cancer-associated fibroblast (CAF) cell, and heparan sulfate proteoglycan (HSPG)], inhibitory cells [regulatory T cells (Tregs), myeloid-derived suppressor cells (MDSCs), immature dendritic cell (iDC), tumor-associated macrophages (TAM), and tumor-associated neutrophils (TAN)], inhibitory enzymes [indoleamine 2,3 dioxygenase (IDO), protein kinase A (PKA), and adenosine], inhibitory cytokines (IL-4, IL-10, and TGF-β), inhibitory checkpoints [cytotoxic T lymphocyte antigen-4 (CTLA-4), B and T lymphocyte attenuators (BTLA), programmed death 1 (PD-1), lymphocyte activation gene 3 (LAG3), T cell immunoglobulin and mucin-3 (TIM-3)], nutrient starvation (tryptophan, lysine, and arginine), and hypoxia are among the essential inhibitory hurdles to CAR-T cells in tumor sites (Junghans 2017).

4 Side Effects of CAR-T Cell

The sustained and drastic proliferation of CAR-T cells can cause critical adverse effects like cytokine release syndrome (CRS), which is one of the most prevalent toxicities detected after CAR-T cell therapy. CRS is a systemic inflammatory phenomenon derived from overproduction of pro-inflammatory cytokines, including tumor necrosis factor-alpha (TNF-α), interferon-gamma (IFN-γ), IL-6, and IL-1β that may lead to tissue injury and multi-organ dysfunction (Shimabukuro-Vornhagen et al. 2018). Moreover, in addition to cancer cells, some target antigens are typically expressed on healthy cells and are targeted by CAR cells. In this case, CAR-T cells lead to normal tissue damage introduced as "on-target/off-tumor" toxicity (Davila and Brentjens 2016). Neurotoxicity is another critical side effect after administration of CAR-T cells and is characterized by aphasia, tremor, changed mental condition, headache, seizures, and life-threatening cerebral edema symptoms. It used to be called "T CAR-associated encephalopathy syndrome" and is now referred to as "immune cell-associated neurotoxicity syndrome (ICANS)." ICANS is related to a disturbance of the blood-brain barrier so that cerebrospinal fluid cytokine levels may rise. It frequently occurs alongside or after CRS (Lee et al. 2019). Anaphylaxis is another crucial adverse effect of CAR-T cell therapy that arises following the prescription of murine ScFv-derived CAR-T cells. Based upon this, murine protein immunogenicity triggers the undesired immune responses and leads to acute anaphylaxis (Maus et al. 2013). As a result, measures must be taken to address the challenges that prevent the best performance of CAR-T cells and to restrict the side effects of these cells. Regarding the importance of this issue, two substantial and practical solutions; engineering armored CAR-T cells and combining CAR-T cells with other cancer treatments, have been developed to improve the efficiency and safety of CAR-T cell therapy in cancer treatment.

5 Efficacy Improvement Strategies of CAR-T Cells

As described previously, numerous factors cause the malfunction of CAR-T cells or reduce their ability to fight the tumors. Based on the importance of this issue, administrating CAR-T cell therapy in combination with other cancer treatments such as chemotherapy, radiotherapy, checkpoint inhibitors, cytokines, cancer vaccines, oncolytic viruses, and immunomodulatory agents (Fig. 2), as well as applying the genetic engineering methods, including gene expression changes with CRISPR/Cas9 mechanism, epigenetic manipulations, programmable and equipped (armored) CAR-T cell engineering, and switch mechanism (Fig. 3), are considered as the novel cutting-edge technologies that have emerged to enhance CAR-T cell efficiency and are discussed in detail below.

5.1 Combination Therapy of CAR-T Cells

5.1.1 CAR-T Cell Therapy with Radiotherapy

As long as antigen presentation by dendritic cells is sustained, tumoricidal responses of T lymphocytes are maintained, and immune system mechanisms are enhanced by radiation. It is reasonable to assume that radiotherapy may have enhancing and even synergistic effects on the treatment regimen (DeSelm et al. 2018). Radiation has been utilized in conjunction with other therapeutics such as checkpoint inhibitors and tumor vaccines as an excellent supplementary treatment (Shevtsov et al. 2019). MHC class I expression is increased by radiotherapy, which boosts peptide production and antigen presentation to maximize cytotoxic T cell identification and enhance the effectiveness of adoptive T cell immunotherapy both locally and remotely (Reits et al. 2006). According to some research, radiotherapy can make tumor cells more sensitive to tumor-specific cytotoxic lymphocytes, which provides feasible access for them. The tumor cells will be eradicated due to this (Sharma et al. 2011a, b).

Radiation not only trigger the secretion of pro-inflammatory cytokines such as IL-6, IL-1α/β, and TNF-α by activating NF-kB and IFN-α/β, but it also aids in the release of IFN-γ and DAMPs (damage-associated molecular patterns), which

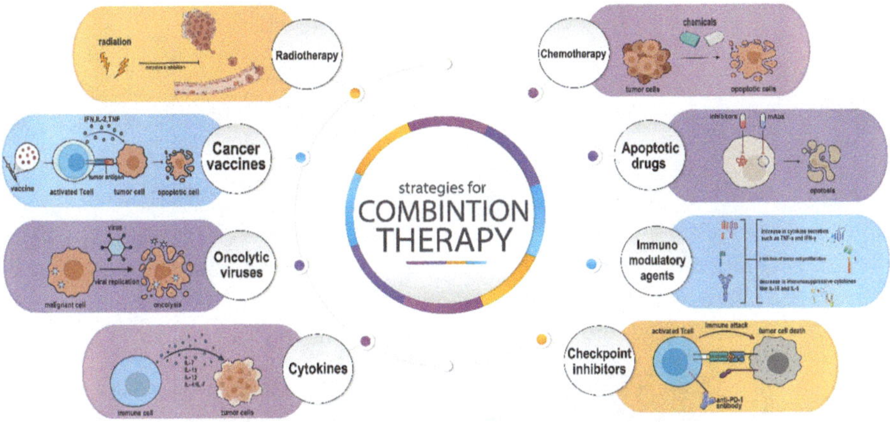

Fig. 2 CAR-T cell combination therapy. Combining CAR-T cell therapy with other cancer treatments enhances the efficacy and safety of CAR-T cells. *Chemotherapy* with CAR strengthens immune system function, reduces tumor burden, increases active dendritic cells (DCs), elevates the migration of DC and T cells to the tumor site, and suppresses immunosuppressive cells. *Radiotherapy* with CAR stimulates the production of inflammatory cytokines, increases the migration of T cells to the tumor site, prevents tumor escape, and inhibits tumor growth and metastasis. *Cancer vaccines* with CAR increase the activation of T cells and their effective function in tumor regression. *Apoptotic drugs* with CAR reduce the tumor cell resistance, induce the TNF-α-dependent apoptosis pathway, and reduce the expression of anti-apoptotic proteins. *Oncolytic viruses* with CAR enhance the migration, accumulation, and function of T cells at the tumor site and reverse the immunosuppressive state of the TME. *Immunomodulatory agents* with CAR trigger immunological synapses, increase CAR persistence and cytotoxicity, inhibit the production of anti-inflammatory cytokines, and induce the production of inflammatory cytokines. *Cytokines* with CAR block anti-inflammatory cytokines and elevate inflammatory cytokines. *Checkpoint inhibitors* with CAR prevent inhibition of T cells and increase the activity of effector cells in TME

stimulate the entry of immune effector cells into the tumor microenvironment and boost their activity (Ganss et al. 2002; Spiotto et al. 2016). In addition, local irradiation may increase the expression of specific chemokines such (CXCL) 1, 2, 9, 10, and 16 in the tumor microenvironment, increasing T cell entrance (Zhang et al. 2007). The dual aspect of radiation against cancers distinguishes it. Radiation not only causes tumor immunity by boosting CTLs on the local level, but it can also have an inhibitory effect on distal cancers. As a result, in addition to the anti-tumor effect at the local level, metastasis suppression can be accomplished remotely (Demaria et al. 2004).

CAR-T cells are now being tested in several clinical trials combined with other therapies. For example, Duke University research examines the safety and efficacy of EGFRvIII CAR-T cells combined with radiation therapy (NCT02664363). According to the authors, radiotherapy had synergistic or additive effects on CAR-T cell therapy and could be a promising treatment for malignancies. The first findings of a study by Weiss et al. (2018) suggest that radiation can improve CAR-T cell activity in solid tumors. In an orthotopic mouse model of glioblastoma, radiation

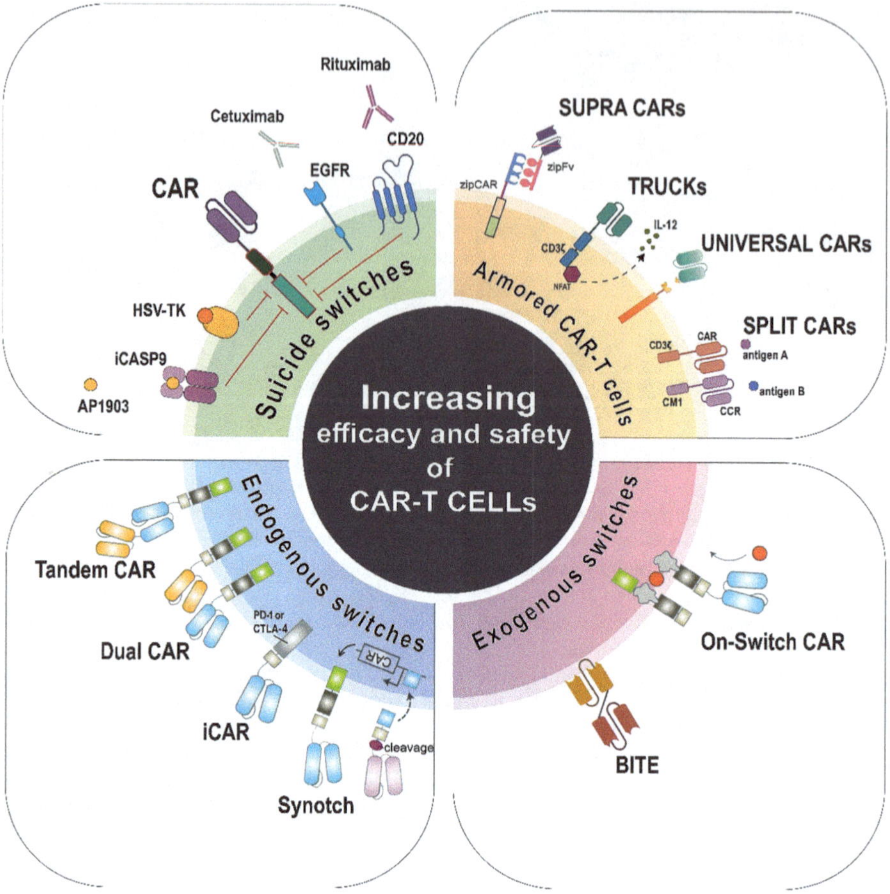

Fig. 3 **Armored and switch-based CAR-T cells.** *Armored CARs* are engineered to express proteins, reduce immunosuppression, and further mediate anti-tumor efficacy. They contain SUPRA CARs (antigen-binding zipFv containing a matching leucine zipper), TRUCKs (CAR-T cells armed with immune-stimulatory cytokines), UNIVERSAL CARs ("off-the-shelf," or allogeneic, CAR-T cells), and SPLIT CARs (a first-generation CAR and a chimeric co-stimulatory CAR (CCR)). *Exogenous switches* consist of on-switch CARs (enabling protein-protein interactions to be regulated by small molecules), and BITE CARs (recombinant proteins made of two scFv from two different antibodies). *Endogenous switches* contain SynNotch receptor CARs (activate a transcriptional output when they recognize their cognate antigen), iCARs (consist of an inhibitory signaling domain of immunoinhibitory receptors (PD-1 and CTLA-4) to restrict T-cell activity), DUAL CARs (consist of two separate CAR constructs), and TANDEM CARs (two tandemly linked scFvs targeting different tumor antigens coupled with one activation domain). *Suicide switches* contain iCasp9 (activates the downstream caspase molecules, resulting in apoptosis of CAR-T cells), HSV-tk (leading to inhibition of DNA synthesis and the cellular death using toxic GCV-triphosphate), and CAR-T cells expressing CD20 or EGFRt which can be targeted by rituximab and cetuximab, respectively

increased NKG2D-expressing CAR-T cells (natural killer group 2D receptor) synergistically. NKG2D connects to a variety of ligands, which may reduce the possibility of antigen escape on the one hand. Still, it exacerbates off-tumor death by attaching to nonmalignant cells.

According to a report by DeSelm et al. (2018), antigen escape can result in monotherapy failure in the treatment of solid malignancies. They looked at an orthotopic pancreatic cancer type with 25% of the cells missing sialyl-Lewis A, the tumor-associated antigen for the CAR-T cells used in the test. Due to the proapoptotic TRAIL ligand released by activated CAR-T cells, combined therapy of low-dose sensitizing radiation and CAR-T cell therapy resulted in better responses, whereas CAR-T cell monotherapy did not. This finding supports the notion that a combination of radiation and CAR-T cells can overcome antigen escape and significantly destroy tumor cells by enhancing antigen expression.

5.1.2 CAR-T Cell Therapy with Chemotherapy

Chemotherapy can augment the effectiveness of CAR-T cell therapy. Clinical trials have indicated that monotherapy is less useful than a combination of chemotherapy and CAR-T cell therapy. Utilizing both of them together has a more noticeable therapeutic impact. They cannot destroy tumor cells and prevent metastasis when used alone, leading to tumor recurrence. According to some research, a combination of chemotherapy and immunotherapy should be used in the near future (Bracci et al. 2014; Anampa et al. 2018). Chemotherapy boosts immune function while also lowering tumor burden. This technique increases the amount of mature and active DCs) in the tumor microenvironment, as well as the migration of DCs and T cells. When chemotherapy is used before other techniques, it can enhance the immunogenicity of T cells and raise the probability of lymphocyte presence in the area (Muranski et al. 2006).

Also, chemotherapy inhibits the activity of immunosuppressive cells such as regulatory T cells (Tregs) and myeloid-derived suppressor cells (MDSCs), as well as immunosuppressive cytokines such as IL-10 and TGF-β. As a result, combining CAR-T cell therapy with chemotherapy can have positive results in improving antitumor efficacy. Maher et al. found that chemotherapy with a standard dose of carboplatin had synergistic effects on CAR-T cells that target Erb-B and sensitized tumor cells in research (Parente-Pereira et al. 2013). According to some studies, chemotherapeutic drugs have a more significant effect on immunosuppressive cells than Tregs and are not toxic (Heylmann et al. 2013). Another effect of chemotherapy is its role in boosting tumor antigen detection and presenting them to T lymphocytes by DCs. According to current research, several chemotherapeutic drugs, such as taxanes and vinca alkaloids, can make tumor cell detection easier by increasing calreticulin exposure and destroying tumor cells by creating a large number of tumor antigens (Paulsson and Micke 2014). Recent research has shown that early CAR-T cell therapy without integrating other approaches results in lower persistence of CAR-T cells and poor tumor treatment outcomes. As a result, combining CAR-T cells with other medicines such as chemotherapy will boost the likelihood of successful treatment. This results in a correct equilibrium that maximizes the efficacy of both medicines (Lamers et al. 2011). So far, the impact of chemotherapy on CAR-T cell therapy has been studied, but a study also showed that CAR-T cells could improve the performance of chemotherapy. According to Wang et al., adaptive T cells can reduce and even eliminate ovarian tumor cell resistance to treatment by producing IFN-γ. They discovered that fibroblast-produced glutathione and cysteine contribute to chemoresistance, and IFN-γ can alter fibroblast metabolism via the Janus kinase 1/signal transducer and transcription 1 signaling pathway activator (JAK-STAT). As a result, CAR-T cells can overcome chemoresistance (Wang et al. 2016). All these studies shed new light on maximizing the potential of CAR-T cells in the treatment of tumors and open new perspectives for further research into the functional significance of these methods.

5.1.3 Cancer Vaccine

Cancer vaccines are immunotherapeutic approaches that can optimize immune response by disposing of tumor-associated epitopes to induce adaptive immune system as a target tool. So, combining cancer vaccines with CAR-T cells can be a proper solution to overcome some limitations of CAR-T cell therapy like downregulation of target antigen, exhaustion, etc. (Bansal and Reshef 2021). Notably, monotherapy of cancer vaccines has shown a small amount of clinical effectiveness, so the attention of the researchers has been focused on combining this approach with other immunotherapeutic methods, such as CAR-T cells. This therapeutic combination technique would enhance CAR-T cell therapy, including direct stimulation of dual/bispecific CAR-T cells and stimulation of CAR-T cells through HLA-dependent pathways (Avigan and Rosenblatt 2018). In the cellular vaccines platform, the whole cell or just cellular components are applied as an antigen source as well as a carrier of antigen to antigen-presenting cells (APCs). To achieve this, different cells can be exploited in cellular vaccine approaches, like tumor cells, irradiated immortalized cell lines, and dendritic cells (DCs) (Le et al. 2010). Accordingly, Caruana et al. (2015) tried to evaluate the combination of CAR-T cell with a whole-cell vaccine by engineering a CAR-redirected virus-specific cytotoxic T cell (CAR-CMV-CTLs). In this case, GD2-specific CAR was transduced into cytomegalovirus (CMV)-cytotoxic T cells (CTLs) to made a dual-specific T cell. As a result, the vaccine led to better in vivo anti-tumor effects of adoptively transferred CAR-CMV-CTLs among xenogeneic models of neuroblastoma without significant side effects. This cellular approach not only benefits from the faster cross-presentation of viral epitopes as MHC on APCs but also can easily be manipulated ex vivo to express co-stimulatory molecules like CD40L and OX40L. The DC-based vaccine has been developed through ex vivo activation of DCs by loading specific antigens to induce immunological memory and prevent relapse (Le et al. 2010). As tumor relapse is one of the obstacles of CAR-T cell therapy in hematological malignancies, it can be overcome via combining CAR-T cell therapy with DC-based vaccines. According to Wu et al. (2019), epidermal growth factor receptor (EGFR) pathway substrate 8 (Eps8)-DC vaccine co-cultured with CD19 CAR-T cells resulted in longer in vitro persistence and better expansion of CARs, synergistic effect on cytolysis of Eps8+ target cells, and increased production of IL-2 and TNF-α upon stimulation with $CD19^+$ leukemia cells.

Different molecules are involved in molecular-based vaccine therapy against cancers, like peptides, RNA, and DNA vaccines. Most of them follow the same mechanism in which they load specific antigens into APCs to induce T cells, and, therefore, CAR-T cell efficacy can be boosted. Based on this, Chan et al. (2020) combined a nanoparticulate vaccination platform with CAR-T cell therapy. They encapsulated ovalbumin (OVA) peptides into Clec9A-tailored nanoemulsion (OVA-Clec9A-TNE) and then combined with the dual-specific CAR, so-called CAROT. It was found that adoptive transfer of CAROT cells in combination with the OVA-Clec9A-TNE vaccine led to durable remission as well as the significant proliferation and anti-tumor activity of CAROT cells, high levels of tumor-infiltrating DCs, and permanent immune response memory.

5.1.4 Apoptotic Agents

One of the current strategies to fight against the tumor microenvironment is to target apoptotic pathways. The anticancer therapeutic agents that attack apoptotic roots are in the pass of further advancements. Then, to improve the clinical outcomes in cancerous patients, the mentioned drugs can be combined with the other anticancer methods, such as radiotherapy, chemotherapy, and immunotherapy (Carneiro and El-Deiry 2020). A study demonstrated that the administration of histone deacetylase inhibitors like suberoylanilide hydroxamic acid (SAHA) and nonsteroidal anti-inflammatory drugs (NSAIDs) like celecoxib along with CD19-CAR-T cells in non-Hodgkin's lymphoma (NHL) could reduce the resistance of tumor cells against CD19-CAR-T cells. The described drugs have shown potent efficacy on the CAR-T cell therapy of NHL; moreover, they have influenced tumor necrosis factor-related apoptosis-inducing ligand (TRAIL) apoptotic pathway to decrease the resistance of the tumor microenvironment (Torres-Collado and Jazirehi 2018). Other studies showed that using B cell lymphoma-2 (BCL-2) inhibitors, such as ABT-263/Navitoclax and ABT-737 with CAR-T cell, could prompt the apoptosis pathway and even be more effective cytotoxicity in B cell malignancies (Wilson et al. 2010; Karlsson et al. 2013). According to research, one of the reasons for the long-lasting survival and apoptosis-resistant state of the cancerous cells is the overexpression of anti-apoptotic proteins like the BCL-2 family members (Mcl-1, Bcl-xl, and Bcl-2). Thus, the tumor cells could be sensitized to apoptosis by administering apoptosis inhibitor blockade agents (AIBAs) like MCl-1, COX, and Bcl-2 inhibitors. Subsequently, combining the CAR-T cells with AIBAs would have better clinical quality and more efficient outcomes in treating cancers (Yang et al. 2019).

5.1.5 Cytokines

As is well-known, the tumor microenvironment makes an immunosuppressive state through secreting some anti-inflammatory cytokines, such as colony-stimulating factor-1 (CSF-1), TGF-β, IL-4, and IL-10. The mentioned cytokine creates an atmosphere to support the growth of the tumor cells and preserve them from devastating by the immune system. Hence, it would be a promising strategy to produce further designs in CAR-T cells to protect them against the immunosuppressive TME (Wang et al. 2020). In a study, it has been demonstrated that secreting

TGF-β DNR II or TGF-β receptors by the CAR-T cells in a melanoma tumor model environment reduced the immunosuppressive potential of TGF-β (Zhang et al. 2013). Other related research had engineered prostate-specific membrane antigen (PSMA) CAR-T cell to express TGF-β DNR, which had improved the secretion of pro-inflammatory cytokines. Also, this engineered CAR-T cell had promoted the innate and acquired immune system responses (Kloss et al. 2018). Thus, designing the CAR structure to express TGF-β DNR would be an optimal strategy for better therapeutic consequences. A study also engineered TGF-β/CD28 CAR-T cells, which contained CD28-CD3ζ signaling and TGF-β binding domains. According to their results, TGF-β/CD28 CAR-T cells demonstrated the reassuring anti-tumor function (Chang et al. 2018). Additionally, some researches have represented principles to generate IL-4-enhanced CAR-T cells (Wilkie et al. 2010; Mohammed et al. 2017). One of the studies had created a co-expressed IL-4-/IL-7-inverted cytokine receptor (4/7 ICR), which was the fusion of the IL-7 receptor endodomain with the IL-4 exodomain receptor on the PSCA-CAR-T cells. This engineered CAR-T cell proved the anti-tumor efficacy in pancreatic cancer (Mohammed et al. 2017). It is worth considering that the administration of some pro-inflammatory cytokines, including IL-15, IL-12, IL-7, and IL-23 in CAR structures, is another way to engineer cytokine-armored CAR-T cells (Singh et al. 2016; Huang et al. 2020; Ma et al. 2020). Overall, combining the CAR-T cells with the tumor-derived cytokines would remain a promising approach to improve the anti-tumor efficacy of the CAR-T cells. Importantly, we should notice the cytokines that somehow deteriorated the CAR-T cell-induced CRS. Some cytokines like IL-15 and IL-12, which affect the production of IFN-γ, IL-1, or IL-6, could worsen the CRS. Hence, the researchers should consider the toxicity levels of the cytokine-secreting CAR-T cells to reduce the CRS occurrence (Bell and Gottschalk 2021).

5.1.6 Immune Checkpoint Inhibitors

If the excessive functions of the immune system occur, checkpoint signaling routes will balance it by suppressing the extreme immune activities. Notably, cancerous cells abuse the ability of immune checkpoints to run away from immune system surveillance. Nowadays, one of the immunotherapeutic methods is to inhibit immune checkpoints from amplifying the anti-tumor immune responses (Ribas and Wolchok 2018). Due to the low clinical responses of immune checkpoint inhibitors, researchers have decided to combine this strategy with CAR-T cells in cancer treatments.

A study has demonstrated that the programmed cell death protein 1 (PD-1) blockage in the murine breast cancer model could enhance the expression of granzyme B and IFN-γ and develop CAR-T cell therapy's function by promoting the T cell activities in vivo and in vitro (John et al. 2013). The other research has shown that the combined administration of CAR-T cell with pembrolizumab (anti-PD-1 mAb) in metastatic melanoma prolonged the persistence of CAR-T cells and improved the expression of IFN-γ and TNF-α (Gargett et al. 2016). Considerably, obtaining the therapeutic amount of PD-1 inhibitor agents in the tumor microenvironment is infrequent. Hence, the systemic administration of these factors is required. After that, the systemic infusion of PD-1 blockade would have some adverse effects in multi-organs, including nephritis, hepatitis, hypothyroidism, dermatitis, etc. Thus, besides the beneficial outcomes of combining CAR-T cells and anti-PD-1 agents, they would have deteriorating consequences that should be notified (Hofmann et al. 2016; Shivaji et al. 2019).

Furthermore, inhibiting the other checkpoints such as T cell immunoglobulin and mucin-domain-containing-3 (TIM3), cytotoxic T lymphocyte-associated protein 4 (CTLA-4; CD154), and lymphocyte activation gene 3 (LAG3; CD223) also could be combined with CAR-T cell in treating cancers (Grosser et al. 2019). Interestingly, the administration of CRISPR/Cas9 is one of the latest novel strategies in inhibiting immune checkpoints. This technique can delete the gene loci that participate in the expression of immune checkpoint receptors. A study has shown the extreme activity of CAR-T cells in vitro and in vivo in the lymphoma xenograft model, followed by knocking out the lymphocyte activation gene 3 (LAG3) (Zhang et al. 2017). Research in 2019 demonstrated that targeting the PDCD1 and mesothelin gene loci by CRISPR/Cas9 elicited the improvement of cytotoxicity and cytokine secretion of modified CAR-T cells. Moreover, tumor relapse was decreased in vivo (Steinfeld et al. 2015).

5.1.7 Oncolytic Viruses

Oncolytic virotherapy is one of the recent immunotherapeutic approaches, which administrates cancer killer cells to target tumor cells and induce adaptive and acquired immune system responses at a significant level. This method can also be combined with other strategies, such as CAR-T cell therapy. This approach could develop the persistence of CAR-T cells in the tumor site through reversing the tumor-associated immunosuppression, preventing antigen loss, and arming with the therapeutic agents like chemokines (Russell et al. 2012; Zhang et al. 2021).

One research reported the enhanced accumulation of CAR-T cells in the tumor site and increased susceptibility of tumor cells to the anti-cancerous effects of CAR-T cells by combining the oncolytic adenovirus expressing IL-15 and CCL5 (RANTES) with GD2-CAR-T cells in neuroblastoma xenograft mouse model (Nishio et al. 2014). Another study represented the promising results following the combined administration of engineered oncolytic virus expressing IL-12 and TNF-α with CAR-T cells in the pancreatic ductal adenocarcinoma murine model. After that, this method resulted in the polarization of M1 macrophage and the maturation of dendritic cells, which could overcome the immunosuppressive environment. Also, this combining strategy prevented cancer metastasis by inhibiting anti-inflammatory cytokines and promoting inflammatory cytokine expression (Watanabe et al. 2018). In another study, researchers have combined three treatment approaches, including immune checkpoint inhibitors, oncolytic virus, and CAR-T cell, which led to the prolonged survival in xenograft prostate cancer mouse model compared to the prescription of monotherapy (Tanoue et al. 2017).

It has been proved that intratumoral injection of oncolytic viruses could be implied in nonmetastatic cancers. Considerably, the systemic utilization of oncolytic viruses has some circumscriptions and pitfalls like being identified by the host immune system and being neutralized. Therefore, a study recommended loading oncolytic viruses into human and murine CAR-T cells in vitro. The following demonstrated that oncolytic viruses were delivered appropriately by the abovementioned method, and there was no alteration of CAR expression. Moreover, this approach enhanced the anti-tumor function of CAR-T cells (Van Seggelen et al. 2015; Slaney et al. 2017). Of note, the therapeutic dose of oncolytic viruses would be high due to the host immune response against them. In vitro research has been designed to solve this problem by combining CAR-T cells with low-dose oncolytic viruses. Study findings indicated that CAR-T cells transferred the oncolytic viruses to the tumor cells (Van Seggelen et al. 2015). Also, the researchers have combined oncolytic viruses with CAR-T cells in treating neuroblastoma and head and neck cancers in animal studies. They have administrated CAR-T cells along with the Ad5Δ24 virus, leading to prolonged survival of CAR-T cells in the neuroblastoma environment (Nishio et al. 2014).

5.1.8 Immunomodulatory Agents

One of the current methods in cancer treatment is to combine the CAR-T cells with immunomodulatory drugs. This strategy assists CAR-T cells in increasing their persistence, proliferation, and cytokine secretion in the tumor microenvironment (Schafer et al. 2003). Based on the recent study (Wang et al. 2018), the co-treatment of CAR-T cells and lenalidomide as an immunomodulatory agent showed promising results in treating multiple myeloma mice cancer models. Accordingly, lenalidomide strengthened the formation of immunological synapses between CAR-T cells and myeloma cells, improved the cytotoxicity and persistence of CAR-T cells, increased the proliferation of CTLs, enhanced the secretion of cytokines such as TNF-α and IFN-γ, and also inhibited the expression of immunosuppressive cytokines like IL-10 and IL-4. Moreover, in the colon cancer xenograft model, the co-administration of CAR-T cells and IDO enzyme inhibitors (miR-153) represented efficient outcomes in eradicating tumor cells (Hornyák et al. 2018; Huang et al. 2018). Additionally, another research reported an impressive remission of ALL patients following the co-treatment of CD19-CAR-T cells and decitabine (Li et al. 2019). Moreover, co-treating of CD33-CAR-T cells and decitabine has eradicated tumor cells through upregulating CD33 in AML cell lines (Xue et al. 2019). The study represented the prolonged survival and increased cytotoxicity of CAR-T cells in Burkitt's lymphoma mouse model due to co-treating with CD20-CAR-T cell and romidepsin, a histone deacetylase inhibitor (HDACis) agent (Xu et al. 2019). According to research (Laurent et al. 2015), γ-secretase complex (GS), an intramembrane protease, is releasing the soluble B cell maturation antigen (BCMA) to the circulation through cleaving the BCMA. In the following, GS decreases the function of CAR-T cells. Thus, administrating γ-secretase inhibitors (GSIs) would be a potent strategy to enhance the effectiveness of CAR-T cells. Pont et al. exhibited the enhancement of BCMA levels and reduced sBCMA levels via utilizing BCMA-CAR-T cells and GSIs in preclinical cancer models. Their research showed the notable anti-tumor effect of CAR-T cells (Pont et al. 2019). Furthermore, other studies have notified the combination therapy of CAR-T cells with the second mitochondrial-derived activator caspase (SMAC) mimetics to obtain impressive outcomes in cancer therapeutic methods (Petersen et al. 2007; Michie et al. 2019).

5.2 Armored CAR-T Cells

5.2.1 TRUCKs

The fourth generation of CAR-T cells, so-called T cell redirected for antigen-unrestricted cytokine-initiated killing (TRUCK), a specific type of armored CAR-T cells, is designed to produce transgenic cytokines or various biological molecules via transduction of relevant encoding genes into CAR structure. TRUCK can modulate the cytokine profile in TME, generate the immune-activating conditions, and augment the anti-tumor activity of CAR-T cells as well as resident immune cells in the tumor site (Chmielewski and Abken 2020). Previously published reports documented that CAR-T cells producing IL-12 reduced tumor cell growth and led to antigen-independent anti-tumor activity by accumulating the macrophages in the tumor site (Chmielewski et al. 2011). Furthermore, CAR-T cells, along with the inducible secretion of IL-15, exhibited boosted tumor cytotoxicity in vitro and in vivo, as well as potent protection against tumor in vivo. IL-15 could also increase the proliferation, expansion, and persistence of T cells in vitro, independently of the antigen (Hurton et al. 2016; Chen et al. 2019). Similarly, CAR-T cells with the inducible secretion of IL-18 effectively mitigated tumor cell growth and improved survival in the pancreatic cancer mice model (Chmielewski and Abken 2017). Armored CAR-T cell releasing IL-7 has also been found to be resistant to immunosuppressive effects of TGF-β in addition to amplified proliferation and cytotoxicity (Golumba-Nagy et al. 2018). Interestingly, the CAR-T cell expressing the dominant-negative TGF-β receptor II (dnTGF-βRII) has been found to prevent the immunosuppressive function of TGF-β, increasing the persistence and proliferation of CAR-T cell, decrease the CAR-T cell exhaustion, and improve the anti-tumor cytotoxicity in vivo (Kloss et al. 2018). In the same way, altering the CAR-T cell response to IL-4, another immunosuppressive cytokine, via designing a CAR expressing the hybrid IL-4/IL-7 receptor (the exodomain of the IL-4 receptor that was fused to the IL-7 intracellular domain) indicated the augmented proliferation, persistence, and cytotoxicity of CAR-T cells as well as effective tumor cell eradication (Mohammed et al. 2017). Based on the abovementioned details, TRUCK CAR-T cells exhibit potent capabilities in stimulating the bystander anti-tumor immune responses, increased cytotoxicity, proliferation, and persistence in TME, which can be more effective in combating tumors than other generations.

5.2.2 Universal CARs

The universal CAR-T cell is formed by combining the conventional CAR structure with a separate system consisting of an extracellular adapter. In response to a soluble tumor antigen-targeting ligand bound to the tumor antigen, the extracellular adaptor is linked to the intracellular signaling domain of T cell that leads to synapses and

CAR-T cell activation (Zhao et al. 2018). Anti-tag CARs, antibody-dependent cellular cytotoxicity (ADCC), mediating immune receptors, tag-specific interaction receptors, and bispecific protein engaging immune receptors are the different kinds of universal CARs developed to improve CAR-T cell performance (Tahmasebi et al. 2021). Using the allogeneic healthy donor T cells instead of autologous cells with low cost and short time without complex equipment is one of the main benefits of the universal CAR structure. The sufficient number of allogeneic derived CAR-T cells provides the appropriate therapeutic choice for patients with severe diseases and require immediate treatment (Schmidts and Maus 2018; Zhao et al. 2018). The risk of graft-versus-host disease (GVHD) has also been resolved by removing the allogenic T cell TCR gene or HLA-A locus from T cells (Torikai et al. 2013). As another advantage, the split structure of universal CAR paves the way to target the multiple different antigens on the tumor cell surface without requiring to design new CAR-T cell and overcomes the antigen heterogeneity challenge in most solid cancers (Urbanska et al. 2012). On the other hand, the "on switch" feature of universal CAR has made it more flexible and controllable, resulting in CAR-T cell activation only in the presence of a soluble adaptor molecule. This manageable mechanism brings the targeting antigen specifically and confines the "on-target/off-tumor" toxicity (Cho et al. 2018). The anti-tag-specific universal receptor is the ScFv receptor that recognizes the tumor antigens conjugated with small tags, ligands, or antibodies. CAR-T cell is activated and exerts its cytotoxicity by engaging the anti-tag ScFv receptor with the tag-labeled tumor antigens. The fluorescein isothiocyanate (FITC), the peptide neo-epitope (PNE), and the peptide of nuclear antigen-La-SS-B (E5B9) are the examples of tag molecules used to engineer these types of CAR-T cells (Tamada et al. 2012). In ADCC-mediated universal CAR, engagement of FcgRIIIa (CD16) with an anti-tumor specific IgG, as an extracellular adaptor domain, composes the CAR structure and elicits tumor lysis via antibody-dependent cellular cytotoxicity (ADCC). Promising outcomes have been obtained from investigating the CD16 universal CAR-T cell in HER2-positive cancer, non-Hodgkin's lymphoma, and multiple myeloma undergoing clinical trials (D'Aloia et al. 2016). The tag-specific immune receptor is another type of universal CARs that acts based on ligand-ligand interaction. The biotin-binding immune receptor (BBIR), a tag-specific immune receptor, is bound to the T cell intracellular domain and connects the T cell to tumor antigen via binding to the biotinylated antigen-specific molecules like monoclonal antibodies (mAbs). This armored CAR-T cell provides potent and specific responses to biotinylated tumor antigens without targeting the non-biotinylated antigens; therefore, it prevents bystander cell damage, as well (Lohmueller et al. 2017). Bispecific protein engaging immune receptor is another kind of universal CARs that leads to the engagement of extracellular domain of the universal receptor and target antigen on the tumor cell surface via a bispecific antibody. An example of bispecific immune receptor CAR structure is engineered universal CAR that redirects the T cell to simultaneously target folate receptor (FRa) and CD20 antigens expressing tumor cells (Urbanska et al. 2014).

5.2.3 SUPRA CARs

A split, universal, and programmable (SUPRA) CAR is an armored and multi-targeted-switchable CAR consisting of universal receptor and ScFv adaptor molecule. This type of CAR is specified by the flexible structure and capability of targeting multiple antigens with high efficacy and safety under controllable mechanisms (Tahmasebi et al. 2021). A universal receptor-expressing T cell called zipCAR (intracellular signaling domain linked to an extracellular domain) and a tumor-targeting ScFv adaptor, so-called zipFV (ScFv and cognate leucine) zipper), are two main sections of the SUPRA system. zipFV is responsible for antigen recognition and establishing immunological synapses, which subsequently accompanies CAR activation and signaling mediated by zipCAR. As a prominent feature, SUPRA CAR can lead to tumor cell killing by simultaneously targeting the multiple antigens without reengineering the different CAR-T cells. To target the myelogenous leukemia cells, Cho et al. (2018) designed mad then evaluated a SUPRA CAR system from human primary T CD8+ cells, which was made up of zipCAR (CD3ζ, CD28, and 4-1BB domains) and three different zipFVs targeting the α-Her2, α-Axl, and α-mesothelin antigens. The findings of this study illustrated the fantastic concepts of SUPRA CARs, which are briefly mentioned in the following. As described previously, conventional CAR-T cell acts with no controllable mechanism; however, SUPRA CAR solves this limitation and elicits safe responses. Moreover, the combinational antigen targeting feature of the SUPRA system increases the anti-tumor efficacy of CAR-T cells. In a regulatory manner, to prevent cytokine storm and other related toxicities to conventional CAR-T cells, the SUPRA system is suppressed by prescribing a competitive zipFv, which is bound to other zipFvs and inhibited the CAR-T cell function. The high potential of SUPRA CAR structure in tumor cell eradication with higher cytotoxicity and longer persistence has been demonstrated by administrating the α-Axl zipFv and α-Her2 zipFv into cell culture the Her2/Axl + tumor cells (Cho et al. 2018). Potent tumor cell killing, reducing the tumor burden, overcoming the antigen heterogeneity and antigen losing, preventing the unwanted toxicities, and possessing the excellent specificity and cytotoxicity are the brief advantages of the SUPRA CAR system that it has become a powerful therapeutic choice, especially for solid cancers.

5.2.4 Split CARs (CAR + CCR)

Split CAR structure, or in other words, CAR combined with a chimeric co-stimulatory receptor (CCR), is another potent smart CAR-T cell model. Split CAR has been developed to increase the specificity and safety of CAR-T cells and prevent "on-target/off-tumor" toxicity on bystander tissues. In this structure, T cells express two CARs with different tumor antigen recognition regions (ScFvs); one is specific for tumor antigen A with the CD3ζ main signaling domain (signal 1), and the other is specific for tumor antigen B with the co-stimulatory signaling domain (signal 2). The activation and function of CAR-T cells are the results of the cooperation of both CARs in recognizing both target antigens expressed at the tumor cell surface. In this case, the detection of antigen B stimulates the co-stimulatory CAR signaling, which induces the signaling of the next CAR containing CD3ζ and leads to the recognition of antigen A, the final anti-tumor response (Rafiq et al. 2020; Tahmasebi et al. 2021). Accordingly, the effective tumor destruction of split CAR-T cells has been proved in prostate cancer. It was mediated by the first generation of CAR against prostate-specific membrane antigen (PSMA) in combination with the chimeric co-stimulatory receptor (CCR) against prostate stem cell antigen (PSCA) (Kloss et al. 2013).

6 Safety and Specificity Improvement Strategies of CAR-T Cells

Another important aspect of employing CAR-T cells in cancer treatment is paying more attention to their safety, specifically targeting and minimizing the related adverse effects. On the one hand, CAR-T cell overactivity, the presence of foreign agents in the CAR structure (mice-derived ScFv), and the absence of controlling mechanisms to quench the CAR-T cells after completed anti-tumor function cause cytokine storm, anaphylaxis, and neurotoxicity. Furthermore, less precise tumor antigen targeting as well as damage to healthy cells, which causes on-target/off-tumor toxicity, doubles the importance of designing CAR-T cells with high quality. The following describes the various developed details to improve the safety and specificity of CAR-T cells.

6.1 Suicide Switches

Engineering the CAR-T cells accompanied by suicide switches or off switches has been developed to intensify the safety and efficacy of CAR-T cells. The suicide switches are utilized to inactivate the CAR-T cells and, in this case, prevent the CRS and "on-target/off-tumor" toxicities. Indeed, these controlling regimens optimize the CAR-T cell performance and avoid the exhaustion of these engineered T cells. Based upon this, developing the CAR co-expressing with cell-surface antigens like CD20 and EGFRt to target by FDA-approved mAbs, an apoptosis-triggering fusion protein comprising caspase 9 (iCasp9), and HSV-TK enzyme producing the toxic GCV-triphosphate are the examples of developed suicide switches that have been described briefly in the following sections.

6.1.1 iCasp9

The modified human caspase 9 fused to the human FK506 binding protein (FKBP), is inducible safety switch caspase 9 (iCasp9), which is one of the most utilized suicide switches that manages the CAR-T cell function. To activate, iCasp9 needs to be dimerized via a chemical inducer of dimerization (CID) like AP1903 (Gargett and Brown 2014). After activation and downstream signaling, apoptosis is induced in CAR-T cells expressing the FKBP binding protein. As an excellent example of this approach, it can be referred to as iCasp9/CAR-CD19/IL-15-T cell, the anti-CD19 CAR-T cell co-expressing the IL-15 and iCasp9. Encouragingly, findings exhibited adequate safety and efficacy as well as more significant expansion and survival in vivo and in vitro exploiting the iCasp9/CAR-CD19/IL-15 T cell compared to lonely CD19-CAR-T cell. Besides, the expression of iCasp9 in CAR structure revealed the effective elimination of these modified T cells following their anti-tumor mission (Hoyos et al. 2010). As another example, the anti-CD20 CAR-T cell co-expressing the truncated CD19 (ΔCD19) selectable marker and iCasp9, named iCasp9/CAR-CD20/ΔCD19 T cell, indicated the potent cytotoxicity and cytokine secretion against CD20-expressing tumor cells. It has been obtained that administration of AP1903 led to the elimination of 90% and 98% of modified T cells during 24 h and 72 h, respectively. As an exciting outcome, CID prescription does not affect the non-modified T cells even in high concentrations (Budde et al. 2013). Moreover, the iCasp9/CAR-CD19/ΔNGFR T cells containing iCasp9 and truncated nerve growth factor receptor (ΔNGFR) resulted in effective tumor cell killing in vitro. Similarly, this safety switch regimen elicited the potent cytotoxicity against CD19 expressing tumor cells and prevented B cell aplasia, known as an "on-target/off-tumor" toxicity (Diaconu et al. 2017). The iCasp9/CAR-CD33/ΔCD19 T cells against CD33-positive acute myeloid leukemia (AML) blasts and multipotent myeloid precursors demonstrated potent cytotoxicity and great safety (Minagawa et al. 2016). The iCasp9/CAR-IL-1RAP T cells showed the effective targeting of the interleukin-1 receptor accessory protein (IL-1RAP)-positive chronic myeloid leukemia (CML) cells with great production of pro-inflammatory cytokine in vitro and in vivo, as well (Warda et al. 2019).

6.1.2 HSV.TK

Herpes simplex virus thymidine kinase (HSV-TK) is another useful suicide gene applied for managing the CAR-T cell function alongside ganciclovir (GCV) (Vassaux and Martin-Duque 2004). HSV-TK catalyzes the phosphorylation of GCV and converts it to the toxic component, the so-called GCV-triphosphate. This toxic compound acts as a substrate for the DNA polymerase enzyme with the corporation in the DNA structure, inhibiting DNA synthesis and cell death (Matthews and Boehme 1988). HSV-TK suicide gene is mainly utilized to prevent the GVHD after hematopoietic stem cell transplantation (HSCT) in donor lymphocyte infusion and after haploidentical hematopoietic stem cell transplantation (haplo-HSCT) in leukemia patients (Ciceri et al. 2007, 2009). As an example, it has been reported that CD44 isoform variant 6 (CD44v6)-CAR-T cell that was armored to express HSV-TK indicated the effective anti-tumor cytotoxicity against CD44v6, an overexpressed antigen in multiple myeloma (MM) and acute myeloid leukemia (AML) tumor cells. Interestingly, findings revealed the successful elimination of activated CD44v6-CAR-T cells after the tumor cell killing exposed to GCV (Casucci et al. 2018). Despite the advantages of this HSV-TK enzyme in controlling CAR-T cell activity, it faces limitations, including the possibility of immunogenicity and consequent endangerment of CAR-T cell function and survival due to the viral origin of the enzyme, the need for activation with a prodrug like GCV, and also requiring a long time to remove modified T cells (Tiberghien et al. 2001; Berger et al. 2006).

6.1.3 CD20 and EGFRt

Induction of suicide by elimination genes is another controlling regimen that mediates the depletion of engineered CAR-T cells via expressing the targetable molecules. The gene-based suicide switches consist of the programed CAR-T cells expressing the known cell-surface antigens like CD20 and the truncated epidermal growth factor receptor (EGFRt) (Bonifant et al. 2016). In this strategy, the inactivation of CAR-T cells results from the antigen-antibody interaction following the infusion of specific anti-CD20 mAb (rituximab) or anti-EGFRt mAb (cetuximab). Prescription of the specific mAbs triggers cell death through antibody-dependent cell-mediated cytotoxicity (ADCC) and complement-dependent cytotoxicity (CDC). In this attractive cell control method, Food and Drug Administration (FDA)-approved antibodies are used to ensure safety. Interestingly, known cell-surface antigens expressed on CAR-T cells can be utilized as identification markers to ex vivo selection or in vivo tracking of these modified cells (Wang et al. 2011; Philip et al. 2014). One of the limitations of this strategy is the possibility of on-target toxicity derived from the mAb binding to healthy cells expressing the target antigen and subsequent antibody-dependent cellular cytotoxicity. This limitation also raises concerns in immunocompromised cancer patients who cannot clear modified CAR-T cells, especially in toxic conditions (Jones et al. 2014). In preclinical and clinical studies, mAb-based suicide switches revealed promising efficacy in managing the performance of modified CAR-T cells (Philip et al. 2014; Koneru et al. 2015). A preclinical investigation evaluated the different safety switch methodologies and demonstrated the encouraging outcomes with superior safety and efficacy utilizing the CD20/rituximab and iCap9 technologies, among other ones (Marin et al. 2012).

6.2 Endogenous Switches

The smart-multi-targeted modified CAR structures, including tandem CAR, dual CAR, and synthetic Notch receptor (Synotch) CAR, as well as inhibitory CAR like iCAR, are known as endogenous switches that have been designed to increase the safety and specificity of CAR-T cells. The great applicability of dual and tandem CARs has been highlighted in targeting a border scale of tumor antigens, lowering rate of exhaustion, and overcoming the antigen heterogeneity, antigen losing, and tumor antigen escape challenges. Also, the proficiency of the mentioned switches in alleviating the CAR-T cell side effects, particularly "on-target/off-tumor" toxicity, is another advantage of these mentioned switches.

6.2.1 Dual CARs

Both dual and tandem CAR structures simultaneously recognize the two different tumor antigens, except that the dual CAR has a separate structure with two split ScFvs and signaling domains (Shah et al. 2019). The bispecific CD19-CD22-CAR-T cell is one of the potent dual-CAR structures that has indicated the effective cytotoxicity, proliferation, and IFN-γ cytokine production in targeting the CD19+

and CD22+ tumor cells in immune-deficient mice as well as human adults with relapsed or refractory B cell acute lymphoblastic leukemia (R/R ALL) (Fry et al. 2018; Dai et al. 2020). In addition to hematological malignancies, the applicability of dual-CAR-T cells has been confirmed in solid tumors. It has been reported that dual-receptor CAR-T cell targeting mesothelin (MSLN) and carcinoembryonic antigen (CEA) that are expressed on pancreatic cancer cell lines (AsPC-1) could significantly kill the tumor cells expressing both antigens without affecting the healthy cells or single expressed antigen tumor cells. Besides, findings demonstrated the longitude persistence, increased level of cytokine production, and mitigated "on-target/off-tumor" toxicity using the CEA-MSLN-dual-CAR-T cell (Zhang et al. 2018). Similar promising outcomes were obtained in a pancreatic cancer xenograft model using the dual-CAR-T cell targeting the MUC1 and prostate stem cell antigen (PSCA) (Anurathapan et al. 2014). Interestingly, dual-targeted T cells expressing CD28-MUC1 CAR and CD3ζ-ErbB2 CAR exhibited the effective elimination of ErbB2- and MUC1-positive tumor cells, increased proliferation, and superior production of IFN-γ in the treatment of breast cancer (Wilkie et al. 2012). Similarly, dual-CAR-T cells targeting both mesothelin (Meso) and a-folate receptor (Fra) antigens on tumor cells illustrated the robust anti-tumor activity and higher persistence in an ovarian cancer xenograft model (Lanitis et al. 2013).

6.2.2 Tandem CAR

Tandem CAR (TanCAR) is another smart and bispecific CAR consisting of two sequentially ScFvs against two different target antigens with a single transmembrane and signaling domains. The potent application of TanCAR in increasing the safety and specificity of CAR-T cells has been proved in both hematological and solid cancers. Like the dual CAR, TanCAR activity confines tumor tissues expressing the two target antigens without affecting the normal cells or single positive antigen tumor cells (Grada et al. 2013; Yan and Liu 2019). For example, CD19-CD20-TanCAR exhibited the potent anti-tumor function; higher persistence; increased production of IFN-γ, TNF-α, and GM-CSF cytokines; and decreased rate of "on-target/off-tumor" toxicity in targeting the leukemia cell lines in vivo and in vitro (Zah et al. 2016; Schneider et al. 2017). Evaluating the TanCAR targeting the HER2 and IL13Rα2 antigens in the glioblastoma xenograft model demonstrated the effective interaction between CAR-T cells and tumor cells, resulting in effective tumor cell killing and cytokine production (IL-2 and IFN-γ) compared to applying mono-specific CAR-T cells (Hegde et al. 2016). Interestingly, the diminished rate of CRS and "on-target/off-tumor" toxicity were also reported as the advantages of utilizing CD19-CD133-TanCAR in targeting the positive mixed-lineage leukemia (MLL) cells in a xenograft model in addition to the potent cytotoxicity of TanCAR (Zah et al. 2016). Moreover, successful tumor cell eradication has been observed prescribing the modified CD19/CD22-TanCAR in the B-ALL xenograft model compared to utilizing the monospecific conventional CAR-T cell (Li et al. 2018).

6.2.3 Inhibitory CAR (iCAR)

To prevent the overactivation of CAR-T cells and increase their safety, utilizing inhibitory checkpoints like PD-1 and CTLA-4 would be a contributory strategy. The inhibitory checkpoints have a prominent role in regulating the immune system responses, particularly in suppressing the T cell function (Sharma et al. 2011a, b). In this case, an inhibitory chimeric antigen receptor (iCAR) has been developed to recognize the specific antigen on normal cells that are absent or downregulated in tumor cells, along with an active CAR receptor that recognizes the target antigen on tumor cells. Following the antigen recognition, iCAR suppresses the activated CAR-T cell function via PD-1 or CTLA-4 inhibitory signaling domain and dephosphorylating the activating receptor. iCAR induces inhibitory signaling despite the activated CAR receptor involvement with antigen (Fedorov et al. 2013). To restrict the CAR-T cell function, iCAR inhibits the proliferation, cytotoxicity, and cytokine production of effector CAR, reversibly and temporarily. Consequently, iCAR provides the self-regulating mechanism to enclose the CAR-T cell activity to tumor tissues and mitigate the "on-target/off-tumor" toxicity.

6.2.4 Synthetic Notch Receptor (SynNotch) CAR

Synthetic Notch receptor (SynNotch) CAR, so-called "AND-gate" CAR, is known as other endogenous switches designed for improving the safety and specificity of CAR-T cells (Morsut et al. 2016). The possibility of secreting cytokines or other biological molecules and remodeling the tumor microenvironment to enhance the anti-tumor responses are other applicable capabilities of the SynNotch receptors (Roybal et al. 2016a, b). The SynNotch receptor consists of a ligand-binding extracellular domain containing epidermal growth factor (EGF) sequences, Notch intracellular domain (NICD), and a central core. To trigger the signaling, the extracellular domain recognizes the ligands from Delta family proteins, leading to proteolysis. Subsequently, ligand-induced cleavage elicits the releasing of the intracellular transcription domain, which is activated through the entrance into the nucleus (Gordon et al. 2007; Kopan and Ilagan 2009). Therefore, the modified SynNotch receptor possesses the only central part of the transmembrane region, mediating the proteolysis and the activation of downstream genes (Yuan et al. 2015). Based upon this, SynNotch AND-gate circuits have emerged to induce the activation of CAR-T cells only in the presence of two target antigens on tumor cells, increasing the safety of CAR-T cells and protecting the bystander cells under this controlling manner. In simultaneous exposure to two tumor antigens, firstly, the SynNotch receptor recognizes the antigen A, resulting in the release of a transcriptional effector domain, which subsequently induces the expression of CAR on the T cell surface to recognize the antigen B on tumor cells (Li and Zhao 2017). Accordingly, the efficient tumor cell killing without significant toxicity has been reported as a promising outcome of evaluating the SynNotch receptor CAR in Jurkat T cells to target both CD19 and mesothelin antigens expressed on tumor cells, as well as in the primary T cells to target green fluorescent protein (GFP) and CD19 (Roybal et al. 2016a, b). As another example, anti-ROR1 CAR-T cells engineered with anti-EPCAM or B7-H3-specific SynNotch receptors indicated the selective cytotoxicity in eliminating the ROR1-positive tumor cells with no observational effects on stromal and normal cells expressing the ROR1 (Srivastava et al. 2019).

6.3 Exogenous Switches

6.3.1 Bispecific T Cell Engager

Bispecific T cell engager is a dual-function antibody that consists of two ScFvs originated from different monoclonal antibodies; one specific for a tumor antigen (TAA) and the other specific for a T cell epitope, mostly CD3. This structure can effectively engage the CAR-T cells with tumor cells and boost tumor cell killing. Synergistically, the combination of both BiTE and CAR-T cell therapy strengthens the therapeutic efficacy compared to each treatment lonely. In this case, BiTE-armored-CAR-T cells are generated via transferring the BiTE and CAR encoding gene sequences in the T cell structure, which leads to increased proliferation, persistence, and cytotoxicity of CAR-T cells. Also, this provides effective infiltration and overcoming antigen heterogeneity (de Gruijl et al. 2015; Huang et al. 2020). CD3/EGFR BiTE with the adaption for EGFRIII-CAR-T cell has been introduced to contribute to the CARs targeting the neuroblastoma tumor cells. This combination therapy revealed to facilitate recruitment, infiltration, and activation of CAR-T cells in the tumor site. Choi et al. reported the successful outcomes of tumor cell eradication following the prescription of the secreted EGFR-BiTE-armored EGFRvIII-CAR-T cells in glioblastoma mouse models without any significant toxicities (Choi et al. 2019). In different studies, the potent anti-tumor function of combinatorial treatment consisting of blinatumomab BiTE and CD19- or CD22-targeted CAR-T cells has been highlighted more and more. Published results of these studies reported the enhanced efficiency of CAR-T cells, significant elimination of tumor cells, and increased survival in treated cases. Mechanistically, blinatumomab upregulates the CAR function by inducing proliferation, persistence, and cytokine production (Goebeler and Bargou 2016; Pillai et al. 2019; Shalabi et al. 2019). In another way, bispecific adapters, so-called tags (fluorescein, isothiocyanate, biotin, etc.) composed of conjugated antibody portions, have been developed to increment the anti-tumor activity of CAR-T cells. In this manner, CAR-T cells exert tumor cell killing via the engagement of anti-tag CAR-T cells with specific tags bound to the tumor antigens. It has been shown that biotin-targeted CAR-T cells in combination with anti-CD19 or anti-CD20 biotinylated bispecific antibodies, which were attached to tumor antigens, displayed the potent cytotoxicity and IFN-γ secretion against tumor cells (Lohmueller et al. 2017). Interestingly, combinatorial treatment of FITC-targeted CAR-T cells with the folate-FITC conjugate-bispecific switch can conjugate to different antibodies and bound to folate receptor (FR)-positive tumor cells exhibited the substantial cytotoxicity of CARs and tumor regression (Kim et al. 2015). These CAR-T cells are enclosed to the tumor cells expressing the target antigens as a prominent advantage. They are activated only in the presence of bispecific adapters, thereby resulting in a selectively specific response with limited "on-target/off-tumor" toxicity. Consequently, BiTEs improve the safety and efficacy of CAR-T cells and lead to overcoming the loss of tumor antigens and antigen heterogeneity.

6.3.2 On-Switch CAR

The on-switch strategy is designed to remotely control CAR-T cells and pharmacologically regulate the dose, time, location, and amount of CAR-T cell activity at the tumor site. In an on-switch scheme, CAR-T cell consists of two separate polypeptides, one representing the co-stimulatory signaling molecule attached to the extracellular portion (ScFv) and the other representing the only main signaling domain (CD3ζ) (Li and Zhao 2017; Lanitis et al. 2020). Both split portions possess the binding domain for small dimerizing molecule (drug) or chemical inducer of dimerization (CID). Activation and initiation of the T cell responses occur when tumor antigen is detected, and a small dimerizing molecule is present, which together cause the co-localization of two separate portions into a single signaling structure (Wu et al. 2015). Similarly, in an alternative strategy to control the costimulation of T cells, exploiting the separate signaling portions that a dimerizing small molecule regulates only the co-stimulatory region can be useful, as well. In this regimen, a separate co-stimulatory region (MyD88/CD40) is designed to be linked to FKBP12 ligand-binding domain. As a result, oligomerization and co-stimulatory signaling are initiated via the administration of the small inducer like AP1903, which converts the off-state CAR (inactive) to on-state CAR (active) (Foster et al. 2017; Mata et al. 2017). In a similar strategy, the on-switch CAR is designed to separate the ScFv and the signaling domain. In this scheme, CAR-T cell toxicity is reduced under the controlling mechanisms. The production of pro-inflammatory cytokines that cause cytokine storm is reduced compared to conventional CAR-T cells. Liu et al. engineered and evaluated the hGPC3-CAR-T cell split on-switch structure to target the human glypican-3 (hGPC3) antigen, a highly expressed protein in hepatocellular carcinoma (HCC) (Liu et al. 2020). The hGPC3-CAR-T cell was composed of hGPC3 ScFv-SpyTag containing the anti-hGPC3 ScFv bound to a 13-amino acid peptide SpyTag and SpyCatcher-CAR signaling domain containing the extracellular SpyCatcher bound to the intracellular domains consisting of 4-1BB and CD3ζ molecules. The in vitro and in vivo findings revealed the higher cytotoxicity against HCC tumor cells and improved safety by preventing CRS. So, this mentioned split on-switch hGPC3 CAR structure was introduced as a versatile, practical, and safer treatment choice for HCC treatment (Liu et al. 2020). In this case, two switchable types of HER-2 CAR-T cells were engineered and evaluated in a rodent xenograft model of breast cancer using the FITC. Findings revealed a greater safety and specificity in CAR-T cell performance under a controllable manner (Cao et al. 2016). These strategies provide selectivity tumor identification, increased cytokine production, maximal safety and efficacy, and reduced "on-target/off-tumor" toxicity because the activation and inactivation of CAR-T cells depend on the presence of a dimerizing molecule.

7 Combination and Modification Strategies of CAR-T Cell in Clinics

To date, several preclinical studies have been performed to evaluate the efficacy and safety of genetically engineered CAR-T cells or in combination with other cancer treatments, and their encouraging results have been reported. However, addressing concerns about using this treatment in humans and ensuring their high efficacy requires numerous studies at the clinical trial level. To date, various clinical trial studies have been completed or are underway regarding CAR-T cell combination therapy as well as armored and switch-based CAR-T cells, some of which are summarized in Tables 1 and 2, respectively.

8 Conclusion

CAR-T cell therapy made a dramatic revolution in the treatment of cancers, especially hematological malignancies, and achieved promising outcomes in improving the condition of cancer patients. Engineering the armored CAR-T cells by genetic engineering techniques and combining CAR-T cells with other cancer therapeutic approaches are the effective efforts of the last decade in augmenting the anti-tumor function and safety of CAR-T cell therapy. Designing smart and powerful CAR structures such as TRUCKs, universal CARs, SUPRA CARs, and split CARs with different functional mechanisms such as increasing cytokine production, targeting more tumor antigens simultaneously, and functioning by selectively identifying tumor antigens elicits more notable cytotoxicity with restricted adverse effects in tumor sites. Another solution is to use switching regimens that either on- or off-switch. In this case, on-switches regulate the onset of CAR-T cell activity, requiring the simultaneous identification of two antigens or the presence of small dimerizing molecules; however, off-switches mediate the inactivation of the CAR-T cells to prevent their exhaustion and side effects. These genetic engineering techniques have alleviated mainly concerns about the efficacy and safety of CAR-T cell therapy in tumors. CAR-T cell combination therapy with other cancer treatments, including chemotherapy, radiotherapy, and immune-based therapies, has been developed to improve CAR-T cell function. Accordingly, blocking the immunosuppressive cytokines (TGF-β and IL-4) with CAR-T cells and administrating the anti-tumor inflammatory cytokines (IL-15, IL-12, and IL-7) can increase the anti-tumor function. On the other hand, the use of inhibitory checkpoint blockers like pembrolizumab (anti-PD-1 mAb) can prevent the suppression of effector T cells and CAR-T cells in the tumor microenvironment. Cancer vaccines and oncolytic viruses can also be effectively direct cells to the target tumor site and upregulate their cytotoxicity against tumors. Interestingly, immunomodulatory agents, particularly lenalidomide, have been shown to strengthen the CAR-T cell efficiency by activating T cell signaling pathways and increasing cell proliferation. As a result, with the trend of global science toward the deployment of combination therapies for the treatment of cancers, it can be realized that upgrading research in

Table 1 Summary of clinical trials based on CAR-T cell combination therapy in cancers

Treatment	Combination strategy	CAR-T cell type	Cancer type	Phase	Reference
Immunomodulators	Decitabine	CD19/ CD20 CAR	B-NHL	1 , 2	NCT04697940 NCT04553393
		CD19 PD-1 CAR	B-cell lymphoma	1	NCT04850560
	Lenalidomide	BCMA CAR	MM	1	NCT03070327
BiTEs	Obinutuzumab, glofitamab	CD19 CAR	Lymphomas	2	NCT04703686
	Obinutuzumab, glofitamab, mosunetuzumab	CD19 CAR	DLBCL	2	NCT04889716
PD-1 inhibitor	PD-1 mAb	MUC1 CAR	NSCLC	1, 2	NCT03525782
	Nivolumab Pembrolizumab	CD30 CAR	B-HL	1	NCT04134325
	Pembrolizumab	CD19 CAR	DLBCL and MCL	1, 2	NCT02650999
	Pembrolizumab	EGFRvIII CAR	Glioblastoma	1	NCT03726515
	Durvalumab	CD19 CAR	NHL	1	NCT02706405
	Tislelizumab	CD19/22 CAR	NHL	2	NCT04539444
PD-1 inhibitor CTLA-4 inhibitor	Nivolumab Ipilimumab	IL13Ra2 CAR	Glioblastoma	1	NCT04003649
Vaccine	Imovax rabies	B cell CAR	B-cell neoplasm	1	NCT04410900
	VZV vaccine	GD2 CAR	Neuroblastoma, osteosarcoma	1	NCT01953900
	PCV13 vaccine	CD19 CAR	PMBCL, TFL, HGBCL, DLBCL	2	NCT04745559

Radiation	Apamistamab	CD19 CAR	ALL and DLBCL	1	NCT04512716
	Radiotherapy	CAR-T Cell	HMs	1, 2	NCT04790747
		CAR-T Cell	Lymphoma	NA	NCT04473937
Oncolytic virus	Binary oncolytic adenovirus	HER2 CAR	Solid tumors	1	NCT03740256
Cytokine	IFN-α	CAR-T Cell	ALL	2	NCT04534634
	Aldesleukin (IL-2)	CD19 CAR	DLBCL	1, 2	NCT00924326
		CD19/ CD22 CAR	B-ALL/B-LBL	1, 2	NCT03098355
Chemotherapy Cytokine	Cyclophosphamide, fludarabine, aldesleukin (IL-2)	IL13Rα2 CAR	Melanoma	1	NCT04119024
		EGFRvIII CAR	Glioblastoma	1, 2	NCT01454596
Chemotherapy CRISPR/Cas9	Cyclophosphamide, fludarabine	XYF19 CAR	B-ALL	1	NCT04037566
		CB-010 CAR	B-NHL	1	NCT04637763
Chemotherapy mAb	Cyclophosphamide, fludarabine, ALLO-647 (anti-CD52)	CD19 CAR	LBCL	1	NCT03939026
				1, 2	NCT04416984
		BCMA CAR	MM	1	NCT04706936
				1, 2	NCT05000450
Chemotherapy mAb Immunomodulator	Cyclophosphamide, fludarabine, ALLO-647 (anti-CD52) Nirogacestat	BCMA CAR	MM	1	NCT04093596
Immunomodulator Corticosteroid Antibiotic	Lenalidomide Dexamethasone Clarithromycin	BCMA CAR	MM	3	NCT04287660
Chemotherapy Dimerizer drug	Bendamustine Fludarabine Cyclophosphamide AP1903	iC9-CD19 CAR	Lymphoma	1	NCT03696784
			MM	3	NCT04923893

(continued)

Table 1 (continued)

Treatment	Combination strategy	CAR-T cell type	Cancer type	Phase	Reference
Proteasome inhibitor Immunomodulator Corticosteroid Chemotherapy	Bortezomib Lenalidomide Dexamethasone Fludarabine Cyclophosphamide	BCMA CAR			
LAG3 inhibitor PD-1 inhibitor	Relatlimab Nivolumab Durvalumab	CAR-T cell	NHL, DLBCL	1, 2	NCT03310619

Abbreviations: *CARs* chimeric antigen receptors, *NHL* non-Hodgkin's lymphoma, *MM* multiple myeloma, *DLBCL* diffuse large B-cell lymphoma, *NSCLC* non-small-cell lung carcinoma, *MCL* mantle cell lymphoma, *HMs* hematological malignancies, *ALL* acute lymphocytic leukemia, *BCMA* B-cell maturation antigen, *EGFR* epidermal growth factor receptor, *MUC1* mucin 1, *BiTE* bispecific T-cell engager, *PD-1* programmed death-1, *CTLA-4* cytotoxic T lymphocyte antigen-4, *LAG3* lymphocyte activation gene 3, *PCV* pneumococcal conjugate vaccine, *mAb* monoclonal antibody, *VZV* varicella zoster vaccine, *IFN-α* interferon alfa

Table 2 Summary of clinical trials based on CAR-T cell therapy with switches genes in cancers

Switches	CAR-T cell type	Phase	Cancer type	References
iCasp9-AP1903	IL-15/GPC3 CAR	1	Pediatric solid tumors Hepatocellular carcinoma	NCT04377932 NCT05103631
	iCasp9 (BPZ-1001) CAR	1, 2	Leukemia, myeloma, myeloproliferative diseases	NCT01875237
Anti PD-L1	PD-L1/CD22 CAR	1	Solid tumor, adult cervical cancer sarcoma, NSCLC	NCT04556669
EGFRt Suicide switch	B7H3 CAR	1	Refractory solid tumors in children and young adults	NCT04483778
			DIPG, DMG	NCT04185038
	EGFR806 CAR	1	Refractory pediatric CNS tumors	NCT03638167
			Refractory solid tumors in children and young adults	NCT03618381
	HER2/EGFRt CAR	1	Refractory pediatric CNS tumors	NCT03500991
CD20 Suicide switch	CD19/CD20 CAR	1	Refractory hematological malignancies	NCT04700319
			B-cell malignancies, HL	NCT04160195
	CD20/CD22 CAR	1	Refractory lymphoid malignancies	NCT04283006
Dual CAR	BCMA/CD19 CAR	1	BCMA+ R/R MM	NCT04236011
	CD38/BCMA CAR	1, 2	R/R MM	NCT03767751
	HER2-dual switch CAR	1	HER2-positive solid tumors	NCT04650451
	CD19/CD22 CAR	1	B-cell leukemia	NCT03330691
	CD19/CD20 CAR	1	B-cell leukemia	NCT04260945
Tandem CAR	CD19/CD20 CAR	1, 2	R/R NHL	NCT04553393 NCT04697940
			Refractory B-cell malignancy	NCT03097770
iCAR	PD-L1 CAR Plus Pembrolizumab	2	Recurrent/metastatic gastric or head and neck cancer	NCT04847466
	PD-L1/CD22 CAR	1	Solid tumors	NCT04556669

Abbreviations: *CARs* chimeric antigen receptors, *iCasp9* inducible caspase 9, *NHL* non-Hodgkin's lymphoma, *MM* multiple myeloma, *NSCLC* non-small-cell lung carcinoma, *DIPG* diffuse intrinsic pontine glioma, *DMG* diffuse midline gliomas, *HL* Hodgkin's lymphoma, *GPC3* glypican 3, *BCMA* B-cell maturation antigen, *EGFR* epidermal growth factor receptor, *PD-1* programmed death-1, *iCAR* inhibitory CAR, *R/R* relapsed/refractory

genetic engineering approaches to produce smart and programmable CAR-T cells with functional aspects and practical anti-tumor function, as well as acceptable safety, can figure out a bright and promising future in the field of cancer treatment.

Acknowledgments None.

Compliance with Ethical Standards The authors declare that there is no conflict of interest.

References

Abramson JS, Palomba ML, Gordon LI, Lunning MA, Wang M, Arnason J, Mehta A, Purev E, Maloney DG, Andreadis C, Sehgal A, Solomon SR, Ghosh N, Albertson TM, Garcia J, Kostic A, Mallaney M, Ogasawara K, Newhall K, Kim Y, Li D, Siddiqi T (2020) Lisocabtagene maraleucel for patients with relapsed or refractory large B-cell lymphomas (TRANSCEND NHL 001): a multicentre seamless design study. Lancet 396:839–852

Anampa J, Chen A, Wright J, Patel M, Pellegrino C, Fehn K, Sparano JA, Andreopoulou E (2018) Phase I trial of Veliparib, a poly ADP ribose polymerase inhibitor, plus metronomic cyclophosphamide in metastatic HER2-negative breast cancer. Clin Breast Cancer 18:e135–e142

Anurathapan U, Chan RC, Hindi HF, Mucharla R, Bajgain P, Hayes BC, Fisher WE, Heslop HE, Rooney CM, Brenner MK, Leen AM, Vera JF (2014) Kinetics of tumor destruction by chimeric antigen receptor-modified T cells. Mol Ther 22:623–633

Avigan D, Rosenblatt J (2018) Vaccine therapy in hematologic malignancies. Blood 131:2640–2650

Bach PB, Giralt SA, Saltz LB (2017) FDA approval of Tisagenlecleucel: promise and complexities of a $475 000 cancer drug. JAMA 318:1861–1862

Bansal R, Reshef R (2021) Revving the CAR - combination strategies to enhance CAR T cell effectiveness. Blood Rev 45:100695

Bell M, Gottschalk S (2021) Engineered cytokine signaling to improve CAR T cell effector function. Front Immunol 12:684642

Berger C, Flowers ME, Warren EH, Riddell SR (2006) Analysis of transgene-specific immune responses that limit the in vivo persistence of adoptively transferred HSV-TK-modified donor T cells after allogeneic hematopoietic cell transplantation. Blood 107:2294–2302

Bonifant CL, Jackson HJ, Brentjens RJ, Curran KJ (2016) Toxicity and management in CAR T-cell therapy. Mol Ther Oncolytics 3:16011

Bouchkouj N, Kasamon YL, de Claro RA, George B, Lin X, Lee S, Blumenthal GM, Bryan W, McKee AE, Pazdur R (2019) FDA approval summary: Axicabtagene Ciloleucel for relapsed or refractory large B-cell lymphoma. Clin Cancer Res 25:1702–1708

Bracci L, Schiavoni G, Sistigu A, Belardelli F (2014) Immune-based mechanisms of cytotoxic chemotherapy: implications for the design of novel and rationale-based combined treatments against cancer. Cell Death Differ 21:15–25

Bridgeman JS, Hawkins RE, Bagley S, Blaylock M, Holland M, Gilham DE (2010) The optimal antigen response of chimeric antigen receptors harboring the CD3zeta transmembrane domain is dependent upon incorporation of the receptor into the endogenous TCR/CD3 complex. J Immunol 184:6938–6949

Budde LE, Berger C, Lin Y, Wang J, Lin X, Frayo SE, Brouns SA, Spencer DM, Till BG, Jensen MC, Riddell SR, Press OW (2013) Combining a CD20 chimeric antigen receptor and an inducible caspase 9 suicide switch to improve the efficacy and safety of T cell adoptive immunotherapy for lymphoma. PLoS One 8:e82742

Cao Y, Rodgers DT, Du J, Ahmad I, Hampton EN, Ma JS, Mazagova M, Choi SH, Yun HY, Xiao H, Yang P, Luo X, Lim RK, Pugh HM, Wang F, Kazane SA, Wright TM, Kim CH, Schultz PG, Young TS (2016) Design of Switchable Chimeric Antigen Receptor T Cells Targeting Breast Cancer. Angew Chem Int Ed Engl 55:7520–7524

Carneiro BA, El-Deiry WS (2020) Targeting apoptosis in cancer therapy. Nat Rev Clin Oncol 17: 395–417

Caruana I, Weber G, Ballard BC, Wood MS, Savoldo B, Dotti G (2015) K562-derived whole-cell vaccine enhances antitumor responses of CAR-redirected virus-specific cytotoxic T lymphocytes in vivo. Clin Cancer Res 21:2952–2962

Casucci M, Falcone L, Camisa B, Norelli M, Porcellini S, Stornaiuolo A, Ciceri F, Traversari C, Bordignon C, Bonini C, Bondanza A (2018) Extracellular NGFR spacers allow efficient tracking and enrichment of fully functional CAR-T cells co-expressing a suicide gene. Front Immunol 9:507

Chan JD, von Scheidt B, Zeng B, Oliver AJ, Davey AS, Ali AI, Thomas R, Trapani JA, Darcy PK, Kershaw MH, Dolcetti R, Slaney CY (2020) Enhancing chimeric antigen receptor T-cell immunotherapy against cancer using a nanoemulsion-based vaccine targeting cross-presenting dendritic cells. Clin Transl Immunol 9:e1157

Chang ZL, Lorenzini MH, Chen X, Tran U, Bangayan NJ, Chen YY (2018) Rewiring T-cell responses to soluble factors with chimeric antigen receptors. Nat Chem Biol 14:317–324

Chen Y, Sun C, Landoni E, Metelitsa L, Dotti G, Savoldo B (2019) Eradication of neuroblastoma by T cells redirected with an optimized GD2-specific chimeric antigen receptor and Interleukin-15. Clin Cancer Res 25:2915–2924

Chmielewski M, Abken H (2015) TRUCKs: the fourth generation of CARs. Expert Opin Biol Ther 15:1145–1154

Chmielewski M, Abken H (2017) CAR T cells releasing IL-18 convert to T-bet(high) FoxO1(low) effectors that exhibit augmented activity against advanced solid tumors. Cell Rep 21:3205–3219

Chmielewski M, Abken H (2020) TRUCKS, the fourth-generation CAR T cells: current developments and clinical translation. Adv Cell Gene Ther 3:e84

Chmielewski M, Hombach A, Heuser C, Adams GP, Abken H (2004) T cell activation by antibody-like immunoreceptors: increase in affinity of the single-chain fragment domain above threshold does not increase T cell activation against antigen-positive target cells but decreases selectivity. J Immunol 173:7647–7653

Chmielewski M, Kopecky C, Hombach AA, Abken H (2011) IL-12 release by engineered T cells expressing chimeric antigen receptors can effectively Muster an antigen-independent macrophage response on tumor cells that have shut down tumor antigen expression. Cancer Res 71: 5697–5706

Cho JH, Collins JJ, Wong WW (2018) Universal chimeric antigen receptors for multiplexed and logical control of T cell responses. Cell 173:1426–1438.e1411

Choi BD, Yu X, Castano AP, Bouffard AA, Schmidts A, Larson RC, Bailey SR, Boroughs AC, Frigault MJ, Leick MB, Scarfò I, Cetrulo CL, Demehri S, Nahed BV, Cahill DP, Wakimoto H, Curry WT, Carter BS, Maus MV (2019) CAR-T cells secreting BiTEs circumvent antigen escape without detectable toxicity. Nat Biotechnol 37:1049–1058

Ciceri F, Bonini C, Marktel S, Zappone E, Servida P, Bernardi M, Pescarollo A, Bondanza A, Peccatori J, Rossini S, Magnani Z, Salomoni M, Benati C, Ponzoni M, Callegaro L, Corradini P, Bregni M, Traversari C, Bordignon C (2007) Antitumor effects of HSV-TK-engineered donor lymphocytes after allogeneic stem-cell transplantation. Blood 109:4698–4707

Ciceri F, Bonini C, Stanghellini MT, Bondanza A, Traversari C, Salomoni M, Turchetto L, Colombi S, Bernardi M, Peccatori J, Pescarollo A, Servida P, Magnani Z, Perna SK, Valtolina V, Crippa F, Callegaro L, Spoldi E, Crocchiolo R, Fleischhauer K, Ponzoni M, Vago L, Rossini S, Santoro A, Todisco E, Apperley J, Olavarria E, Slavin S, Weissinger EM, Ganser A, Stadler M, Yannaki E, Fassas A, Anagnostopoulos A, Bregni M, Stampino CG, Bruzzi P, Bordignon C (2009) Infusion of suicide-gene-engineered donor lymphocytes after family haploidentical haemopoietic stem-cell transplantation for leukaemia (the TK007 trial): a non-randomised phase I-II study. Lancet Oncol 10:489–500

Dai H, Wu Z, Jia H, Tong C, Guo Y, Ti D, Han X, Liu Y, Zhang W, Wang C, Zhang Y, Chen M, Yang Q, Wang Y, Han W (2020) Bispecific CAR-T cells targeting both CD19 and CD22 for therapy of adults with relapsed or refractory B cell acute lymphoblastic leukemia. J Hematol Oncol 13:30

D'Aloia MM, Caratelli S, Palumbo C, Battella S, Arriga R, Lauro D, Palmieri G, Sconocchia G, Alimandi M (2016) T lymphocytes engineered to express a CD16-chimeric antigen receptor redirect T-cell immune responses against immunoglobulin G-opsonized target cells. Cytotherapy 18:278–290

Davila ML, Brentjens RJ (2016) CD19-targeted CAR T cells as novel cancer immunotherapy for relapsed or refractory B-cell acute lymphoblastic leukemia. Clin Adv Hematol Oncol 14:802–808 de Gruijl TD, Janssen AB, van Beusechem VW (2015) Arming oncolytic viruses to leverage antitumor immunity. Expert Opin Biol Ther 15:959–971

Demaria S, Ng B, Devitt ML, Babb JS, Kawashima N, Liebes L, Formenti SC (2004) Ionizing radiation inhibition of distant untreated tumors (abscopal effect) is immune mediated. Int J Radiat Oncol Biol Phys 58:862–870

DeSelm C, Palomba ML, Yahalom J, Hamieh M, Eyquem J, Rajasekhar VK, Sadelain M (2018) Low-dose radiation conditioning enables CAR T cells to mitigate antigen escape. Mol Ther 26: 2542–2552

Diaconu I, Ballard B, Zhang M, Chen Y, West J, Dotti G, Savoldo B (2017) Inducible Caspase-9 selectively modulates the toxicities of CD19-specific chimeric antigen receptor-modified T cells. Mol Ther 25:580–592

Elahi R, Khosh E, Tahmasebi S, Esmaeilzadeh A (2018) Immune cell hacking: challenges and clinical approaches to create smarter generations of chimeric antigen receptor T cells. Front Immunol 9:1717

Esmaeilzadeh A, Tahmasebi S, Athari SS (2020) Chimeric antigen receptor -T cell therapy: applications and challenges in treatment of allergy and asthma. Biomed Pharmacother 123: 109685

Fedorov VD, Themeli M, Sadelain M (2013) PD-1- and CTLA-4-based inhibitory chimeric antigen receptors (iCARs) divert off-target immunotherapy responses. Sci Transl Med 5:215ra172

Feins S, Kong W, Williams EF, Milone MC, Fraietta JA (2019) An introduction to chimeric antigen receptor (CAR) T-cell immunotherapy for human cancer. Am J Hematol 94:S3–s9

Foster AE, Mahendravada A, Shinners NP, Chang WC, Crisostomo J, Lu A, Khalil M, Morschl E, Shaw JL, Saha S, Duong MT, Collinson-Pautz MR, Torres DL, Rodriguez T, Pentcheva-Hoang T, Bayle JH, Slawin KM, Spencer DM (2017) Regulated expansion and survival of chimeric antigen receptor-modified T cells using small molecule-dependent inducible MyD88/CD40. Mol Ther 25:2176–2188

Fry TJ, Shah NN, Orentas RJ, Stetler-Stevenson M, Yuan CM, Ramakrishna S, Wolters P, Martin S, Delbrook C, Yates B, Shalabi H, Fountaine TJ, Shern JF, Majzner RG, Stroncek DF, Sabatino M, Feng Y, Dimitrov DS, Zhang L, Nguyen S, Qin H, Dropulic B, Lee DW, Mackall CL (2018) CD22-targeted CAR T cells induce remission in B-ALL that is naive or resistant to CD19-targeted CAR immunotherapy. Nat Med 24:20–28

Ganss R, Ryschich E, Klar E, Arnold B, Hämmerling GJ (2002) Combination of T-cell therapy and trigger of inflammation induces remodeling of the vasculature and tumor eradication. Cancer Res 62:1462–1470

Gargett T, Brown MP (2014) The inducible caspase-9 suicide gene system as a "safety switch" to limit on-target, off-tumor toxicities of chimeric antigen receptor T cells. Front Pharmacol 5:235

Gargett T, Yu W, Dotti G, Yvon ES, Christo SN, Hayball JD, Lewis ID, Brenner MK, Brown MP (2016) GD2-specific CAR T cells undergo potent activation and deletion following antigen encounter but can be protected from activation-induced cell death by PD-1 blockade. Mol Ther 24:1135–1149

Goebeler ME, Bargou R (2016) Blinatumomab: a CD19/CD3 bispecific T cell engager (BiTE) with unique anti-tumor efficacy. Leuk Lymphoma 57:1021–1032

Golumba-Nagy V, Kuehle J, Hombach AA, Abken H (2018) CD28-ζ CAR T cells resist TGF-β repression through IL-2 signaling, which can be mimicked by an engineered IL-7 autocrine loop. Mol Ther 26:2218–2230

Gordon WR, Vardar-Ulu D, Histen G, Sanchez-Irizarry C, Aster JC, Blacklow SC (2007) Structural basis for autoinhibition of notch. Nat Struct Mol Biol 14:295–300

Grada Z, Hegde M, Byrd T, Shaffer DR, Ghazi A, Brawley VS, Corder A, Schönfeld K, Koch J, Dotti G, Heslop HE, Gottschalk S, Wels WS, Baker ML, Ahmed N (2013) TanCAR: a novel bispecific chimeric antigen receptor for cancer immunotherapy. Mol Ther Nucleic Acids 2:e105

Grosser R, Cherkassky L, Chintala N, Adusumilli PS (2019) Combination immunotherapy with CAR T cells and checkpoint blockade for the treatment of solid tumors. Cancer Cell 36:471–482

Guest RD, Hawkins RE, Kirillova N, Cheadle EJ, Arnold J, O'Neill A, Irlam J, Chester KA, Kemshead JT, Shaw DM, Embleton MJ, Stern PL, Gilham DE (2005) The role of extracellular spacer regions in the optimal design of chimeric immune receptors: evaluation of four different scFvs and antigens. J Immunother 28:203–211

Hegde M, Mukherjee M, Grada Z, Pignata A, Landi D, Navai SA, Wakefield A, Fousek K, Bielamowicz K, Chow KK, Brawley VS, Byrd TT, Krebs S, Gottschalk S, Wels WS, Baker ML, Dotti G, Mamonkin M, Brenner MK, Orange JS, Ahmed N (2016) Tandem CAR T cells targeting HER2 and IL13Rα2 mitigate tumor antigen escape. J Clin Invest 126:3036–3052

Heylmann D, Bauer M, Becker H, van Gool S, Bacher N, Steinbrink K, Kaina B (2013) Human CD4+CD25+ regulatory T cells are sensitive to low dose cyclophosphamide: implications for the immune response. PLoS One 8:e83384

Hofmann L, Forschner A, Loquai C, Goldinger SM, Zimmer L, Ugurel S, Schmidgen MI, Gutzmer R, Utikal JS, Göppner D, Hassel JC, Meier F, Tietze JK, Thomas I, Weishaupt C, Leverkus M, Wahl R, Dietrich U, Garbe C, Kirchberger MC, Eigentler T, Berking C, Gesierich A, Krackhardt AM, Schadendorf D, Schuler G, Dummer R, Heinzerling LM (2016) Cutaneous, gastrointestinal, hepatic, endocrine, and renal side-effects of anti-PD-1 therapy. Eur J Cancer 60:190–209

Hornyák L, Dobos N, Koncz G, Karányi Z, Páll D, Szabó Z, Halmos G, Székvölgyi L (2018) The role of Indoleamine-2,3-dioxygenase in cancer development, diagnostics, and therapy. Front Immunol 9:151

Hoyos V, Savoldo B, Quintarelli C, Mahendravada A, Zhang M, Vera J, Heslop HE, Rooney CM, Brenner MK, Dotti G (2010) Engineering CD19-specific T lymphocytes with interleukin-15 and a suicide gene to enhance their anti-lymphoma/leukemia effects and safety. Leukemia 24:1160–1170

Huang Q, Xia J, Wang L, Wang X, Ma X, Deng Q, Lu Y, Kumar M, Zhou Z, Li L, Zeng Z, Young KH, Yi Q, Zhang M, Li Y (2018) miR-153 suppresses IDO1 expression and enhances CAR T cell immunotherapy. J Hematol Oncol 11:58

Huang R, Li X, He Y, Zhu W, Gao L, Liu Y, Gao L, Wen Q, Zhong JF, Zhang C, Zhang X (2020) Recent advances in CAR-T cell engineering. J Hematol Oncol 13:86

Hurton LV, Singh H, Najjar AM, Switzer KC, Mi T, Maiti S, Olivares S, Rabinovich B, Huls H, Forget MA, Datar V, Kebriaei P, Lee DA, Champlin RE, Cooper LJ (2016) Tethered IL-15 augments antitumor activity and promotes a stem-cell memory subset in tumor-specific T cells. Proc Natl Acad Sci U S A 113:E7788–E7797

John LB, Devaud C, Duong CP, Yong CS, Beavis PA, Haynes NM, Chow MT, Smyth MJ, Kershaw MH, Darcy PK (2013) Anti-PD-1 antibody therapy potently enhances the eradication of established tumors by gene-modified T cells. Clin Cancer Res 19:5636–5646

Jones BS, Lamb LS, Goldman F, Di Stasi A (2014) Improving the safety of cell therapy products by suicide gene transfer. Front Pharmacol 5:254

Junghans RP (2017) The challenges of solid tumor for designer CAR-T therapies: a 25-year perspective. Cancer Gene Ther 24:89–99

Karlsson H, Lindqvist AC, Fransson M, Paul-Wetterberg G, Nilsson B, Essand M, Nilsson K, Frisk P, Jernberg-Wiklund H, Loskog A (2013) Combining CAR T cells and the Bcl-2 family apoptosis inhibitor ABT-737 for treating B-cell malignancy. Cancer Gene Ther 20:386–393

Khalil DN, Budhu S, Gasmi B, Zappasodi R, Hirschhorn-Cymerman D, Plitt T, De Henau O, Zamarin D, Holmgaard RB, Murphy JT (2015) The new era of cancer immunotherapy: manipulating T-cell activity to overcome malignancy. Adv Cancer Res 128:1–68

Kim MS, Ma JS, Yun H, Cao Y, Kim JY, Chi V, Wang D, Woods A, Sherwood L, Caballero D, Gonzalez J, Schultz PG, Young TS, Kim CH (2015) Redirection of genetically engineered CAR-T cells using bifunctional small molecules. J Am Chem Soc 137:2832–2835

Kloss CC, Condomines M, Cartellieri M, Bachmann M, Sadelain M (2013) Combinatorial antigen recognition with balanced signaling promotes selective tumor eradication by engineered T cells. Nat Biotechnol 31:71–75

Kloss CC, Lee J, Zhang A, Chen F, Melenhorst JJ, Lacey SF, Maus MV, Fraietta JA, Zhao Y, June CH (2018) Dominant-negative TGF-β receptor enhances PSMA-targeted human CAR T cell proliferation and augments prostate cancer eradication. Mol Ther 26:1855–1866

Koneru M, O'Cearbhaill R, Pendharkar S, Spriggs DR, Brentjens RJ (2015) A phase I clinical trial of adoptive T cell therapy using IL-12 secreting MUC-16(ecto) directed chimeric antigen receptors for recurrent ovarian cancer. J Transl Med 13:102

Kopan R, Ilagan MX (2009) The canonical notch signaling pathway: unfolding the activation mechanism. Cell 137:216–233

Lamers CH, Willemsen R, van Elzakker P, van Steenbergen-Langeveld S, Broertjes M, Oosterwijk-Wakka J, Oosterwijk E, Sleijfer S, Debets R, Gratama JW (2011) Immune responses to transgene and retroviral vector in patients treated with ex vivo-engineered T cells. Blood 117: 72–82

Lanitis E, Poussin M, Klattenhoff AW, Song D, Sandaltzopoulos R, June CH, Powell DJ Jr (2013) Chimeric antigen receptor T cells with dissociated signaling domains exhibit focused antitumor activity with reduced potential for toxicity in vivo. Cancer Immunol Res 1:43–53

Lanitis E, Coukos G, Irving M (2020) All systems go: converging synthetic biology and combinatorial treatment for CAR-T cell therapy. Curr Opin Biotechnol 65:75–87

Laurent SA, Hoffmann FS, Kuhn PH, Cheng Q, Chu Y, Schmidt-Supprian M, Hauck SM, Schuh E, Krumbholz M, Rübsamen H, Wanngren J, Khademi M, Olsson T, Alexander T, Hiepe F, Pfister HW, Weber F, Jenne D, Wekerle H, Hohlfeld R, Lichtenthaler SF, Meinl E (2015) γ-Secretase directly sheds the survival receptor BCMA from plasma cells. Nat Commun 6:7333

Le DT, Pardoll DM, Jaffee EM (2010) Cellular vaccine approaches. Cancer J 16:304–310

Lee DW, Santomasso BD, Locke FL, Ghobadi A, Turtle CJ, Brudno JN, Maus MV, Park JH, Mead E, Pavletic S, Go WY, Eldjerou L, Gardner RA, Frey N, Curran KJ, Peggs K, Pasquini M, DiPersio JF, van den Brink MRM, Komanduri KV, Grupp SA, Neelapu SS (2019) ASTCT consensus grading for cytokine release syndrome and neurologic toxicity associated with immune effector cells. Biol Blood Marrow Transplant 25:625–638

Li H, Zhao Y (2017) Increasing the safety and efficacy of chimeric antigen receptor T cell therapy. Protein Cell 8:573–589

Li D, Hu Y, Jin Z, Zhai Y, Tan Y, Sun Y, Zhu S, Zhao C, Chen B, Zhu J, Chen Z, Chen S, Li J, Liu H (2018) TanCAR T cells targeting CD19 and CD133 efficiently eliminate MLL leukemic cells. Leukemia 32:2012–2016

Li S, Xue L, Wang M, Qiang P, Xu H, Zhang X, Kang W, You F, Xu H, Wang Y, Liu X, Yang L, Wang X (2019) Decitabine enhances cytotoxic effect of T cells with an anti-CD19 chimeric antigen receptor in treatment of lymphoma. Onco Targets Ther 12:5627–5638

Liu J, Zhong JF, Zhang X, Zhang C (2017) Allogeneic CD19-CAR-T cell infusion after allogeneic hematopoietic stem cell transplantation in B cell malignancies. J Hematol Oncol 10:35

Liu X, Wen J, Yi H, Hou X, Yin Y, Ye G, Wu X, Jiang X (2020) Split chimeric antigen receptor-modified T cells targeting glypican-3 suppress hepatocellular carcinoma growth with reduced cytokine release. Ther Adv Med Oncol 12:1758835920910347

Lohmueller JJ, Ham JD, Kvorjak M, Finn OJ (2017) mSA2 affinity-enhanced biotin-binding CAR T cells for universal tumor targeting. Onco Targets Ther 7:e1368604

Ma X, Shou P, Smith C, Chen Y, Du H, Sun C, Porterfield Kren N, Michaud D, Ahn S, Vincent B, Savoldo B, Pylayeva-Gupta Y, Zhang S, Dotti G, Xu Y (2020) Interleukin-23 engineering improves CAR T cell function in solid tumors. Nat Biotechnol 38:448–459

Marin V, Cribioli E, Philip B, Tettamanti S, Pizzitola I, Biondi A, Biagi E, Pule M (2012) Comparison of different suicide-gene strategies for the safety improvement of genetically manipulated T cells. Hum Gene Ther Methods 23:376–386

Marofi F, Motavalli R, Safonov VA, Thangavelu L, Yumashev AV, Alexander M, Shomali N, Chartrand MS, Pathak Y, Jarahian M, Izadi S, Hassanzadeh A, Shirafkan N, Tahmasebi S, Khiavi FM (2021a) CAR T cells in solid tumors: challenges and opportunities. Stem Cell Res Ther 12:81

Marofi F, Rahman HS, Al-Obaidi ZMJ, Jalil AT, Abdelbasset WK, Suksatan W, Dorofeev AE, Shomali N, Chartrand MS, Pathak Y, Hassanzadeh A, Baradaran B, Ahmadi M, Saeedi H, Tahmasebi S, Jarahian M (2021b) Novel CAR T therapy is a ray of hope in the treatment of seriously ill AML patients. Stem Cell Res Ther 12:465

Marofi F, Tahmasebi S, Rahman HS, Kaigorodov D, Markov A, Yumashev AV, Shomali N, Chartrand MS, Pathak Y, Mohammed RN, Jarahian M, Motavalli R, Motavalli Khiavi F (2021c) Any closer to successful therapy of multiple myeloma? CAR-T cell is a good reason for optimism. Stem Cell Res Ther 12:217

Mata M, Gerken C, Nguyen P, Krenciute G, Spencer DM, Gottschalk S (2017) Inducible activation of MyD88 and CD40 in CAR T cells results in controllable and potent antitumor activity in preclinical solid tumor models. Cancer Discov 7:1306–1319

Matthews T, Boehme R (1988) Antiviral activity and mechanism of action of ganciclovir. Rev Infect Dis 10(Suppl 3):S490–S494

Maude SL, Laetsch TW, Buechner J, Rives S, Boyer M, Bittencourt H, Bader P, Verneris MR, Stefanski HE, Myers GD, Qayed M, De Moerloose B, Hiramatsu H, Schlis K, Davis KL, Martin PL, Nemecek ER, Yanik GA, Peters C, Baruchel A, Boissel N, Mechinaud F, Balduzzi A, Krueger J, June CH, Levine BL, Wood P, Taran T, Leung M, Mueller KT, Zhang Y, Sen K, Lebwohl D, Pulsipher MA, Grupp SA (2018) Tisagenlecleucel in children and Young adults with B-cell lymphoblastic leukemia. N Engl J Med 378:439–448

Maus MV, Haas AR, Beatty GL, Albelda SM, Levine BL, Liu X, Zhao Y, Kalos M, June CH (2013) T cells expressing chimeric antigen receptors can cause anaphylaxis in humans. Cancer Immunol Res 1:26–31

Michie J, Beavis PA, Freeman AJ, Vervoort SJ, Ramsbottom KM, Narasimhan V, Lelliott EJ, Lalaoui N, Ramsay RG, Johnstone RW, Silke J, Darcy PK, Voskoboinik I, Kearney CJ, Oliaro J (2019) Antagonism of IAPs enhances CAR T-cell efficacy. Cancer Immunol Res 7:183–192

Miliotou AN, Papadopoulou LC (2018) CAR T-cell therapy: a new era in cancer immunotherapy. Curr Pharm Biotechnol 19:5–18

Minagawa K, Jamil MO, Al-Obaidi M, Pereboeva L, Salzman D, Erba HP, Lamb LS, Bhatia R, Mineishi S, Di Stasi A (2016) In vitro pre-clinical validation of suicide gene modified anti-CD33 redirected chimeric antigen receptor T-cells for acute myeloid leukemia. PLoS One 11: e0166891

Mohammed S, Sukumaran S, Bajgain P, Watanabe N, Heslop HE, Rooney CM, Brenner MK, Fisher WE, Leen AM, Vera JF (2017) Improving chimeric antigen receptor-modified T cell function by reversing the immunosuppressive tumor microenvironment of pancreatic cancer. Mol Ther 25:249–258

Morsut L, Roybal KT, Xiong X, Gordley RM, Coyle SM, Thomson M, Lim WA (2016) Engineering customized cell sensing and response behaviors using synthetic notch receptors. Cell 164: 780–791

Muranski P, Boni A, Wrzesinski C, Citrin DE, Rosenberg SA, Childs R, Restifo NP (2006) Increased intensity lymphodepletion and adoptive immunotherapy--how far can we go? Nat Clin Pract Oncol 3:668–681

Nishio N, Diaconu I, Liu H, Cerullo V, Caruana I, Hoyos V, Bouchier-Hayes L, Savoldo B, Dotti G (2014) Armed oncolytic virus enhances immune functions of chimeric antigen receptor-modified T cells in solid tumors. Cancer Res 74:5195–5205

Oiseth SJ, Aziz MS (2017) Cancer immunotherapy: a brief review of the history, possibilities, and challenges ahead. J Cancer Metastasis Treat 3:250–261

Parente-Pereira AC, Whilding LM, Brewig N, van der Stegen SJ, Davies DM, Wilkie S, van Schalkwyk MC, Ghaem-Maghami S, Maher J (2013) Synergistic Chemoimmunotherapy of epithelial ovarian cancer using ErbB-retargeted T cells combined with carboplatin. J Immunol 191:2437–2445

Paulsson J, Micke P (2014) Prognostic relevance of cancer-associated fibroblasts in human cancer. Semin Cancer Biol 25:61–68

Petersen SL, Wang L, Yalcin-Chin A, Li L, Peyton M, Minna J, Harran P, Wang X (2007) Autocrine TNFalpha signaling renders human cancer cells susceptible to Smac-mimetic-induced apoptosis. Cancer Cell 12:445–456

Philip B, Kokalaki E, Mekkaoui L, Thomas S, Straathof K, Flutter B, Marin V, Marafioti T, Chakraverty R, Linch D, Quezada SA, Peggs KS, Pule M (2014) A highly compact epitope-based marker/suicide gene for easier and safer T-cell therapy. Blood 124:1277–1287

Pillai V, Muralidharan K, Meng W, Bagashev A, Oldridge DA, Rosenthal J, Van Arnam J, Melenhorst JJ, Mohan D, DiNofia AM, Luo M, Cherian S, Fromm JR, Wertheim G, Thomas-Tikhonenko A, Paessler M, June CH, Luning Prak ET, Bhoj VG, Grupp SA, Maude SL, Rheingold SR (2019) CAR T-cell therapy is effective for CD19-dim B-lymphoblastic leukemia but is impacted by prior blinatumomab therapy. Blood Adv 3:3539–3549

Pont MJ, Hill T, Cole GO, Abbott JJ, Kelliher J, Salter AI, Hudecek M, Comstock ML, Rajan A, Patel BKR, Voutsinas JM, Wu Q, Liu L, Cowan AJ, Wood BL, Green DJ, Riddell SR (2019) γ-Secretase inhibition increases efficacy of BCMA-specific chimeric antigen receptor T cells in multiple myeloma. Blood 134:1585–1597

Rafiq S, Hackett CS, Brentjens RJ (2020) Engineering strategies to overcome the current roadblocks in CAR T cell therapy. Nat Rev Clin Oncol 17:147–167

Ramos CA, Rouce R, Robertson CS, Reyna A, Narala N, Vyas G, Mehta B, Zhang H, Dakhova O, Carrum G, Kamble RT, Gee AP, Mei Z, Wu MF, Liu H, Grilley B, Rooney CM, Heslop HE, Brenner MK, Savoldo B, Dotti G (2018) In vivo fate and activity of second- versus third-generation CD19-specific CAR-T cells in B cell non-Hodgkin's lymphomas. Mol Ther 26: 2727–2737

Reits EA, Hodge JW, Herberts CA, Groothuis TA, Chakraborty M, Wansley EK, Camphausen K, Luiten RM, de Ru AH, Neijssen J, Griekspoor A, Mesman E, Verreck FA, Spits H, Schlom J, van Veelen P, Neefjes JJ (2006) Radiation modulates the peptide repertoire, enhances MHC class I expression, and induces successful antitumor immunotherapy. J Exp Med 203:1259–1271

Ribas A, Wolchok JD (2018) Cancer immunotherapy using checkpoint blockade. Science 359: 1350–1355

Roybal KT, Rupp LJ, Morsut L, Walker WJ, McNally KA, Park JS, Lim WA (2016a) Precision tumor recognition by T cells with combinatorial antigen-sensing circuits. Cell 164:770–779

Roybal KT, Williams JZ, Morsut L, Rupp LJ, Kolinko I, Choe JH, Walker WJ, McNally KA, Lim WA (2016b) Engineering T cells with customized therapeutic response programs using synthetic notch receptors. Cell 167:419–432.e416

Russell SJ, Peng KW, Bell JC (2012) Oncolytic virotherapy. Nat Biotechnol 30:658–670

Sadelain M, Brentjens R, Rivière I (2013) The basic principles of chimeric antigen receptor design. Cancer Discov 3:388–398

Schafer PH, Gandhi AK, Loveland MA, Chen RS, Man HW, Schnetkamp PP, Wolbring G, Govinda S, Corral LG, Payvandi F, Muller GW, Stirling DI (2003) Enhancement of cytokine production and AP-1 transcriptional activity in T cells by thalidomide-related immunomodulatory drugs. J Pharmacol Exp Ther 305:1222–1232

Schmidts A, Maus MV (2018) Making CAR T cells a solid option for solid tumors. Front Immunol 9:2593

Schneider D, Xiong Y, Wu D, Nölle V, Schmitz S, Haso W, Kaiser A, Dropulic B, Orentas RJ (2017) A tandem CD19/CD20 CAR lentiviral vector drives on-target and off-target antigen modulation in leukemia cell lines. J Immunother Cancer 5:42

Shah NN, Maatman T, Hari P, Johnson B (2019) Multi targeted CAR-T cell therapies for B-cell malignancies. Front Oncol 9:146

Shalabi H, Koegel A, Ponduri A, Qin H, Salem D, Stetler-Stevenson M, Yuan C, Yates B, Delbrook C, Loh M (2019) Case report: impact of BITE on CAR-T cell expansion. Adv Cell Gene Ther 2:e50

Sharma A, Bode B, Wenger RH, Lehmann K, Sartori AA, Moch H, Knuth A, Boehmer L, Broek M (2011a) γ-Radiation promotes immunological recognition of cancer cells through increased expression of cancer-testis antigens in vitro and in vivo. PLoS One 6:e28217

Sharma P, Wagner K, Wolchok JD, Allison JP (2011b) Novel cancer immunotherapy agents with survival benefit: recent successes and next steps. Nat Rev Cancer 11:805–812

Shevtsov M, Sato H, Multhoff G, Shibata A (2019) Novel approaches to improve the efficacy of Immuno-radiotherapy. Front Oncol 9:156

Shimabukuro-Vornhagen A, Gödel P, Subklewe M, Stemmler HJ, Schlößer HA, Schlaak M, Kochanek M, Böll B, von Bergwelt-Baildon MS (2018) Cytokine release syndrome. J Immunother Cancer 6:56

Shivaji UN, Jeffery L, Gui X, Smith SCL, Ahmad OF, Akbar A, Ghosh S, Iacucci M (2019) Immune checkpoint inhibitor-associated gastrointestinal and hepatic adverse events and their management. Ther Adv Gastroenterol 12:1756284819884196

Singh N, Perazzelli J, Grupp SA, Barrett DM (2016) Early memory phenotypes drive T cell proliferation in patients with pediatric malignancies. Sci Transl Med 8:320ra323

Slaney CY, von Scheidt B, Davenport AJ, Beavis PA, Westwood JA, Mardiana S, Tscharke DC, Ellis S, Prince HM, Trapani JA, Johnstone RW, Smyth MJ, Teng MW, Ali A, Yu Z, Rosenberg SA, Restifo NP, Neeson P, Darcy PK, Kershaw MH (2017) Dual-specific chimeric antigen receptor T cells and an indirect vaccine eradicate a variety of large solid tumors in an immunocompetent, self-antigen setting. Clin Cancer Res 23:2478–2490

Spiotto M, Fu YX, Weichselbaum RR (2016) The intersection of radiotherapy and immunotherapy: mechanisms and clinical implications. Sci Immunol 1:EAAG1266

Srivastava S, Salter AI, Liggitt D, Yechan-Gunja S, Sarvothama M, Cooper K, Smythe KS, Dudakov JA, Pierce RH, Rader C, Riddell SR (2019) Logic-gated ROR1 chimeric antigen receptor expression rescues T cell-mediated toxicity to Normal tissues and enables selective tumor targeting. Cancer Cell 35:489–503.e488

Steinfeld B, Scott J, Vilander G, Marx L, Quirk M, Lindberg J, Koerner K (2015) The role of lean process improvement in implementation of evidence-based practices in behavioral health care. J Behav Health Serv Res 42:504–518

Tahmasebi S, Elahi R, Esmaeilzadeh A (2019) Solid tumors challenges and new insights of CAR T cell engineering. Stem Cell Rev Rep 15:619–636

Tahmasebi S, Elahi R, Khosh E, Esmaeilzadeh A (2021) Programmable and multi-targeted CARs: a new breakthrough in cancer CAR-T cell therapy. Clin Transl Oncol 23:1003–1019

Tamada K, Geng D, Sakoda Y, Bansal N, Srivastava R, Li Z, Davila E (2012) Redirecting gene-modified T cells toward various cancer types using tagged antibodies. Clin Cancer Res 18: 6436–6445

Tanoue K, Rosewell Shaw A, Watanabe N, Porter C, Rana B, Gottschalk S, Brenner M, Suzuki M (2017) Armed oncolytic adenovirus-expressing PD-L1 mini-body enhances antitumor effects of chimeric antigen receptor T cells in solid tumors. Cancer Res 77:2040–2051

Tasian SK, Gardner RA (2015) CD19-redirected chimeric antigen receptor-modified T cells: a promising immunotherapy for children and adults with B-cell acute lymphoblastic leukemia (ALL). Ther Adv Hematol 6:228–241

Tiberghien P, Ferrand C, Lioure B, Milpied N, Angonin R, Deconinck E, Certoux JM, Robinet E, Saas P, Petracca B, Juttner C, Reynolds CW, Longo DL, Hervé P, Cahn JY (2001) Administration of herpes simplex-thymidine kinase-expressing donor T cells with a T-cell-depleted allogeneic marrow graft. Blood 97:63–72

Torikai H, Reik A, Soldner F, Warren EH, Yuen C, Zhou Y, Crossland DL, Huls H, Littman N, Zhang Z, Tykodi SS, Kebriaei P, Lee DA, Miller JC, Rebar EJ, Holmes MC, Jaenisch R, Champlin RE, Gregory PD, Cooper LJ (2013) Toward eliminating HLA class I expression to generate universal cells from allogeneic donors. Blood 122:1341–1349

Torres-Collado AX, Jazirehi AR (2018) Overcoming resistance of human non-Hodgkin's lymphoma to CD19-CAR CTL therapy by celecoxib and histone deacetylase inhibitors. Cancers (Basel) 10:200

Urbanska K, Lanitis E, Poussin M, Lynn RC, Gavin BP, Kelderman S, Yu J, Scholler N, Powell DJ Jr (2012) A universal strategy for adoptive immunotherapy of cancer through use of a novel T-cell antigen receptor. Cancer Res 72:1844–1852

Urbanska K, Lynn RC, Stashwick C, Thakur A, Lum LG, Powell DJ Jr (2014) Targeted cancer immunotherapy via combination of designer bispecific antibody and novel gene-engineered T cells. J Transl Med 12:347

van der Stegen SJ, Hamieh M, Sadelain M (2015) The pharmacology of second-generation chimeric antigen receptors. Nat Rev Drug Discov 14:499–509

Van Seggelen H, Tantalo DG, Afsahi A, Hammill JA, Bramson JL (2015) Chimeric antigen receptor-engineered T cells as oncolytic virus carriers. Mol Ther Oncolytics 2:15014

Vassaux G, Martin-Duque P (2004) Use of suicide genes for cancer gene therapy: study of the different approaches. Expert Opin Biol Ther 4:519–530

Wang X, Chang WC, Wong CW, Colcher D, Sherman M, Ostberg JR, Forman SJ, Riddell SR, Jensen MC (2011) A transgene-encoded cell surface polypeptide for selection, in vivo tracking, and ablation of engineered cells. Blood 118:1255–1263

Wang W, Kryczek I, Dostál L, Lin H, Tan L, Zhao L, Lu F, Wei S, Maj T, Peng D, He G, Vatan L, Szeliga W, Kuick R, Kotarski J, Tarkowski R, Dou Y, Rattan R, Munkarah A, Liu JR, Zou W (2016) Effector T cells abrogate stroma-mediated Chemoresistance in ovarian cancer. Cell 165: 1092–1105

Wang X, Walter M, Urak R, Weng L, Huynh C, Lim L, Wong CW, Chang WC, Thomas SH, Sanchez JF, Yang L, Brown CE, Pichiorri F, Htut M, Krishnan AY, Forman SJ (2018) Lenalidomide enhances the function of CS1 chimeric antigen receptor-redirected T cells against multiple myeloma. Clin Cancer Res 24:106–119

Wang X, Wu Z, Qiu W, Chen P, Xu X, Han W (2020) Programming CAR T cells to enhance anti-tumor efficacy through remodeling of the immune system. Front Med 14:1–20

Warda W, Larosa F, Neto Da Rocha M, Trad R, Deconinck E, Fajloun Z, Faure C, Caillot D, Moldovan M, Valmary-Degano S, Biichle S, Daguindau E, Garnache-Ottou F, Tabruyn S, Adotevi O, Deschamps M, Ferrand C (2019) CML hematopoietic stem cells expressing IL1RAP can be targeted by chimeric antigen receptor-engineered T cells. Cancer Res 79:663–675

Watanabe K, Luo Y, Da T, Guedan S, Ruella M, Scholler J, Keith B, Young RM, Engels B, Sorsa S, Siurala M, Havunen R, Tähtinen S, Hemminki A, June CH (2018) Pancreatic cancer therapy with combined mesothelin-redirected chimeric antigen receptor T cells and cytokine-armed oncolytic adenoviruses. JCI Insight 3:e99573

Weinkove R, George P, Dasyam N, McLellan AD (2019) Selecting costimulatory domains for chimeric antigen receptors: functional and clinical considerations. Clin Transl Immunol 8:e1049

Weiss T, Weller M, Guckenberger M, Sentman CL, Roth P (2018) NKG2D-based CAR T cells and radiotherapy exert synergistic efficacy in glioblastoma. Cancer Res 78:1031–1043

Wilkie S, Burbridge SE, Chiapero-Stanke L, Pereira AC, Cleary S, van der Stegen SJ, Spicer JF, Davies DM, Maher J (2010) Selective expansion of chimeric antigen receptor-targeted T-cells with potent effector function using interleukin-4. J Biol Chem 285:25538–25544

Wilkie S, van Schalkwyk MC, Hobbs S, Davies DM, van der Stegen SJ, Pereira AC, Burbridge SE, Box C, Eccles SA, Maher J (2012) Dual targeting of ErbB2 and MUC1 in breast cancer using chimeric antigen receptors engineered to provide complementary signaling. J Clin Immunol 32: 1059–1070

Wilson WH, O'Connor OA, Czuczman MS, LaCasce AS, Gerecitano JF, Leonard JP, Tulpule A, Dunleavy K, Xiong H, Chiu YL, Cui Y, Busman T, Elmore SW, Rosenberg SH, Krivoshik AP, Enschede SH, Humerickhouse RA (2010) Navitoclax, a targeted high-affinity inhibitor of BCL-2, in lymphoid malignancies: a phase 1 dose-escalation study of safety, pharmacokinetics, pharmacodynamics, and antitumour activity. Lancet Oncol 11:1149–1159

Wu CY, Roybal KT, Puchner EM, Onuffer J, Lim WA (2015) Remote control of therapeutic T cells through a small molecule-gated chimeric receptor. Science 350:aab4077

Wu M, Zhang L, Zhang H, Ning J, Tu S, He Y, Li Y (2019) CD19 chimeric antigen receptor-redirected T cells combined with epidermal growth factor receptor pathway substrate 8 peptide-derived dendritic cell vaccine in leukemia. Cytotherapy 21:659–670

Xu Y, Li S, Wang Y, Liu J, Mao X, Xing H, Tian Z, Tang K, Liao X, Rao Q, Xiong D, Wang M, Wang J (2019) Induced CD20 expression on B-cell malignant cells heightened the cytotoxic activity of chimeric antigen receptor engineered T cells. Hum Gene Ther 30:497–510

Xue T, Del Real M, Marcucci E, Toribio C, Setayesh SM, Forman SJ, Horne DA, Budde LE (2019) Checkpoint blockade in combination with CD33 chimeric antigen receptor T cell therapy and hypomethylating agent against acute myeloid leukemia. American Society of Hematology, Washington, DC

Yan L, Liu B (2019) Critical factors in chimeric antigen receptor-modified T-cell (CAR-T) therapy for solid tumors. Onco Targets Ther 12:193–204

Yang M, Wang L, Ni M, Schubert M-L, Neuber B, Hückelhoven-Krauss A, Gößmann RA, Kleist C, Eckstein V, Müller-Tidow C (2019) The effect of apoptosis inhibitor blockade agents on the third generation CD19 CAR T cells. American Society of Hematology, Washington, DC

Yuan X, Wu H, Xu H, Xiong H, Chu Q, Yu S, Wu GS, Wu K (2015) Notch signaling: an emerging therapeutic target for cancer treatment. Cancer Lett 369:20–27

Zah E, Lin MY, Silva-Benedict A, Jensen MC, Chen YY (2016) T cells expressing CD19/CD20 bispecific chimeric antigen receptors prevent antigen escape by malignant B cells. Cancer Immunol Res 4:498–508

Zhang B, Bowerman NA, Salama JK, Schmidt H, Spiotto MT, Schietinger A, Yu P, Fu YX, Weichselbaum RR, Rowley DA, Kranz DM, Schreiber H (2007) Induced sensitization of tumor stroma leads to eradication of established cancer by T cells. J Exp Med 204:49–55

Zhang L, Yu Z, Muranski P, Palmer D, Restifo N, Rosenberg S, Morgan R (2013) Inhibition of TGF-β signaling in genetically engineered tumor antigen-reactive T cells significantly enhances tumor treatment efficacy. Gene Ther 20:575–580

Zhang Y, Zhang X, Cheng C, Mu W, Liu X, Li N, Wei X, Liu X, Xia C, Wang H (2017) CRISPR-Cas9 mediated LAG-3 disruption in CAR-T cells. Front Med 11:554–562

Zhang E, Yang P, Gu J, Wu H, Chi X, Liu C, Wang Y, Xue J, Qi W, Sun Q, Zhang S, Hu J, Xu H (2018) Recombination of a dual-CAR-modified T lymphocyte to accurately eliminate pancreatic malignancy. J Hematol Oncol 11:102

Zhang Y, Li Y, Chen K, Qian L, Wang P (2021) Oncolytic virotherapy reverses the immunosuppressive tumor microenvironment and its potential in combination with immunotherapy. Cancer Cell Int 21:262

Zhao J, Lin Q, Song Y, Liu D (2018) Universal CARs, universal T cells, and universal CAR T cells. J Hematol Oncol 11:132

Zhong XS, Matsushita M, Plotkin J, Riviere I, Sadelain M (2010) Chimeric antigen receptors combining 4-1BB and CD28 signaling domains augment PI3kinase/AKT/Bcl-XL activation and CD8+ T cell-mediated tumor eradication. Mol Ther 18:413–420

An Updated Focus on Immune Checkpoint Inhibitors and Tubulointerstitial Nephritis

Daniela Picciotto, Carlo Genova, Francesca Costigliolo, Annarita Bottini, Giacomo Garibotto, Francesca Viazzi, and Pasquale Esposito

Abstract

One of the most relevant achievements in oncological research is represented by the development of a new category of anticancer drugs, the immune checkpoint inhibitors (ICIs), which are currently widely used as new efficient therapeutic weapons in medical oncology. ICIs are monoclonal antibodies specifically designed to disrupt the inhibitory activity of immune checkpoints to enable the T lymphocyte-mediated recognition and elimination of tumor cells. However, the activation of the immune system may cause immune-mediated specific target organ toxicity, leading to so-called immune-related adverse events (irAEs).

Here, we review the available evidence on kidney damage in the course of ICIs treatment, focusing on acute tubulointerstitial nephritis (ATIN), the most common clinical presentation of ICI-related nephrotoxicity. Therefore, we present an updated excursus on the epidemiology, the clinical relevance, and the physio-pathological mechanisms leading to ICI-related ATIN.

Moreover, we describe the diagnostic approach to adopt in case of acute kidney injury onset in a patient in treatment with ICIs, pinpointing the importance

D. Picciotto · F. Costigliolo
Nephrology Unit, IRCCS Ospedale Policlinico San Martino, Genoa, Italy

C. Genova
UOC Clinica di Oncologia Medica; IRCCS Ospedale Policlinico San Martino, Genoa, Italy

Department of Internal Medicine, University of Genova, Genoa, Italy

A. Bottini · G. Garibotto (✉)
Department of Internal Medicine, University of Genova, Genoa, Italy
e-mail: gari@unige.it

F. Viazzi · P. Esposito
Nephrology Unit, IRCCS Ospedale Policlinico San Martino, Genoa, Italy

Department of Internal Medicine, University of Genova, Genoa, Italy

Interdisciplinary Cancer Research, https://doi.org/10.1007/16833_2022_80
Published online: 18 November 2022

of histopathology which enables a certain differential diagnosis between ATIN and other rare, underrated but clinically relevant forms of kidney involvement in course of ICIs therapy.

Therapeutic approaches suggested by oncological guidelines are reported bearing in mind that while responsiveness to steroids is ascertained, the role and benefit of using other immunosuppressants have still to be clarified.

Finally, the clinical conundrums represented by the possibility of rechallenging patients with ICIs after an ICI-related ATIN episode and ICIs treatment in the kidney transplanted patient are discussed.

Keywords

Acute kidney injury · Acute tubulo-interstitial nephritis · Biomarkers · Immune checkpoint inhibitors · Kidney biopsy · Nephrotoxicity · Onconephrology

1 Introduction

The kidney has a crucial role in regulating the metabolism and excretion of numerous medications; so, it is not surprising that nephrotoxicity is one of the most common adverse effects (AE) of several drugs (Perazella 2009).

The mechanisms of renal toxicity may be various ranging from direct tubular toxicity to vascular injury or alterations in glomerular hemodynamics (Perazella 2019). Clinically, nephrotoxicity may present as acute or chronic impairment of the kidney function, urinary alterations, electrolyte, and acid-base disorders, or a combination of them (Naughton 2008). Theoretically, most of the medications available on the market may present renal AE, but the drugs more commonly associated with nephrotoxicity include some categories of antibiotics, such as aminoglycosides, non-steroidal anti-inflammatory drugs, and iodinated contrast agents (Geenen et al. 2013).

Chemotherapeutic agents used in the treatment of cancer constitute an important group of drugs potentially linked to renal AE. Indeed, beyond the well-known nephrotoxic platinum-based drugs, continuous research in the oncological field has led to the development of novel therapeutic approaches, such as monoclonal antibodies acting on different biological targets (i.e., growth factors, B cells, tumor antigens, etc.), that add new questions about the kidney safety of anticancer drugs (Izzedine and Perazella 2017).

It is also important to bear in mind that kidney function is one of the main factors influencing the prescription and dosage of agents used in the treatment of cancer (Stengel 2010). More importantly, data from large cohorts demonstrate that patients with cancer developing kidney disease have a worse outcome (Guo et al. 2022).

The complexity of the interactions between kidney function and management of the oncological disease has led to the development of a new subspecialty of nephrology, the so-called onconephrology (Rosner et al. 2021; Perazella 2012). Onconephrology, which implies collaborative care between oncologists and nephrologists, is a clear example of the utility of a multidisciplinary method for complex conditions.

The need for this approach has been recently put in the spotlight after the introduction of a new category of anticancer drugs, the immune checkpoint inhibitors (ICIs), that are opening a new era of immune therapy (O'Donnell et al. 2019).

Indeed, these drugs, through mechanisms that will be better explained in the following paragraphs of this chapter, activate the immune system to recognize and eliminate the tumor cells.

This peculiar mechanism, although effective, is not risk-free. In fact, the activation of the immune system may also lead to immune-mediated damage of distant organs, depicting the condition of the so-called immune-related adverse events (irAEs) (Das and Johnson 2019). irAEs may interest many organs or tissues, including endocrine glands, skin, gastrointestinal apparatus, and, less frequently, the lung and kidney.

The most common presentation of ICI-related nephrotoxicity is acute kidney injury (AKI), due to acute tubulointerstitial nephritis (ATIN), a histological picture characterized by edema, and interstitial inflammation, infiltration of T lymphocytes, eosinophils, and plasma cells (Franzin et al. 2020). The occurrence of ATIN and the associated kidney function impairment in patients on ICIs may significantly impact the management of cancer and the prognosis of these patients (Murakami et al. 2016).

Therefore, the awareness of this complication may be helpful for both nephrologists and oncologists. For this purpose, in this chapter, we provide a comprehensive overview of ICI-related nephrotoxicity, focusing on ATIN. We will discuss the available evidence derived from studies addressed to evaluate pathogenetic mechanisms, characterize early biomarkers, and define specific management and therapeutic strategies for this condition.

2 ICI Classes and Mechanism of Action

2.1 Rationale and Mechanisms of Action

ICIs are monoclonal antibodies specifically designed to disrupt the inhibitory activity of immune checkpoints, which normally act as regulatory pathways with the function of ensuring self-tolerance. While the physiological activity of immune checkpoints prevents the development of autoimmune diseases, tumor cells might exploit these mechanisms to avoid detection and elimination by T cells (Farkona et al. 2016). In the last years, ICIs have acquired increasing relevance in medical oncology, both as single therapeutic approach and as part of combinations (i.e., with chemotherapy).

To date, the most relevant immune checkpoints from a therapeutic perspective are represented by cytotoxic T lymphocyte antigen 4 (CTLA-4) and the axis constituted by programmed death protein 1 (PD-1) and its ligand (PD-L1). In short terms, once administered via intravenous route, ICIs bind their designated immune checkpoint molecules and disrupt their inhibitory effect, thus favoring the activation of immune cells, with specific reference to T cells, which in turn exert cytotoxic activity on neoplastic cells (Wei et al. 2018). While CTLA-4 and PD-1/PD-L1 share an inhibitory role, they exert their activity in a slightly different way; indeed, CTLA-4, which is expressed on T cells, can bind ligands of the B7 family expressed on antigen-presenting cells, and their interaction might take place in lymph nodes during the priming phase, thus resulting in T cell anergic state; by contrast, the PD-1/PD-L1 interaction occurs when T cells infiltrate tumor tissue, with PD-1 expressed on T cells and PD-L1 expressed on tumor cells, respectively. This difference might appear trivial at first glance; however, CTLA-4 inhibitors act at an early phase of immune response within lymph nodes, while PD-1/PD-L1 inhibitors act in a later phase, within tumor microenvironment. Indeed, on one hand, this difference results in the possibility to concurrently use both ICIs with synergic, non-redundant effect; on the other hand, CTLA-4 blockade usually results in a more challenging safety profile compared to PD-1/PD-L1 inhibitors, as reported in the following sections (Franzin et al. 2020).

Finally, a synergic effect of ICIs and other treatment modalities, including chemotherapy and targeted agents, has been demonstrated across different solid tumors, based on the ability of chemotherapy to induce immune response and enroll T cells and the ability of specific inhibitors, such as the multi-target tyrosine kinase inhibitor axitinib, to influence tumor microenvironment towards a pro-immunogenic phenotype (Wei et al. 2018; Genova et al. 2021).

2.2 Currently Available ICIs in Solid Tumors

Starting from their inception in the oncology field, increasing ICI-based regimens have become available throughout different tumors and various settings; notably, the available ICIs are directed against CTLA-4, PD-1, and PD-L1. Ipilimumab is the only currently employed CTLA-4 inhibitor and has shown to be effective in metastatic melanoma as single agent, thus representing the first approved ICI in oncology (Hodi et al. 2010). The first approved PD-1 inhibitor was nivolumab, initially registered for metastatic melanoma and for previously treated NSCLC. In the following years, the combination of ipilimumab and nivolumab showed efficacy in multiple neoplasms, including melanoma, renal cell carcinoma, non-small cell lung cancer (NSCLC), malignant pleural mesothelioma, colorectal cancer, and esophageal squamous cell carcinoma (EMA 2018a, b; Shiravand et al. 2022; Jin and Sinicrope 2022; Kim et al. 2022). Pembrolizumab is another effective ICI directed against PD-1, and it was the first agent approved for first-line treatment of advanced NSCLC; subsequently, pembrolizumab was approved across multiple solid tumors as single agent. Notably, pembrolizumab demonstrated strong synergy with chemotherapy, with particular reference to platinum-based regimens in various tumors, including triple-negative breast cancer (EMA 2018c; Agostinetto et al. 2022). The most recently introduced anti-PD-1 ICI, cemiplimab, was initially approved as the first agent of its class active on basal cell carcinoma and squamous cell carcinoma of the skin, although its indications are rapidly expanding (Boutros et al. 2021; EMA

2019). In addition to the aforementioned agents, also specific PD-L1 inhibitors have been developed. The first of such agents, atezolizumab, is acquiring increasing relevance both as single agent and as part of combination regimens, and indeed it represents the first ICI approved in combination with chemotherapy for the treatment of advanced small cell lung cancer and triple-negative breast cancer (EMA 2018d). The other available PD-L1 inhibitor, durvalumab, has a narrower spectrum of indication, compared to other agents; however, it was the first agent showing to be effective as maintenance treatment after a concurrent chemo-radiation approach with curative intent for locally advanced, non-metastatic NSCLC (EMA 2018e). An up-to-date list of the current indications for ICIs according to the European Medicines Agency has been reported in Table 1.

At present, other immune checkpoints are being explored in clinical trials as potential exploitable targets (Jiang et al. 2021). Notably, several clinical trials investigating the use of PD-1/PD-L1 inhibitors have shown increasing anti-neoplastic activity when treated tumors had a strong PD-L1 expression (≥50% evaluated at immunohistochemistry on tumor samples); this occurrence is especially relevant in trials assessing the use of ICIs as single agent in specific settings (i.e., first line for advanced NSCLC), although such findings were not always consistent across different tumors and lines of treatment; furthermore, the use of PD-1/PD-L1 inhibitors within combinations generally appears less dependent from PD-L1 expression. In this regard, colorectal cancer represents an intriguing exception, since ICIs are effective in presence of mismatch repair deficiency or microsatellite instability. A detailed description of the pivotal trials for each solid tumor and the current prescribing indication of each ICI-based regimen falls beyond the scope of this text.

3 Immune-Related Adverse Events

3.1 Safety Profiles of ICIs

Based on the available literature, ICIs are generally well tolerated; however, such agents are characterized by a peculiar safety profile, strictly associated with their mechanism of action. Indeed, since ICIs disrupt the mechanisms of immune tolerance, it is possible that the consequent accentuated immune response may cause damage to different organs and apparatus, an occurrence collectively known as irAEs. Although virtually any district might be involved in irAEs, some are more prone than others to develop this immune-mediated damage. The most frequent irAEs include endocrinologic events, skin toxicity, and hepatitis, while less frequent events include pneumonitis and renal toxicity. Approximate incidence values for relevant irAEs were collected from pivotal studies and prescribing information and reported in Table 2. Notably, the onset time for each event may vary across different irAEs, and the same applies to their duration (Genova et al. 2017), and while most events, if adequately treated, are resolved after few weeks, some irAEs, such as endocrinopathies, are persistent and require long-term hormonal replacement.

Table 1 List of the most relevant ICIs currently employed in solid tumors based on the prescribing information of the European Medicines Agency. The setting refers to advanced/metastatic disease unless otherwise specified

Agent	Immune checkpoint(s)	Regimen	Setting
Atezolizumab	PD-L1	Single agent	NSCLC[a]
		Combination with chemotherapy	TNBC[a] NSCLC SCLC Urothelial carcinoma[a]
Cemiplimab	PD-1	Single agent	NSCLC, including locally advanced disease Cutaneous squamous cell carcinoma Basal cell carcinoma
Durvalumab	PD-L1	Combination with chemotherapy	SCLC
		Maintenance after chemo-radiation	Locally advanced NSCLC[a]
Ipilimumab	CTLA-4	Single agent	Melanoma
		Combination with nivolumab	RCC Melanoma Malignant pleural mesothelioma dMMR MSI-H CRC Esophageal squamous cell carcinoma[a]
		Combination with nivolumab and chemotherapy	NSCLC
Nivolumab	PD-L1	Single agent	Resected melanoma NSCLC RCC SCCHN Urothelial carcinoma (including resected urothelial carcinoma)[a] Esophageal squamous cell carcinoma[a] GEJ or esophageal carcinoma after chemo-radiation
		Combination with ipilimumab	See ipilimumab in combination with nivolumab
		Combination with chemotherapy	Esophageal squamous cell carcinoma[a] Gastric carcinoma[a] GEJ carcinoma[a]

(continued)

Table 1 (continued)

Agent	Immune checkpoint(s)	Regimen	Setting
		Combination with ipilimumab and chemotherapy	NSCLC
		Combination with cabozantinib	RCC
Pembrolizumab	PD-1	Single agent	NSCLC[a] Melanoma (including stage III resected melanoma) Urothelial carcinoma SCCHN[a] Resected RCC dMMR MSI-H CRC
		Combination with chemotherapy	NSCLC SCCHN[a] Esophageal carcinoma[a] TNBC[a] (including neoadjuvant treatment) Cervical cancer[a]
		Combination with chemotherapy and bevacizumab	Cervical cancer[a]
		Combination with axitinib	RCC
		Combination with lenvatinib	RCC Endometrial carcinoma

Reference can be found in the text

Legend: *CRC* colorectal cancer; *dMMR* mismatch repair deficient; *HCC* hepatocellular carcinoma; *GEJ*: gastro-esophageal junction; *ICI* immune checkpoint inhibitor; *MSI-H* microsatellite instability-high; *NSCLC* non-small cell lung cancer; *PD-1* programmed death protein 1; *PD-L1* PD-1 ligand; *RCC* renal cell carcinoma; *SCCHN* squamous cell carcinoma of the head and neck; *SCLC* small cell lung cancer; *TNBC* triple-negative breast cancer

[a]Indications for which PD-L1 is relevant

Additionally, as previously stated, the specific ICI regimen may influence the frequency and severity of observed irAEs, with regimens containing ipilimumab alone or in combination generally being characterized by worse toxicities. Interestingly, clinical trials involving ipilimumab plus nivolumab have shown that patients who had severe irAEs which forced them to treatment discontinuation subsequently achieved sustained clinical and radiological benefit, even with survival advantage, in spite of early immunotherapy discontinuation; these data suggest that the stimulated immune system remained active against tumor cells (Reck et al. 2021; Paz-Ares et al. 2022; Baas et al. 2021).

Table 2 Main irAEs associated with ICIs alone or in combination, extrapolated from prescribing information and relevant pivotal trials, including frequency range across multiple pivotal studies

irAE	CTLA-4		PD-1/PD-L1		PD-1/PD-L1 plus chemotherapy		PD-1 plus CTLA-4	
	Any	Gr 3–4	Any	Gr 3–4	Any	Gr 3–4	Any	Gr 3–4
Skin toxicity	40–56%	2–3%	46%	2–6%	20%	2%	20–62%	1–6%
Diarrhea/colitis	32–38%	5–12%	7–22%	1–4%	30%	5%	21–48%	4–15%
Endocrinopathies	4–12%	1–3%	4–17%	1–2%	6–7%	0–1%	16–34%	1–6%
Hepatic toxicity	2–7%	1–2%	1–8%	1–3%	2%	2%	6–33%	4–20%
Pulmonary toxicity	2%	<1%	1–8%	<1–3%	4–6%	2–3%	6–8%	1–3%
Renal toxicity	3%	<1%	0–1%	<1%	0–2%	0–1%	1–7%	<1–2%

Note: Ipilimumab-containing regimens significantly varied in terms of dose across studies, potentially influencing the safety profile
Reference can be found in the text

The timely treatment of irAEs might significantly influence the outcomes, especially for potentially life-threatening events; hence, prompt recognition of said events represents the first step of an appropriate management of the irAE, and it starts with educating the patient and her/his caregivers, with clear instructions for irAEs recognition. The therapeutic approach to irAEs strictly depends on the specific event and its severity, defined according to common terminology criteria for adverse events (CTCAE). To date, multiple guidelines for the management of immunotherapy-induced toxicities have been developed and are currently accessible by healthcare professionals (Schneider et al. 2021; Brahmer et al. 2021).

Generally speaking, mild events (CTCAE Gr 1) usually do not require treatment interruption and can be managed with loco-regional approaches, such as topical corticosteroids; moderate events (CTCAE Gr 2) might still benefit from local treatments but often require systemic corticosteroids and ICI interruption. Severe events (CTCAE ≥3) typically require high doses of corticosteroids (up to 2 mg/Kg of prednisone or equivalent on a daily basis) with slow steroid tapering; such events, based on the specific site of toxicity, might make permanent treatment discontinuation necessary. While most irAEs respond to corticosteroids, in some cases other treatments might be required. Such agents may include immunosuppressant commonly employed as treatment for autoimmune of bowel inflammatory diseases (i.e., infliximab) or for transplant rejection (i.e., mycophenolate); in extreme circumstances, life-threatening irAEs might be managed with plasmapheresis or the use of intravenous immunoglobulins. Notably, most available evidence of immunosuppression for irAEs beyond the use of corticosteroids is generally limited and often depending on expert opinions or case reports (Schneider et al. 2021; Haanen et al. 2017).

4 Spectrum of the Kidney Involvement in ICI-Related Toxicities: From Acute Kidney Injury to Electrolyte Disorders

4.1 Acute Kidney Injury: Epidemiology and Histopathological Findings

Among the different organs potentially involved in irAE, the kidneys have a relevant role since the impairment of the kidney function may have a significant impact on the general patient condition and cancer management.

ICI-related nephrotoxicity is associated with different clinical presentations that may recognize various pathogenetic mechanisms (Perazella 2020). Overall, the data on the incidence of nephrotoxicity are limited and derived largely from small case series and oncologic studies. In early clinical trials, the rate of ICI-related nephrotoxicity ranged from as low as 2% with a single agent and up to 4.5% when a combination of agents was used (Cortazar et al. 2016).

So, it seems that renal involvement is relatively rare when compared to AE involving other districts, such as skin or gastrointestinal tract (where ICI-related toxicity may occur in about 15% of the patients) (Champiat et al. 2016). However, the results of recent studies suggest that the incidence rates of renal toxicities in the real-world use of these agents might be significantly higher (from 10% to 30% of cases) (Wanchoo et al. 2017).

The most common clinical presentation of ICI nephrotoxicity is AKI, characterized by an abrupt reduction of the renal function, as proven by the rapid increase in serum creatinine levels (>50% of the basal value), in absence of other evident causes of kidney damage (Schneider et al. 2021).

Nevertheless, it should be also recognized that patients with active cancer may present several reasons to develop kidney injury, including volume depletion, obstructive nephropathy, hypercalcemia, and nephrotoxicity from other drugs. So, the establishment of a clear causal effect of ICI in the pathogenesis of AKI may be challenging in this clinical setting.

A peculiar characteristic of ICI-related AKI, which may help in diagnostic workup, is the latency between ICI-based therapy initiation and the onset of kidney damage. Indeed, differently from the other forms of AKI that classically occur immediately after the injury, AKI associated with ICI may develop after a long interval (ranging from 6 weeks to 12 months) from the exposure to the medication (Seethapathy et al. 2021a, b).

Regarding the specific causes of ICI-related AKI, the most reliable data come from studies evaluating kidney biopsies.

In the large series, Cortazar et al. evaluated 138 patients with a diagnosis of ICI-AKI, 43% of whom (60 patients) underwent a kidney biopsy (Cortazar et al. 2020).

They found that >90% of these patients had ATIN as a dominant histological picture, while only four patients presented other lesions, including minimal change disease with tubular damage, antineutrophil cytoplasmic antibody (ANCA)-negative pauci-immune crescentic glomerulonephritis, anti-glomerular basement membrane disease, and C3 glomerulonephritis.

Similarly, Mamlouk et al. evaluated 16 cases of patients with advanced solid or hematologic malignancy on anti-PD-1-based therapy who underwent kidney biopsies because of AKI.

They found in 14/16 biopsies histological findings of ATIN alone or in association with other glomerular pathological patterns, such as pauci-immune glomerulonephritis, membranous glomerulonephritis, C3 glomerulonephritis, and immunoglobulin A (IgA) (Mamlouk et al. 2019).

Lastly, in a smaller study by Meraz-Muñoz et al. involving a total of 309 patients on ICI, the authors evaluated 51 cases of AKI that occurred after a median time from ICI initiation of 30 (IQR 21 to 79) days. Among them, kidney biopsies were performed in 12 patients (Meraz-Muñoz et al. 2020). Also in this case series, histological evaluations confirmed that ATIN was the most common finding (50% of the biopsies), but a significant incidence of glomerular lesions, including cases of minimal change disease and membranous nephropathy, was also found. Interestingly, as expected, patients with glomerular disease, apart from AKI, presented significant alterations of urinalysis, often characterized by high-grade proteinuria.

Therefore, the overall analysis of these data suggests that, although predominant, ATIN is not the only kidney manifestation of ICIs and other compartments of the kidney may be involved in ICI-related nephrotoxicity (Izzedine et al. 2017).

As for as non-ATIN kidney lesions, Kitchlu et al. examined 27 papers reporting a total of 45 biopsy-proven cases of glomerular disease occurring in patients on ICIs (Kitchlu et al. 2020).

They found that the most common glomerular alterations were pauci-immune-glomerulonephritis/vasculitis (27%), podocytopathies (20%), and C3 glomerulopathy (11%). However, it should be emphasized that 40% of these patients had concomitant ATIN.

Moreover, the median time to glomerular disease was 3 months after ICI initiation, which is similar to ICI-induced ATIN. Most importantly, the outcomes of patients with de novo ICI-related glomerular diseases were poor; indeed, despite 98% receiving corticosteroid treatment, 20% of the patients progressed to end-stage kidney disease, and one-third died.

The exact pathogenesis of ICI-related glomerular disease is unknown, even if it has been hypothesized that immune hyperactivity elicited by ICI and the consequent T cell activation may trigger an inflammatory response and cause cytotoxic injury to the kidney (Kitchlu et al. 2020; Keir et al. 2006).

A counterproof of these mechanisms comes from experimental models of PD-1-knockout mice which spontaneously develop glomerulonephritis, mediated by the activation of cells of hematopoietic origin (Menke et al. 2007). In addition to triggering the onset of de novo glomerulonephritis, it should be noticed that ICIs may also reactivate preexisting autoimmune diseases. So, similar to what reported in patients with rheumatic disease, it is tempting to hypothesize that initiation of ICI treatment may exacerbate preexisting glomerulonephritis (Johnson et al. 2018). Furthermore, apart from the interstitium (involved in ATIN) and glomeruli, also other compartments of the kidney could be affected by ICI-related nephrotoxicity, as proven by the cases of acute tubular necrosis, thrombotic microangiopathy, and distal renal tubular acidosis that have been occasionally found in patients on ICI (Cortazar et al. 2020).

Finally, despite the variability of histological lesions found in patients with ICI-related nephrotoxicity, the indication of kidney biopsy in this population is still under debate.

Indeed, some authors suggest that considering the high prevalence of ATIN and its responsiveness to corticosteroids, initial empirical therapy is possible, and kidney biopsy should be performed only on a case-by-case basis (Gutgarts and Glezerman 2020).

However, due to heterogeneity of histological pictures and their potential impact on renal prognosis, a wider use of kidney biopsy in case of ICI-related AKI is often recommended (Perazella 2020).

4.2 Electrolyte Disorders

Beyond structural kidney alterations, a specific feature of the kidney involvement in ICI-related AE is the occurrence of electrolyte disorders (Tinawi and Bastani 2020).

Indeed, both clinical experience and literature data have shown that multiple electrolyte disorders may develop in patients on ICI, including hyponatremia, hypocalcemia, hypercalcemia, hypomagnesemia, hypokalemia, hyperkalemia, hypophosphatemia, and Fanconi syndrome.

In a cohort study involving a total of 2458 patients, Seethapathy et al. observed that within the first year after starting ICIs, 62% of the patients experienced hyponatremia (plasma sodium <134 mEq/L), which was severe (<124 mEq/L) in the 6% of the cases (Seethapathy et al. 2021a, b).

Development of hyponatremia was correlated with the use of ipilimumab (a cytotoxic T lymphocyte antigen-4 inhibitor), diuretic use, and non-White race. In addition, other electrolyte abnormalities were also observed, including hypophosphatemia (phosphorus <2 mg/dL) and hypokalemia (potassium <3.0 mEq/L). Similar data come from the analysis of the FDA adverse events database. Among 312 cases of electrolyte disorders associated with the use of ipilimumab, nivolumab, and pembrolizumab, hyponatremia was the most common (61.5%), followed by hypokalemia (23%) and hyperkalemia (8%) (Wanchoo et al. 2017).

Manohar et al. performed a different approach designing a meta-analysis that included five randomized controlled trials (RCTs) to assess the association between PD-1 inhibitors and electrolyte disorders (Manohar et al. 2019). They found an overall pooled risk of electrolyte disorders of 1.67 (95% CI 0.89–3.12), which rose to 3.91 (95% CI 1.22–12.56) in studies comparing PD-1 inhibitors with ipilimumab (used as control).

However, when the authors looked at the relationship of single electrolyte alteration with ICI-based therapy, they observed that only hypocalcemia was significantly associated with the treatment.

Apart from data on large cohorts that allow focusing on the more common forms of electrolyte disorders, some insight into the possibility of different manifestations comes from the description of singular clinical cases. So, for example, there are reports on the association of ICI treatment with rare conditions, such as renal tubular acidosis and Fanconi syndrome (Balakrishna and Villegas 2017; Farid et al. 2020). The exact mechanisms of electrolyte disorders occurring as a sequela of ICI treatment are largely unknown. It has been hypothesized that analogously to other irAEs related to ICI, also electrolyte disorders may be the expression of autoimmune response elicited by the treatment. So, hypophysitis and secondary adrenal insufficiency, such as immune-mediated alterations of thyroid or parathyroid, may constitute the underlying conditions leading to dysregulation of serum electrolyte levels (Barnard et al. 2012).

Of note, the effectiveness of steroid treatment to treat electrolyte disorders in patients on ICI may provide a further clue to support the involvement of autoimmune mechanisms in the pathogenesis of these complications (Balakrishna and Villegas 2017).

5 Tubulointerstitial Nephritis

5.1 Epidemiology

AKI consequent to ICIs treatment has been described early after inclusion of these drugs in clinical practice. As above reported, the actual incidence of AKI in course of ICIs treatment is still an open issue, since there is a discrepancy between data coming from clinical trials (reporting AKI incidence of 2–5%) and data from real-life studies (where an incidence of 15–17% is reported) (Seethapathy et al. 2019). A common finding in the different studies is that ATIN represents the histological diagnosis in the majority (till 80%) of the cases (Perazella and Shirali 2020).

However, it is conceivable that due to a probable more diffuse use of these chemotherapeutics in the future, the incidence of both AKI and ATIN related to ICIs treatment will further increase in the following years.

5.2 Pathophysiology

IrAEs are off-target effects caused by the activation of the immune system against non-tumor cells, but the exact mechanisms underlying ICI-related ATIN development are yet not fully understood. Various research groups have dealt with this issue and formulated valid hypothesis (Nussbaum and Perazella 2018; Seethapathy et al. 2019; Seethapathy et al. 2021a, b; Sury et al. 2018).

Some authors have found activation of inflammatory pathways due to molecular target recognition (CTLA4, PD-1, PD-L1) in non-tumoral tissues as one of the main causative mechanisms of irAEs (Sury et al. 2018; Ding et al. 2005). Notably, PD-L1 is expressed in renal tubular cells and upregulated in case of inflammation (Sury et al. 2018). Moreover, ICIs therapy may lead to loss of tolerance and activation of T cells directed against renal self-antigens or to the reactivation of dormant effector T lymphocytes directed against specific nephrotoxins (Spanou et al. 2006).

There is evidence that ICIs may break tolerance to non-steroidal anti-inflammatory drugs (NSAIDs) and proton pump inhibitors (PPIs) (Seethapathy et al. 2019; Seethapathy et al. 2021a, b; Kato et al. 2021). In fact, in a wide patient cohort, Cortazar et al. highlighted how patients developing ICIs AIN had higher rates of complete recovery in case of NSAIDs and PPIs discontinuation (Cortazar et al. 2020). Furthermore, circulating T lymphocytes with TCR restriction of patients affected by ICI-induced ATIN were exposed in vitro to specific drugs with subsequent activation (Spanou et al. 2006). Finally, inhibition of immune checkpoints is associated with an increase in circulating and tissue pro-inflammatory cytokines which may further contribute to organ damage (Sury et al. 2018) (for a summary of the main pathogenic mechanisms, see Fig. 1).

For what concerns the risk factors identified for the development of ICI-associated ATIN, a low basal eGFR, combined dual checkpoint inhibition, and PPI use were identified as the main ones in various studies (Seethapathy et al. 2019; Kato et al. 2021; Cortazar et al. 2020; Gupta et al. 2021).

5.3 Clinical Presentation

Oncology societies have developed a staging of ICIs AKI based on creatinine values in analogy to the criteria used for the staging of AKI by the Kidney Disease: Improving Global Outcomes (KDIGO). Stages 1–3 are graded on behalf of increasing creatinine values, and stage 4 is represented by the need of replacement renal therapy and stage 5 by the death of the patient (Sise et al. 2019). It is important to underline that oncologic patients often have a reduced muscular mass and therefore serum creatinine values may underestimate the degree of kidney injury.

The mean creatinine peak reported in various papers in ICI-induced ATIN is 4.5 mg/dl (Cortazar et al. 2020; Draibe et al. 2020).

ICI-induced ATIN has no pathognomonic clinical features which can help to distinguish it from acute nephritis caused by other drugs (Cortazar et al. 2016; Oleas et al. 2020). In various reports the most frequent findings were sub-nephrotic proteinuria and sterile pyuria which was found in nearly 50% of the patients. The classic triad of fever, rash, and eosinophilia is nonspecific and rarely reported in ICI-associated ATIN as well as in ATIN related to other nephrotoxins (Moledina and Parikh 2019). The delayed onset of AKI reported in some studies (Cortazar et al. 2020; Draibe et al. 2020) compared to other drug-induced ATIN could be explained by the prolonged activity of effector T lymphocytes in the absence of a mechanism of direct toxicity (Franzin et al. 2020).

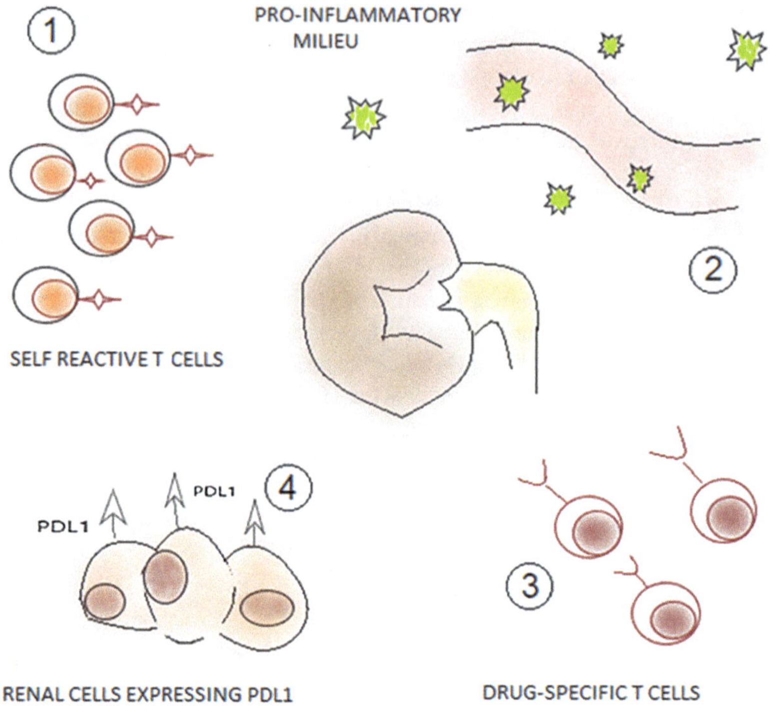

Fig. 1 Physiopathological mechanisms associated with ICI-related ATIN. (1) Loss of immunotolerance due to self-reactive T cell activation and differentiation. (2) Increased production and release of cytokines. (3) Reactivation of dormant effector T lymphocytes directed against specific nephrotoxins. (4) Molecular target recognition of PD-L1 overexpressed by tubular cells

Mortality rates in patients with ICIs associated ATIN appear to be lower compared to patients affected by AKI from other causes. This was shown by Baker et al. in a recent study in which patients with ICI-induced ATIN exhibited lower mortality than those suffering from AKI unrelated to ICIs therapy in univariable analysis (HR 0.43 (95% CI 0.21 to 0.89)) as well as after adjusting for confounders (adjusted HR 0.44 (95% CI 0.21 to 0.93)) (Baker et al. 2022).

6 Diagnosis

The main challenge to face in the management of AKI in a patient on ICIs is to make a correct differential diagnosis, taking into account that the discontinuation of the treatment may be a double-edged sword by implying a risk of progression of the oncological disease.

A patient affected by cancer may develop AKI as a result of multiple causes like dehydration due to gastrointestinal side effects of chemotherapy, severe infections, and urinary obstruction caused by intra-abdominal masses.

Moreover, oncologic patients have complex therapies which often include potential nephrotoxic drugs which may be responsible of ATIN as much as ICIs.

The first required step in the diagnostic workup is therefore to exclude other alternative etiologies as well as to consider the presence of risk factors linked to ICI-associated ATIN like PPI use, ICIs combined therapy, or a low eGFR at baseline (Seethapathy et al. 2021a, b).

A significant clue that suggests ICI-induced ATIN rather than other types of AKI is the coexistence of irAEs which were reported in 43% of patients suffering from ICI-related acute kidney failure in a large multicenter analysis by Cortazar et al. (Cortazar et al. 2020).

As previously mentioned, the clinical presentation of ICI-related ATIN, being rather nonspecific, is of limited usefulness in the diagnostic process.

Performing a urinalysis with sediment examination is nevertheless mandatory in order to find those alterations as sterile pyuria, leukocytes casts, or tubular proteinuria that might, though not specific nor sensitive, orient the clinician towards ICI-induced ATIN (Perazella and Sprangers 2021).

Moreover, some authors have tried to define the main characteristics which may help to differentiate between ICIs associated versus "classical" ATIN. Recently, Draibe et al. analyzed the clinical and laboratoristic features of 47 patients affected by ATIN. Patients with ICIs nephritis showed lower serum creatinine values at diagnosis and a higher leukocytes count compared with patients with non-ICI-related nephritis. They confirmed a longer latency in the onset of ATIN induced by immunotherapy, whereas a faster creatinine decrease was observed in patients with ATIN from other nephrotoxins. No difference in the degree of proteinuria was found among the two cohorts (Draibe et al. 2020).

Performing a kidney biopsy surely represents the mean to obtain a sure diagnosis. It namely allows to differentiate between classical forms and ICI-induced ATIN due to the presence of specific hallmarks associated with these clinical entities.

Interstitial nephritis is the most recognized histopathologic lesion on kidney biopsy from patients with AKI related to ICIs. The term interstitial nephritis is used to describe an inflammatory condition of the kidney where the interstitium and the tubules are the most involved compartments, with relative sparing of glomeruli and vessels.

Because both interstitium and tubules are often involved, the terms acute tubulointerstitial nephritis (ATIN) and acute interstitial nephritis (AIN) are mostly interchangeable.

The main histologic feature is a diffuse interstitial inflammation with mononuclear cells, neutrophils, plasma cells, and usually eosinophils, especially when the etiology is related to a medication. Mononuclear cells are usually CD3 T lymphocytes. Tubulitis with infiltrating mononuclear inflammatory cells and disruption of tubular basement membrane are also frequent. Interstitial edema is a common finding, and interstitial fibrosis can be observed as part of the regenerative process (Fig. 2). Immunofluorescence can be helpful to define the etiology of the process, revealing deposits of immunoglobulin and complement indicating an

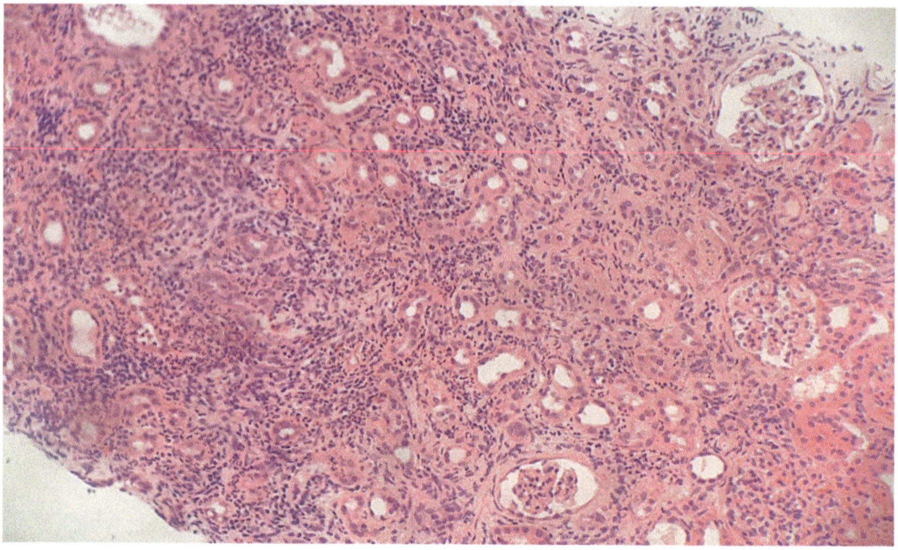

Fig. 2 Kidney biopsy findings in a patient with ICI-related ATIN: interstitial nephritis with severe interstitial inflammation including neutrophils, plasma cells, and mononuclear cells; tubulitis is also present. H&E 40x

immune complex pathogenesis. However, this is usually not observed when interstitial nephritis is secondary to a medication, and immunofluorescence in these cases is usually nonspecific.

Electron microscopy is of less relevance in the diagnosis of interstitial nephritis.

Interestingly, PD-L1 by has been recently tested by IHC on kidney biopsies (Cassol et al. 2019), and among 15 patients, only the patients with acute interstitial nephritis stained positive for PD-L1 along tubular epithelial cell membrane, whereas patients with acute tubular necrosis stained negative (Fig. 3). Despite the small study group, this finding might point out PD-L1 as a useful marker to diagnose AIN related to anti-PD-1 therapy, and further research in this field is much needed. Although interstitial nephritis is the most common lesion described in renal biopsies of patients with AKI due to ICI, several series and case reports are emerging with other findings on kidney biopsies (Wanchoo et al. 2017; Mamlouk et al. 2019). In the largest review published so far, pauci-immune vasculitis, mostly ANCA negative, is the most common pathologic finding. The second most common lesions are podocytopathies, minimal change disease, and focal segmental glomerulosclerosis, and the third most frequent is C3 glomerulonephritis. Cases of AA amyloid, IgA nephropathy, thrombotic microangiopathy, and membranous nephropathy are also reported.

Kidney biopsy is the gold standard to identify an ICI as the main culprit for renal injury; nevertheless, it is challenging to decide which patients with acute kidney injury should receive a kidney biopsy and which is the best time to perform it, and guidelines lack a definitive strategy in this regard (Thompson et al. 2019; Brahmer

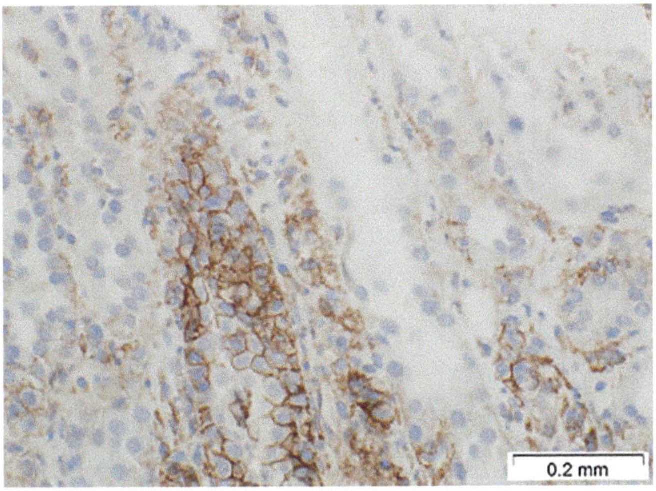

Fig. 3 Immunohistochemistry staining with an antibody to PD-L1 shows positive membrane staining in tubular epithelial cells. Original magnification ×400. (Reproduced by permission from Elsevier Inc. Cassol et al. 2019)

et al. 2018). However, an early renal biopsy could point out an alternative diagnosis for renal injury, not necessarily related to ICIs, and this might allow to pursue the oncological treatment and to spare unnecessary and potentially toxic corticosteroids (Perazella and Shirali 2020).

Figure 4 the diagnostic workup for ICI-associated AKI is reported

6.1 Role of Biomarkers

Kidney biopsy represents the gold standard for ICI-induced ATIN, but it is not always feasible, and it is not a riskless procedure. Therefore, much effort has been recently put in trying to find biomarkers which can aid in the noninvasive diagnosis of this disease.

irAEs are associated with deranged immune and inflammatory responses as well as with a pro-inflammatory milieu in the affected non-tumoral tissues. As a matter of fact, elevated blood interleukin-17 (IL-17) levels were found in patients with ICIs associated immune colitis (Tarhini et al. 2015). Of note, increased IL-17 levels were also found in various settings of AKI as septic shock or delayed graft function and were associated with unfavorable outcomes (Loverre et al. 2011; Maravitsa et al. 2016). Moledina and colleagues have looked at the expression of various urinary and plasmatic cytokines comparing their levels in patients affected by ATIN and acute tubular injury (ATI). In ATIN patients, tumor necrosis factor alpha (TNFα) and interleukin-9 (IL-9) were found significantly higher than in patients with a diagnosis of ATI (Moledina and Parikh 2019).

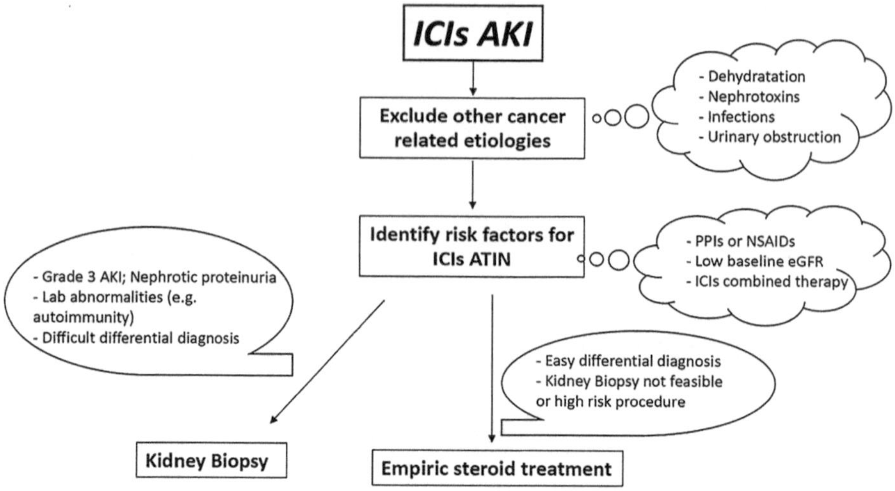

Fig. 4 Diagnostic workup for immune checkpoint inhibitors (ICIs)-associated acute kidney injury (AKI). Legend: *ATIN* acute tubulointerstitial nephritis, *PPIs* proton pump inhibitors, *NSAIDs* non-steroidal anti-inflammatory drugs, *eGFR* estimated glomerular filtration rate

Moreover, in an interesting case report of a melanoma-affected patient on combined immunotherapy, a significant upregulation of serum circulating TNF-α, interleukin-1Ra, CXC-chemokine ligand 10 (CXCL10), and soluble interleukin-2 receptor was observed (Murakami et al. 2016). The anti-inflammatory M2 macrophage phenotype is over represented in tumoral tissues. The overexpression of the soluble form of the M2 macrophages receptor CD163 (sCD163) was reported in melanoma affected patients with irAEs associated with nivolumab treatment (Fujimura et al. 2018). Notably, increased levels of urinary sCD163 were also found in AKI with a good diagnostic and prognostic value (Su et al. 2012).

For what concerns potential biomarkers which may be of easier application in clinical practice, Isik et al. recently found that serum C-reactive protein (CRP) and urine retinol binding protein/urine creatinine (uRBP/Cr) levels in patients affected by ICI-associated AKI were increased compared to non-ICI-AKI patients (Isik et al. 2021).

Although nonspecific for ICI-associated ATIN or AKI and based on limited evidence, all these findings are encouraging and deserve to be further deepened.

As previously mentioned, the overexpression of PD-L1 in renal tubular cells was identified as one of the pathogenic mechanisms of ICI-induced ATIN, and it was further hypothesized that PD-L1 positivity could reflect a susceptibility to develop this complication (Cassol et al. 2019).

It is important to underline that PD-L1 in murine models was found overexpressed also in various kidney diseases independent of immunotherapy with a distinct expression in different renal compartments according to the type of renal damage (Hakroush et al. 2021).

Of note, in this recent paper, Hakroush et al. have also found a correlation between PD-L1 tubular positivity in tissue specimens and the detection of urinary PD-L1 positive tubular epithelial cells. This could lead to a noninvasive identification of patients at risk of ICI-related ATIN and their monitoring during treatment or rechallenge with ICIs (Hakroush et al. 2021).

Finally, gut microbiome composition as well as immune senescence was reported to be associated on the one hand with ICIs oncological response but on the other hand also with irAEs development and ICI-associated AKI hopefully leading to new research scenarios in this field (Franzin et al. 2020). Table 3 sums up some of the abovementioned potential biomarkers and their clinical relevance.

Table 3 Biomarkers of potential clinical utility in the diagnosis of immune checkpoint inhibitors ICI-related ATIN

Biomarker	Setting and clinical relevance		
	irAEs	AKI	ICIs AKI
IL 17	Circulating levels predictive of immune colitis in melanoma patients treated with ipilimumab (Tarhini et al. 2015)	High circulating levels in course of AKI associated with septic shock and DGF (Loverre et al. 2011; Maravitsa et al. 2016)	
Soluble CD163	Predictive role in melanoma patients treated with Nivolumab (Fujimura et al. 2018)	Diagnostic value in AKI associated with sepsis (Su et al. 2012)	
TNFα		Higher in ATIN vs. ATI (Moledina and Parikh 2019)	High circulating levels in course of severe ICI-related ATIN (Murakami et al. 2016)
PD-L1			Renal tubular expression of PD-L1 means susceptibility for ATIN (Cassol et al. 2019) Urinary PD-L1-positive tubular cells associated with tubular PD-L1 expression (Hakroush et al. 2021)
CRP uRBP/ creatinine levels			Increased levels in ICIs AKI vs. non-ICI-AKI (Isik et al. 2021)

Legend: *irAEs* immune-related adverse effects, *IL17* interleukin 17, *CRP* C-reactive protein, *TNFα* tumor necrosis factor alpha, *uRBP* urinary retinol-binding protein, *PD-L1* programmed death-ligand 1

7 Management and Treatment

In recent years, renal involvement is increasingly acknowledged as a relevant adverse effect observed in oncologic patients on immunotherapy, and several guidelines regarding the clinical management of acute kidney failure during ICIs treatment have been released (Thompson et al. 2019; Brahmer et al. 2018).

The cornerstone of the therapy is represented by corticosteroids; their use is suggested at an initial dose of 0.5–1 mg/kg/day for grade 2 and 1–2 mg/kg/day for grade 3–4 ICI-associated AKI. Tapering over 4–6 weeks once creatinine values return to 1.5–2 × baseline (grade 1) is recommended. Both NCCN and the American Society of Clinical Oncology Clinical Practice Guideline (ASCO) guidelines consider the use of other immunosuppressive drugs (without a preference for a specific therapeutic agent) if renal improvement is not observed after 1 week.

This approach is largely adopted with good results taking into account that in multiple series recovery (partial or complete) is reported to range between 60% and 80% (Seethapathy et al. 2021a, b; Gupta et al. 2021). In particular higher odds of renal recovery are observed if steroids are started early (Gupta et al. 2021), and this is of relevance bearing in mind that AKI non-recovery is associated with a higher mortality (Seethapathy et al. 2021a, b). Conversely, data on long-term outcomes after partial or complete recovery are lacking.

Of interest, steroids were reported to be associated with a reduced response to cancer immunotherapy (Petrelli et al. 2020; Faje et al. 2018); for this reason and for the well-known corticosteroid-related adverse effects, Lee et al. have conducted a single-center retrospective cohort study (Lee et al. 2021) in which cases of ICI-induced AKI treated with a shorter course of prednisone showed analogous kidney outcomes as patients treated with a standard tapering protocol. This result has to be obviously confirmed in larger studies and may be considered for selected patients. Interestingly, Sise et al. have suggested to discontinue PPIs and trimethoprim/sulfamethoxazole, both associated with ATIN development and usually prescribed as prophylactic drug in case of treatment with high doses of steroids, and to replace them, respectively, with H2 antagonists and atovaquone (Sise et al. 2019). A second line of immunosuppression is rarely needed with rates reported to be about 5% and with mycophenolate mofetil being the most frequently used drug in case of steroid-resistant ICI-associated AKI (Gupta et al. 2021).

Interestingly, the anti-TNF monoclonal antibody infliximab was also used with promising results in case of persistent or recurrent AKI (Seethapathy et al. 2021a, b).

In the large multicenter study by Cortazar et al., 22% of patients with grade 2 or 3 ICI-induced AKI were rechallenged with a recurrence rate of 23% (Cortazar et al. 2020), and similar rates were reported in other studies (Gupta et al. 2021). Once rechallenged patients are often preemptively treated with steroids, but documented and evidence-based benefits from applying this strategy are lacking. In most of the cases, patients with recurrent AKI during rechallenge are treated with a second course of corticosteroids with good results in terms of recovery (Gupta et al. 2021).

Until now no significant differences between patients who relapsed and those who did not nor definite risk factors for recurrence were found; therefore, more studies are much needed in order to better define patients at higher risk for recurrent AKI.

8 ICI and Kidney Transplantation

After cardiovascular disease, cancer is the second cause of death among kidney transplant recipients (KTRs). Of note, KTRs have a two- to threefold augmented risk of developing cancer compared to the general population (Al-Adra et al. 2022).

The clinical management of malignancies in KTRs is of extreme complexity because the reduction of immunosuppression required to limit oncological progression represents a threat for the allograft possibly leading to rejection. KTRs were not included in the clinical trials which lead to ICIs commercialization, but immunotherapy was soon introduced as a promising weapon to use in their oncological management. Nevertheless, besides the risk of ICI-induced ATIN, in organ-transplanted patients, an augmented risk of allograft rejection associated with the specific mechanism of action of ICIs was reported (Lai et al. 2019). Following PD-1 inhibition, activated T lymphocytes may be not only specifically directed against tumoral cells but also against donor antigens in the graft. Moreover, the PD-1/PD-L1 axis is involved in the activation of regulatory T cells with consequent suppression of alloreactive T lymphocytes (Kean et al. 2017).

A reduced risk of rejection was observed with anti-CTLA4 monoclonal antibodies compared to PD-1/PD-L1 blockade (Regalla et al. 2018); it has been suggested that the PD-1-PD-L1 axis acts not only in the induction but also in the maintenance of allograft tolerance and most importantly PD-L1 tubular expression has been observed to be linked to suppression of alloreactive T cells (Chae et al. 2018). With the aim of better defining the incidence and outcome of acute rejection associated with immunotherapy, case reports and case series reporting the follow-up of kidney transplant recipients treated with ICIs have been recently analyzed in systematic reviews and multicenter retrospective studies have been conducted.

Overall, the studies reported very similar results with a rate of rejection between 41% and 48% (Murakami et al. 2021; Rossi et al. 2022; Kumar et al. 2020; Abdel-Wahab et al. 2019) and of graft loss between 65% and 80% (Murakami et al. 2021; Kumar et al. 2020; Abdel-Wahab et al. 2019); the onset was reported to occur after a median time of 21–24 days after the beginning of ICIs (Murakami et al. 2021; Rossi et al. 2022; Abdel-Wahab et al. 2019), and a T cell-mediated rejection (TCMR) was reported in half of the cases (Murakami et al. 2021; Abdel-Wahab et al. 2019). Abdel Wahab et al. observed that the majority of antibody-mediated rejections (ABMR) is associated with both negative DSA and C4d and hypothesized triggering of the humoral immune system by activated T lymphocytes as the etiopathogenetic mechanism (Abdel-Wahab et al. 2019).

For what concerns the efficacy of ICIs in immunocompromised patients, the disease control rate and partial or complete response rate to immunotherapy were reported to range between 20% and 50% (Kumar et al. 2020). Data are still lacking regarding the definite risk factors for rejection occurrence in KTRs taking ICIs, including type of cancer, time since transplantation, or prior rejection (Kumar et al. 2020).

There is conflicting evidence about the benefit of an immunosuppressive regimen comprehensive of a mammalian target of rapamycin inhibitor (mTORi) in KTRs affected by malignancies, with some authors reporting a better overall survival and others limiting a favorable effect only in case of non-melanoma skin cancers and in particular cutaneous squamous cell carcinoma (Rousseau et al. 2019; de Fijter 2017).

The *rationale* beyond the favorable anti-tumoral effect of mTORi is that the mTOR pathway is involved in tumor progression (Tian et al. 2019).

Indeed Vanasek et al. have shown T cell anergy with the association of mTORi with ICIs (Vanasek et al. 2001), and in an international multicenter retrospective study, patients on mTORi showed a reduced risk of rejection (Murakami et al. 2021).

Nevertheless, further investigation is needed in order to support and confirm these findings.

Regarding the diagnostic process, a recent paper by Adam et al. identified a biopsy-based measurement with nanostring technology of IFI27, an IFN-α-induced transcript, as a potential biomarker able to differentiate between ICI-induced ATIN and TCMR which could be useful considering the histological analogies shared by these clinical entities (Adam et al. 2021).

Bearing in mind that KTRs are at highest risk for malignancies and therefore ideally represent the population who would benefit the most from the good oncological results obtained with ICIs, preclinical studies are urgently needed in order to better understand how to uncouple allograft tolerance from their anti-tumoral action.

In the meantime, treatment with ICIs in a transplanted patient needs a thorough and multidisciplinary evaluation of the risk-benefit ratio of this therapeutic choice and an honest and precise doctor-patient communication.

9 Conclusions and Perspectives

In this chapter, we aimed at reviewing the available evidence on the kidney damage in the course of ICIs treatment, focusing on ATIN, the most common clinical presentation of ICI-related nephrotoxicity. The potential high clinical impact of this complication, also due to the rapid implementation of ICIs in the clinical practice, has represented the reason for the design of many experimental and clinical trials. These studies explored the pathogenesis, the diagnostic and therapeutic approaches, and the impact of this condition on the general management of patients affected by cancer. The results of these studies have been included in the oncological guidelines that currently recognize kidney damage as one of the most important ICI-related AEs.

However, although these recent advances rapidly increased our awareness and knowledge about ICI-related kidney damage, many issues remain open and still need to be investigated.

While the involvement of the immune system has been ascertained, the exact mechanisms underlying ICI-related ATIN are not fully understood. In particular, the biological basis of the interaction of ICI treatment with other concomitant drugs is not clear. This could be a crucial point to focus on, also in order to identify patients at higher risk and try to prevent kidney damage. In addition, the actual role of biomarkers in the prediction and management of ATIN in patients on ICIs is still far to be elucidated. In this regard, it could be interesting to evaluate the correlation between pathological findings on kidney biopsies and noninvasive biomarkers, also to permit a longitudinal control of the renal effects of these drugs. Regarding the treatment of ICI-related ATIN, while responsiveness to steroids is a characteristic feature, it is not clear if the addition of other immunosuppressants may be useful, especially in patients with concomitant glomerular damage. Most importantly, determining which patients may be safe for a rechallenge of ICIs and if preemptive steroid/immunosuppressive treatments are effective in preventing AKI recurrence are questions without a clear response.

Finally, we need data on long-term follow-up of patients experiencing AKI and ATIN due to ICI therapy to quantitatively estimate the impact of this condition on patient survival.

From this brief excursus, it is evident that much work has to be done in order to improve our biological and clinical knowledge of renal irAEs. These efforts are necessary to improve the quality of care provided to a fragile population, such as patients with cancer, and constitute a further step on the way to developing a multidisciplinary and personalized approach.

References

Abdel-Wahab N, Safa H, Abudayyeh A et al (2019) Checkpoint inhibitor therapy for cancer in solid organ transplantation recipients: an institutional experience and a systematic review of the literature. J Immunother Cancer 7(1):106. https://doi.org/10.1186/s40425-019-0585-1

Adam BA, Murakami N, Reid G et al (2021) Gene expression profiling in kidney transplants with immune checkpoint inhibitor-associated adverse events. Clin J Am Soc Nephrol 16(9): 1376–1386. https://doi.org/10.2215/CJN.00920121

Agostinetto E, Losurdo A, Nader-Marta G et al (2022) Progress and pitfalls in the use of immunotherapy for patients with triple negative breast cancer. Expert Opin Investig Drugs 31: 567–591. https://doi.org/10.1080/13543784.2022.2049232

Al-Adra D, Al-Qaoud T, Fowler K, Wong G (2022) De novo malignancies after kidney transplantation. Clin J Am Soc Nephrol 17(3):434–443. https://doi.org/10.2215/CJN.14570920

Baas P, Scherpereel A, Nowak AK et al (2021) First-line nivolumab plus ipilimumab in unresectable malignant pleural mesothelioma (CheckMate 743): a multicentre, randomised, open-label, phase 3 trial. Lancet 397:375–386. https://doi.org/10.1016/S0140-6736(20)32714-8

Baker ML, Yamamoto Y, Perazella MA et al (2022) Mortality after acute kidney injury and acute interstitial nephritis in patients prescribed immune checkpoint inhibitor therapy. J Immunother Cancer 10:e004421. https://doi.org/10.1136/jitc-2021-004421

Balakrishna P, Villegas A (2017) Hypokalemic paralysis secondary to immune checkpoint inhibitor therapy. Case Rep Oncol Med 2017:5063405. https://doi.org/10.1155/2017/5063405

Barnard ZR, Walcott BP, Kahle KT et al (2012) Hyponatremia associated with Ipilimumab-induced hypophysitis. Med Oncol 29:374–377. https://doi.org/10.1007/s12032-010-9794-7

Boutros A, Cecchi F, Tanda ET et al (2021) Immunotherapy for the treatment of cutaneous squamous cell carcinoma. Front Oncol 11:733917. https://doi.org/10.3389/fonc.2021.733917

Brahmer JR, Lacchetti C, Schneider BJ et al (2018) Management of immune-related adverse events in patients treated with immune checkpoint inhibitor therapy: American Society of Clinical Oncology Clinical Practice Guideline. J Clin Oncol 36:1714–1768. https://doi.org/10.1200/JCO.21.01440

Brahmer JR, Abu-Sbeih H, Ascierto PA et al (2021) Society for Immunotherapy of cancer (SITC) clinical practice guideline on immune checkpoint inhibitor-related adverse events. J Immunother Cancer 9:e002435. https://doi.org/10.1136/jitc-2021-002435

Cassol C, Satoskar A, Lozanski G et al (2019) Anti-PD-1 immunotherapy may induce interstitial nephritis with increased tubular epithelial expression of PD-L1. Kidney Int Rep 4(8): 1152–1160. https://doi.org/10.1016/j.ekir.2019.06.001

Chae YK, Galvez C, Anker JF et al (2018) Cancer immunotherapy in a neglected population: the current use and future of T-cell-mediated checkpoint inhibitors in organ transplant patients. Cancer Treat Rev 63:116–121. https://doi.org/10.1016/j.ctrv.2017.1

Champiat S, Lambotte O, Barreau E et al (2016) Management of immune checkpoint blockade dysimmune toxicities: a collaborative position paper. Ann Oncol 27(4):559–574. https://doi.org/10.1093/annonc/mdv623

Cortazar FB, Marrone KA, Troxell ML et al (2016) Clinicopathological features of acute kidney injury associated with immune checkpoint inhibitors. Kidney Int 90(3):638–647. https://doi.org/10.1016/j.kint.2016.04.008

Cortazar FB, Kibbelaar ZA, Glezerman IG et al (2020) Clinical features and outcomes of immune checkpoint inhibitor-associated AKI: a multicenter study. J Am Soc Nephrol 31(2):435–446. https://doi.org/10.1681/ASN.2019070676

Das S, Johnson DB (2019) Immune-related adverse events and anti-tumor efficacy of immune checkpoint inhibitors. J Immunother Cancer 7:306. https://doi.org/10.1186/s40425-019-0805-8

de Fijter JW (2017) Cancer and mTOR inhibitors in transplant recipients. Transplantation 101(1): 45–55. https://doi.org/10.1097/TP.0000000000001447

Ding H, Wu X, Gao W (2005) PD-L1 is expressed by human renal tubular epithelial cells and suppresses T cell cytokine synthesis. Clin Immunol 115(2):184–191. https://doi.org/10.1016/j.clim.2005.01.005

Draibe JB, García-Carro C, Martinez-Valenzuela L et al (2020) Acute tubulointerstitial nephritis induced by checkpoint inhibitors versus classical acute tubulointerstitial nephritis: are they the same disease? Clin Kidney J 14(3):884–890. https://doi.org/10.1093/ckj/sfaa027

EMA (2018a) Yervoy. In: European Medicines Agency. https://www.ema.europa.eu/en/medicines/human/EPAR/yervoy. Accessed 16 June 2022

EMA (2018b) Opdivo. In: European Medicines Agency. https://www.ema.europa.eu/en/medicines/human/EPAR/opdivo. Accessed 16 June 2022

EMA (2018c) Keytruda. In: European Medicines Agency. https://www.ema.europa.eu/en/medicines/human/EPAR/keytruda. Accessed 16 June 2022

EMA (2018d) Tecentriq. In: European Medicines Agency. https://www.ema.europa.eu/en/medicines/human/EPAR/tecentriq. Accessed 16 June 2022

EMA (2018e) Imfinzi. In: European Medicines Agency. https://www.ema.europa.eu/en/medicines/human/EPAR/imfinzi. Accessed 16 June 2022

EMA (2019) Libtayo. In: European Medicines Agency. https://www.ema.europa.eu/en/medicines/human/EPAR/libtayo. Accessed 16 June 2022

Faje AT, Lawrence D, Flaherty K et al (2018) High-dose glucocorticoids for the treatment of ipilimumab-induced hypophysitis is associated with reduced survival in patients with melanoma. Cancer 124(18):3706–3714. https://doi.org/10.1002/cncr.31629

Farid S, Latif H, Nilubol C, Kim C (2020) Immune checkpoint inhibitor-induced Fanconi syndrome. Cureus 12(4):e7686. https://doi.org/10.7759/cureus.7686

Farkona S, Diamandis EP, Blasutig IM (2016) Cancer immunotherapy: the beginning of the end of cancer? BMC Med 14:73. https://doi.org/10.1186/s12916-016-0623-5

Franzin R, Netti GS, Spadaccino F et al (2020) The use of immune checkpoint inhibitors in oncology and the occurrence of AKI: where do we stand? Front Immunol 11:574271. https://doi.org/10.3389/fimmu.2020.574271

Fujimura T, Sato Y, Tanita K et al (2018) Serum levels of soluble CD163 and CXCL5 may be predictive markers for immune-related adverse events in patients with advanced melanoma treated with nivolumab: a pilot study. Oncotarget 9:15542–15551. https://doi.org/10.18632/oncotarget.24509

Geenen RW, Kingma HJ, van der Molen AJ (2013) Contrast-induced nephropathy: pharmacology, pathophysiology and prevention. Insights Imaging 4(6):811–820. https://doi.org/10.1007/s13244-013-0291-3

Genova C, Rossi G, Rijavec E et al (2017) Releasing the brake: safety profile of immune checkpoint inhibitors in non-small cell lung cancer. Expert Opin Drug Saf 16:573–585. https://doi.org/10.1080/14740338.2017.1313228

Genova C, Dellepiane C, Carrega P et al (2021) Therapeutic implications of tumor microenvironment in lung cancer: focus on immune checkpoint blockade. Front Immunol 12:799455. https://doi.org/10.3389/fimmu.2021.799455

Guo K, Wang Z, Luo R et al (2022) Association between chronic kidney disease and cancer including the mortality of cancer patients: national health and nutrition examination survey 1999-2014. Am J Transl Res 14(4):2356–2366

Gupta S, Short SAP, Sise ME et al (2021) Acute kidney injury in patients treated with immune checkpoint inhibitors. J Immunother Cancer 9(10):e003467. https://doi.org/10.1136/jitc-2021-003467

Gutgarts V, Glezerman IG (2020) Kidney biopsy should be performed to document the cause of immune checkpoint inhibitor-associated acute kidney injury: CON. Kidney360 1(3):162–165. https://doi.org/10.34067/KID.0000132020

Haanen JBAG, Carbonnel F, Robert C et al (2017) Management of toxicities from immunotherapy: ESMO clinical practice guidelines for diagnosis, treatment and follow-up. Ann Oncol 28:iv119–iv142. https://doi.org/10.1093/annonc/mdx225

Hakroush S, Kopp SB, Tampe D et al (2021) Variable expression of programmed cell death protein 1-ligand 1 in kidneys independent of immune checkpoint inhibition. Front Immunol 11:624547. https://doi.org/10.3389/fimmu.2020.624547

Hodi FS, O'Day SJ, McDermott DF et al (2010) Improved survival with ipilimumab in patients with metastatic melanoma. N Engl J Med 363:711–723. https://doi.org/10.2217/imt-2021-0195

Isik B, Alexander MP, Manohar S et al (2021) Biomarkers, clinical features, and Rechallenge for immune checkpoint inhibitor renal immune-related adverse events. Kidney Int Rep 6(4):1022–1031. https://doi.org/10.1016/j.ekir.2021.01.013

Izzedine H, Perazella MA (2017) Anticancer drug-induced acute kidney injury. Kidney Int Rep 2(4):504–514. https://doi.org/10.1016/j.ekir.2017.02.008

Izzedine H, Mateus C, Boutros C et al (2017) Renal effects of immune checkpoint inhibitors. Nephrol Dial Transplant 32(6):936–942. https://doi.org/10.1093/ndt/gfw382

Jiang X, Liu G, Li Y, Pan Y (2021) Immune checkpoint: the novel target for antitumor therapy. Genes Dis 8:25–37. https://doi.org/10.1016/j.gendis.2019.12.004

Jin Z, Sinicrope FA (2022) Mismatch repair-deficient colorectal cancer: building on checkpoint blockade. J Clin Oncol:JCO2102691. https://doi.org/10.1200/JCO.21.02691

Johnson DB, Beckermann KE, Wang DY (2018) Immune checkpoint inhibitor therapy in patients with autoimmune disease. Oncology (Williston Park) 32(4):190–194

Kato K, Mizuno T, Koseki T et al (2021) Concomitant proton pump inhibitors and immune checkpoint inhibitors increase nephritis frequency. In Vivo 35(5):2831–2840. https://doi.org/10.21873/invivo.12570

Kean LS, Turka LA, Blazar BR (2017) Advances in targeting co-inhibitory and co-stimulatory pathways in transplantation settings: The Yin to the Yang of cancer immunotherapy. Immunol Rev 276:192–212. https://doi.org/10.1111/imr.12523

Keir ME, Liang SC, Guleria I et al (2006) Tissue expression of PD-L1 mediates peripheral T cell tolerance. J Exp Med 203(4):883–895. https://doi.org/10.1084/jem.20051776

Kim H, Choi JM, Lee K (2022) Immune checkpoint blockades in triple-negative breast cancer: current state and molecular mechanisms of resistance. Biomedicine 10:1130. https://doi.org/10.3390/biomedicines10051130

Kitchlu A, Jhaveri KD, Wadhwani S et al (2020) A systematic review of immune checkpoint inhibitor-associated glomerular disease. Kidney Int Rep 6(1):66–77. https://doi.org/10.1016/j.ekir.2020.10.002

Kumar V, Shinagare AB, Rennke HG et al (2020) The safety and efficacy of checkpoint inhibitors in transplant recipients: a case series and systematic review of literature. Oncologist 25(6):505–514. https://doi.org/10.1634/theoncologist

Lai HC, Lin JF, Hwang TIS et al (2019) Programmed cell death 1 (PD-1) inhibitors in renal transplant patients with advanced cancer: a double-edged sword? Int J Mol Sci 20(9):2194. https://doi.org/10.3390/ijms20092194

Lee MD, Seethapathy H, Strohbehn IA et al (2021) Rapid corticosteroid taper versus standard of care for immune checkpoint inhibitor induced nephritis: a single-center retrospective cohort study. J Immunother Cancer 9(4):e002292. https://doi.org/10.1136/jitc-2020-002292

Loverre A, Divella C, Castellano G et al (2011) T helper 1, 2 and 17 cell subsets in renal transplant patients with delayed graft function. Transpl Int 24:233–242. https://doi.org/10.1111/j.1432-2277.2010.01157.x

Mamlouk O, Selamet U, Machado S et al (2019) Nephrotoxicity of immune checkpoint inhibitors beyond tubulointerstitial nephritis: single-center experience. J Immunother Cancer 7(1):2. https://doi.org/10.1186/s40425-018-0478-8

Manohar S, Kompotiatis P, Thongprayoon C et al (2019) Programmed cell death protein 1 inhibitor treatment is associated with acute kidney injury and hypocalcemia: a meta-analysis. Nephrol Dial Transplant 34(1):108–117. https://doi.org/10.1093/ndt/gfy105

Maravitsa P, Adamopoulou M, Pistiki A et al (2016) Systemic over-release of interleukin-17 in acute kidney injury after septic shock: clinical and experimental evidence. Immunol Lett 178:68–76. https://doi.org/10.1016/j.imlet.2016.08.002

Menke J, Lucas JA, Zeller GC et al (2007) Programmed death 1 ligand (PD-L) 1 and PD-L2 limit autoimmune kidney disease: distinct roles. J Immunol 179:7466–7477. https://doi.org/10.4049/jimmunol.179.11.7466

Meraz-Muñoz A, Amir E, Ng P et al (2020) Acute kidney injury associated with immune checkpoint inhibitor therapy: incidence, risk factors and outcomes. J Immunother Cancer 8(1):e000467. https://doi.org/10.1136/jitc-2019-000467

Moledina DG, Parikh CR (2019) Differentiating acute interstitial nephritis from acute tubular injury: a challenge for clinicians. Nephron 143(3):211–216. https://doi.org/10.1159/000501207

Murakami N, Borges TJ, Yamashita M, Riella LV (2016) Severe acute interstitial nephritis after combination immune-checkpoint inhibitor therapy for metastatic melanoma. Clin Kidney J 9(3):411–417. https://doi.org/10.1093/ckj/sfw024

Murakami N, Mulvaney P, Danesh M et al (2021) A multi-center study on safety and efficacy of immune checkpoint inhibitors in cancer patients with kidney transplant. Kidney Int 100(1):196–205. https://doi.org/10.1016/j.kint.2020.12.015

Naughton CA (2008) Drug-induced nephrotoxicity. Am Fam Physician 78(6):743–750

Nussbaum EZ, Perazella MA (2018) Update on the nephrotoxicity of novel anticancer agents. Clin Nephrol 89(3):149–165. https://doi.org/10.5414/CN109371

O'Donnell JS, Teng MWL, Smyth MJ (2019) Cancer immunoediting and resistance to T cell-based immunotherapy. Nat Rev Clin Oncol 16(3):151–167. https://doi.org/10.1038/s41571-018-0142-8

Oleas D, Bolufer M, Agraz I et al (2020) Acute interstitial nephritis associated with immune checkpoint inhibitors: a single-centre experience. Clin Kidney J 14(5):1364–1370. https://doi.org/10.1093/ckj/sfaa008

Paz-Ares LG, Ramalingam SS, Ciuleanu T-E et al (2022) First-line Nivolumab plus Ipilimumab in advanced NSCLC: 4-year outcomes from the randomized, open-label, phase 3 CheckMate 227 part 1 trial. J Thorac Oncol 17:289–308. https://doi.org/10.1016/j.jtho.2021.09.010

Perazella MA (2009) Renal vulnerability to drug toxicity. Clin J Am Soc Nephrol 4:1275–1283. https://doi.org/10.2215/CJN.02050309

Perazella MA (2012) Onco-nephrology: renal toxicities of chemotherapeutic agents. Clin J Am Soc Nephrol 7(10):1713–1721. https://doi.org/10.2215/CJN.02780312

Perazella MA (2019) Drug-induced acute kidney injury: diverse mechanisms of tubular injury. Curr Opin Crit Care 25(6):550–557. https://doi.org/10.1097/MCC.0000000000000653

Perazella MA (2020) Kidney biopsy should be performed to document the cause of immune checkpoint inhibitor-associated acute kidney injury: commentary. Kidney360 1(3):166–168. https://doi.org/10.34067/KID.0001072019

Perazella MA, Shirali AC (2020) Immune checkpoint inhibitor nephrotoxicity: what do we know and what should we do? Kidney Int 97(1):62–74. https://doi.org/10.1016/j.kint.2019.07.022

Perazella MA, Sprangers B (2021) Checkpoint inhibitor therapy-associated acute kidney injury: time to move on to evidence-based recommendations. Clin Kidney J 14(5):1301–1306. https://doi.org/10.1093/ckj/sfab052

Petrelli F, Signorelli D, Ghidini M et al (2020) Association of steroids use with survival in patients treated with immune checkpoint inhibitors: a systematic review and meta-analysis. Cancers (Basel) 12(3):546. https://doi.org/10.3390/cancers12030546

Reck M, Ciuleanu T-E, Cobo M et al (2021) First-line nivolumab plus ipilimumab with two cycles of chemotherapy versus chemotherapy alone (four cycles) in advanced non-small-cell lung cancer: CheckMate 9LA 2-year update. ESMO Open 6:100273. https://doi.org/10.1016/j.esmoop.2021.100273

Regalla DKR, Williams GR, Paluri RK (2018) Immune checkpoint inhibitors in the management of malignancies in transplant recipients. Postgrad Med J 94:704–708. https://doi.org/10.1136/postgradmedj-2018-136081

Rosner MH, Jhaveri KD, McMahon BA, Perazella MA (2021) Onconephrology: the intersections between the kidney and cancer. CA Cancer J Clin 202171(1):47–77. https://doi.org/10.3322/caac.21636

Rossi E, Schinzari G, Maiorano BA et al (2022) Immune-checkpoint inhibitors in renal transplanted patients affected by melanoma: a systematic review. Immunotherapy 14(1):65–75. https://doi.org/10.2217/imt-2021-0195

Rousseau B, Guillemin A, Duvoux C et al (2019) Optimal oncologic management and mTOR inhibitor introduction are safe and improve survival in kidney and liver allograft recipients with de novo carcinoma. Int J Cancer 144:886–896. https://doi.org/10.1002/ijc.3176

Schneider BJ, Naidoo J, Santomasso BD et al (2021) Management of immune-related adverse events in patients treated with immune checkpoint inhibitor therapy: ASCO guideline update. J Clin Oncol. https://doi.org/10.1200/JCO.21.01440

Seethapathy H, Zhao S, Chute DF et al (2019) The incidence, causes, and risk factors of acute kidney injury in patients receiving immune checkpoint inhibitors. Clin J Am Soc Nephrol 14(12):1692–1700. https://doi.org/10.2215/CJN.00990119

Seethapathy H, Herrmann SM, Sise ME (2021a) Immune checkpoint inhibitors and kidney toxicity: advances in diagnosis and management. Kidney Med 3(6):1074–1081. https://doi.org/10.1016/j.xkme.2021.08.008

Seethapathy H, Rusibamayila N, Chute DF et al (2021b) Hyponatremia and other electrolyte abnormalities in patients receiving immune checkpoint inhibitors. Nephrol Dial Transplant 36(12):2241–2247. https://doi.org/10.1093/ndt/gfaa272

Shiravand Y, Khodadadi F, Kashani SMA et al (2022) Immune checkpoint inhibitors in cancer therapy. Curr Oncol 29:3044–3060. https://doi.org/10.3390/curroncol29050247

Sise ME, Seethapathy H, Reynolds KL (2019) Diagnosis and management of immune checkpoint inhibitor-associated renal toxicity: illustrative case and review. Oncologist 24(6):735–742. https://doi.org/10.1634/theoncologist.2018-0764

Spanou Z, Keller M, Britschgi M et al (2006) Involvement of drug-specific T cells in acute drug-induced interstitial nephritis. J Am Soc Nephrol 17(10):2919–2927. https://doi.org/10.1681/ASN.2006050418

Stengel B (2010) Chronic kidney disease and cancer: a troubling connection. J Nephrol 23(3): 253–262

Su L, Feng L, Liu C et al (2012) Diagnostic value of urine sCD163 levels for sepsis and relevant acute kidney injury: a prospective study. BMC Nephrol 13:123. https://doi.org/10.1186/1471-2369-13-123

Sury K, Perazella MA, Shirali AC (2018) Cardiorenal complications of immune checkpoint inhibitors. Nat Rev Nephrol 14(9):571–588. https://doi.org/10.1038/s41581-018-0035-1

Tarhini AA, Zahoor H, Lin Y et al (2015) Baseline circulating IL-17 predicts toxicity while TGF-beta1 and IL-10 are prognostic of relapse in ipilimumab neoadjuvant therapy of melanoma. J Immunother Cancer 3:39. https://doi.org/10.1186/s40425-015-0081-1

Thompson JA, Schneider BJ, Brahmer J et al (2019) Management of immunotherapy-related toxicities, version 1. J Natl Compr Cancer Netw 17:255–289. https://doi.org/10.6004/jnccn.2019.0013

Tian T, Li X, Zhang J (2019) mTOR signaling in cancer and mTOR inhibitors in solid tumor targeting therapy. Int J Mol Sci 20(3):755. https://doi.org/10.3390/ijms20030755

Tinawi M, Bastani B (2020) Nephrotoxicity of immune checkpoint inhibitors: acute kidney injury and beyond. Cureus 12(12):e12204. https://doi.org/10.7759/cureus.12204

Vanasek TL, Khoruts A, Zell T, Mueller DL (2001) Antagonistic roles for CTLA-4 and the mammalian target of rapamycin in the regulation of clonal anergy: enhanced cell cycle progression promotes recall antigen responsiveness. J Immunol 167:5636–5644. https://doi.org/10.4049/jimmunol.167.10.5636

Wanchoo R, Karam S, Uppal NN et al (2017) Cancer and kidney international network workgroup on immune checkpoint inhibitors adverse renal effects of immune checkpoint inhibitors: a narrative review. Am J Nephrol 45(2):160–169. https://doi.org/10.1159/000455014

Wei SC, Duffy CR, Allison JP (2018) Fundamental mechanisms of immune checkpoint blockade therapy. Cancer Discov 8:1069–1086. https://doi.org/10.1158/2159-8290.CD-18-0367

Cancer Stem Cell as a Target for Immunotherapeutic Approach

Kimia Kazemzadeh and Nima Rezaei

Abstract

In today's world, immunotherapy is known as revolutionary in cancer treatment. Until now, many clinical trials tried to find different targets for immunotherapeutic approaches. Cancer stem cells are a group of tumor cells with the ability to self-renewal and initiation of cancer growth. In this chapter, we try to demonstrate the immunological features and pathways of cancer stem cells which open up a way to consider them as a therapeutic target. Although these cells are highly resistant to traditional treatments, there are some immunotherapeutic methods such as oncolytic viruses, dendritic cell-based vaccines, and adaptive T-cells that can efficiently eliminate CSCs which will be discussed in continue. More investigation on CSCs will definitely illustrate a promising perspective in cancer therapy.

Keywords

Cancer · Cancer stem cell · Immunotherapy · Stem cell · Tumor-initiating cell

K. Kazemzadeh
Students' Scientific Research Center, Tehran University of Medical Sciences, Tehran, Iran

Cancer Immunology Project (CIP), Universal Scientific Education and Research Network (USERN), Tehran, Iran

N. Rezaei (✉)
Research Center for Immunodeficiencies, Pediatrics Center of Excellence, Children's Medical Center, Tehran University of Medical Sciences, Tehran, Iran

Department of Immunology, School of Medicine, Tehran University of Medical Sciences, Tehran, Iran

Cancer Immunology Project (CIP), Universal Scientific Education and Research Network (USERN), Stockholm, Sweden
e-mail: rezaei_nima@tums.ac.ir

Interdisciplinary Cancer Research, https://doi.org/10.1007/16833_2023_166
Published online: 28 June 2023

1 Introduction

Cancer stem cells (CSCs) are a group of tumor cells that arise in a variable manner based on epigenetic and genetic changes during cancer development (stochastic theory). From another point of view, they are single cells with a unique ability to self-renewal and initiating tumor growth (hierarchical theory). Experimental evidence proving the existence of CSCs was first provided in 1964. A group of cells with $CD34^{high}$ $CD32^{low}$ phenotype in acute myeloid leukemia was reported to be extremely capable of embedding leukemia in immunodeficient mice (Lapidot et al. 1994). Cancer stem cells are the main reason for cancer relapse and metastasis. Drug resistance against chemotherapeutic drugs was reported among these cells. Cancer immunotherapy is revolutionary in cancer treatment and uses different methods to boost the human body's immune system. CSCs are capable of expressing various immune markers and presenting particular immune characteristics in different tumors. These features are used in immunotherapeutic approaches to target CSCs. Currently, oncolytic viruses, dendritic cell-based vaccines, adaptive T-cells, and combination therapy are being used to target CSCs. This method shows a promising perspective for cancer treatment (Codd et al. 2018; Badrinath and Yoo 2019).

Hereafter, we will discuss the main characteristics of CSCs to illustrate an immunological view of their role in cancer initiation and growth. Then we will discuss immunotherapy as a novel method of cancer treatment. Finally, we will elucidate different ways of targeting CSCs in tumor immunotherapy.

2 What Are CSCs?

The concept of CSC, also known as tumor-initiating cells (TICs) or stem-like cells, has first developed about four decades ago (Batlle and Clevers 2017; Codd et al. 2018). CSCs are a small subpopulation of tumor cells that are significantly characterized by their special capabilities of differentiation (rising into mature cell types), self-renewal (generating more SCs in order to maintain an undifferentiated status), and tumor growth initiation (Yu et al. 2012). Based on these features, it was hypothesized that CSCs originated from normal progenitor cells/SCs of tumor tissue (Ayob and Ramasamy 2018). Eradicating CSCs is one of the most important therapeutic struggles with cancer. Presentation of CSCs in tumors can lead to metastasis, minimal residual disease, relapse of tumor cells, and cancer cell heterogeneity. Escaped CSCs can cause tumor formation unexpectedly after the complete removal of adult cancer cells (Pattabiraman and Weinberg 2014; Kaiser 2015; Kaur et al. 2018). The main reason for CSCs' resistance to therapies might be based on interleukin-4 (IL-4) signaling, epithelial-mesenchymal transition, and drug efflux proteins (Doherty et al. 2016). The principal CSC markers which are used to recognize these cells from just cancer cells are aldehyde dehydrogenase (ALDH), IL-6 receptor, CD44, and CD133 (Codd et al. 2018).

2.1 CSC in Tumor Initiations

Based on CSC theory, these cells are hidden in tumors and present as fuel for cancer growth (Batlle and Clevers 2017). Carcinogenesis contains various events which are initiated with loss of cell growth control due to accumulated mutations and lead to uncontrolled proliferation. This process is usually based on gene alternations including tumor suppressor genes and oncogenes as well as genes involved in the deoxyribonucleic acid (DNA) repair mechanisms (Tysnes and Bjerkvig 2007).

2.2 History of CSC

In 1994, different studies by Dick group indicates that when leukemia-initiating stem cells in acute myeloid leukemia (AML) in humankind are transplanted into severe combined immunodeficient mice, AML can be induced (Lapidot et al. 1994). Over time, the presence of SCs in breast and brain cancer was supported by different studies, respectively (Al-Hajj et al. 2003; Singh et al. 2004).

2.3 Association Between CSCs and Normal SCs (NSCs)

CD133, CD44, and CD29 are some similar surface markers among CSCs and NSCs. Various mutations in NSCs can lead to CSC formation (Kim and Ryu 2017). This transformation might be associated with mechanisms of tumor suppression and genomic instability. Also, environmental abnormalities while embryonic SCs differentiation can lead to CSCs formation with apoptosis resistance (Fujimori et al. 2012; Yoshioka et al. 2015).

3 Immunological Landscape on CSCs

3.1 CSCs in Different Types of Cancer

Various immune receptors are expressed on CSCs' surface that play a key role in the metastasis and therapeutic resistance of tumors. For instance, the leucine-rich repeat-containing G-protein-coupled receptor 5 (Lgr5) is recognized in colorectal cancer. These receptors promote tumor growth re-initiation after treatment (de Sousa e Melo et al. 2017; Badrinath and Yoo 2019). CD95 expression is related to gastrointestinal cancer and its stimulation can increase the number of tumor cells with SCs features (Ceppi et al. 2014). CD133+ is expressed on the colon cancer cell's surface. These cells produce IL-4 which makes them resistant to apoptosis (Todaro et al. 2007). $\alpha2\beta1$ integrin, Trop-2, and CD133 are the three main receptors identified in prostate cancer (Trerotola et al. 2010). Invasion is promoted by expressing receptor tyrosine kinase-like orphan receptor 1 (ROR1) in ovarian CSCs that can be inhibited by humanized monoclonal antibodies (mAbs) (Zhang et al. 2014). Poor prognosis and migration of hepatocellular carcinoma (HCC) are related to the expression of toll-like receptors 4 (TLR-4) on CSCs (Liu et al. 2015). Programmed death ligand-1 (PD-L1), vascular endothelial growth factor receptor type 2 (VEGFR2), and CD24 expression in epithelial CSCs can lead to rapid tumorigenesis, transformation, and increased calcium signaling in patients suffering from bladder cancer (Jinesh et al. 2017). Expression of PD-L1 on CSCs in breast cancer can sustain its stemness as a result of Nanog transcription factors and octamer-binding transcription factor-4A (OCT-4A) expression and phosphatidylinositol 3-kinase (PI3K)/protein kinase B (AKT) signaling pathway activation (Almozyan et al. 2017).

Check out Fig. 1 (Zhang et al. 2016; Nguyen et al. 2017; Curtarelli et al. 2018; Muinao et al. 2018; Badrinath and Yoo 2019) for more information on CSCs in different types of cancer.

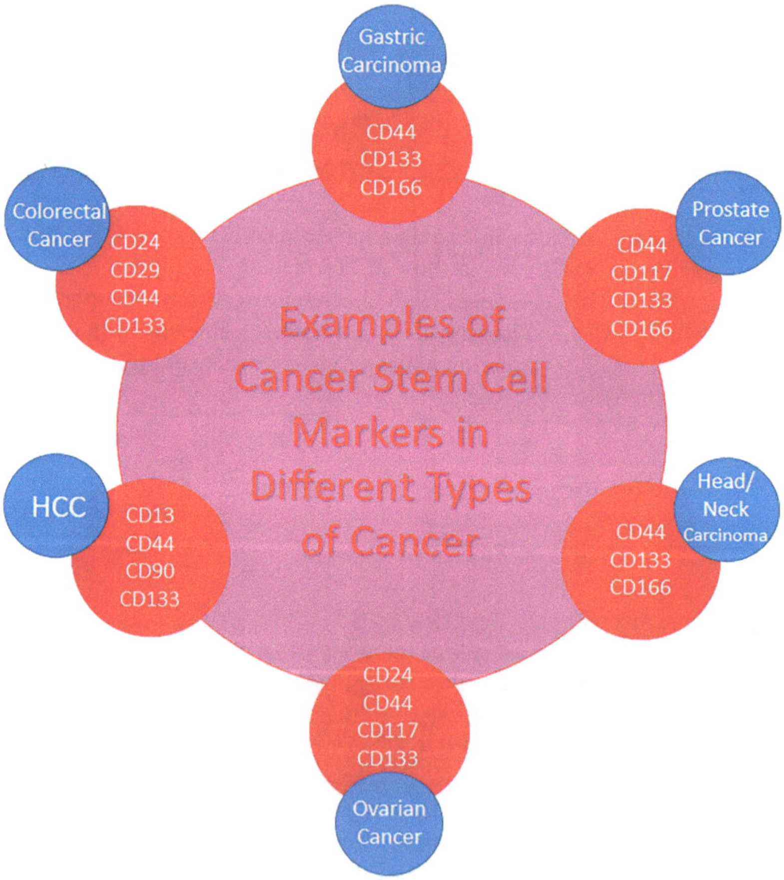

Fig. 1 Examples of CSC markers in different types of cancer

3.2 Developmental Pathways

The notch signaling pathway plays a significant role in the proliferation, cell fate specification, hemostasis, and differentiation of multicellular organisms. Also, it is one of the most important activated signaling pathways in cancer cells related to cancer metastasis and illustrates the linkage between SCs' self-renewal and angiogenesis. Inhibiting this signaling pathway might be considered as a therapeutic method for cancer by CSCs eradication (Al-Hajj et al. 2003; Patel et al. 2005; Venkatesh et al. 2018).

Hedgehog (Hh) signaling is an essential pathway for cell fate and self-renewal determination. Abnormal Hh signaling including ligands overexpression, transcription factors dysregulation, and loss of receptor function is related to the progression and devolvement of different types of cancer as well as tumorigenesis such as CSCs maintenance (Cochrane et al. 2015; Codd et al. 2018).

3.3 CSCs Escaping

CSCs can escape from cancer-killer cells including T-cells and natural killer (NK) cells due to their low expression of innate immune receptors. The majority of signaling pathways participating in typical SCs are dysregulated in CSCs as ligands, receptors, or oncogenes based on the cancer type. It was reported that the markers of normal stem cells such as Nanog and octamer-binding transcription factor 4 (Oct-4) are overexpressed in CSCs that cause resistance against anticancer immunity (Doherty et al. 2017; Zhang et al. 2018). Additionally, stromal cells in a tumor microenvironment consist of cancer-associated fibroblasts and endothelial cells secreting different cytokines and chemokines to suppress anticancer immunity (Klemm and Joyce 2015; Relation et al. 2017).

4 CSCs as a Target for Human Immune System

The expression of histocompatibility complex (MHC) class I in CSCs is often lower than in other tumor cells. As a result, CSCs are more susceptible to natural killer (NK) cells. CSCs in breast and some brain cancers lack NK-activating ligands; nonetheless, those in colorectal cancer and glioblastoma express different ligands for NK cells including poliovirus receptor (PVR) which are extremely susceptible to NK cells (Wu et al. 2007; Castriconi et al. 2009; Tallerico et al. 2013; Wang et al. 2014).

CSCs in solid tumors can express human leucocyte antigen (HLA) class I which is associated with efficient targeting by CD8+ T-cells. According to tumor type and cell origins, susceptibility or resistance to T-cells might be seen. For example, CSCs of colon cancers express lower levels of MHC class I compared to non-stem-like cells (Tallerico et al. 2013).

Some tumor-associated antigens (TAA) such as centrosomal protein 55 (CEP55) and mucin 1 (MUC-1) are expressed equally in CSCs and non-CSCs. Others including olfactory receptor family 7 subfamily C member 1 (OR7C1) are expressed more in CSCs. T-cell responses to TAA can lead to temporary tumor control. Despite that, it may cause tumor escape by inducing the loss of antigens which are not essential for cellular fitness (Engelmann et al. 2008; Inoda et al. 2011; Morita et al. 2016; Verdegaal et al. 2016).

5 Efficacy of Different Treatments on CSCs

Radiation therapy: CSCs were reported to be highly resistant to radiation therapy. At least some of the CSCs remain in the tumor after radiation therapy and cause cancer recurrence. Radiation therapy directly causes DNA damage including single-strand breaks. It may also cause indirect damage to the DNA by reactive oxygen species (ROS) which are highly radioresistant. As a result, the cell cycle is interrupted permanently or temporarily, mainly by checkpoint kinase activity that provides time for repairing DNA damage. Irreparable DNA damage can lead to cell death or senescence. Additionally, the localization of CSCs can be considered as another important feature in radioresistance. It was claimed that CSCs located in hypoxic areas are significantly more resistant to radiation therapy in comparison to CSCs in normoxic areas. Hypoxia-inducing factors are able to activate the Hh and Notch signaling pathways that are necessary for CSCs maintenance (de Jong et al. 2010; Krause et al. 2017). However, high-dose radiation might lonely eliminate CSCs; for instance, lung and prostate cancers are cured by radiation therapy alone based on generating immunogenic cell death (Salimu et al. 2015).

Chemotherapy: The adenosine triphosphate (ATP)-binding cassette (ABC) transporter family of proteins is active in CSCs and switched off while cell differentiation. They are well organized for pumping out molecules from the cytoplasm. This process leads to cell protection from toxins such as chemotherapeutic drugs (Hirschmann-Jax et al. 2004; Davidson et al. 2008). From another point of view, ABCB proteins play a significant role in peptide trafficking across the cell membranes that leads to the presentation of MHC class I antigen and dendritic cell (DC) function which eventually results in effective anti-tumor T-cell responses (van de Ven et al. 2009).

6 Immunotherapy for Cancer

6.1 Historical View

In the nineteenth century, the idea of deploying the immune system as a method for treating neoplastic disease was first developed. Friedrich Fehleisen and Wilhelm Busch illustrated an epidemiological association between cancer and immune status. They noted spontaneous tumor regression following the erysipelas development caused by Streptococcus pyogenes. Then, William coley, known as the father of immunotherapy, noticed that erysipelas was related to a better outcome in patients suffering from sarcoma. At that time, he aimed to treat cancer patients using extracts of heat-inactivated Serratia marcescens and Streptococcus pyogenes to boost immunity. This extract was called "Coley's toxins" and achieved promising responses in many types of cancer. Anyway, the discovery of chemotherapeutic drugs and radiation therapy in concert with a lack of scientific rigor prevented this treatment from becoming a standard approach (Decker and Safdar 2009; Decker et al. 2017; Oiseth and Aziz 2017).

In the early twentieth century, the concept of cancer immunotherapy resurfaced with the development of technology. Sir Frank Macfarlane Burnet and Lewis Thomas proposed the "cancer immunosurveillance" hypothesis in which tumor-associated neoantigens are identified and targeted by the human body's immune system to avoid carcinogenesis similar to graft rejection. There were some pieces of evidence to support this hypothesis as follows: (1) tumoral adoptive transfer led to productive immune responses in mice, and (2) there were some reports of melanoma recurrence in patients suffering from autoimmune disease (Smith Jr and Stehlin Jr 1965; Oiseth and Aziz 2017; Waldman et al. 2020). Further biochemical and molecular advances consequenced in the recognization of the cancer-specific immune response. This prepared clear evidence that the immune system (especially T-cells) was able to wage war on tumor tissue (Halliday et al. 1995).

In the 1970s, immunologists investigated for antibodies able to bind to tumors in cancer patients, and lymphocytes activated with IL-2 or lectins were found to target cancer cells in vitro (Strausser et al. 1981; Grimm et al. 1982; Mazumder et al. 1982). Then, cytokines were searched in various clinical trials for renal cell and breast cancer, lymphoma, melanoma, and glioblastoma. At this time, immunologists also worked on the clinical use of interferon-α (IFN-α) which obviously showed antitumor activity in some solid tumors like melanoma and hairy cell leukemia. For instance, IFN-α2 was expressed to be highly antiproliferative, apoptotic, differentiation-inducing, and pleiotropic in multiple malignancies. In 1986, IFN-α2 was approved as a therapy for hairy cell leukemia and in 1995 it was approved as the adjuvant therapy for stage IIB/III melanoma by US Food and Drug Administration (FDA) (Kirkwood and Ernstoff 1984; Krown et al. 1984; Kirkwood et al. 2012).

6.2 Immunotherapy in Brief

Generally, immunotherapy is a therapeutic method to boost the body's immune system to fight against cancer cells. There are many types of immunotherapy with different success rates, benefits, and side effects based on the patient's condition and cancer type. However, the overall response rate for immunotherapeutic drugs is approximately 15–20% (Cancer Center 2022; Medicine 2023).

Herein, we discuss some types of immunotherapy in brief. Monoclonal antibodies are injected into the body to mark cancer cells. In this way, the immune system can better recognize and destroy them. Immune checkpoint inhibitors (ICIs) can remove natural blockades in the human body which are often used by cancer cells to hide from the immune system. In chimeric antigen receptor (CAR)-T-cell therapy, white blood cells (WBC) are harvested from the patient's tumor and grown in the lab to boost their natural ability to fight cancer. Then, they will be injected back into the patient's body. Cancer vaccines can provide immune cells with a specific target found on tumor cells and stimulate the creation of antibodies against them (Cancer Center 2022).

In the world today, cancer immunotherapy has revolutionized the field of oncology by improving the survival time of patients suffering from fatal cancers. The number of patients permitted to receive immune-based cancer therapies as their first line of treatment has increased rapidly. Also, novel combination therapies show a promising perspective in cancer treatment for decades to come (Waldman et al. 2020).

7 CSCs as a Target for Immunotherapy

Immunotherapy can target CSCs in different ways as follows:

7.1 DC-Based Vaccines

DCs pulsed with CSC lysates or cancer cell lines can be used as a cancer vaccine. In a study, CSCs lysate-pulsed DCs induced IL-4 and IFN-γ secretion resulted in tumor (malignant melanoma) growth suppression and increased survival time in vaccinated mice (Dashti et al. 2016). Chemokine receptor (CCR) downregulation was related to therapeutic efficacy in squamous cell carcinoma and melanoma (Lu et al. 2015). DCs loaded with NANOG peptides can cause specific anti-cancer T-cell responses in ovarian cancer (Wefers et al. 2018). Another study reported that inhibiting primary cancer growth can reduce lung metastasis. This result is related to CCR10 downregulation on $ALDH^{high}$ D5 CSCs in lung tissue (Hu et al. 2016). *Pellegatta* et al. claimed that DCs loaded with GL261-neurospheres (NS) lysates can save mice against gliomas from GL261-adherent cells (AC) and GL261-NS by tumor growth prevention (Pellegatta and Finocchiaro 2009).

7.2 Adaptive T-cell Therapy (ACT)

ACT is a personalized cancer immunotherapy using host immune cancer-bearing cells. In this method, the patient's tumor-infiltrating lymphocytes (TIL) are isolated in the presence of IL-2. After evaluating specific tumor recognition, selected TILs will be reinjected into a similar patient (Rosenberg and Restifo 2015). Lately, CAR T-cells have been used against CSCs' antigens. In prostate cancer, they are targeted against epithelial cells adhesion molecules (EpCAM) antigens leading to the elimination of CSCs (Deng et al. 2015). Adoptively transferred CD8+ cytotoxic T-cells can selectively kill CSCs in colon cancer (Miyamoto et al. 2018). CAR T-cells with cytokine-induced killer (CIK) cells are able to kill CD123+ cell lines in acute myeloid leukemia (Tettamanti et al. 2013). In nasopharyngeal carcinoma, CIK cells can recognize NKG2D-ligands on CSCs causing efficient therapy (Wei et al. 2015). In invasive bladder cancer, the adoptive transfer of NK cells from a healthy donor consequenced in killing CSCs by activation with IL-15 and IL-2 (Ferreira-Teixeira et al. 2016). In oral squamous carcinoma, the adoptive transfer of NK cells activates super-charged NK cells (mediated with IL-12 and IL-15) against CSCs (Kaur et al. 2017).

7.3 Oncolytic Virotherapy (OVT)

T-cells activation and immunogenic cell death are the results of using OVT as an immunotherapeutic method. For example, in glioblastoma, the oncolytic herpes simplex virus marked with IL-12 led to IFN-γ release, reducing the number of regulatory T-cells, and inhibiting angiogenesis (Cheema et al. 2013). In breast cancer, killing CSCs by the oncolytic vaccinia virus was reported (Wang et al. 2012). Chemokine C-X-C-Motif receptor 4 (CXCR4) antagonist expressed-oncolytic vaccinia virus $CD44^{+}$ $CD117^{+}$ cells of ovarian cancer (Gil et al. 2014). Also, lysing $CD133^{+}$ cells in hepatocellular carcinoma by oncolytic measles viruses were reported (Bach et al. 2013).

7.4 Combination Therapy

In recent years, combined immunotherapy has developed for the complete elimination of CSCs. In mouse melanoma, eradication of $ALDH^{high}$ CSCs, elevated IFN-γ secretion, and increased $CD8^{+}$ T-cells are the results of using cytotoxic anti-T-lymphocyte associated antigen 4 (CTLA-4) and anti-PD-L1 in combination with a DC-based vaccine (Zheng et al. 2018). A triple combination of an oncolytic herpes simplex virus expressing IL-12, anti-CTLA-4, and anti-programmed cell death 1 (PD-1) can eliminate CSCs in glioblastoma (Saha et al. 2017). In bladder cancer, a strong anti-tumor immune response is induced by increasing the number of $CD4^{+}$ and $CD8^{+}$ cells as a result of combination therapy with anti-PD-1 and streptavidin-granulocyte-macrophage-colony triggering factor surface-modified CSCs vaccine (Shi et al. 2018).

8 Conclusion

In this chapter, we tried to illustrate obvious imaging of the role of CSCs in tumor initiation, metastasis, and cancer's resistance to immune responses. Then, we elucidated the role of immunotherapy in cancer treatment in recent decades to show its importance in increasing the survival time of patients suffering from rapidly fatal cancers. CSC can be considered as a significant immunotherapeutic approach and some advancements were discussed herein. However, more large-scale clinical trials are required in the future to better evaluate CSCs as a target for immunotherapy which will definitely show a promising perspective in cancer treatment.

Acknowledgments None.

Ethical Statement The manuscript does not contain clinical studies or patient data.

Conflict of Interest The authors declare that they have no conflict of interest.

References

Al-Hajj M, Wicha MS, Benito-Hernandez A, Morrison SJ, Clarke MF (2003) Prospective identification of tumorigenic breast cancer cells. Proc Natl Acad Sci U S A 100(7):3983–3988

Almozyan S, Colak D, Mansour F, Alaiya A, Al-Harazi O, Qattan A, Al-Mohanna F, Al-Alwan M, Ghebeh H (2017) PD-L1 promotes OCT4 and Nanog expression in breast cancer stem cells by sustaining PI3K/AKT pathway activation. Int J Cancer 141(7):1402–1412

Ayob AZ, Ramasamy TS (2018) Cancer stem cells as key drivers of tumour progression. J Biomed Sci 25(1):20

Bach P, Abel T, Hoffmann C, Gal Z, Braun G, Voelker I, Ball CR, Johnston IC, Lauer UM, Herold-Mende C (2013) Specific elimination of CD133+ tumor cells with targeted oncolytic measles virus. Cancer Res 73(2):865–874

Badrinath N, Yoo SY (2019) Recent advances in cancer stem cell-targeted immunotherapy. Cancers (Basel) 11(3):310

Batlle E, Clevers H (2017) Cancer stem cells revisited. Nat Med 23(10):1124–1134

Cancer Center (2022) Immunotherapy. 2023, from https://www.cancercenter.com/treatment-options/precision-medicine/immunotherapy

Castriconi R, Daga A, Dondero A, Zona G, Poliani PL, Melotti A, Griffero F, Marubbi D, Spaziante R, Bellora F (2009) NK cells recognize and kill human glioblastoma cells with stem cell-like properties. J Immunol 182(6):3530–3539

Ceppi P, Hadji A, Kohlhapp FJ, Pattanayak A, Hau A, Liu X, Liu H, Murmann AE, Peter ME (2014) CD95 and CD95L promote and protect cancer stem cells. Nat Commun 5(1):5238

Cheema TA, Wakimoto H, Fecci PE, Ning J, Kuroda T, Jeyaretna DS, Martuza RL, Rabkin SD (2013) Multifaceted oncolytic virus therapy for glioblastoma in an immunocompetent cancer stem cell model. Proc Natl Acad Sci 110(29):12006–12011

Cochrane CR, Szczepny A, Watkins DN, Cain JE (2015) Hedgehog signaling in the maintenance of cancer stem cells. Cancers (Basel) 7(3):1554–1585

Codd AS, Kanaseki T, Torigo T, Tabi Z (2018) Cancer stem cells as targets for immunotherapy. Immunology 153(3):304–314

Curtarelli RB, Gonçalves JM, Dos Santos LGP, Savi MG, Nör JE, Mezzomo LAM, Rodriguez Cordeiro MM (2018) Expression of cancer stem cell biomarkers in human head and neck carcinomas: a systematic review. Stem Cell Rev Rep 14:769–784

Dashti A, Ebrahimi M, Hadjati J, Memarnejadian A, Moazzeni SM (2016) Dendritic cell based immunotherapy using tumor stem cells mediates potent antitumor immune responses. Cancer Lett 374(1):175–185

Davidson AL, Dassa E, Orelle C, Chen J (2008) Structure, function, and evolution of bacterial ATP-binding cassette systems. Microbiol Mol Biol Rev 72(2):317–364

de Jong MC, Pramana J, van der Wal JE, Lacko M, Peutz-Kootstra CJ, de Jong JM, Takes RP, Kaanders JH, van der Laan BF, Wachters J (2010) CD44 expression predicts local recurrence after radiotherapy in larynx CancerCD44 predicts outcome after radiotherapy in larynx cancer. Clin Cancer Res 16(21):5329–5338

de Sousa e Melo F, Kurtova AV, Harnoss JM, Kljavin N, Hoeck JD, Hung J, Anderson JE, Storm EE, Modrusan Z, Koeppen H (2017) A distinct role for Lgr5+ stem cells in primary and metastatic colon cancer. Nature 543(7647):676–680

Decker WK, Safdar A (2009) Bioimmunoadjuvants for the treatment of neoplastic and infectious disease: Coley's legacy revisited. Cytokine Growth Factor Rev 20(4):271–281

Decker WK, da Silva RF, Sanabria MH, Angelo LS, Guimarães F, Burt BM, Kheradmand F, Paust S (2017) Cancer immunotherapy: historical perspective of a clinical revolution and emerging preclinical animal models. Front Immunol 8:829

Deng Z, Wu Y, Ma W, Zhang S, Zhang Y-Q (2015) Adoptive T-cell therapy of prostate cancer targeting the cancer stem cell antigen EpCAM. BMC Immunol 16(1):1–9

Doherty MR, Smigiel JM, Junk DJ, Jackson MW (2016) Cancer stem cell plasticity drives therapeutic resistance. Cancers 8(1):8

Doherty MR, Cheon H, Junk DJ, Vinayak S, Varadan V, Telli ML, Ford JM, Stark GR, Jackson MW (2017) Interferon-beta represses cancer stem cell properties in triple-negative breast cancer. Proc Natl Acad Sci 114(52):13792–13797

Engelmann K, Shen H, Finn OJ (2008) MCF7 side population cells with characteristics of cancer stem/progenitor cells express the tumor antigen MUC1. Cancer Res 68(7):2419–2426

Ferreira-Teixeira M, Paiva-Oliveira D, Parada B, Alves V, Sousa V, Chijioke O, Münz C, Reis F, Rodrigues-Santos P, Gomes C (2016) Natural killer cell-based adoptive immunotherapy eradicates and drives differentiation of chemoresistant bladder cancer stem-like cells. BMC Med 14(1):1–13

Fujimori H, Shikanai M, Teraoka H, Masutani M, Yoshioka K (2012) Induction of cancerous stem cells during embryonic stem cell differentiation. J Biol Chem 287(44):36777–36791

Gil M, Komorowski MP, Seshadri M, Rokita H, McGray AR, Opyrchal M, Odunsi KO, Kozbor D (2014) CXCL12/CXCR4 blockade by oncolytic virotherapy inhibits ovarian cancer growth by decreasing immunosuppression and targeting cancer-initiating cells. J Immunol 193(10): 5327–5337

Grimm EA, Mazumder A, Zhang H, Rosenberg S (1982) Lymphokine-activated killer cell phenomenon. Lysis of natural killer-resistant fresh solid tumor cells by interleukin 2-activated autologous human peripheral blood lymphocytes. J Exp Med 155(6):1823–1841

Halliday GM, Patel A, Hunt MJ, Tefany FJ, Barnetson RSC (1995) Spontaneous regression of human melanoma/nonmelanoma skin cancer: association with infiltrating CD4+ T cells. World J Surg 19:352–358

Hirschmann-Jax C, Foster AE, Wulf GG, Nuchtern JG, Jax TW, Gobel U, Goodell MA, Brenner MK (2004) A distinct "side population" of cells with high drug efflux capacity in human tumor cells. Proc Natl Acad Sci 101(39):14228–14233

Hu Y, Lu L, Xia Y, Chen X, Chang AE, Hollingsworth RE, Hurt E, Owen J, Moyer JS, Prince ME (2016) Therapeutic efficacy of cancer stem cell vaccines in the adjuvant setting. Cancer Res 76(16):4661–4672

Inoda S, Hirohashi Y, Torigoe T, Morita R, Takahashi A, Asanuma H, Nakatsugawa M, Nishizawa S, Tamura Y, Tsuruma T (2011) Cytotoxic T lymphocytes efficiently recognize human colon cancer stem-like cells. Am J Pathol 178(4):1805–1813

Jinesh GG, Manyam GC, Mmeje CO, Baggerly KA, Kamat AM (2017) Surface PD-L1, E-cadherin, CD24, and VEGFR2 as markers of epithelial cancer stem cells associated with rapid tumorigenesis. Sci Rep 7(1):1–12

Kaiser J (2015) The cancer stem cell gamble. American Association for the Advancement of Science, Washington, DC

Kaur K, Cook J, Park S-H, Topchyan P, Kozlowska A, Ohanian N, Fang C, Nishimura I, Jewett A (2017) Novel strategy to expand super-charged NK cells with significant potential to lyse and differentiate cancer stem cells: differences in NK expansion and function between healthy and cancer patients. Front Immunol 8:297

Kaur G, Sharma P, Dogra N, Singh S (2018) Eradicating cancer stem cells: concepts, issues, and challenges. Curr Treat Options in Oncol 19:1–23

Kim W-T, Ryu CJ (2017) Cancer stem cell surface markers on normal stem cells. BMB Rep 50(6): 285

Kirkwood JM, Ernstoff M (1984) Interferons in the treatment of human cancer. J Clin Oncol 2(4): 336–352

Kirkwood JM, Butterfield LH, Tarhini AA, Zarour H, Kalinski P, Ferrone S (2012) Immunotherapy of cancer in 2012. CA Cancer J Clin 62(5):309–335

Klemm F, Joyce JA (2015) Microenvironmental regulation of therapeutic response in cancer. Trends Cell Biol 25(4):198–213

Krause M, Dubrovska A, Linge A, Baumann M (2017) Cancer stem cells: radioresistance, prediction of radiotherapy outcome and specific targets for combined treatments. Adv Drug Deliv Rev 109:63–73

Krown SE, Burk MW, Kirkwood JM, Kerr D, Morton DL (1984) American Cancer Society phase II trial 1, 2. Cancer Treat Rep 68(5):723

Lapidot T, Sirard C, Vormoor J, Murdoch B, Hoang T, Caceres-Cortes J, Minden M, Paterson B, Caligiuri MA, Dick JE (1994) A cell initiating human acute myeloid leukaemia after transplantation into SCID mice. Nature 367(6464):645–648

Liu W-T, Jing Y-Y, Yu G-f, Han Z-p, Yu D-d, Fan Q-M, Ye F, Li R, Gao L, Zhao Q-D (2015) Toll like receptor 4 facilitates invasion and migration as a cancer stem cell marker in hepatocellular carcinoma. Cancer Lett 358(2):136–143

Lu L, Tao H, Chang AE, Hu Y, Shu G, Chen Q, Egenti M, Owen J, Moyer JS, Prince ME (2015) Cancer stem cell vaccine inhibits metastases of primary tumors and induces humoral immune responses against cancer stem cells. Onco Targets Ther 4(3):e990767

Mazumder A, Grimm EA, Zhang HZ, Rosenberg SA (1982) Lysis of fresh human solid tumors by autologous lymphocytes activated in vitro with lectins. Cancer Res 42(3):913–918

Medicine JH (2023) Immunotherapy: precision medicine in action. 2023, from https://www.hopkinsmedicine.org/inhealth/about-us/immunotherapy-precision-medicine-action-policy-brief.html#:~:text=Immunotherapy%20drugs%20work%20better%20in,are%20about%2015%20to%2020%25

Miyamoto S, Kochin V, Kanaseki T, Hongo A, Tokita S, Kikuchi Y, Takaya A, Hirohashi Y, Tsukahara T, Terui T (2018) The antigen ASB4 on cancer stem cells serves as a target for CTL immunotherapy of colorectal cancer. Cancer Immunol Res 6(3):358–369

Morita R, Hirohashi Y, Torigoe T, Ito-Inoda S, Takahashi A, Mariya T, Asanuma H, Tamura Y, Tsukahara T, Kanaseki T (2016) Olfactory receptor family 7 subfamily C member 1 is a novel marker of colon cancer-initiating cells and is a potent target of immunotherapy. Clin Cancer Res 22(13):3298–3309

Muinao T, Boruah HPD, Pal M (2018) Diagnostic and prognostic biomarkers in ovarian cancer and the potential roles of cancer stem cells – an updated review. Exp Cell Res 362(1):1–10

Nguyen PH, Giraud J, Chambonnier L, Dubus P, Wittkop L, Belleannée G, Collet D, Soubeyran I, Evrard S, Rousseau B (2017) Characterization of biomarkers of tumorigenic and chemoresistant cancer stem cells in human gastric carcinoma. Clin Cancer Res 23(6):1586–1597

Oiseth SJ, Aziz MS (2017) Cancer immunotherapy: a brief review of the history, possibilities, and challenges ahead. J Cancer Metastasis Treat 3:250–261

Patel NS, Li J-L, Generali D, Poulsom R, Cranston DW, Harris AL (2005) Up-regulation of delta-like 4 ligand in human tumor vasculature and the role of basal expression in endothelial cell function. Cancer Res 65(19):8690–8697

Pattabiraman DR, Weinberg RA (2014) Tackling the cancer stem cells—what challenges do they pose? Nat Rev Drug Discov 13(7):497–512

Pellegatta S, Finocchiaro G (2009) Dendritic cell vaccines for cancer stem cells. Methods Mol Biol 568:233–247

Relation T, Dominici M, Horwitz EM (2017) Concise review: an (im)penetrable shield: how the tumor microenvironment protects cancer stem cells. Stem Cells 35(5):1123–1130

Rosenberg SA, Restifo NP (2015) Adoptive cell transfer as personalized immunotherapy for human cancer. Science 348(6230):62–68

Saha D, Martuza RL, Rabkin SD (2017) Macrophage polarization contributes to glioblastoma eradication by combination immunovirotherapy and immune checkpoint blockade. Cancer Cell 32(2):253–267. e255

Salimu J, Spary LK, Al-Taei S, Clayton A, Mason MD, Staffurth J, Tabi Z (2015) Cross-presentation of the oncofetal tumor antigen 5T4 from irradiated prostate cancer cells—a key role for heat-shock protein 70 and receptor CD91Antigen cross-presentation from irradiated tumor cells. Cancer Immunol Res 3(6):678–688

Shi X, Zhang X, Li J, Mo L, Zhao H, Zhu Y, Hu Z, Gao J, Tan W (2018) PD-1 blockade enhances the antitumor efficacy of GM-CSF surface-modified bladder cancer stem cells vaccine. Int J Cancer 142(10):2106–2117

Singh SK, Hawkins C, Clarke ID, Squire JA, Bayani J, Hide T, Henkelman RM, Cusimano MD, Dirks PB (2004) Identification of human brain tumour initiating cells. Nature 432(7015): 396–401

Smith JL Jr, Stehlin JS Jr (1965) Spontaneous regression of primary malignant melanomas with regional metastases. Cancer 18(11):1399–1415

Strausser J, Mazumder A, Grimm E, Lotze M, Rosenberg S (1981) Lysis of human solid tumors by autologous cells sensitized in vitro to alloantigens. J Immunol (Baltimore, MD.: 1950) 127(1): 266–271

Tallerico R, Todaro M, Di Franco S, Maccalli C, Garofalo C, Sottile R, Palmieri C, Tirinato L, Pangigadde PN, La Rocca R (2013) Human NK cells selective targeting of colon cancer-initiating cells: a role for natural cytotoxicity receptors and MHC class I molecules. J Immunol 190(5):2381–2390

Tettamanti S, Marin V, Pizzitola I, Magnani CF, Giordano Attianese GM, Cribioli E, Maltese F, Galimberti S, Lopez AF, Biondi A (2013) Targeting of acute myeloid leukaemia by cytokine-induced killer cells redirected with a novel CD 123-specific chimeric antigen receptor. Br J Haematol 161(3):389–401

Todaro M, Alea MP, Di Stefano AB, Cammareri P, Vermeulen L, Iovino F, Tripodo C, Russo A, Gulotta G, Medema JP (2007) Colon cancer stem cells dictate tumor growth and resist cell death by production of interleukin-4. Cell Stem Cell 1(4):389–402

Trerotola M, Rathore S, Goel HL, Li J, Alberti S, Piantelli M, Adams D, Jiang Z, Languino LR (2010) CD133, Trop-2 and α2β1 integrin surface receptors as markers of putative human prostate cancer stem cells. Am J Transl Res 2(2):135

Tysnes BB, Bjerkvig R (2007) Cancer initiation and progression: involvement of stem cells and the microenvironment. Biochim Biophys Acta 1775(2):283–297

van de Ven R, Scheffer GL, Scheper RJ, de Gruijl TD (2009) The ABC of dendritic cell development and function. Trends Immunol 30(9):421–429

Venkatesh V, Nataraj R, Thangaraj GS, Karthikeyan M, Gnanasekaran A, Kaginelli SB, Kuppanna G, Kallappa CG, Basalingappa KM (2018) Targeting notch signalling pathway of cancer stem cells. Stem Cell Invest 5:5

Verdegaal EM, De Miranda NF, Visser M, Harryvan T, Van Buuren MM, Andersen RS, Hadrup SR, Van Der Minne CE, Schotte R, Spits H (2016) Neoantigen landscape dynamics during human melanoma–T cell interactions. Nature 536(7614):91–95

Waldman AD, Fritz JM, Lenardo MJ (2020) A guide to cancer immunotherapy: from T cell basic science to clinical practice. Nat Rev Immunol 20(11):651–668

Wang H, Chen NG, Minev BR, Szalay AA (2012) Oncolytic vaccinia virus GLV-1h68 strain shows enhanced replication in human breast cancer stem-like cells in comparison to breast cancer cells. J Transl Med 10(1):1–15

Wang B, Wang Q, Wang Z, Jiang J, Yu S-C, Ping Y-F, Yang J, Xu S-L, Ye X-Z, Xu C (2014) Metastatic consequences of immune escape from NK cell cytotoxicity by human breast cancer stem cells. Cancer Res 74(20):5746–5757

Wefers C, Schreibelt G, Massuger LF, de Vries IJM, Torensma R (2018) Immune curbing of cancer stem cells by CTLs directed to NANOG. Front Immunol 9:1412

Wei F, Rong X-X, Xie R-Y, Jia L-T, Wang H-Y, Qin Y-J, Chen L, Shen H-F, Lin X-L, Yang J (2015) Cytokine-induced killer cells efficiently kill stem-like cancer cells of nasopharyngeal carcinoma via the NKG2D-ligands recognition. Oncotarget 6(33):35023

Wu A, Wiesner S, Xiao J, Ericson K, Chen W, Hall WA, Low WC, Ohlfest JR (2007) Expression of MHC I and NK ligands on human CD133+ glioma cells: possible targets of immunotherapy. J Neuro-Oncol 83:121–131

Yoshioka K, Atsumi Y, Nakagama H, Teraoka H (2015) Development of cancer-initiating cells and immortalized cells with genomic instability. World J Stem Cells 7(2):483–489

Yu Z, Pestell TG, Lisanti MP, Pestell RG (2012) Cancer stem cells. Int J Biochem Cell Biol 44(12): 2144–2151

Zhang S, Cui B, Lai H, Liu G, Ghia EM, Widhopf GF, Zhang Z, Wu CC, Chen L, Wu R (2014) Ovarian cancer stem cells express ROR1, which can be targeted for anti–cancer-stem-cell therapy. Proc Natl Acad Sci 111(48):17266–17271

Zhang K, Zhou S, Wang L, Wang J, Zou Q, Zhao W, Fu Q, Fang X (2016) Current stem cell biomarkers and their functional mechanisms in prostate cancer. Int J Mol Sci 17(7):1163

Zhang D, Tang DG, Rycaj K (2018) Cancer stem cells: regulation programs, immunological properties and immunotherapy. Semin Cancer Biol 52(Pt 2):94–106. Elsevier

Zheng F, Dang J, Zhang H, Xu F, Ba D, Zhang B, Cheng F, Chang AE, Wicha MS, Li Q (2018) Cancer stem cell vaccination with PD-L1 and CTLA-4 blockades enhances the eradication of melanoma stem cells in a mouse tumor model. J Immunother (Hagerstown, MD.: 1997) 41(8): 361

Immunological Properties of Manipulated Hematopoietic Stem Cell Grafts

Tahereh Rostami, Saeed Mohammadi, and Azadeh Kiumarsi

Abstract

Hematopoietic stem cell (HSC) graft manipulations comprise immunologic laboratory techniques designed for negative selection (i.e., reduction of unwanted cells) and/or positive selection (i.e., enrichment of the desired hematopoietic cells), in order to optimize the cellular composition and immunological properties of stem cell grafts and to improve clinical outcomes of hematopoietic stem cell transplantation (HSCT). In this chapter, the technique of different cellular manipulations on HSC grafts has been explained briefly. The immunological properties of each type of manipulation are discussed separately. An update on the conducted clinical trials implementing various manipulative methods and their outcomes are also provided. Apparently, designed or manipulated grafts have provided a safe platform for improving HSCT outcomes.

Keywords

Enrichment · Graft manipulation · Graft-versus-host disease · Hematopoietic stem cell transplantation · Rejection · T cell depletion

T. Rostami
Hematologic Malignancies Research Center, Research Institute for Oncology, Hematology and Cell Therapy (RIOHCT), Tehran University of Medical Sciences (TUMS), Tehran, Iran

S. Mohammadi
Cell Therapy and Hematopoietic Stem Cell Transplantation Research Center, Research Institute for Oncology, Hematology and Cell Therapy (RIOHCT), Tehran University of Medical Sciences (TUMS), Tehran, Iran

A. Kiumarsi (✉)
Hematology-Oncology and Stem Cell Transplantation Research Center, Department of Pediatric Cell Therapy, Research Institute for Oncology, Hematology and Cell Therapy (RIOHCT), Shariati Hospital, Tehran University of Medical Sciences (TUMS), Tehran, Iran
e-mail: akiumarsi@sina.tums.ac.ir

Interdisciplinary Cancer Research, https://doi.org/10.1007/16833_2022_115
Published online: 31 January 2023

1 Introduction

Hematopoietic stem cell (HSC) graft manipulations comprise immunologic laboratory techniques designed for negative selection (i.e., reduction of unwanted cells) and/or positive selection (i.e., enrichment of the desired hematopoietic cells), in order to optimize the cellular composition and immunological properties of stem cell grafts and to improve clinical outcomes of hematopoietic stem cell transplantation (HSCT).

Successful allogeneic HSCT involves ablation or attenuation of the recipient's blood and immune system by preparative conditioning regimen, ensued by engraftment of donor HSCs in bone marrow niche of the recipient and reconstitution of hematopoietic cell lineages and immune cells (Peci et al. 2022). However, graft rejection, graft-versus-host disease (GvHD), severe infections, and disease relapse remain to be the major complications faced throughout transplant process. Recent progress in understanding the transactions between specific cell subsets in HSC grafts has led to novel strategies of cellular manipulation in transplant platforms, which could allow prevention of graft rejection and GvHD together with increasing graft-versus-tumor/leukemia (GvT/L) effect, more rapid immune reconstitution, and augmented infection protection.

This review aims to summarize the method of different cellular manipulations on HSC grafts and to discuss their immunological properties and clinical effects.

2 Types of Hematopoietic Stem Cell Graft Cellular Manipulation

The main cellular components of an unmanipulated HSC graft include the hematopoietic progenitors, dendritic cells (DCs), monocytes, granulocytes, T and B lymphocytes, natural killer (NK) cells, and so on (Fig. 1) (Biernacki et al. 2020).

Optimization of graft cellular composition has allowed to achieve steady engraftment beyond major HLA barriers, with negligible transplant complications and improved survival rates. In these procedures, anti-HSC, anti-T, and/or anti-B cell antibodies conjugated with superparamagnetic microbeads or immunomagnetic beads cooperate for separating target cells within a strong magnetic separation column (Avecilla et al. 2016).

2.1 Depletion (Targeted Negative Selection)

Depletion of different cellular elements in HSC graft was previously based on agglutination and elimination of unwanted cells (Aversa et al. 1994; Soiffer et al. 1997). Not attaining good manufacturing practice (GMP) standards and being resource-intensive led to introduction of a more efficient immunomagnetic system (CliniMACS system, Miltenyi Biotec, Bergisch-Gladbach, Germany). In this structure, magnetically labeled cells are held in the separation column, while other

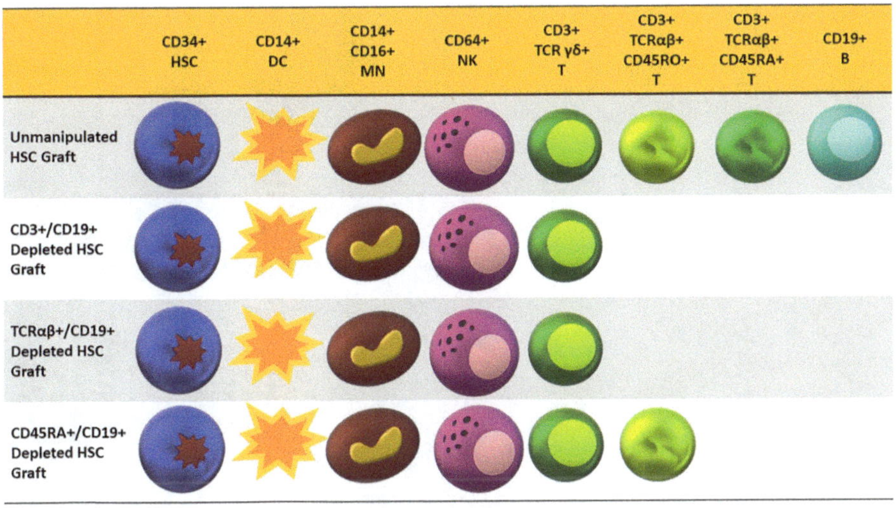

Fig. 1 Cellular composition of unmanipulated and manipulated hematopoietic stem cell grafts. *B* B lymphocyte, *DC* dendritic cell, *HSC* hematopoietic stem cell, *MN* monocyte, *NK* natural killer, *T* T lymphocyte, *TCR* T cell receptor

non-labeled cells stream into the column and are stored up in a collection bag eventually. Likewise, non-labeled cells are let out from the separation column and cumulated in the negative fraction bag (Fig. 2) (CliniMACS 2020).

2.1.1 CD3+ T Cell Depletion

Cluster of differentiation (CD) 3 is a multimeric protein complex, which functions as a T cell co-receptor, expressed with T cell receptor (TCR) α/β or TCR γ/δ heterodimers, crucial for T cell ontogeny (Smith-Garvin et al. 2009). CD3 antigen is a reliable marker for identification of normal T cells and also T cell neoplasms (Salvadori et al. 1994).

Depletion of CD3+ T cells could be conducted by CliniMACS LS or DTS tubing set (Schumm et al. 2013). By this method, a 4.15-log depletion of T cells is reported (Lang et al. 2014).

TCRαβ+ T Cell Depletion

TCRαβ is a heterodimer receptor comprised of the two α and β transmembrane glycoprotein chains, expressed on the majority of peripheral blood T cells. TCRαβ has a variable region which is involved in antigen recognition (CliniMACS 2020).

By means of magnetic microbeads conjugated to a murine monoclonal biotinylated anti-TCRαβ antibody together with an anti-biotin antibody (Fig. 3), TCRαβ+ T cells could be removed from the graft (CliniMACS 2020).

Efficacy of T cell depletion (TCD) with TCRαβ reagent is satisfactory (4.7 log) and is shown to be more effective than CD3+ depletion (4.0 log) and comparable to CD34+ enrichment (4.6 log) (Carreras et al. 2019). By implementation of TCRαβ+

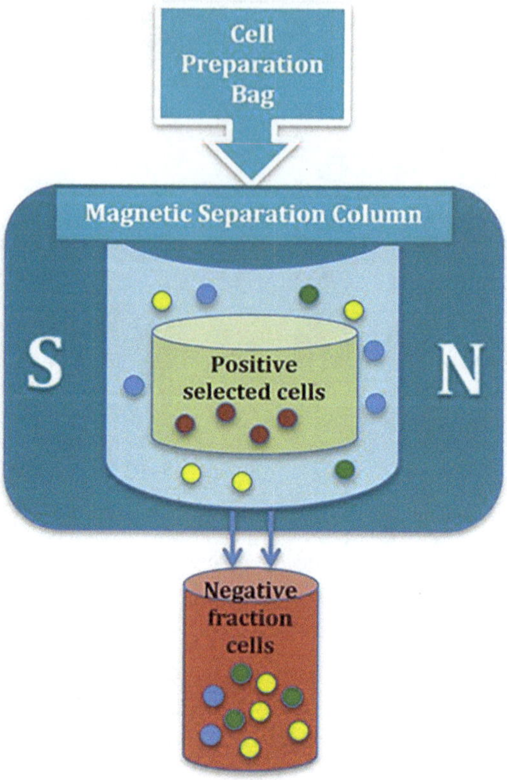

Fig. 2 Magnetic cell separation system

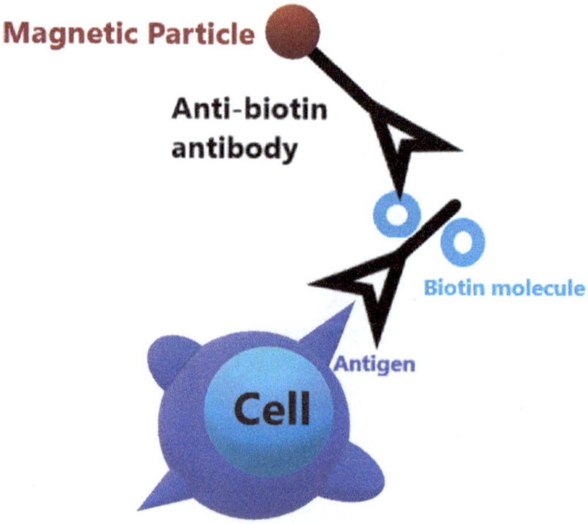

Fig. 3 Structure of TCRαβ depletion reagent

T cell/CD19+ B depletion technique, 0.1–1 × 10^5 αβ T cells/kg is retained together with the preservation of γδ T cells and NK cells (Handgretinger 2012).

Naive CD45RA+ T Cell Depletion

CD45 is a receptor present in all hematopoietic cells except erythrocytes and plasma cells. CD45 mRNA has six isoforms. The suffix RA and RB indicate the requirement of the amino acid residues, and RO indicates a lack of amino acid residues for the CD45 epitope expression. CD45RA+ naive alloreactive T cells are blamed to have a part in GvHD causation (Shlomchik 2007). Thus, their depletion from HSC graft, as a simple and rapid strategy, could lessen the potential complications. In a study after depleting CD45RA+ T cell depletion by magnetic bead technology, a median count of CD45RO+ T cells from the CD34 negative fraction were recovered (Slatter and Gennery 2017).

2.1.2 CD19+ B Cell Depletion

CD19 is a regulatory transmembrane glycoprotein which is involved in B lymphocyte's development and function (Poe et al. 2012; Fujimoto et al. 1998). In all the stages of B cell maturation, from pre-B cells to plasma cells, CD19 is expressed. Therefore, it is considered as a specific surface marker for B cells (Haas and Tedder 2005; Tedder 2009).

The delayed immune reconstitution following TCD is considered as a major risk factor for Epstein-Barr virus (EBV)-associated posttransplantation lymphoproliferative disorders (PTLD); thus, CD19+ B cell depletion is performed concurrently with the depletion of CD3+ or TCRαβ+ T cells.

Labeled CD19+ cells by means of selective CD19 monoclonal antibodies conjugated to superparamagnetic particles pass through and retain in the separation column with strong magnetic gradient (CliniMACS 2020). In one study, following CD19+ B cell depletion of HSC graft using the CliniMACS device, a median of 3.4-log (ranging from 2.0 to 4.7) reduction in B cells was achieved (Pira et al. 2016). In another trial, TCRαβ+/CD19+ depletion in haploidentical HSCT setting led to a median of 3.4-log (ranging from 2.3 to 4.5) depletion of B cells (Bethge et al. 2022).

2.2 Inclusion (Positive Selection/Expansion)

2.2.1 CD34+ Cell Enrichment

At the very least, HSC grafts should include hematopoietic progenitor/stem cells that engraft in recipient's bone marrow and are proven to be CD34 positive (Notta et al. 2011). CD34 is a transmembrane protein that is expressed on early hematopoietic progenitor cells and is used to identify and isolate HSCs (AbuSamra et al. 2017) CD133 is also used as a marker for detection and enrichment of HSCs (Koehl et al. 2002).

When labeled HSCs by superparamagnetic microbeads conjugated to a CD34 monoclonal antibody pass through a cell separation column within a strong magnetic field, they retain in the column and a high level of CD34+ cell enrichment is achieved (Fig. 2). CD34+ stem cell positive selection was the first manipulative technique employed on HSC grafts in order to decrease T cell count and to minimize the rate of GvHD. After using CD34+ cell enrichment method, a 4.5 log of reduction in T cells is attained, indirectly (Schumm et al. 2006).

2.2.2 Regulatory T Cell Expansion

Regulatory T (Treg) cells are a subgroup of CD4+ T cells which are involved in promoting immune reconstitution post-HSCT, and they also have a role in endorsing immune tolerance and limiting GvHD (Lalfer et al. 2019).

Several protocols for expanding pure functional Treg cells have been proposed which generally include cultivation in the presence of rapamycin, interleukin (IL) 2, and anti-CD3/CD28 beads for 3–4 weeks. Through these methods, the number of Treg cells could be amplified up to 20–200-fold while preserving their immunoregulatory activity (Lavazza et al. 2022).

2.2.3 NK Cell Expansion

Allogeneic NK cells are recognized to have a considerable GvT/L effect without playing a significant role in GvHD development. By using the NK MACS Medium kit (Miltenyi, Bergisch Gladbach, Germany), from healthy donors, NK cells become isolated by negative selection and then could be expanded without feeder cells along with IL-15 and IL-2 supplementation. In this technique, the maximum cell number is reachable within 5 weeks, with a median of 14050 ± 302 million NK cells attained from a single donor (Ye et al. 2020). In another study, after 5 weeks, in a GMP-grade feeder-free medium, expansion of NK cells led to a median of $14,050 \times 10^6$ NK cells and an ultimate median number of 7.59×10^8 CD56+/CD3- cells with 94% purity and viability (Handgretinger and Schilbach 2018).

2.2.4 γδ T Cell Expansion

Gammadelta (ϒδ) T lymphocytes are a minor subset of T cells, defined by expression of γ and δ heterodimeric chains of TCR. It is suggested that γδ T cells have a favorable impact in the rebuild of immune system post-HSCT, and they also have a GvT/L effect. Various methods for ϒδ T cell expansion have been established. Coculture of peripheral blood mononuclear cells and ϒδ T cells, incubated with zoledronate, IL-15, and IL-2 combined with aminobisphosphonates, has been shown to enhance the proliferation of purified ϒδ T cells, and an average expansion of 229000-fold from a single donor could be achieved (Landin et al. 2021).

3 Immunological Effects of Manipulated Grafts

After allogeneic HSCT, immune reconstitution occurs through several stages. Recovery of innate immunity takes place during weeks to few months after transplant, while the adoptive immunity reconstitution happens within a longer duration (Storek et al. 2008). Considering the importance of prompt immune recovery following HSCT, strategies to improve immune reconstitution post-HSCT, such as cellular manipulation of HSC grafts, are being more and more employed and have attracted attention.

3.1 Negative Selections

An innovation in the pathway toward successful HSCT was configuring the possibility of GvHD prevention by complete lymphoid cell depletion. However, due to delayed engraftment and immune reconstitution along with higher risk of relapse and infection, more selective depletion methods were brought forward.

3.1.1 CD3+ T Cell /CD19+ B Cell Depletion

T cells (CD3+) are among the main components of HSC graft. Naive T cells (CD45RA+, CD62L+, CCR7+, and CD45RO-) which are produced and released from the thymus proliferate and differentiate into effector T cells (CD45RA+, CD45RO-, CD62L-, and CCR7-) following infection or antigen exposure. After the control of infection, most effector T cells are lost, but a small proportion of them develop into memory T cells (CD45RO+ but CD45RA-), which could be either CD4+ or CD8+ (Mahnke et al. 2013; Farber et al. 2014).

After depletion of CD3+ T cells, although all the abovementioned subtypes of T cells are lost, together with CD34+ progenitors, several graft facilitating cells such as DCs, monocytes, and NK cells remain in the graft (Bader et al. 2011). As the same eliminated alloreactive T cells in charge of GvHD are also advantageous to engraftment and GvT/L effect, following pan-T cell depletion, an increased rate of graft rejection and disease relapse may be observed (Kernan et al. 1989; Ash et al. 1991).

The rationale for co-depletion of CD19+ B cells with CD3+ T cells is that an increased probability of EBV-driven PTLD is mediated by delayed immune reconstitution due to removal of the T cells (Saad and Lamb 2017). After HSCT, EBV-specific T cell responses are weak and impaired, so EBV would be able to apply transforming effects on B cells, leading to proliferation of lymphoblastoid cell lines and oncogenesis of PTLD (Burns and Chaganti 2021). CD19 is expressed by more than 90% of B cell malignancies, so it could act as an attractive target for prevention and treatment of B cell lineage malignancies (Breton et al. 2014).

3.1.2 TCRαβ+ T Cell/CD19+ B Cell Depletion

Double-negative (CD4- and CD8-) thymocytes which are originated from thymus differentiate in to two T cell lineages demarcated by the expression of αβ or γδ heterodimers of TCR. Through further development toward double-positivity (CD4+ and CD8+) stage, mature single positive (CD4+ or CD8+) αβ T cells are produced. However, unlike αβ T cells, γδ T cells do not progress through a double-positive stage, and most γδ T cells remain double-negative (Ciofani and Zúñiga-Pflücker 2010). Hence, CD3+ T cells in peripheral circulation are mostly αβ T cells (95%) and in a smaller extent are γδ T cells (5%). The αβ T cells, as soldiers of adaptive immunity, have a key role in mediating GvHD, while γδ T cells, as a member of innate immunity, do not seem to have a significant influence on GvHD pathogenesis (Drobyski et al. 1999; Carding and Egan 2002; Lamb Jr and Lopez 2005). γδ T cells operate independent from the assistance of MHC molecules, so they are recognized not to trigger alloreactivity.

In an effort to expel the problems of total lymphoid cell depletion, a more selective graft manipulation method based on the specific depletion of TCRαβ+ T cells together with CD19+ B cells has been introduced (Bertaina et al. 2013). Spared γδ T cells following this method provide a more effective antiviral and antitumoral effect without increasing the probability of GvHD. Relapse rate has been reported to be lower after haploidentical HSCT using TCRαβ+ TCD compared to haploidentical CD3+ TCD (Mehta et al. 2004). Improved survival rates are associated with higher peripheral blood γδ T cell counts post-HSCT (Lamb Jr et al. 1999).

3.1.3 Naive CD45RA+ T Cell Depletion

Changes in the expression of CD45 surface molecule occur through the differentiation process of naive T cells toward memory and effector cells (see Sect. 2.1.1.2) (Sallusto et al. 1999). CD45RA is expressed on all naive T cells but is absent on most memory T cells. Depletion of CD45RA+ naive T cells from the graft allows for diminishing the probability of GvHD, while preserving CD45RO+ memory T cells may be effective in prevention of disease relapse and infections (Anderson et al. 2003; Teschner et al. 2014; Bleakley et al. 2014). CD45RO is a suitable marker to characterize the activation status of T cells. As part of adoptive immunity, CD45RO + T cells vigorously activate and proliferate following stimulations and persevere their self-renewal characteristics and stem cell-like multipotency for a lifetime (Woodland and Kohlmeier 2009). These cells also induce their antitumor effect by secretion of granzyme and γ-interferon (Hu and Wang 2017).

Donor lymphocyte infusion (DLI) is commonly used as a way to boost antiviral and/or antitumoral effects posttransplant. However, it could cause a significant risk of inducing severe GvHD. Thus, the depletion of CD45RA+ T cells from DLIs, as a simple and rapid strategy, could lessen the potential complications of DLI (Slatter and Gennery 2017).

3.2 Positive Selections

3.2.1 CD34+ Cell Enrichment

CD34 is a marker almost exclusively expressed on HSC, and its expression is reduced by maturation of hematopoietic cells, becoming entirely absent in fully mature cells (Sidney et al. 2014; McGuckin et al. 2003). CD34+ HSCs have the capacity of proliferation and also differentiation into all cells of the hematopoietic lineage (Servida et al. 1996; Huss 2000). It is suggested that CD34 is able to promote engraftment and homing of HSC by binding to a receptor on endothelial cells of bone marrow (Healy et al. 1995). Enrichment of CD34+ cells has been established to be a safe process that permits fast and durable hematological engraftment. However, following the enrichment technique, due to loss of antigen-presenting cells (APCs) and mature lymphocytes, impairment of immune reactivity and increase in infections and relapse may occur (Damiani et al. 2003).

In CD34+ selected transplantation, T cell reconstitution completely depends on the generation of naive T cells. Specifically, rebuild of CD4+ T cell repertoire is reliant on production of CD4+ CD45RA+ naive T cells in the thymus (Huttunen et al. 2015; Vescio et al. 1999). It is possible that following the selection procedure, mature committed dendritic progenitors with low CD34 expression drop out and lead to a slower recovery of circulating DCs posttransplant compared to unmanipulated grafts (Damiani et al. 2003).

NK cell recovery does not seem to be impacted in CD34+ enriched HSCT, but as more than 6 to 8 weeks is mandatory for the first appearance of functional alloreactive NK cells after transplant, their advantageous GvT/L effect is somewhat delayed (Locatelli et al. 2013a).

3.2.2 Regulatory T Cell Expansion

Treg cells are capable of suppressing immune responses, sustaining a state of self-tolerance and inhibition of self-directed immunity. In allogeneic HSCT setting, Treg cells have the potential to resolve tissue inflammation and mediate tissue repair. They also promote immune reconstitution and prevent GvHD, due to their immunosuppressive capacities. It has been proven that CD4+/CD25+/FoxP3+ Treg cells are effective in the prevention of conventional T cell-mediated GvHD without hampering GvT/L effect (Edinger et al. 2003; Pierini et al. 2019). They also facilitate donor engraftment by regulating bone marrow microenvironment and boosting donor immune reconstitution after transplant. Adoptive transfer of ex vivo expanded Treg cells within HSCT process could provide a strong GvT/L effect and promote engraftment (Fujisaki et al. 2011; Pierini et al. 2017).

3.2.3 NK Cell Expansion

Donor NK cells not only play a role in assisting engraftment, but they are also crucial players in relapse prevention after transplant (Murphy et al. 1992; Ruggeri et al. 2002, 2007). It has been demonstrated that adoptive transfer of expanded NK cells is a safe procedure and it does not induce GvHD. Even so, this method could prevent the development of T cell-mediated GvHD (Ruggeri et al. 2002). Numerous studies have advocated that higher number of donor NK cells in the graft could reduce GvHD occurrence (Soiffer et al. 1993; Yamasaki et al. 2003; Abrahamsen et al. 2005; Larghero et al. 2007; Sivori et al. 2011; Tanaka et al. 2012; Kim et al. 2016). Alloreactive NK cells eliminate APCs through their cytolytic activity and indirectly suppress T cells' proliferation and T cell-mediated GvHD (Meinhardt et al. 2015). In addition to the aforementioned indirect mechanism, NK cells could also hamper GvHD by lysing activated T cells directly at effector sites (Ghadially et al. 2014). Moreover, in the presence of NK cells, the ratio of donor Treg cells to total donor conventional CD4+ and CD8+ T cells is increased, which makes an immune-modulated environment contributing to suppression of GvHD (Olson et al. 2010). Increased NK cell count early post-HSCT is a powerful determinant of GvT/L effect, resulting in lower incidence of relapse and better transplant outcomes (Leung 2011; Locatelli et al. 2013b; Pieterse and van der Vlag 2014; Maggs et al. 2017).

3.2.4 γδ T Cell Expansion

Recently, unconventional T cells and their immunologic function in transplant have attracted attention. γδ T cells as one of unconventional T cells have the properties of both innate and adaptive immunity (i.e., prompt response and no donor MHC restriction, similar to innate immunity elements, and TCR-dependent activation alike conventional T cells) (Godfrey et al. 2015).

Following allogenic HSCT, adoptive transfer of expanded γδ T cells could exert antitumoral and anti-infectious effects. γδ T cells are capable of identification and reactivity against multiple ligands on tumor cells, and they also have the ability of early sensing the metabolic changes in malignant-transformed cells (Sebestyen et al. 2020). Moreover, γδ T cells express Fc receptor γIII (CD16) which binds to the Fc portion of immunoglobulins and mediate antitumor effects via antibody-dependent cellular cytotoxicity, similar to NK cells (Lafont et al. 2001). γδ T cells also employ strong antiviral and antibacterial effects. It has been shown that increased number of γδ T cells in the early post-HSCT period is associated with less CMV reactivation compared to patients with lower number of γδ T cell (Park et al. 2018; Gaballa et al. 2019).

4 Clinical Impacts of Manipulated Grafts

Allogeneic HSCT remains to be the best potentially curative option for a diversity of conditions including malignant and nonmalignant disorders (Bertaina et al. 2014). However, due to the absence of an available HLA-matched donor for many patients, a progressive shift toward alternative donors especially HLA-haploidentical relatives has occurred. Nevertheless, significant HLA disparities between recipient and donor trigger development of GvHD and GF, mediated by alloreactive T cell responses (Rocha and Gluckman 2006; Locatelli et al. 2009). In such a case, in vitro TCD of HSC grafts has raised as a safe and efficient method to reduce alloreactivity (Lazzari et al. 2022; Bethge et al. 2022).

Clinical application of CD3+/CD19+ depleted haploidentical HSCT has been reported in patients with hematological malignancies with acceptable GvHD incidence and low TRM, together with comparable survival outcomes to those of conventional HSCT (Bader et al. 2011; Palma et al. 2012; Pérez-Martínez et al. 2012). In a prospective study, in acute leukemia pediatric patients who underwent CD3+/CD19+ depleted allografts from their haploidentical family donors, 88% primary engraftment, 7% grade III–IV acute GvHD, 21% chronic GvHD, and 46% 3-year event-free survival (EFS) were reported (Lang et al. 2014).

Following TCRαβ+/CD19+ depleted haploidentical HSCT in malignant disease, a German group has reported promising results including 88% primary engraftment and 15% acute GvHD grades III–IV. Median time to recovery of CD3+, CD4+, and CD56+ cells was significantly faster in patients who received TCRαβ+/CD19+

depleted allograft compared with historical control group of patients who had received CD34+ selected grafts (Lang et al. 2015).

In a study by Bethge et al., pediatric and adult patients with mostly malignant disorders received TCRαβ+/CD19+ depleted peripheral blood stem cell transplantation from haploidentical family donors with reduced intensity preparative regimen, and none of the patients developed grade III/IV acute GvHD. Estimated probabilities of 2-year overall survival (OS) and disease-free survival (DFS) were 63% and 50%, respectively (Bethge et al. 2022).

In a single-arm clinical trial conducted by Bleakley et al., all of the high-risk leukemia patients who received naive T cell depleted HSCT engrafted successfully. Grades II–IV acute GVHD were developed in 66% of patients that was similar to T cell-replete HSCT recipients. However, chronic GVHD was less frequent in comparison with T cell-replete transplantation. Rate of infection was not so high due to rapid T cell recovery and transfer of functional memory T cells (Bleakley et al. 2015).

In a trial in pediatric and young adult patients with high-risk hematologic malignancies who received ex vivo T cell depleted haploidentical allogeneic HSCT, an increase in the 3-year OS and EFS was observed in recipients of CD45RA+ depleted grafts compared with historical T cell depleted group (Mamcarz et al. 2020).

In the absence of a fully HLA-matched donor, mismatched and haploidentical HSCT has also been considered for patients with nonmalignant diseases. However, the high rate of GF and GvHD, delayed immune recovery, and severe infections still remain the main obstacles of successful outcome.

In patients with Fanconi anemia, following T cell depleted, CD34+ selected haploidentical HSCT, graft rejection has been reported to be 17%. Cumulative incidences of grades II–IV acute and chronic GvHD were 17% and 35%, respectively, and the 5-year OS and DFS were 83% (95% CI, 62% to 100%) and 83% (95% CI, 62% to 100%), respectively (Zecca et al. 2014).

TCRαβ+/CD19+ depleted haploidentical HSCT has also been conducted in patients with primary immunodeficiency and has resulted in a high OS (96.7%) (Bertaina et al. 2014). CD45RA+ T cell depleted mismatched HSCT in patients with severe aplastic anemia and congenital amegakaryocytic thrombocytopenia has been associated with rapid myeloid and platelet recovery and no severe infections within the first hundred days post-HSCT (Gasior Kabat et al. 2021).

In the early posttransplant period, immature and poorly functional NK cells predominate, and mature functional donor derived NK cells emerge in the patient peripheral blood several weeks after transplantation (Pende et al. 2009). NK cell reconstitution and its function are mainly impacted by GvHD prophylaxis, especially by posttransplant cyclophosphamide that abolishes majority of mature donor NK cells including alloreactive NK cells (Russo et al. 2018). Accordingly NK cell-mediated GvT/L effect in the early posttransplant period seems non-efficacious to prevent relapse and provides the rationale for adoptive infusion of ex vivo activated NK cells during this time window especially in haploidentical HSCT setting (Stern et al. 2013; Locatelli et al. 2013b). So it seems that the use of fresh or IL-15 stimulated NK cell infusion early after haploidentical stem cell transplant might enhance GvT/L effect without increasing the risk of GvHD (Leung 2011; Moretta et al. 2011; Maggs et al. 2017).

Doubtlessly, future of transplant therapy will involve more cellular manipulative strategies; thus, more clinical trials with larger study population will be needed to establish the optimal interventions and to maximize the advantages of these novel procedures.

References

Abrahamsen IW, Somme S, Heldal D, Egeland T, Kvale D, Tjonnfjord GE (2005) Immune reconstitution after allogeneic stem cell transplantation: the impact of stem cell source and graft-versus-host disease. Haematologica 90(1):86–93

AbuSamra DB, Aleisa FA, Al-Amoodi AS, Jalal Ahmed HM, Chin CJ, Abuelela AF, Bergam P, Sougrat R, Merzaban JS (2017) Not just a marker: CD34 on human hematopoietic stem/progenitor cells dominates vascular selectin binding along with CD44. Blood Adv 1(27): 2799–2816

Anderson BE, McNiff J, Yan J, Doyle H, Mamula M, Shlomchik MJ, Shlomchik WD (2003) Memory CD4+ T cells do not induce graft-versus-host disease. J Clin Invest 112(1):101–108

Ash RC, Horowitz MM, Gale RP, Van Bekkum DW, Casper JT, Gordon-Smith EC, Henslee PJ, Kolb HJ, Lowenberg B, Masaoka T (1991) Bone marrow transplantation from related donors other than HLA-identical siblings: effect of T cell depletion. Bone Marrow Transplant 7(6): 443–452

Avecilla ST, Goss C, Bleau S, Tonon JA, Meagher RC (2016) How do I perform hematopoietic progenitor cell selection? Transfusion 56(5):1008–1012

Aversa F, Tabilio A, Terenzi A, Velardi A, Falzetti F, Giannoni C, Zei T, Martelli MP, Gambelunghe C, Rossetti M, Caputo P (1994) Successful engraftment of T-cell–depleted haploidentical "three-loci" incompatible transplants in leukemia patients by addition of recombinant human granulocyte colony-stimulating factor–mobilized peripheral blood progenitor cells to bone marrow inoculum. Blood 84(11):3948–3955

Bader P, Soerensen J, Jarisch A, Ponstingl E, Krenn T, Faber J, Dürken M, Reinhardt H, Willasch A, Esser R, Bönig H (2011) Rapid immune recovery and low TRM in haploidentical stem cell transplantation in children and adolescence using CD3/CD19-depleted stem cells. Best Pract Res Clin Haematol 24(3):331–337

Bertaina A, Pagliara D, Pende D, Rutella S, Falco M, Bauquet A, Contoli B, Lucarelli B, Brescia LP, Merli P, Andreani M (2013) Removal of alpha/beta+ T cells and of CD19+ B cells from the graft translates into rapid engraftment, absence of visceral graft-versus-host disease and low transplant-related mortality in children with acute leukemia given HLA-haploidentical hematopoietic stem cell transplantation. Blood 122(21):157

Bertaina A, Merli P, Rutella S, Pagliara D, Bernardo ME, Masetti R, Pende D, Falco M, Handgretinger R, Moretta F, Lucarelli B (2014) HLA-haploidentical stem cell transplantation after removal of αβ+ T and B cells in children with nonmalignant disorders. Blood 124(5): 822–826

Bethge WA, Eyrich M, Mielke S, Meisel R, Niederwieser D, Schlegel PG, Schulz A, Greil J, Bunjes D, Brecht A, Kuball J (2022) Results of a multicenter phase I/II trial of TCRαβ and CD19-depleted haploidentical hematopoietic stem cell transplantation for adult and pediatric patients. Bone Marrow Transplant 57(3):423–430

Biernacki MA, Sheth VS, Bleakley M (2020) T cell optimization for graft-versus-leukemia responses. JCI Insight 5(9):e134939

Bleakley M, Heimfeld S, Jones LA, Turtle C, Krause D, Riddell SR, Shlomchik W (2014) Engineering human peripheral blood stem cell grafts that are depleted of naive T cells and retain functional pathogen-specific memory T cells. Biol Blood Marrow Transplant 20(5): 705–716

Bleakley M, Heimfeld S, Loeb KR, Jones LA, Chaney C, Seropian S, Gooley TA, Sommermeyer F, Riddell SR, Shlomchik WD (2015) Outcomes of acute leukemia patients transplanted with naive T cell–depleted stem cell grafts. J Clin Invest 125(7):2677–2689

Breton CS, Nahimana A, Aubry D, Macoin J, Moretti P, Bertschinger M, Hou S, Duchosal MA, Back J (2014) A novel anti-CD19 monoclonal antibody (GBR 401) with high killing activity against B cell malignancies. J Hematol Oncol 7(1):1–3

Burns DM, Chaganti S (2021) Epstein-Barr virus-associated lymphoproliferative disorders in immunosuppressed patients

Carding SR, Egan PJ (2002) γδ T cells: functional plasticity and heterogeneity. Nat Rev Immunol 2(5):336–345

Carreras E, Dufour C, Mohty M, Kröger N (2019) The EBMT handbook: hematopoietic stem cell transplantation and cellular therapies. Springer, Cham, pp 137–142

Ciofani M, Zúñiga-Pflücker JC (2010) Determining γδ versus αβ T cell development. Nat Rev Immunol 10(9):657–663

CliniMACS® Plus System User Manual (Canadian edition). 37091/04 – ch20 (Issued: 2020–06)

Damiani D, Stocchi R, Masolini P, Michelutti A, Geromin A, Sperotto A, Skert C, Michieli M, Baccarani M, Fanin R (2003) CD34+-selected versus unmanipulated autologous stem cell transplantation in multiple myeloma: impact on dendritic and immune recovery and on complications due to infection. Ann Oncol 14(3):475–480

Drobyski WR, Majewski D, Hanson G (1999) Graft-facilitating doses of ex vivo activated gammadelta T cells do not cause lethal murine graft-vs.-host disease. Biol Blood Marrow Transplant 5(4):222–230

Edinger M, Hoffmann P, Ermann J, Drago K, Fathman CG, Strober S, Negrin RS (2003) CD4+ CD25+ regulatory T cells preserve graft-versus-tumor activity while inhibiting graft-versus-host disease after bone marrow transplantation. Nat Med 9(9):1144–1150

Farber DL, Yudanin NA, Restifo NP (2014) Human memory T cells: generation, compartmentalization and homeostasis. Nat Rev Immunol 14(1):24–35

Fujimoto M, Poe JC, Inaoki M, Tedder TF (1998) CD19 regulates B lymphocyte responses to transmembrane signals. Semin Immunol 10(4):267–277

Fujisaki J, Wu J, Carlson AL, Silberstein L, Putheti P, Larocca R, Gao W, Saito TI, Celso CL, Tsuyuzaki H, Sato T (2011) In vivo imaging of Treg cells providing immune privilege to the haematopoietic stem-cell niche. Nature 474(7350):216–219

Gaballa A, Stikvoort A, Önfelt B, Mattsson J, Sundin M, Watz E, Uhlin M (2019) T-cell frequencies of CD8+ γδ and CD27+ γδ cells in the stem cell graft predict the outcome after allogeneic hematopoietic cell transplantation. Bone Marrow Transplant 54(10):1562–1574

Gasior Kabat M, Bueno D, Sisinni L, De Paz R, Mozo Y, Perona R, Arias-Salgado EG, Rosich B, Marcos A, Romero AB, Constanzo A (2021) Selective T-cell depletion targeting CD45RA as a novel approach for HLA-mismatched hematopoietic stem cell transplantation in pediatric nonmalignant hematological diseases. Int J Hematol 114(1):116–123

Ghadially H, Ohana M, Elboim M, Gazit R, Gur C, Nagler A, Mandelboim O (2014) NK cell receptor NKp46 regulates graft-versus-host disease. Cell Rep 7(6):1809–1814

Godfrey DI, Uldrich AP, Mccluskey J, Rossjohn J, Moody DB (2015) Erratum: the burgeoning family of unconventional T cells. Nature Immunol 16:1114–1123. Nature Immunology. 2016;17(4)

Haas KM, Tedder TF (2005) Role of the CD19 and CD21/35 receptor complex in innate immunity, host defense and autoimmunity. In: Mechanisms of Lymphocyte Activation and Immune Regulation X, pp 125–139

Handgretinger R (2012) Negative depletion of CD3+ and TcRαβ+ T cells. Curr Opin Hematol 19(6):434–439

Handgretinger R, Schilbach K (2018) The potential role of γδ T cells after allogeneic HCT for leukemia. Blood 131(10):1063–1072

Healy L, May G, Gale K, Grosveld F, Greaves M, Enver T (1995) The stem cell antigen CD34 functions as a regulator of hemopoietic cell adhesion. Proc Natl Acad Sci 92(26):12240–12244

Hu G, Wang S (2017) Tumor-infiltrating CD45RO+ memory T lymphocytes predict favorable clinical outcome in solid tumors. Sci Rep 7(1):1

Huss R (2000) Isolation of primary and immortalized CD34− hematopoietic and mesenchymal stem cells from various sources. Stem Cells 18(1):1–9

Huttunen P, Taskinen M, Siitonen S, Saarinen-Pihkala UM (2015) Impact of very early CD4+/CD8+ T cell counts on the occurrence of acute graft-versus-host disease and NK cell counts on outcome after pediatric allogeneic hematopoietic stem cell transplantation. Pediatr Blood Cancer 62(3):522–528

Kernan NA, Bordignon C, Heller G, Cunningham I, Castro-Malaspina H, Shank B, Flomenberg N, Burns J, Yang SY, Black P (1989) Graft failure after T-cell-depleted human leukocyte antigen identical marrow transplants for leukemia: I. Analysis of risk factors and results of secondary transplants. Blood 74(6):2227

Kim SY, Lee H, Han MS, Shim H, Eom HS, Park B, Kong SY (2016) Post-transplantation natural killer cell count: a predictor of acute graft-versus-host disease and survival outcomes after allogeneic hematopoietic stem cell transplantation. Clin Lymphoma Myeloma Leuk 16(9): 527–535

Koehl U, Zimmermann S, Esser R, Sörensen J, Grüttner HP, Duchscherer M, Seifried E, Klingebiel T, Schwabe D (2002) Autologous transplantation of CD133 selected hematopoietic progenitor cells in a pediatric patient with relapsed leukemia. Bone Marrow Transplant 29(11): 927–930

Lafont V, Liautard J, Liautard JP, Favero J (2001) Production of TNF-α by human Vγ9Vδ2 T cells via engagement of FcγRIIIA, the low affinity type 3 receptor for the fc portion of IgG, expressed upon TCR activation by nonpeptidic antigen. J Immunol 166(12):7190–7199

Lalfer M, Chappert P, Carpentier M, Urbain D, Davoust JM, Gross DA (2019) Foxp3+ regulatory and conventional CD4+ T cells display similarly high frequencies of alloantigen-reactive cells. Front Immunol 10:521

Lamb LS Jr, Lopez RD (2005) γδ T cells: a new frontier for immunotherapy? Biol Blood Marrow Transplant 11(3):161–168

Lamb LS Jr, Gee AP, Hazlett LJ, Musk P, Parrish RS, O'Hanlon TP, Geier SS, Folk RS, Harris WG, McPherson K, Lee C (1999) Influence of T cell depletion method on circulating γδ T cell reconstitution and potential role in the graft-versus-leukemia effect. Cytotherapy 1(1):7–19

Landin AM, Cox C, Yu B, Bejanyan N, Davila M, Kelley L (2021) Expansion and enrichment of gamma-delta (γδ) T cells from apheresed human product. JoVE 175:e62622

Lang P, Teltschik HM, Feuchtinger T, Müller I, Pfeiffer M, Schumm M, Ebinger M, Schwarze CP, Gruhn B, Schrauder A, Albert MH (2014) Transplantation of CD 3/CD 19 depleted allografts from haploidentical family donors in paediatric leukaemia. Br J Haematol 165(5):688–698

Lang P, Feuchtinger T, Teltschik HM, Schwinger W, Schlegel P, Pfeiffer M, Schumm M, Lang AM, Lang B, Schwarze CP, Ebinger M (2015) Improved immune recovery after transplantation of TCRαβ/CD19-depleted allografts from haploidentical donors in pediatric patients. Bone Marrow Transplant 50(2):S6–S10

Larghero J, Rocha V, Porcher R, Filion A, Ternaux B, Lacassagne MN, Robin M, Peffault de Latour R, Devergie A, Biscay N, Ribaud P (2007) Association of bone marrow natural killer cell dose with neutrophil recovery and chronic graft-versus-host disease after HLA identical sibling bone marrow transplants. Br J Haematol 138(1):101–109

Lavazza C, Budelli S, Montelatici E, Viganò M, Ulbar F, Catani L, Cannone MG, Savelli S, Groppelli E, Lazzari L, Lemoli RM (2022) Process development and validation of expanded regulatory T cells for prospective applications: an example of manufacturing a personalized advanced therapy medicinal product. J Transl Med 20(1):1–21

Lazzari L, Balaguer-Roselló A, Montoro J, Greco R, Hernani R, Lupo-Stanghellini MT, Villalba M, Giglio F, Facal A, Lorentino F, Guerreiro M (2022) Post-transplant cyclophosphamide and sirolimus based graft-versus-host disease prophylaxis after allogeneic stem cell transplantation for acute myeloid leukemia. Bone Marrow Transplant 57:1389–1398

Leung W (2011) Use of NK cell activity in cure by transplant. Br J Haematol 155(1):14–29

Locatelli F, Pende D, Maccario R, Mingari MC, Moretta A, Moretta L (2009) Haploidentical hemopoietic stem cell transplantation for the treatment of high-risk leukemias: how NK cells make the difference. Clin Immunol 133(2):171–178

Locatelli F, Merli P, Rutella S (2013a) At the bedside: innate immunity as an immunotherapy tool for hematological malignancies. J Leukoc Biol 94(6):1141–1157

Locatelli F, Pende D, Mingari MC, Bertaina A, Falco M, Moretta A, Moretta L (2013b) Cellular and molecular basis of haploidentical hematopoietic stem cell transplantation in the successful treatment of high-risk leukemias: role of alloreactive NK cells. Front Immunol 4:15

Maggs L, Kinsella F, Chan YT, Eldershaw S, Murray D, Nunnick J, Bird J, Craddock C, Zuo J, Malladi R, Moss P (2017) The number of CD56dim NK cells in the graft has a major impact on risk of disease relapse following Allo-HSCT. Blood Adv 1(19):1589–1597

Mahnke YD, Brodie TM, Sallusto F, Roederer M, Lugli E (2013) The who's who of T-cell differentiation: human memory T-cell subsets. Eur J Immunol 43(11):2797–2809

Mamcarz E, Madden R, Qudeimat A, Srinivasan A, Talleur A, Sharma A, Suliman A, Maron G, Sunkara A, Kang G, Leung W (2020) Improved survival rate in T-cell depleted haploidentical hematopoietic cell transplantation over the last 15 years at a single institution. Bone Marrow Transplant 55(5):929–938

McGuckin CP, Pearce D, Forraz N, Tooze JA, Watt SM, Pettengell R (2003) Multiparametric analysis of immature cell populations in umbilical cord blood and bone marrow. Eur J Haematol 71(5):341–350

Mehta J, Singhal S, Gee AP, Chiang KY, Godder K, Van Rhee F, DeRienzo S, O'Neal W, Lamb L, Henslee-Downey PJ (2004) Bone marrow transplantation from partially HLA-mismatched family donors for acute leukemia: single-center experience of 201 patients. Bone Marrow Transplant 33(4):389–396

Meinhardt K, Kroeger I, Bauer R, Ganss F, Ovsiy I, Rothamer J, Büttner M, Atreya I, Waldner M, Bittrich M, Lehmann CH (2015) Identification and characterization of the specific murine NK cell subset supporting graft-versus-leukemia-and reducing graft-versus-host-effects. Onco Targets Ther 4(1):e981483

Moretta L, Locatelli F, Pende D, Sivori S, Falco M, Bottino C, Mingari MC, Moretta A (2011) Human NK receptors: from the molecules to the therapy of high risk leukemias. FEBS Lett 585(11):1563–1567

Murphy WJ, Bennett M, Kumar V, Longo DL (1992) Donor-type activated natural killer cells promote marrow engraftment and B cell development during allogeneic bone marrow transplantation. J Immunol 148(9):2953–2960

Notta F, Doulatov S, Laurenti E, Poeppl A, Jurisica I, Dick JE (2011) Isolation of single human hematopoietic stem cells capable of long-term multilineage engraftment. Science 333(6039): 218–221

Olson JA, Leveson-Gower DB, Gill S, Baker J, Beilhack A, Negrin RS (2010) NK cells mediate reduction of GVHD by inhibiting activated, alloreactive T cells while retaining GVT effects. Blood 115(21):4293–4301

Palma J, Salas L, Carrión F, Sotomayor C, Catalán P, Paris C, Turner V, Jorquera H, Handgretinger R, Rivera GK (2012) Haploidentical stem cell transplantation for children with high-risk leukemia. Pediatr Blood Cancer 59(5):895–901

Park M, Im HJ, Lee YJ, Park N, Jang S, Kwon SW, Park CJ, Choi ES, Koh KN, Seo JJ (2018) Reconstitution of T and NK cells after haploidentical hematopoietic cell transplantation using αβ T cell–depleted grafts and the clinical implication of γδ T cells. Clin Transpl 32(1):e13147

Peci F, Dekker L, Pagliaro A, van Boxtel R, Nierkens S, Belderbos M (2022) The cellular composition and function of the bone marrow niche after allogeneic hematopoietic cell transplantation. Bone Marrow Transplant 57:1357–1364

Pende D, Marcenaro S, Falco M, Martini S, Bernardo ME, Montagna D, Romeo E, Cognet C, Martinetti M, Maccario R, Mingari MC (2009) Anti-leukemia activity of alloreactive NK cells in KIR ligand-mismatched haploidentical HSCT for pediatric patients: evaluation of the functional role of activating KIR and redefinition of inhibitory KIR specificity. Blood 113(13): 3119–3129

Pérez-Martínez A, González-Vicent M, Valentín J, Aleo E, Lassaletta A, Sevilla J, Vicario JL, Ramírez M, Díaz MA (2012) Early evaluation of immune reconstitution following allogeneic CD3/CD19-depleted grafts from alternative donors in childhood acute leukemia. Bone Marrow Transplant 47(11):1419–1427

Pierini A, Nishikii H, Baker J, Kimura T, Kwon HS, Pan Y, Chen Y, Alvarez M, Strober W, Velardi A, Shizuru JA (2017) Foxp3+ regulatory T cells maintain the bone marrow microenvironment for B cell lymphopoiesis. Nat Commun 8(1):1–3

Pierini A, Ruggeri L, Mancusi A, Carotti A, Falzetti F, Terenzi A, Martelli MF, Velardi A (2019) T cell depletion and no post transplant immune suppression allow separation of graft versus leukemia from graft versus host disease. Bone Marrow Transplant 54(2):775–779

Pieterse E, van der Vlag J (2014) Breaking immunological tolerance in systemic lupus erythematosus. Front Immunol 5:164

Pira GL, Malaspina D, Girolami E, Biagini S, Cicchetti E, Conflitti G, Broglia M, Ceccarelli S, Lazzaro S, Pagliara D, Meschini A (2016) Selective depletion of αβ T cells and B cells for human leukocyte antigen–haploidentical hematopoietic stem cell transplantation. A three-year follow-up of procedure efficiency. Biol Blood Marrow Transplant 22(11):2056–2064

Poe JC, Minard-Colin V, Kountikov EI, Haas KM, Tedder TF (2012) A c-Myc and surface CD19 signaling amplification loop promotes B cell lymphoma development and progression in mice. J Immunol 189(5):2318–2325

Rocha V, Gluckman E (2006) Clinical use of umbilical cord blood hematopoietic stem cells. Biol Blood Marrow Transplant 12(1):34–41

Ruggeri L, Capanni M, Urbani E, Perruccio K, Shlomchik WD, Tosti A, Posati S, Rogaia D, Frassoni F, Aversa F, Martelli MF (2002) Effectiveness of donor natural killer cell alloreactivity in mismatched hematopoietic transplants. Science 295(5562):2097–2100

Ruggeri L, Mancusi A, Capanni M, Urbani E, Carotti A, Aloisi T, Stern M, Pende D, Perruccio K, Burchielli E, Topini F (2007) Donor natural killer cell allorecognition of missing self in haploidentical hematopoietic transplantation for acute myeloid leukemia: challenging its predictive value. Blood 110(1):433–440

Russo A, Oliveira G, Berglund S, Greco R, Gambacorta V, Cieri N, Toffalori C, Zito L, Lorentino F, Piemontese S, Morelli M (2018) NK cell recovery after haploidentical HSCT with posttransplant cyclophosphamide: dynamics and clinical implications. Blood 131(2): 247–262

Saad A, Lamb LS (2017) Ex vivo T-cell depletion in allogeneic hematopoietic stem cell transplant: past, present and future. Bone Marrow Transplant 52(9):1241–1248

Sallusto F, Kremmer E, Palermo B, Hoy A, Ponath P, Qin S, Förster R, Lipp M, Lanzavecchia A (1999) Switch in chemokine receptor expression upon TCR stimulation reveals novel homing potential for recently activated T cells. Eur J Immunol 29(6):2037–2045

Salvadori S, Gansbacher B, Pizzimenti AM, Zier KS (1994) Abnormal signal transduction by T cells of mice with parental tumors is not seen in mice bearing IL-2-secreting tumors. J Immunol 153(11):5176–5182

Schumm M, Handgretinger R, Pfeiffer M, Feuchtinger T, Kuci S, Faul C, Vogel W, Bethge W, Lang P (2006) Determination of residual T-and B-cell content after immunomagnetic depletion: proposal for flow cytometric analysis and results from 103 separations. Cytotherapy 8(5): 465–472

Schumm M, Lang P, Bethge W, Faul C, Feuchtinger T, Pfeiffer M, Vogel W, Huppert V, Handgretinger R (2013) Depletion of T-cell receptor alpha/beta and CD19 positive cells from apheresis products with the CliniMACS device. Cytotherapy 15(10):1253–1258

Sebestyen Z, Prinz I, Déchanet-Merville J, Silva-Santos B, Kuball J (2020) Translating gammadelta (γδ) T cells and their receptors into cancer cell therapies. Nat Rev Drug Discov 19(3):169–184

Servida F, Soligo D, Caneva L, Bertolini F, De Harven E, Campiglio S, Corsini C, Deliliers GL (1996) Functional and morphological characterization of immunomagnetically selected CD34+ hematopoietic progenitor cells. Stem Cells 14(4):430–438

Shlomchik WD (2007) Graft-versus-host disease. Nat Rev Immunol 7(5):340–352

Sidney LE, Branch MJ, Dunphy SE, Dua HS, Hopkinson A (2014) Concise review: evidence for CD34 as a common marker for diverse progenitors. Stem Cells 32(6):1380–1389

Sivori S, Carlomagno S, Falco M, Romeo E, Moretta L, Moretta A (2011) Natural killer cells expressing the KIR2DS1-activating receptor efficiently kill T-cell blasts and dendritic cells: implications in haploidentical HSCT. Blood 117(16):4284–4292

Slatter MA, Gennery AR (2017) Approaches to the removal of T-lymphocytes to minimize graft-versus-host disease in patients with primary immunodeficiencies who do not have a matched sibling donor. Curr Opin Allergy Clin Immunol 17(6):414–420

Smith-Garvin JE, Koretzky GA, Jordan MS (2009) T cell activation. Annu Rev Immunol 27:591

Soiffer RJ, Gonin R, Murray C, Robertson MJ, Cochran K, Chartier S, Cameron C, Daley J, Levine H, Nadler LM (1993) Prediction of graft-versus-host disease by phenotypic analysis of early immune reconstitution after CD6-depleted allogeneic bone marrow transplantation

Soiffer RJ, Mauch P, Fairclough D, Alyea E, Anderson K, Fisher D, Freedman A, Bartlett-Pandite L, Robertson M, Schlossman R, Gollob J (1997) CD6+ T cell depleted allogeneic bone marrow transplantation from genotypically HLA nonidentical related donors. Biol Blood Marrow Transplant 3(1):11–17

Stern M, Passweg JR, Meyer-Monard S, Esser R, Tonn T, Soerensen J, Paulussen M, Gratwohl A, Klingebiel T, Bader P, Tichelli A (2013) Pre-emptive immunotherapy with purified natural killer cells after haploidentical SCT: a prospective phase II study in two centers. Bone Marrow Transplant 48(3):433–438

Storek J, Geddes M, Khan F, Huard B, Helg C, Chalandon Y, Passweg J, Roosnek E (2008) Reconstitution of the immune system after hematopoietic stem cell transplantation in humans. Semin Immunopathol 30(4):425–437

Tanaka M, Kobayashi S, Numata A, Tachibana T, Takasaki H, Maruta A, Ishigatsubo Y, Kanamori H (2012) The impact of the dose of natural killer cells in the graft on severe acute graft-versus-host disease after unrelated bone marrow transplantation. Leuk Res 36(6):699–703

Tedder TF (2009) CD19: a promising B cell target for rheumatoid arthritis. Nat Rev Rheumatol 5(10):572–577

Teschner D, Distler E, Wehler D, Frey M, Marandiuc D, Langeveld K, Theobald M, Thomas S, Herr W (2014) Depletion of naive T cells using clinical grade magnetic CD45RA beads: a new approach for GVHD prophylaxis. Bone Marrow Transplant 49(1):138–144

Vescio R, Schiller G, Stewart AK, Ballester O, Noga S, Rugo H, Freytes C, Stadtmauer E, Tarantolo S, Sahebi F, Stiff P (1999) Multicenter phase III trial to evaluate CD34+ selected versus unselected autologous peripheral blood progenitor cell transplantation in multiple myeloma. Blood 93(6):1858–1868

Woodland DL, Kohlmeier JE (2009) Migration, maintenance and recall of memory T cells in peripheral tissues. Nat Rev Immunol 9:153–161. https://doi.org/10.1038/nri2496

Yamasaki S, Henzan H, Ohno Y, Yamanaka T, Iino T, Itou Y, Kuroiwa M, Maeda M, Kawano N, Kinukawa N, Miyamoto T (2003) Influence of transplanted dose of CD56+ cells on development of graft-versus-host disease in patients receiving G-CSF-mobilized peripheral blood progenitor cells from HLA-identical sibling donors. Bone Marrow Transplant 32(5):505–510

Ye W, Kong X, Zhang W, Weng Z, Wu X (2020) The roles of γδ T cells in hematopoietic stem cell transplantation. Cell Transplant 29:0963689720966980

Zecca M, Strocchio L, Pagliara D, Comoli P, Bertaina A, Giorgiani G, Perotti C, Corbella F, Brescia L, Locatelli F (2014) HLA-Haploidentical T cell–depleted allogeneic hematopoietic stem cell transplantation in children with Fanconi anemia. Biol Blood Marrow Transplant 20(4): 571–576

Recent Development of Quinoline Derivatives as Anticancer Agents: 2015–2022

Komalpreet Kaur, Nitish Kumar, Jatinder Vir Singh, Preet Mohinder Singh Bedi, and Harbinder Singh

Abstract

Increased rate of emergence of cancer cases has led to increased demand of new molecules that have low toxicity profile and high efficiency. Therefore, in pursuit of new molecules scientists came across quinoline, a privileged scaffold that has been associated with multiple biological activities like antiviral, antibacterial, antimalarial, antifungal, antitubercular, antileishmanial, anti-inflammatory, anti-HIV, and anticancer. This multifarious profile helped quinoline to gain attention of researchers to develop new anticancer moieties by sequential modification of the substituents attached to it. This chapter provides brief knowledge about the recent developments of quinoline derivatives as anticancer drugs, which includes structure activity relationship, molecular docking studies and their mechanism. Therefore, this compilation could assist the global researchers to develop novel and potent quinolone-based therapeutics to treat various cancerous conditions.

Keywords

Anticancer · Design strategies · Lead modification · Molecular docking · Quinoline

1 Introduction

Cancer, an uncontrolled cell growth, has capability to infect nearby tissues and can spread to other parts of the body via blood or lymphatic system. Their capability to spread and infect other body tissues makes cancer a serious challenge for the medical

K. Kaur · N. Kumar · J. V. Singh · P. M. S. Bedi · H. Singh (✉)
Department of Pharmaceutical Sciences, Guru Nanak Dev University, Amritsar, Punjab, India
e-mail: singh.harbinder40@gmail.com; singhh@westernu.edu

Interdisciplinary Cancer Research, https://doi.org/10.1007/16833_2023_125
Published online: 2 February 2023

practitioner and researcher to find their treatment. Cancer cells are highly affected by genetic changes as compared to normal cells (Cheung et al. 2009). Usually, cancer is asymptomatic, but symptoms can vary from patient to patient and depending on the type of cancer. Nevertheless, a few signs and symptoms can be observed such as fatigue, recurrent fever, irregular loss of weight, pain in certain areas of the body, pigmentation, unusual growth of hairs, red or yellow skin, changes in shape of breast, menorrhagia, sore throat, unusual constipation or diarrhoea, loss of appetite, headache, bloody urine, or blurry vision (John et al. 2011).

Cancer has tendency to affect any age group, but sedentary lifestyle and environment changes have caused a surge in the number of cases all over the world. After United States and China, India is also observing a sudden rise in cancer patients, which can be due to large population, poor environment or living style, or lack of diagnostic tools. Nearly 1.4 million cancer cases (692,704 males and 695,693 females) were estimated in India in 2015 and significant rise in cases were observed in 2020, i.e., 1.74 million cancer cases (871, 756 males and 871, 756 females).

This increased rate of emergence of cancer cases has led to increased demand of new molecules that have low toxicity profile and high efficiency. Therefore, in the pursuit of new molecules, scientists came across Quinoline (C_9H_7N, 129.16 Da), a privileged scaffold that has been associated with multiple biological activities like antiviral, antibacterial, antimalarial, antifungal, antitubercular, antileishmanial, anti-inflammatory, anti-HIV, and anticancer. Quinoline has pKa of 4.85, log P value of 2.04, B.P. of 237 °C and is an oily hygroscopic liquid that darkens upon exposure to light. Quinoline has a stable nucleus but a basic nature and abilities to form salts and show reaction similar to benzene and pyridine. Quinoline accepts both nucleophilic and electrophilic substitution reactions. Among natural sources of quinoline are Cinchona alkaloids that possess antimalarial and antiarrhythmic activity, whereas Camptothecin has a good anticancer activity. This multifarious profile helped quinoline gain attention of researchers to develop new anticancer moieties by sequential modification of the substituents attached to it as shown in Fig. 1. Therefore, this chapter provides brief knowledge about the recent developments of quinoline derivatives as anticancer drugs that include structure activity relationship, molecular docking studies, and their mechanism, thus helping new researchers to design their molecules accordingly.

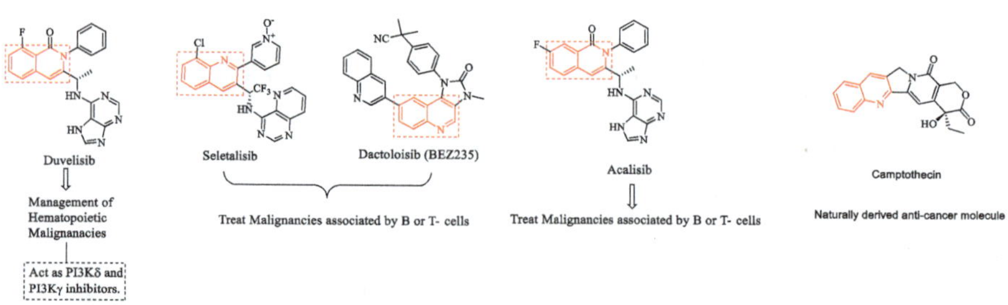

Fig. 1 Quinoline derivatives as potent anticancer agents

2 Recent Discoveries of Quinoline Derivatives as Anticancer Agents

2.1 Quinoline Derivatives

Lee et al. synthesized 2-(Phenylsulfonyl)quinoline N-hydroxyacrylamides as anticancer agents. All the series was evaluated for their anticancer potential. Among them **compound 1** was found to be the most potent and showed antiproliferative action against HL-60 ($GI_{50} = 0.29 \pm 0.06$), HCT116 ($GI_{50} = 0.08 \pm 0.001$), PC-3 ($GI_{50} = 0.15 \pm 0.01$), and A549 ($GI_{50} = 0.27 \pm 0.02$). In addition, mechanistic studies elucidated the capabilities of **compound 1** to inhibit histone deacetylase isoforms with IC_{50} value of 14 to 130 nM (Fig. 2) (Lee et al. 2016).

In 2016, Ge et al. synthesized 6-fluoro-3-phenyl-7-piperazinyl quinolone derivatives as topoisomerase-I inhibitors. After in vitro evaluation of the synthesized series, **compound 2** inhibited the cell proliferation in Hela (IC_{50}: 0.89 ± 0.04 μM), BGC-823 (IC_{50}: 0.61 ± 0.08 μM), HepG2 (IC_{50}: 0.86 ± 0.10 μM), A549 (IC_{50}: 0.11 ± 0.01 μM). Structure activity relationship suggests that 3-chlorophenyl substitution was more active at 3-position of the quinoline nucleus prior to the ketone group in the structure for antitumor potential (Fig. 3) (Ge et al. 2016).

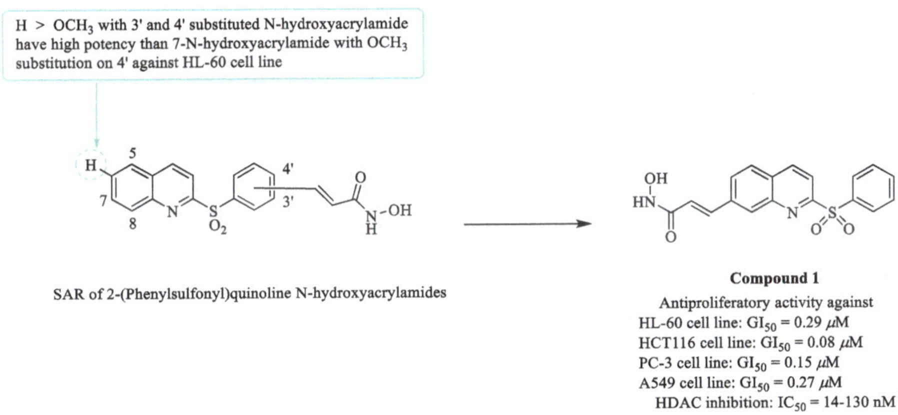

Fig. 2 2-(Phenylsulfonyl)quinoline N-hydroxyacrylamides as anticancer agents

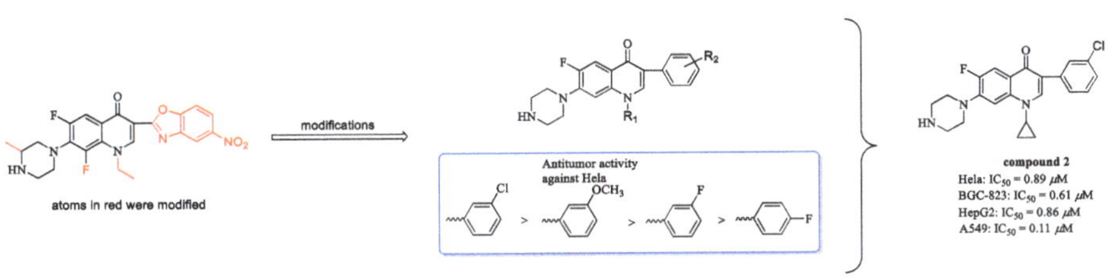

Fig. 3 6-fluoro-3-phenyl-7-piperazinyl quinolone as topoisomerase-I inhibitors

In 2016, Shobeiri et al. synthesized and evaluated quinoline analogues of flavones for their tubulin polymerization inhibitory potential. Among them **compound 3** was the most potent against MCF-7 (IC_{50} = 16.28 μM), MCF-7/MX (IC_{50} = 14.06 μM), A2780 (IC_{50} = 11.44 μM), A2780RCIS (IC_{50} = 8.15 μM) cell lines. Structure activity pattern suggests that 3,4,5-trimethoxyphenyl substitution was more active at second position of the quinoline nucleus in the structure for human cancer cell lines (Fig. 4) (Shobeiri et al. 2016).

In 2016, Perin et al. synthesized amino substituted benzimidazo[1,2-a]quinolines and evaluated them for their antiproliferative potential. Among them, **compound 4** was the most potent by inhibiting proliferation of HCT 116 (IC_{50} = 0.3 ± 0.08 μM), MCF-7 (IC_{50} = 0.6 ± 0.2 μM), H460 (IC_{50} = 0.5 ± 0.04 μM), HMLE (IC_{50} = 0.2 ± 0.03 μM) cell lines. Further, 3,5 dimethylpiperazinyl substitution on the quinoline moiety in the structure was most suitable for antiproliferative potential (Fig. 5) (Perin et al. 2016).

In 2016, Palluotto et al. designed and synthesized heterocyclic compounds quinolino[3,4-b] quinolines N-5 or C-6 and pyridazino [4,3-C] quinoline N-6 candidates against cancer cell lines (HeLA and MCF-7). From all the synthesized compounds, **compound 5** was found to be the most potent with an IC_{50} value of

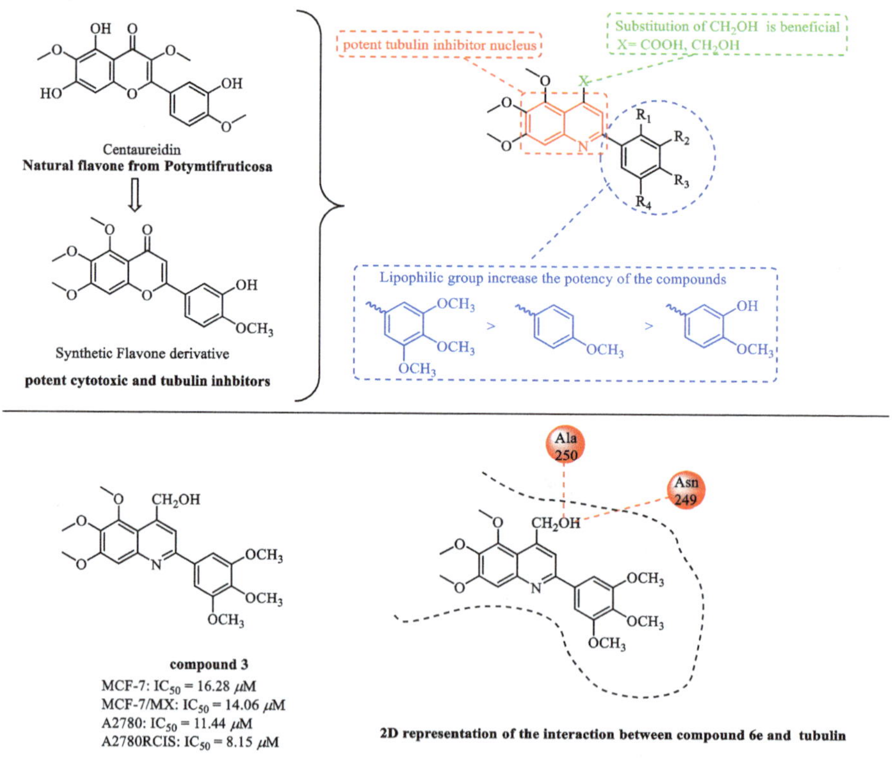

Fig. 4 Quinoline analogues of flavones as tubulin polymerization inhibitors

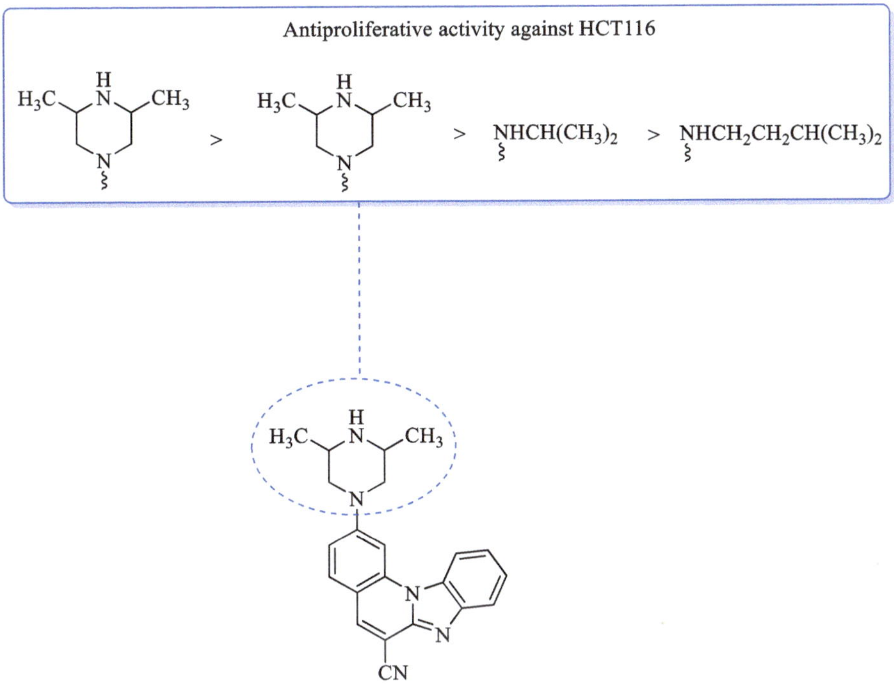

compound 4
Antiproliferative activity against
HCT116 cell line: $IC_{50} = 0.3\ \mu M$
MCF-7 cell line: $IC_{50} = 0.6\ \mu M$
H460 cell line: $IC_{50} = 0.5\ \mu M$
HMLE cell line: $IC_{50} = 0.2\ \mu M$

Fig. 5 Amino substituted benzimidazo[1,2-a]quinolines as antiproliferative agents

5.14 ± 0.32 μM and 2.32 ± 0.26 μM against Topo II α and HeLA, respectively. Moreover, **compound 6** has the maximum ability to interact with G-quadruplex sequences and has an IC_{50} value of 2.04 ± 0.87 μM and > 100 μM against HeLA and Topo II α, respectively. SAR revealed that substitution at C-6 position with different basic chains potency of inhibition of Topo-II α. Increase in chain length affects the inhibitory activity, i.e., $(CH_2)_4N(CH_3)_2 > (CH_2)_3N(CH_3)_2 > (CH_2)_2N(CH_3)_2$ (Fig. 6) (Palluotto et al. 2016).

In 2017, Khelifi et al. designed and synthesized a novel series of iso-combreta quinolines as tubulin inhibitors by replacement of ring-A with nitrogen containing compounds to form iso CA-4 derivatives. These synthesized compounds exhibited significant antimitotic and cytotoxicity effects toward different tumor cells with $IC_{50} \leq 10$ Nm. Among synthesized compounds, **compound 7** was found to be the most potent tubulin inhibitor with IC_{50} value of 1.5 ± 0.05 nM and 0.4 ± 0.04 nM against U87 and A549 cells, respectively. Structure activity relationship revealed

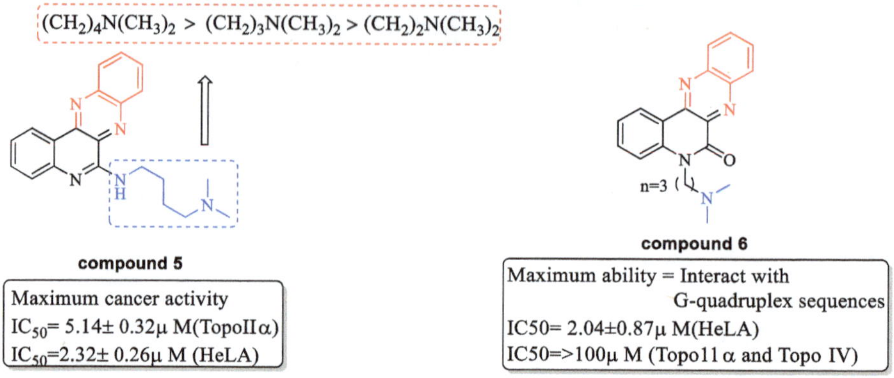

Fig. 6 Quinolino[3,4-b] quinolines N-5 or C-6 and pyridazino [4,3-C] quinoline N-6 derivatives as anticancer agents

that fluorine substituents at meta position on ring B leads to significant potential of cytotoxic effects with $IC_{50} = 5$ nM. 4-methoxy substituents on ring-B leads to significant antiproliferative activity toward U87 cells with $IC_{50} = 21$ nM, while 2-methylquinazolinic derivatives exhibit least cytotoxicity effect. Conversion of methyl group by CN group at C-2 position would be responsible for significant anti-tubulin effect. Molecular docking studies of **compound 7** suggest that binding interaction with β-tubulin shows same action with iso CA-4. **Compound 7** forms hydrogen bonding interaction with Cys-β-241 and Thr-α-179 in the binding site of β-tubulin. (Fig. 7) (Khelifi et al. 2017).

In 2017, Joshi et al. synthesized 4-phenyl quinoline derivatives and evaluated them as serotonin receptor ligands with antiproliferative activity. Of the three most active compounds, **compound 8** with the IC_{50} value of 6.15 ± 1.55 μM was the most potent for the antiproliferative activity. Structure activity pattern suggests that alkyl substitution at 3-position of the quinoline ring is much more active than aromatic substitution in the structure (Fig. 8) (Joshi et al. 2017).

Jitender Dev et al. synthesized a series of novel pyrazolo[3,4-b] quinolinyl acetamide analogues and evaluated them for their anticancer, antimicrobial, and COMFA analysis. Among them, **compound 9** was the most potent against Hela ($IC_{50} = 13.6 \pm 0.28$ μM), HepG2 ($IC_{50} = 11.2 \pm 0.25$ μM), A549 ($IC_{50} = 10.6 \pm 0.24$ μM), COLO 205 ($IC_{50} = 12.2 \pm 0.28$ μM). Structure activity pattern suggests that ethylpiperazine substitution on methylamide linkage in the structure was suitable for anticancer potential (Fig. 9) (Jitender Dev et al. 2017).

Almansour et al. synthesized a series of decarbonyl luotonin analogues and evaluated them for their antiproliferative activity. Among all, **compound 10** was the most potent against cell lines KB ($IC_{50} = 10.9 \pm 0.8$ μM), MDA-MD231 ($IC_{50} = 12 \pm 0.8$ μM), LNCap ($IC_{50} = 11.3 \pm 1.04$ μM), HT1080 ($IC_{50} = 52.9 \pm 6.1$ μM) (Fig. 10) (Almansour et al. 2017).

Kwon et al. synthesized a novel mitochondria-targeting [3,2-c] quinolines photosensitizers and characterized for their photodynamic anticancer activity.

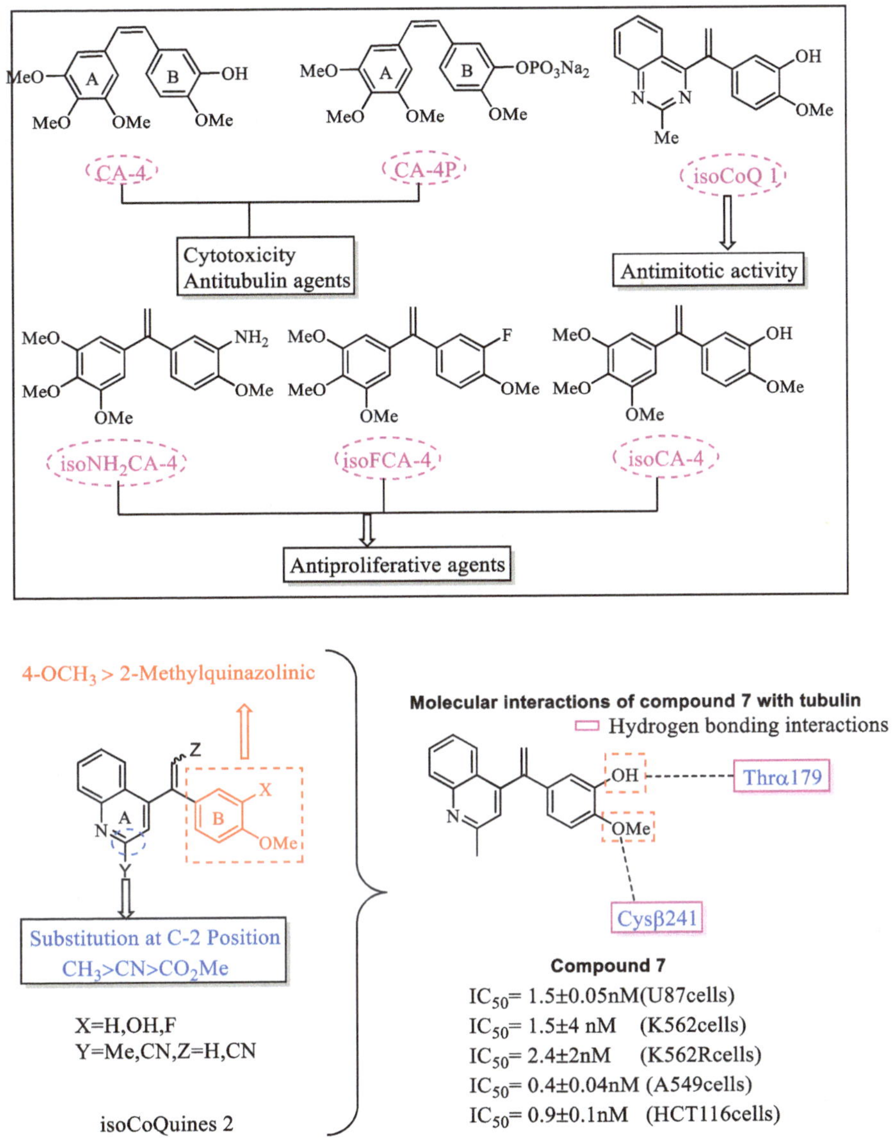

Fig. 7 Novel series of iso-combreta quinolines as tubulin inhibitors

Among them **compound 11** was the most potent and showed higher phototoxicity toward HeLa cell line (IC_{50} = 0.49 ± 0.08 μM) with 5 min of irradiation compared to other two cell lines A549 (IC_{50} = 1.33 ± 0.73 μM) and MCF7 (IC_{50} = 1.68 ± 1.67 μM). Structure activity pattern suggests that substitution of 2-chlorothiophene on the carbon atom next to the nitrogen atom of the quinoline moiety in the structure was most suitable for anticancer activity (Fig. 11) (Kwon et al. 2018).

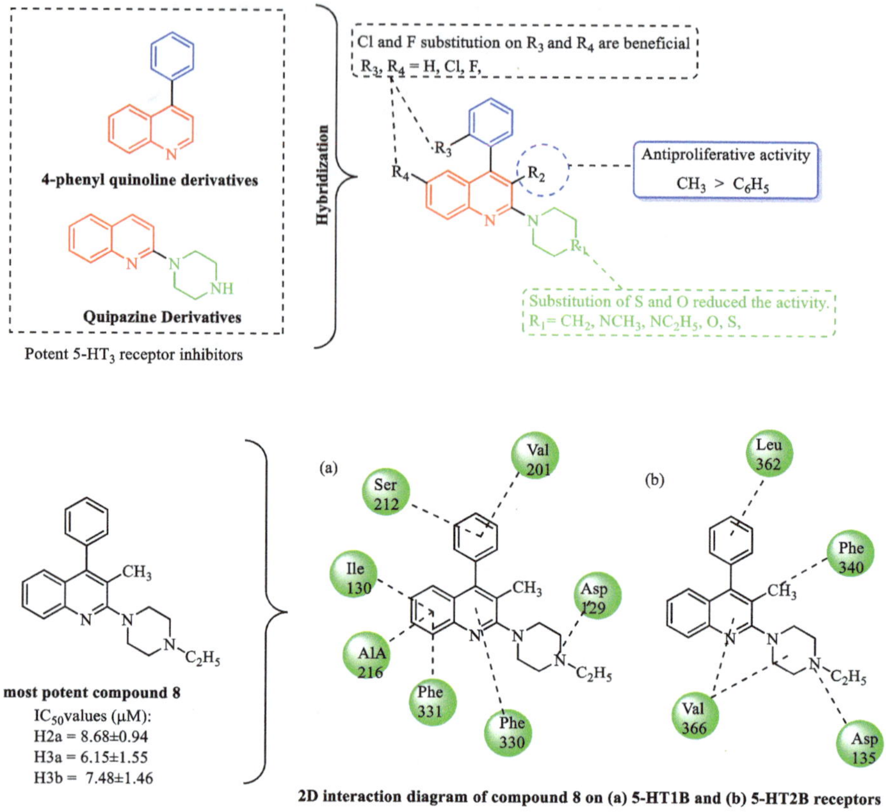

Fig. 8 4-phenyl quinoline derivatives as antiproliferative agents

Fig. 9 Novel pyrazolo[3,4-b] quinolinyl acetamide analogues as anticancer agents

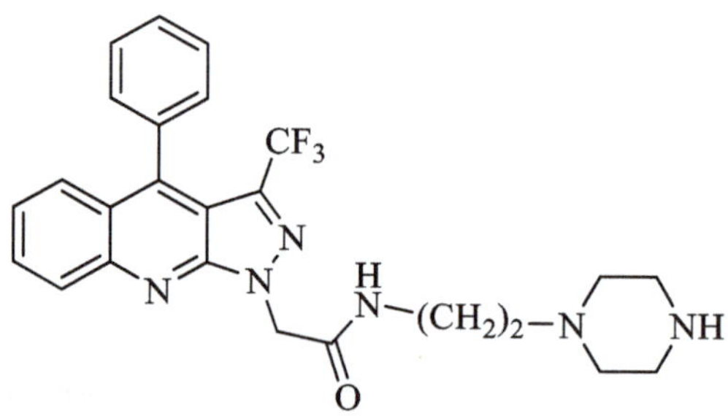

Compound 9

Anticancer activity against

HeLa: $IC_{50} = 13.6\ \mu M$

HepG2: $IC_{50} = 11.2\ \mu M$

A549: $IC_{50} = 10.6\ \mu M$

COLO 205: $IC_{50} = 12.2\ \mu M$

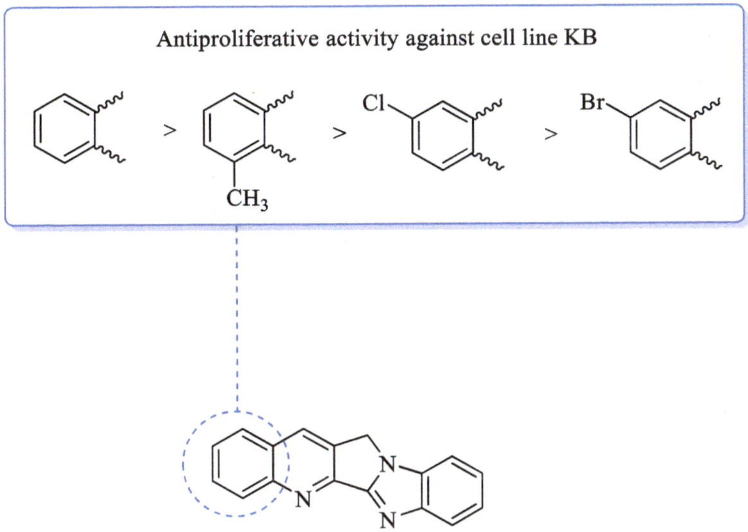

Compound 10

KB: IC_{50} = 10.9 μM
MDA-MD231: IC_{50} = 12 μM
LNCap: IC_{50} = 11.3 μM
HT1080: IC_{50} = 52.9 μM

Fig. 10 Series of decarbonyl luotonin analogues as antiproliferative agents

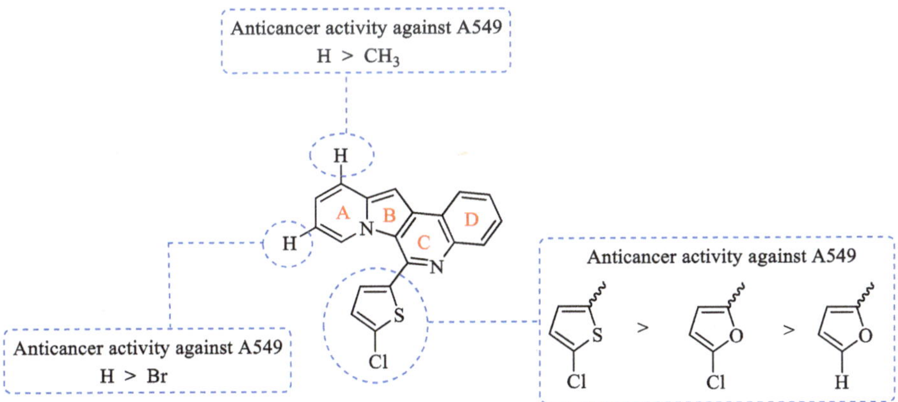

Compound 11
Anticancer activity
HeLa cell line: IC_{50} = 0.49 μM
A549 cell line: IC_{50} = 1.33 μM
MCF7 cell line: IC_{50} = 1.68 μM

Fig. 11 Novel mitochondria-targeting [3,2-c] quinolines photosensitizers as anticancer agents

Alonso et al. synthesized a series of phosphorous-substituted quinoline derivatives and evaluated them for their antiproliferation activity. Among them, **compound 12** was the most potent against cell line lung A549 ($IC_{50} = 0.03–0.02$ μM) but it was less active toward ovarian SKOVO3 ($IC_{50} > 50$ μM), kidney HEK293 ($IC_{50} > 50$ μM), and MRC-5 ($IC_{50} > 50$ μM) for antiproliferation activity. Structure activity pattern suggests that substitution of 4-fluorophenyl on the second and fourth carbon next to nitrogen atom of the tetrahydroquinoline moiety in the structure was most suitable for cytotoxicity toward antiproliferation activity (Fig. 12) (Alonso et al. 2018).

In 2018, Kwak et al. designed and synthesized a novel series of quinolinone and quinoline derivatives as P2X7 receptor antagonists. From all the synthesized compounds, **compounds 13 and 14** possess antagonist activity with % inhibition at 1 μM of 4 ± 5% (P2X4R) and 3.0 ± 0.8% (P2X3R), respectively. In addition, **compounds 13 and 14** inhibited the liberation of pro-inflammatory cytokine against IL-1β in THP1 cells from LPS/IFN-γ/BzATP with IC_{50} values of 7 ± 2 nM and 12 ± 1 nM, respectively. **Compound 13** significantly reduced the growth of TS15–88 glioma cells at 50 μM. Furthermore, **compound 13** has ability to cross blood–brain barrier and has weak metabolic stability in liver (major drawback). SAR

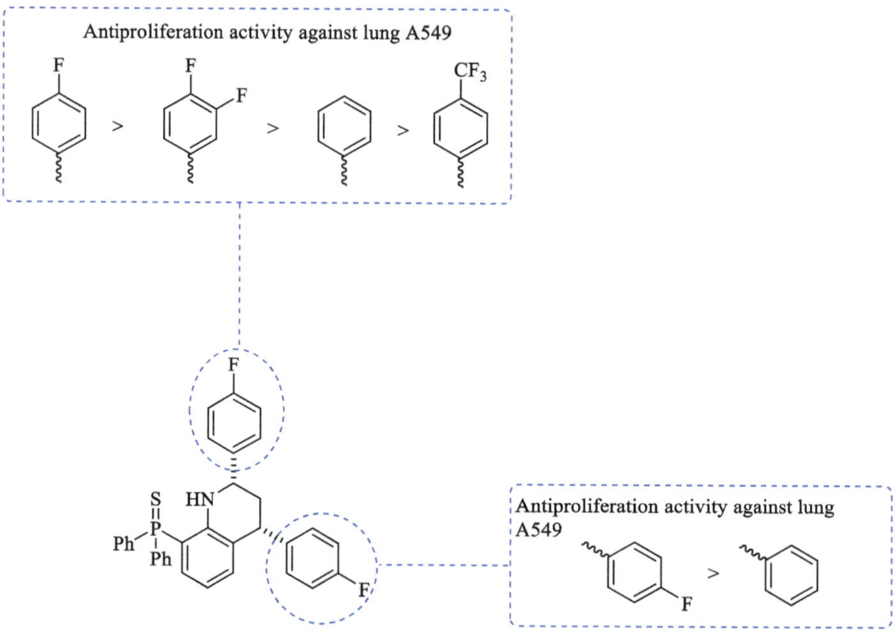

Compound 12
Antiproliferatory activity against
lung A549 cell line: $IC_{50} = 0.03$ μM
ovarian SKOVO3 cell line: $IC_{50} > 50$ μM
kidney HEK293 cell line: $IC_{50} > 50$ μM
MRC-5 cell line: $IC_{50} > 50$ μM

Fig. 12 Phosphorous-substituted quinoline derivatives as antiproliferative agents

study revealed that substitution on R_1, R_2, and R_3 positions of quinoline gave best results. Enlargement of carbon chain length enhanced the antagonist activity. Demethylation on para-phenyl leads to improved antagonist effect (Fig. 13) (Kwak et al. 2018).

In 2018, Crespo et al. designed and synthesized a novel series of 1-oxopyrimido [4,5-c] quinoline-2-acetic acid analogues as aldose reductase (AKR1B1) inhibitors. After successful evaluation, **compound 15** was the most active compound with $K_i = 0.07 \pm 0.010$ μM, IC_{50} value of 0.12 ± 0.004 μM against inhibition of AKR1B1 and was adhering to Lipinski's rule of five. **Compound 15** also showed anti-mitotic activity, but they are not suitable for inhibition of HT-1080 fibrosarcoma

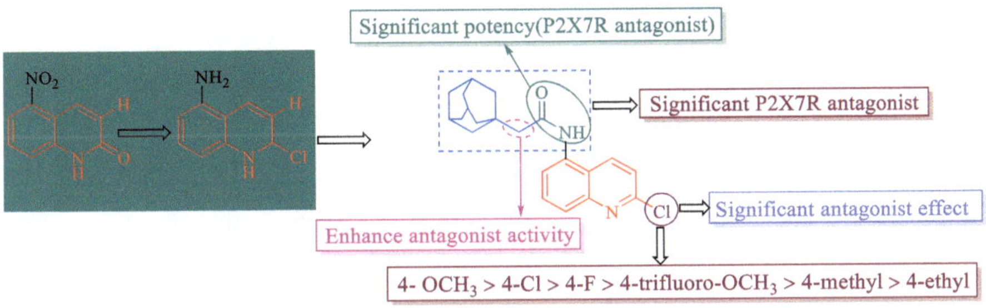

Compound 13

% inhibition against
P2X4R = 4±5% (P2X4R)
Cytokine inhibition against
IL-1β: IC_{50} = 7±2 nM

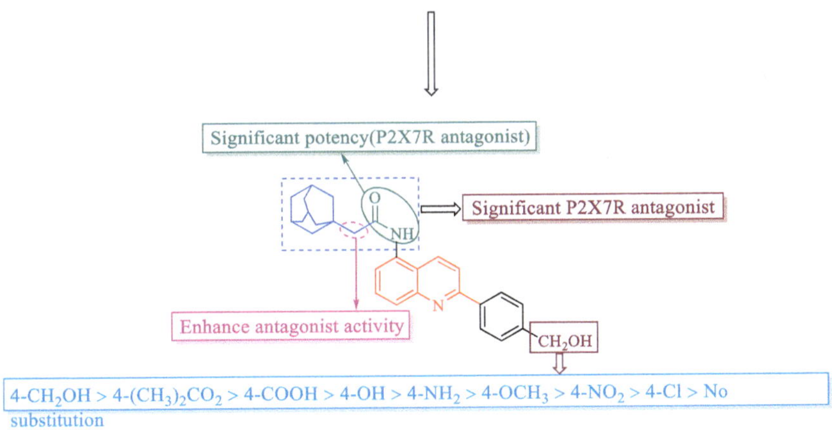

Compound 14

% inhibition against
P2X4R = 3.0±0.8 %
Cytokine inhibition against
IL-1β: IC_{50} = 12±1 nM

Fig. 13 Quinolinone and quinoline derivatives as P2X7 receptor antagonists

cell line. SAR study revealed that conversion of amino with acetic acid enhanced inhibitory action, substitution of aryl group reduced activity, substitution of fluorine on C-5 position of quinoline reduced the activity and 2-amino, acetic acid groups are necessary for inhibition of AKR1B1. Molecular docking studies suggest that **compound 15** interacts with AKR1B1 with Leu300 (Fig. 14) (Crespo et al. 2018).

In 2019, Li et al. designed and synthesized a novel series of quinoline-indole analogues as anti-tubulin agents. After in vitro analysis of all the synthesized compounds, **compound 16 and 17** were found to be the most potent against different cancer cells with IC_{50} values of 0.002 ± 0.001 μM (K562), 0.011 ± 0.002 μM (HepG2), 0.008 ± 0.001 μM (KB), 0.009 ± 0.001 μM (HCT-8), 0.009 ± 0.002 μM (MDA-MB-231), 0.008 ± 0.001 μM (H22), 0.088 ± 0.021 μM (LO2) and 0.002 ± 0.001 μM (K562), 0.006 ± 0.001 μM (HepG2), 0.005 ± 0.001 μM (KB), 0.009 ± 0.001 μM (HCT-8), 0.006 ± 0.001 μM (MDA-MB231), 0.006 ± 0.001 μM (H22), 0.048 ± 0.001 μM (LO2), respectively. **Compound 17** arrested cell cycle arrest in G2/M phase and caused apoptosis and stiffened mitochondria of K562 cell line. SAR study suggests that introduction of olefin group on C-3, C-5 of indole ring reduced activity as compared to substitution on C-4 of indole ring. Substitution of methyl, hydroxymethyl on N-1 of indole ring significantly higher potency than ethyl, acetyl

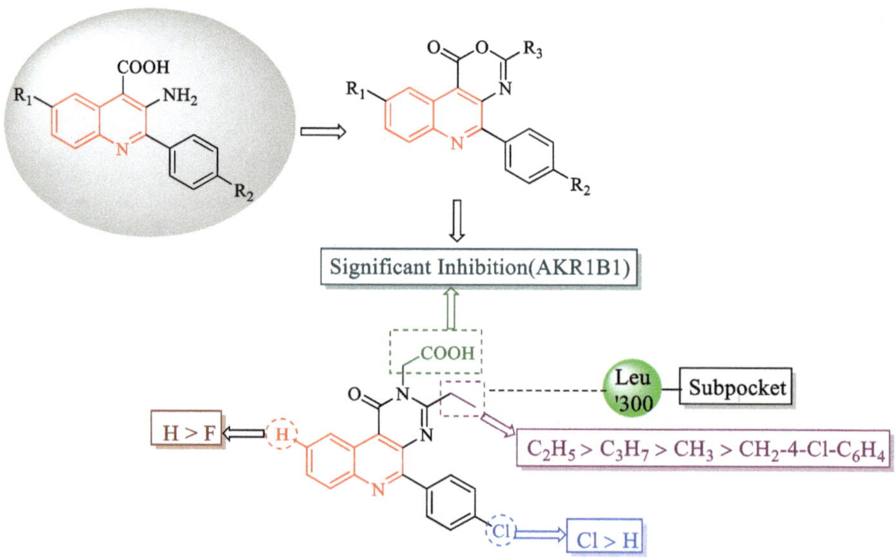

Compound 15

AKR1B1inhibition

$IC_{50} = 0.12 \pm 0.004\ \mu M$

$K_i = 0.073 \pm 0.010\ \mu M$

Fig. 14 1-oxopyrimido[4,5-c] quinoline-2-acetic acid analogues as aldose reductase (AKR1B1) inhibitors

and fluoro-methyl substitutions. Substitution of CHO, CH_2OH, OCH_3, CF_3, $CONH_2$, $NHCH_3$, H, CN groups on C-2 of quinoline moiety reduced potency as compared CH_3. Molecular docking studies suggest that **compounds 16 and 17** form hydrogen-bonding interactions with Cys241. Moreover, hydrophobic interactions with Val312, Thr179, Asn350, Val351 were observed (Fig. 15) (Li et al. 2019).

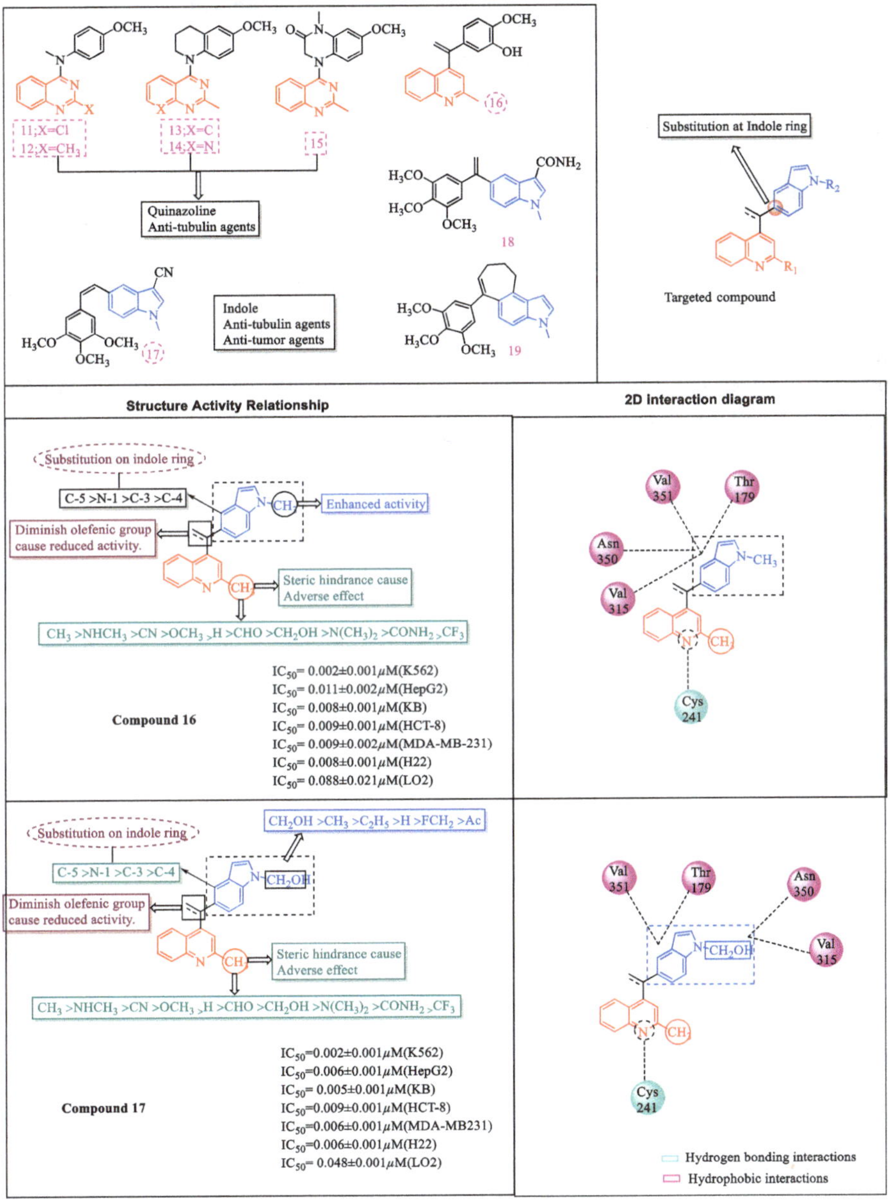

Fig. 15 Quinoline-indole analogues as anti-tubulin agents

In 2022, Soliman et al. synthesized a series of novel quinoline derivatives and screened them against HepG2 cells to assess their antitumor inhibitory activity. Among these, **compound 18** showed most potent inhibitory activity with IC_{50} value of 6.529 μg/ml along with highest binding affinity of −34.478 kcal/mol. Further, structure activity relationship of this potent compound suggested that thio linkage was far more suitable than oxo linkage at ortho position of quinoline moiety in the structure. Moreover, molecular docking study revealed that **compound 18** exhibits hydrogen bond interaction with Trp388 and Asn 288 in the active site of HepG2 cells (Fig. 16) (Soliman et al. 2022).

In 2022, Hauguel et al. designed and synthesized a series of quinoline-2-carbonitrile-based hydroxamic acids and screened them for their tubulin polymerization and histone deacetylase inhibition. Among these, **compound 19** emerged as most potent inhibitor against HCT116 cell line with GI_{50} value of 0.5 ± 0.002 nM and against HDACs with IC_{50} value of 150 ± 10 to 1900 ± 100 nM. Further, structure activity pattern suggested quinoline nucleus was most suitable against HCT116 for cytotoxicity compared to isoquinoline in the structure. Molecular docking studies revealed that **compound 19** was capable of forming hydrogen bond interactions (Asnβ316, Alaα180) and CH/π interaction (Asnβ258, Ala β316) into the binding site of tubulin; however, **compound 19** also possesses hydrogen bond, π/π-stacking, CH/π and CH/CH interactions with Gly151, Phe152, Phe208, and Met274, respectively, in the catalytic site of HDAC8 (Fig. 17) (Hauguel et al. 2022).

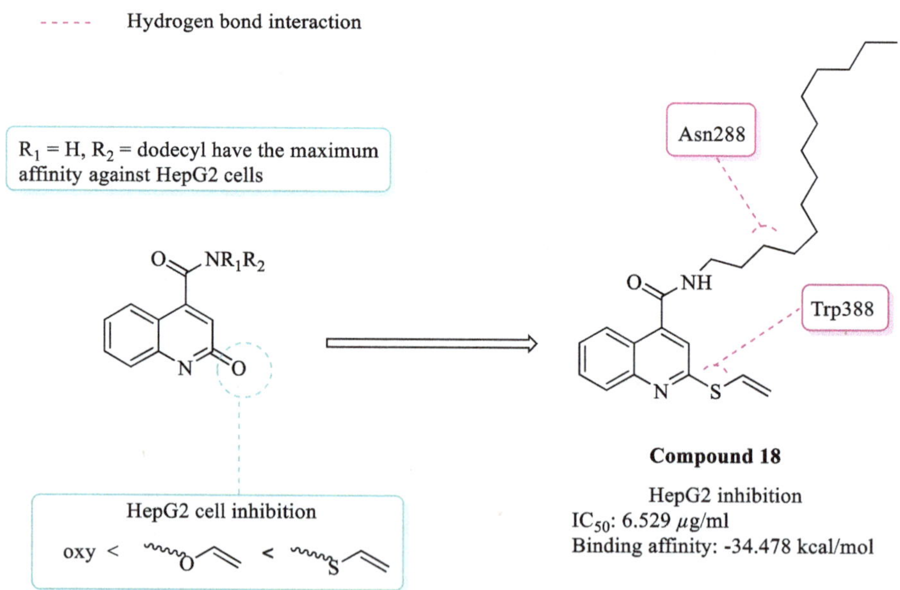

Fig. 16 Quinoline derivatives as antitumor agents

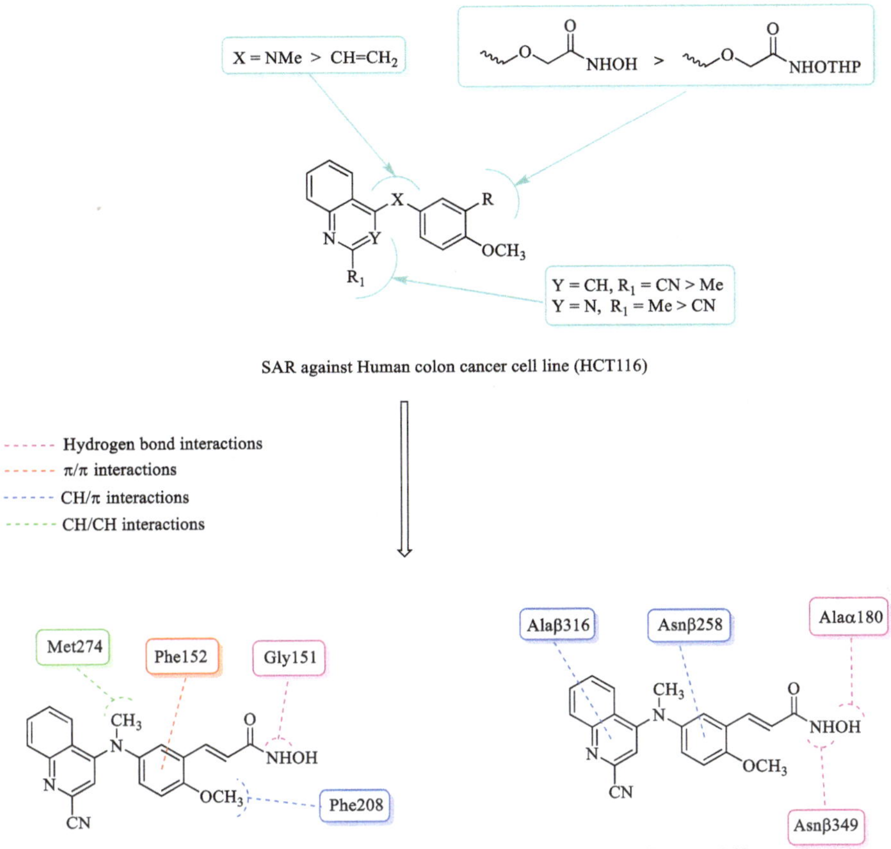

Compound 19
HDAC8 inhibition: IC_{50} =150 ±10 - 1900 ± 100 nM

Compound 19
HCT116 cell line inhibition: GI_{50} = 0.5 ± 0.002 nM

Fig. 17 Quinoline-2-carbonitrile-based hydroxamic acids as tubulin polymerization and histone deacetylase inhibitors

2.2 Quinoline Hybrids

In 2016, Liu et al. discovered novel 6,7-disubstituted-4-(2-fluorophenoxy)quinolines bearing 1,2,3-triazole-4-carboxamide moiety as c-Met kinase inhibitors. Among them, **compound 20** was the most potent and showed cytotoxic activity against HT-29 (IC_{50} = 0.10 ± 0.003 μmol/L), H460 (IC_{50} = 0.18 ± 0.03 μmol/L), A549 (IC_{50} = 0.07 ± 0.01 μmol/L), MKN-45 (IC_{50} = 0.03 ± 0.01 μmol/L) cell lines. Structure activity pattern suggests that N-2-chlorophenyl substitution was more active on the triazole ring in the structure. In addition, **compound 20** also showed c-Met kinase inhibitory potential with the IC_{50} value of 2.27 nM. Molecular docking studies revealed that **compound 20** was capable of hydrogen bond interaction with Met1160, π-π hydrophobic interaction with Tyr1159, conventional hydrogen bond with Lys1110 and π-sigma interaction with Ile1130 in the active site of c-Met (Fig. 18) (Liu et al. 2016a).

In 2016, Liu et al. also designed and synthesized novel 4-phenoxyquinoline derivatives with 1,2,4-triazolone moiety and evaluated them for their anticancer potential. Among them, **compound 21** was the most potent and was cytotoxic against HT-29 ($IC_{50} = 0.08 \pm 0.05$ µmol/L), H460 ($IC_{50} = 0.14 \pm 0.08$ µmol/L), A540 ($IC_{50} = 0.11 \pm 0.06$ µmol/L), MKN-45 ($IC_{50} = 0.03 \pm 0.03$ µmol/L) cell lines. On further evaluation, **compound 21** also showed high potency toward c-Met kinase inhibition with the IC_{50} value of 1.57 nM. Structure activity pattern suggests that 4-methylpiperazinyl substitution on the propanoxyl linkage attached to quinoline moiety in the structure was most suitable for cytotoxic activity. Molecular docking studies reveal that **compound 21** was capable of hydrogen bond interaction with

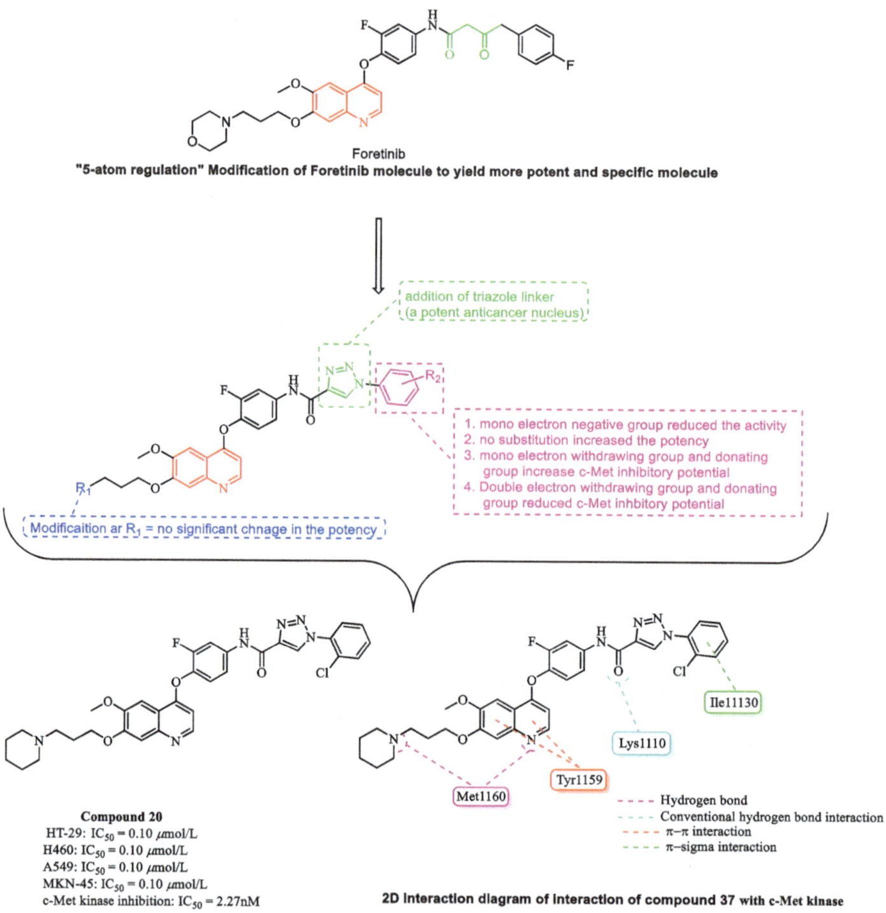

Fig. 18 Novel 6,7-disubstituted-4-(2-fluorophenoxy)quinolines bearing 1,2,3-triazole-4-carboxamide moiety as c-Met kinase inhibitors

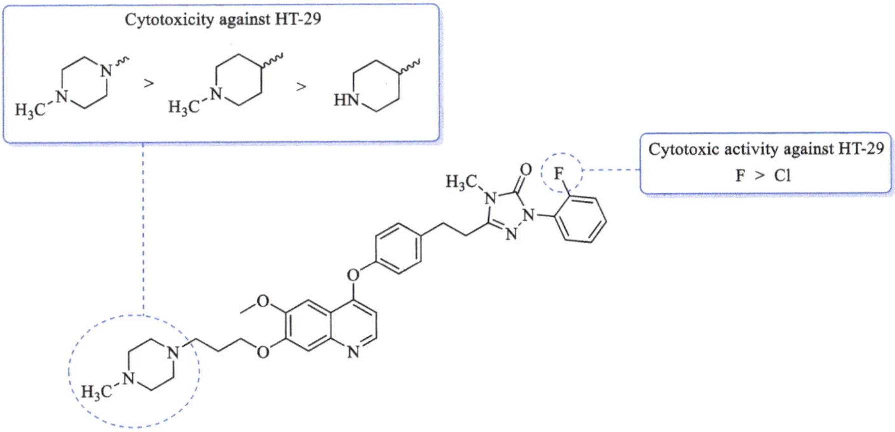

Compound 21

Cytotoxicity against
HT-29 cell line: $IC_{50} = 0.080$ μmol/L
H460 cell line: $IC_{50} = 0.14$ μmol/L
A540 cell line: $IC_{50} = 0.11$ μmol/L
MKN-45 cell line: $IC_{50} = 0.030$ μmol/L
c-Met kinase inhibition: $IC_{50} = 1.57$ nM

Fig. 19 Novel 4-phenoxyquinoline derivatives 1,2,4-triazolone moiety as anticancer agent

Asp1222, Met 1160, Ala1221, and π-π interaction with Phe1134 in the active site of c-Met kinase (Fig. 19) (Liu et al. 2016b).

In 2017, Zhang et al. designed and synthesized a novel series of N-(5-quinollin-6-yl) pyridine-3-yl) benzenesulfonamides and evaluated them against PI3K (Phosphoinositide3-kinase) and mTOR (Mammalian target of rapamycin). In vitro study revealed that **compound 22** was the most potent dual inhibitor (PI3K/mTOR) with $IC_{50} = 3.9$ nM (PI3Kβ), $IC_{50} = 8.4$ nM (PI3Kγ), $IC_{50} = 0.87$ nM (PI3Kδ), $IC_{50} = 10.0$ nM (mTOR). Structure activity relationship revealed that substitution of morpholine, polar group at C-3 of quinoline leads to significant inhibitions of PI3K. Docking studies revealed that nonappearance of H-bond acceptor and donor between oxygen of morpholine and residue Arg770 leads to reduction of potency. **Compound 22** was selected for pharmacokinetic study on fasted mice and oral administration of drug showed good bioavailability with plasma clearance (0.42 L/h/Kg) (Fig. 20) (Zhang et al. 2017).

Shaikh et al. designed and synthesized tetrazolylmethyl quinolines and evaluated them for their anticancer and antifungal activity. Among them, **compound 23** was the most potent for breast cancer cell line against MCF7 (GI = 72.06%), MDA-MB-231/ATCC (GI = 49.28%), HS 578 T (GI = 31.08%), BT-549 (GI = 79.66%), T-47D (GI = 97.56%), and MDA-MB-468 (GI = 70.08%). Structure activity pattern suggests that methoxy group on the 6th position on the quinoline ring in the structure was most suitable for anticancer activity. Molecular docking studies reveal that **compound 23** was capable of interacting with B/DA14.H62, B/DC12.H42, B/DA11.H62 in the active site of PDB 1 AU5 (Fig. 21) (Shaikh et al. 2017).

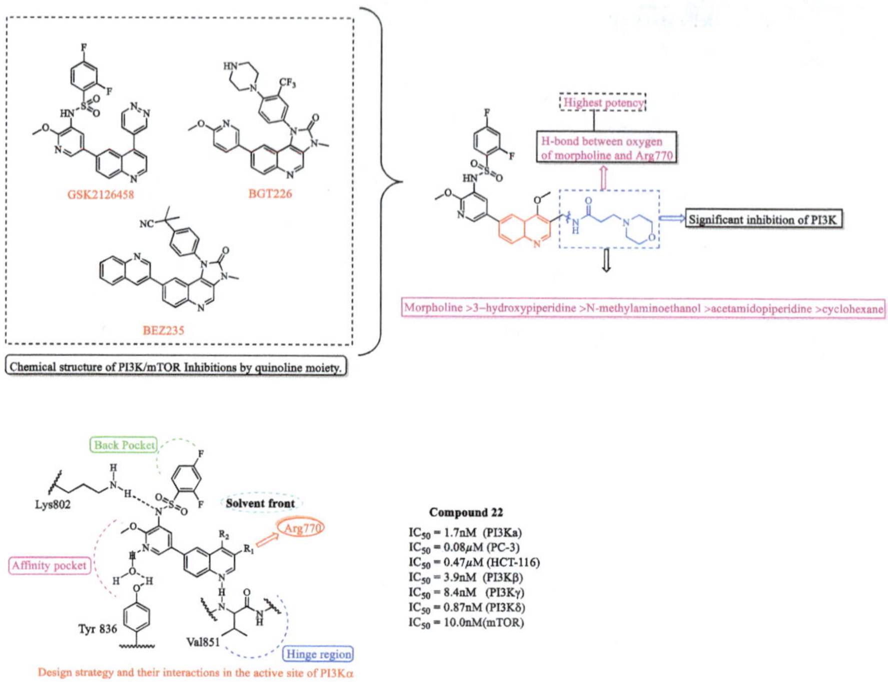

Fig. 20 N-(5-quinollin-6-yl) pyridine-3-yl) benzenesulfonamide derivatives as Phosphoinositide3-kinase inhibitors

Fig. 21 Tetrazolylmethyl quinolines as anticancer agents

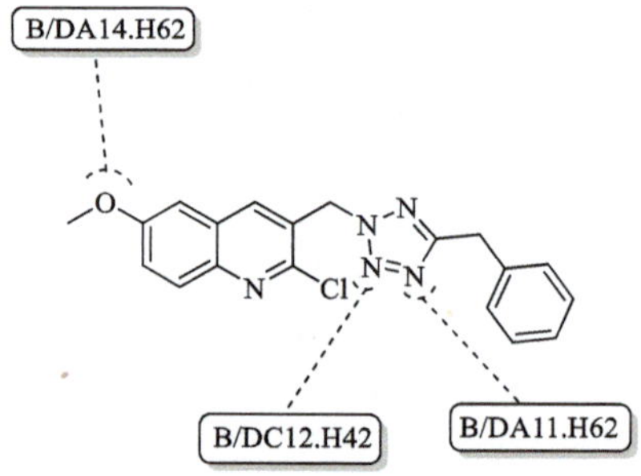

Compound 23

Antibreast cancer activity against-

MCF7: GI = 72.06 %

MDA-MB-231/ATCC: GI = 49.28 %

HS 578T: GI = 31.08 %

BT-549: GI = 79.66 %

T-47D: GI = 97.56 %

MDA-MB-468: GI = 70.08 %

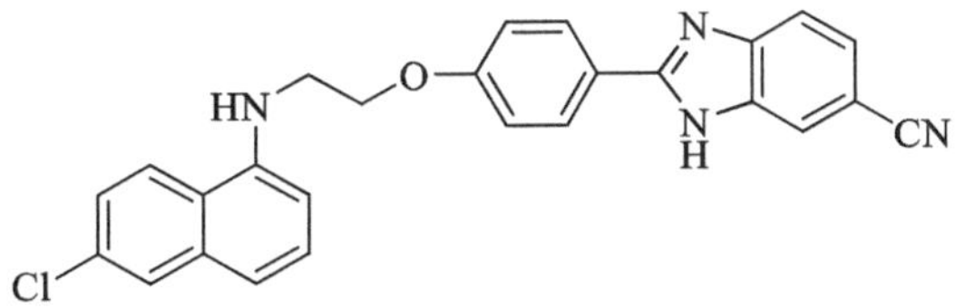

Fig. 22 New quinoline–arylamidine hybrids as antitumor agents

Compound 24

Antitumor activity against-
MDCK1cell line: $GI_{50} = 22.1$ mol dm^{-3}
HeLa cell line: $GI_{50} = 56.6$ mol dm^{-3}
CaCo-2: $GI_{50} = 28.3$ mol dm^{-3}
K562 cell line: $GI_{50} = 7.8$ mol dm^{-3}
Raji: $GI_{50} = 5.2$ mol dm^{-3}

Krstulovic et al. synthesized new quinoline–arylamidine hybrids and evaluated them for their antitumor activity. Among all, **compound 24** was the most potent against cell line MDCK1 ($GI_{50} = 22.1 \pm 8.1$ mol dm^{-3}), HeLa ($GI_{50} = 56.6 \pm 22.1$ mol dm^{-3}), CaCo-2 ($GI_{50} = 28.3 \pm 11.3$ mol dm^{-3}), K562 ($GI_{50} = 7.8 \pm 3.3$ mol dm^{-3}), Raji ($GI_{50} = 5.2 \pm 1.1$ mol dm^{-3}) for antitumor activity. Structure activity pattern suggests that substitution of cyanide on **7-benzimidazole** in the structure was most suitable for antitumor activity (Fig. 22) (Krstulović et al. 2017).

In 2017, Chen et al. designed and synthesized a novel series of quinoline-based N-hydroxycinnaamides and N-hydroxy benzamides analogues as anticancer agent specifically as histone deacetylase (HDAC) inhibitors. In vitro study revealed that these compounds exhibit good antiproliferative action and have inhibitory action against various cancer cells such as MOLT – 4 (acute lymphoblastic leukaemia cell), HEL (erythrocyte leukaemia cell), K562 (chronic myelogenous leukaemia cell), PC-3 (prostatic cancer cell), and HeLa (Cervical carcinoma cell). Among them, **compound 26** was found to be the most potent and was active against 5-cancer cell line with $IC_{50} = 0.16 \pm 0.02$ μM (MOLT- 4), $IC_{50} = 0.11 \pm 0.01$ μM (HEL), $IC_{50} = 0.36 \pm 0.02$ μM (K562), $IC_{50} = 2.92 \pm 0.35$ μM (PC-3), $IC_{50} = 1.82 \pm 0.16$ μM (HeLa). Furthermore, in vitro study suggested that **compounds 25 and 26** exhibit significant programmed cell death confirmed by flow cytometry examination. Moreover, **compound 25** showed significant inhibitory action against HDAC1 and HDAC8 with $IC_{50} = 72.5 \pm 0.5$ μM and $IC_{50} = 442.0 \pm 72.0$ μM, respectively. **Compounds 25 and 26** were selected for cell enzyme test and results suggested that **compounds 25 and 26** have greater penetration power across K562 (chronic myelogenous leukaemia cell) and showed inhibition with IC_{50} values of 108 ± 13 μM and 5213 ± 563 μM against Class I HDAC and Class II HDAC. On exploring SAR, substitution on meta-position of N-hydroxycinnamide increased potency; replacement of amine with amide between quinoline and N-hydroxycinnamide reduced potency; introduction of amine group at C-2 position of quinoline reduced inhibitory action against HDAC than C-6 and C-8 position of quinoline. No substitution at C-2, C-6, and C-8 increased potency against cellular

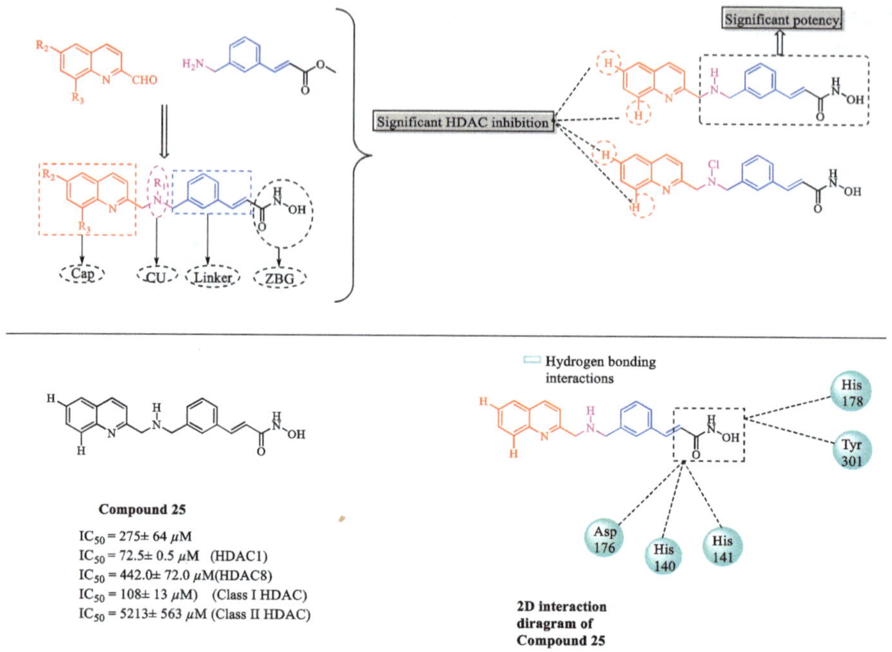

Fig. 23 Novel series of quinoline analogues N-hydroxycinnaamides and N-hydroxy benzamides as histone deacetylase inhibitors

enzyme. Molecular docking studies suggest that **compound 25** made hydrogen bond interactions with His140, His141, Asp176, His178, Tyr301 in the active site of HDAC1 (Fig. 23) (Chen et al. 2017).

In 2017, Zhou et al. replaced coumarin ring with quinoline moiety and synthesized a novel series of 4-anilinoquinoline analogues as tubulin polymerization inhibitors. After evaluation, all the compounds possessed antiproliferative effects but among them **compound 27** was found to be the most potent and showed cytotoxicity activity against different cancer cell lines with $IC_{50} = 1.5–3.9$ nM and favorable potency of multidrug resistance with resistance index = 1.0 (HCT-8/T), 1.0 (HCT-8/V), 2.3 (MCF-7/ADR), 1.7 (A2780/T). SAR study revealed that substitution of CH_3 at C-2 of A-ring increased inhibitory action; substitution of 2-chloro, 2-H showed least inhibition; introduction of 4-methylthio on p-B-ring leads to inhibition of O-demethylation metabolic route; Substitution of CH_3 at C-2 of ring A. NH_2 at C-3 and methoxy at C-4 of B ring showed excellent antiproliferative effect against MDA-MB-231 (breast cancer cells), but were having poor water solubility. For enhancement of water dispersibility, substitution of NH_2 at C-3 position of B-ring with aliphatic chain was done, but this reduced inhibitory action. Moreover, **compound 27** arrested the cell cycle at G2/M phase, inhibited tubulin polymerization and showed its antitumor effect by efficiently reducing body weight via HCT116 xenograft model. Molecular docking studies suggest that **compound 27**

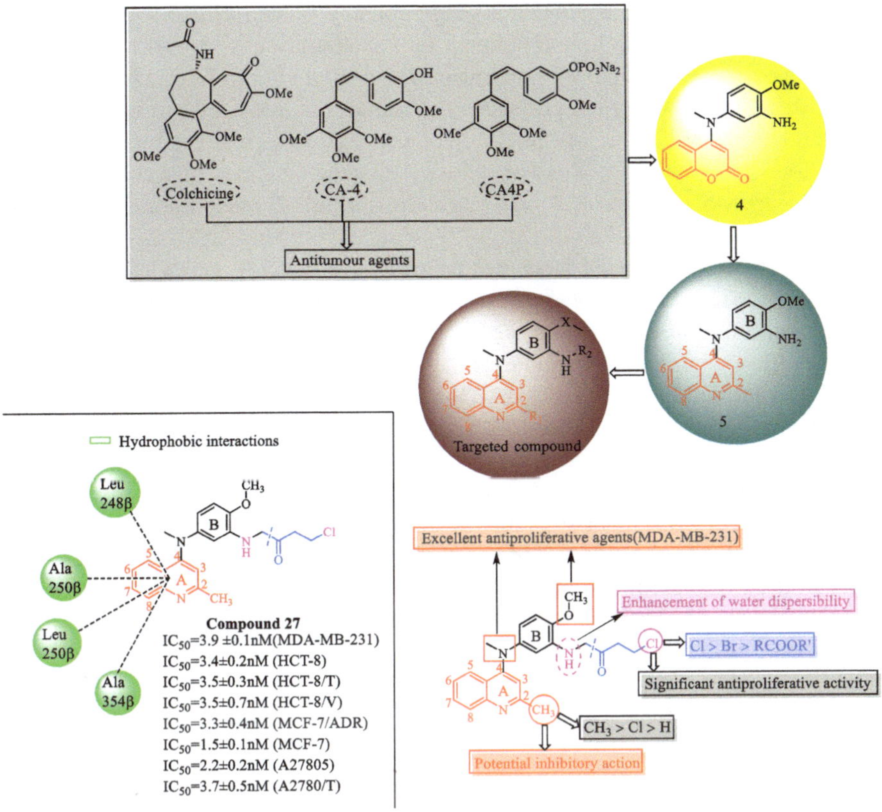

Fig. 24 Novel series of 4-anilinoquinoline analogues as tubulin polymerization inhibitors

made hydrophobic interactions with leu248β, Leu250β, Ala250β, and Ala354β. The novel 4-anilinoquinoline analogues have been remarkably proved as anticancer agents (Fig. 24) (Zhou et al. 2017).

In 2018, Ma et al. designed and synthesized a new series of quinazolinone analogues Pyrazolo[3,4-d] pyrimidin-4-amine for the management of cell-moderate immunity and hematological malignancies. These compounds exhibited their inhibitory action against PI3Kδ and PI3Kδ/γ at a concentration of 1 μM and IC_{50} values ranging between 8.4 nM and 106 nM. Among all the synthesized compounds, **compounds 28 and 29** showed the maximum inhibitory potential against PI3Kδ above PI3Kα, β and γ with $IC_{50} = 8.6 \pm 0.72$ nM and $IC_{50} = 8.4 \pm 0.65$ nM with 97% inhibition at 1 μM. In addition, **compounds 28 and 29** inhibited proliferative activity toward SU-DHL-6 with $GI_{50} = 0.14 \pm 0.01$ μM and $GI_{50} = 0.22 \pm 0.01$ μM. Compound 10e exhibited best plasma exposure $AUC_{Last} = 3527 \pm 287$ h.ng/mL, low volume distribution $V_{ss} = 0.45 \pm 0.1$ L/Kg, low clearance $= 0.99 \pm 0.1$ L/h/Kg, and good oral bioavailability $F\% = 34.9 \pm 2.64\%$, respectively. SAR study revealed that substitution of o-tolyl quinazolines, 6-hydroxy-2-naphthalenyl at C-3 of pyrazolo[3,4-d] pyrimidine showed average potency toward PI3Kδ with 70% inhibition; substitution of 2,6-dimethylphenyl quinazolinones at C-3 position of quinoline group increased the activity as compared to o-tolyl quinazolines; substitution of bulkier trifluoromethoxy phenyl or electron-withdraw group lead to least activity; substitution of 5-indolyl or 3,4-dimethoxyphenyl lead to significant potential inhibitory action against PI3Kδ. Molecular docking studies suggest that **compound 28** made hydrogen-bonding with Asp787 and **compound 29** made hydrogen bonding interactions with Tyr813, Asp911, Lys779, respectively (Fig. 25) (Ma et al. 2018).

Zhang et al. discovered and synthesized a series of [1,2,4]triazolo[1,3,4] thiadiazole derivatives and evaluated for their c-Met kinase inhibitory activity. Among them, **compound 30** was the most potent with the IC_{50} value of 0.002 μM for c-Met kinase inhibitory potential. In addition, **compound 30** was active against SNU-5 (% inhibition = 68.7%)**,** MKN45 (% inhibition = 71.9%), EBC-1 (% inhibition = 84.4%) cell lines at 5 μM and showed high efficacy against EBC-1cell line with IC_{50} value of 88 nM for antiproliferative activity. Furthermore, **compound 30** also inhibited c-Met phosphorylation in MKN45 cell line. Structure activity pattern suggests that substitution of N-methylpyrazole ring attached to the carbon atom next to the sulfur atom of thiadiazole ring in the structure was most suitable for antiproliferatory activity. Molecular docking studies revealed that **compound 30** was capable of forming hydrogen bonds with Met1160 and Tyr1159 in the active site of c-Met kinase (Fig. 26) (Zhang et al. 2018).

In 2019, Khelifi et al. designed and synthesized a novel series of N, N-Bis heteroaryl methylamines 1 like isoazaerianin derivatives as anticancer compounds with anti-mitotic activity. After evaluation, **compound 31** was the most potent

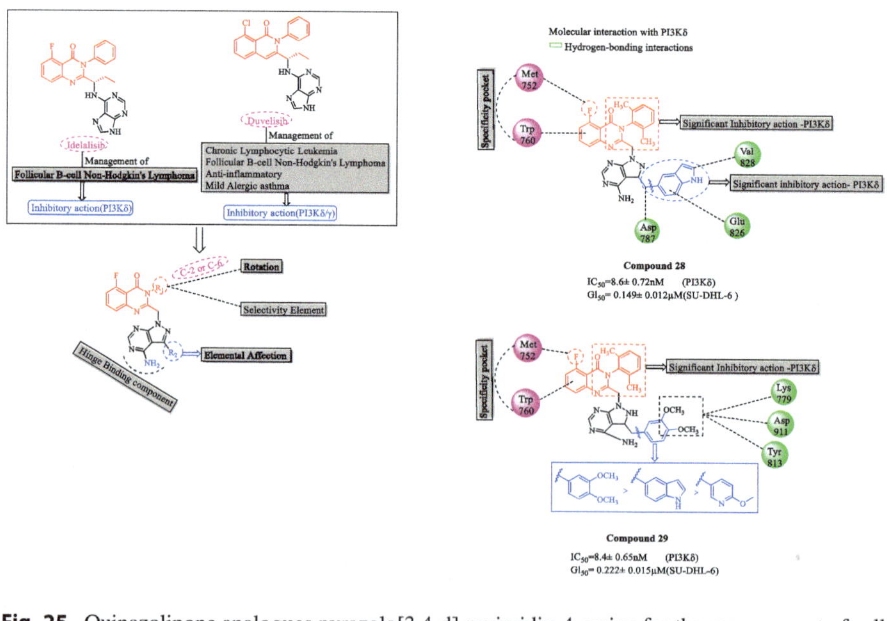

Fig. 25 Quinazolinone analogues pyrazolo[3,4-d] pyrimidin-4-amine for the management of cell-moderate immunity and hematological malignancies

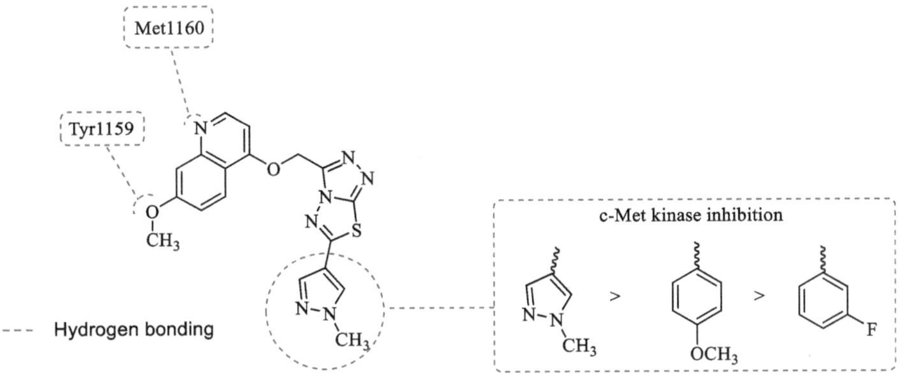

Compound 30

Antiproliferatory activity against
c-Met kinase cell line: IC_{50} = 0.00202 μM
c-Met phosphorylation in MKN45: IC_{50} = 88 nM
SNU-5 cell line: %inhibition = 68.7%
MKN_{45} cell line: %inhibition = 71.9%
EBC-1 cell line: %inhibition = 84.4%

Fig. 26 [1,2,4]triazolo[1,3,4]thiadiazole derivatives as c-Met kinase inhibitors

inhibitor of tubulin at a concentration of 1 μM and showed cytotoxic activity with IC_{50} value of 0.07 ± 0.001 μM, 0.53 ± 0.0 μM, 0.28 ± 0.02 μM, 0.54 ± 0.09 μM, 0.36 ± 0.02 μM, 0.47 ± 0.01 μM, 0.6 ± 0.08 μM against HCT116, A2780, K562R, A2780R, JIM-T1, HCT116, and K562 cell lines, respectively. Moreover, **compound 31** arrested cell cycle in G2/M phase and caused apoptosis of HCT116 cell line at 5 μM concentration. SAR study revealed that conversion of CH_3 group with electron-withdraw such as CN, CF_3, and Cl group at C-2 caused reduction of cytotoxicity effect. Substitution at quinoline and carbazole reduced cytotoxicity effects (Fig. 27) (Khelifi et al. 2019).

In 2020, Teng et al. designed and synthesized a novel series of quinazoline analogues as PI3kδ inhibitors. After evaluation of compounds, **compound 32** was the most potent inhibitor of PI3Kδ with an IC_{50} value of 27.5 nM and also exhibited antiproliferation properties against Raji and Ramos cells with IC_{50} values 8.5 and 5.4 nM. **Compound 32** shows fatality rate > inhibition after 24 h on 10 μM concentration against Raji cells and possesses least metabolic stability. Molecular docking studies revealed that **compound 32** interacts with non-conversed residue Asp832 and Val828 in the binding site of PI3Kδ rather than PI3K (Fig. 28) (Teng et al. 2020).

In 2020, Antoni et al. designed and synthesized a novel series of tariquidar-based triazoles derivatives as breast cancer resistance protein inhibitors. From all the synthesized compounds, the **compounds 33** and **34** significantly inhibited ABCG2 cell growth with IC_{50} value of 79 ± 5 nM and 81 ± 16 nM, respectively. Moreover, at a concentration of 1 nM, **compound 33** was nontoxic whereas **compound 34** on excess concentration shows cytotoxic effect. SAR study revealed that substitution on benzamide group increased activity against ABCG2 and ABCB1, substitution of

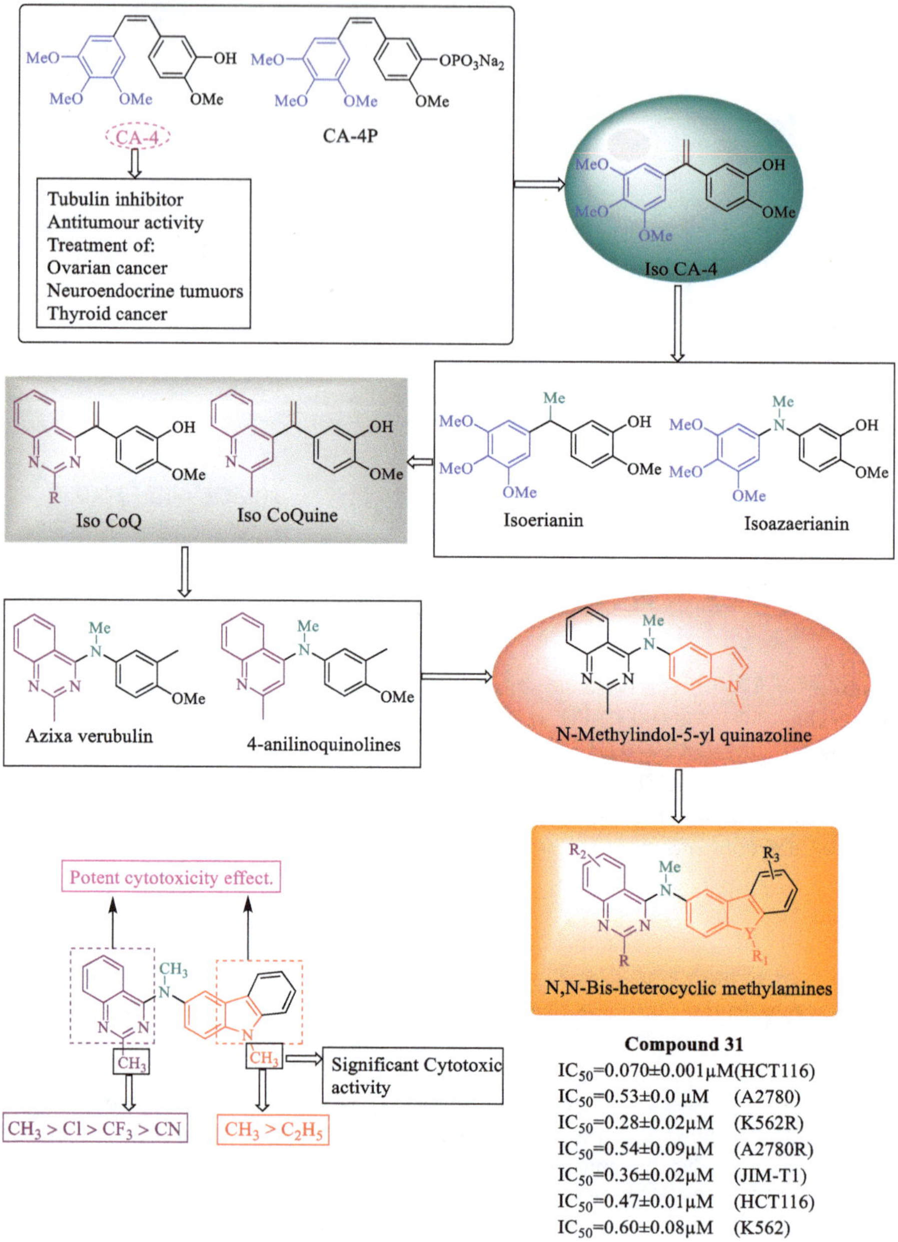

Fig. 27 N, N-Bis heteroaryl methylamines 1 like isoazaerianin derivatives as anticancer agents

2-methylene group on tetrahydroisoquinoline group causes inactivation of the compound and substitution of propionyl was more potent at acetyl group (Fig. 29) (Antoni et al. 2020).

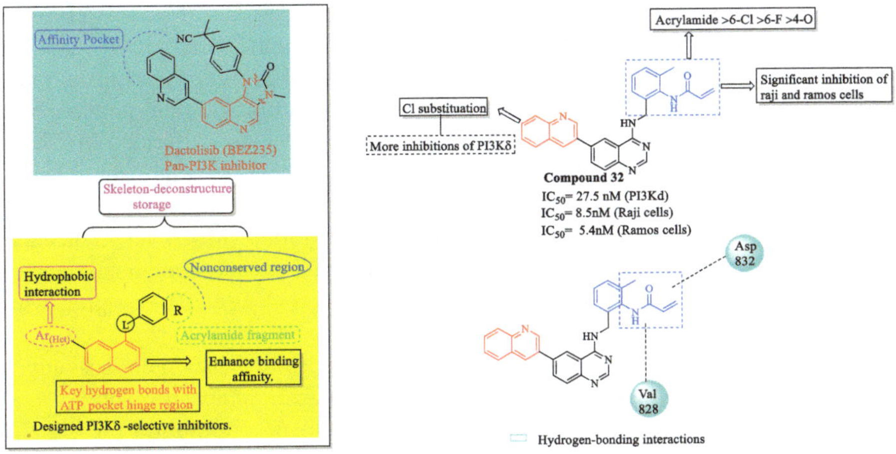

Fig. 28 Quinazoline analogues as PI3kδ inhibitors

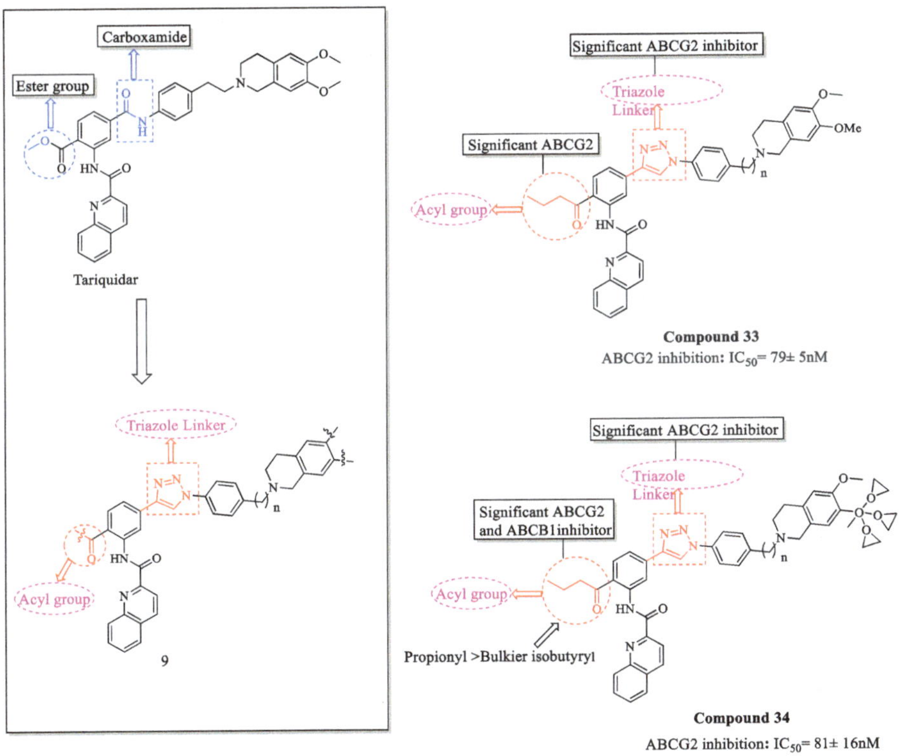

Fig. 29 Novel series of tariquidar-based triazoles derivatives as breast cancer resistance protein inhibitors

In 2022, Nippu et al. designed and synthesized a series of novel tetrazolo quinoline-isatin scaffold derivatives to determine the anticancer activity against MIA PaCa-2 cancer cell line. Among these, **compound 35** was found to be most active with IC_{50} value of 60.17 ± 3.12 μM, respectively. In addition, pharmacokinetic studies like ADMET screening and Lipinski rule were performed in which potent compound showed considerable drug ability. Further, structure activity pattern suggested that both unsubstituted benzene rings in the structure were most favorable for inhibitory potential than halogen substitution. Moreover, molecular docking studies revealed that **compound 35** is stabilized via hydrogen bond interaction with His207, Trp387, Gln203, π-alkyl with Val444, Val291, π-sigma with Trp387 (Fig. 30) (Nippu et al. 2022).

In 2022, Omidkhah et al. synthesized a novel series of benzamide derivatives containing quinoline nucleus to evaluate them for their anticancer activity and evaluated them against histone deacetylase. Among them, **compound 36** was the most potent against HT-29 (IC_{50}: 14.5 ± 1.5 μM), HCT116 (IC_{50}: 8.6 ± 0.8 μM) cell line for cytotoxicity and HCT116 (IC_{50}: 1.1 ± 0.1 μM), HT-29 (IC_{50}: 2.9 ± 0.38 μM) cell line to determine HDAC inhibitory potential. Structure activity pattern suggested that only methyl group next to nitrogen in quinoline structure was sufficient for antiproliferatory and HDAC inhibitory activity. Moreover, molecular dynamic simulations revealed that **compound 36** of both HDAC1 and HDAC3 complexes possess H-bonding interaction of Gly149 and Gly143 with carbonyl group in the active site of COX-2 (Fig. 31) (Omidkhah et al. 2022).

In 2022, Zaraei et al. designed and synthesized a series of new quinoline derivatives and assessed their C-RAF kinase inhibition and anticancer activity. Among these, **compound 37** exhibited most potent inhibitory activity against 53 cancer cell lines (TGI = 1.18–12.80) and **compound 38** showed most effective inhibition against C-RAF kinase (IC_{50} = 0.067 μM). Structure activity pattern of

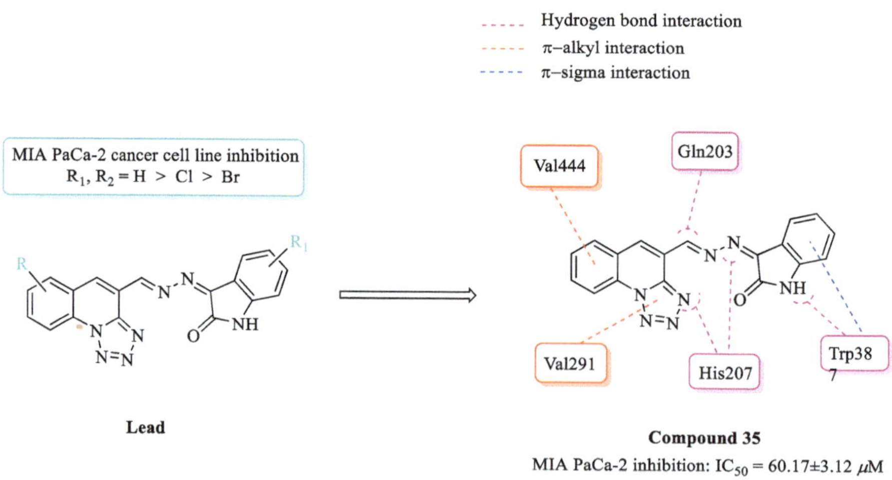

Fig. 30 Novel tetrazolo quinoline-isatin scaffold derivatives as anticancer agents

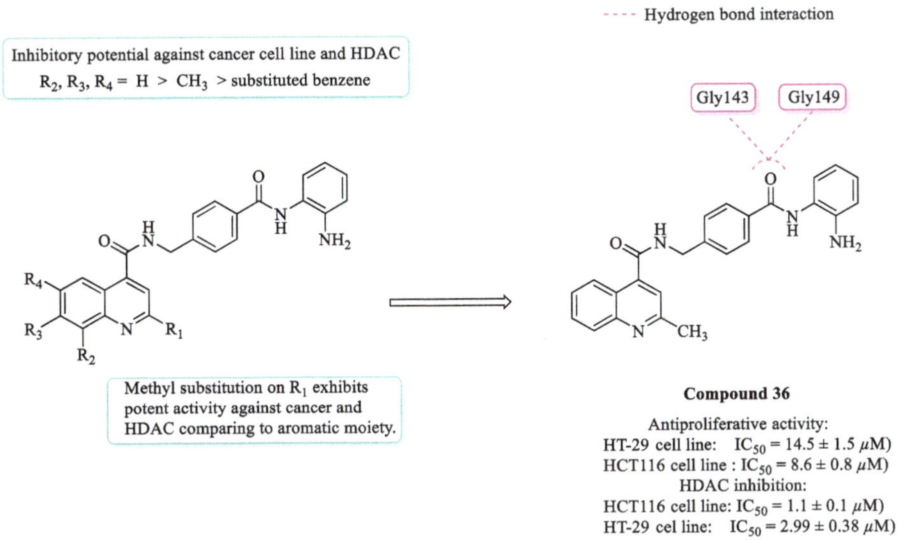

Fig. 31 Benzamide derivatives containing quinoline nucleus as histone deacetylase inhibitors

compound 37 and **38** suggested that both 4-fluoro-3-(trifluoromethyl) phenyl moiety for **compound 38** and 6-methoxy-7-(morpholinomethoxy) quinoline in **compound 37** have significant impact on antiproliferative activity and C-RAF kinase inhibition, respectively. Further, ligand–receptor interactions revealed that **compound 38** was capable of forming hydrogen bond interactions (Asn472, Asp486, Phe487, Gly485), π-sigma interactions (Val363, Thr421), π-alkyl interactions (Phe475, Ile419, Lys375), and alkyl interactions (Leu406, Leu397, Phe408) in the active site of C-RAF (Fig. 32) (Zaraei et al. 2022).

In 2022, He et al. synthesized a series of β-methyl-4-acrylamido quinoline derivatives as PI3K/mTOR dual inhibitor and evaluated to improve its anticancer activity by structure modification. Among these, **compound 39** displayed most potent antiproliferative activity against PI3K(α to δ) cell lines ($IC_{50} = 0.67 \pm 0.11$ to 1.30 ± 0.15 nM) and mTOR ($IC_{50} = 5.0 \pm 0.39$ nM). Structure activity pattern suggested that substitution of 1-methyl group at alkylcarbonyl linkage along with *N*-methyl pyridazine moiety of this linkage in *E*-configuration attached to quinoline nucleus was most favorable for improved antiproliferatory activity (Fig. 33) (He et al. 2021).

2.3 Organo-Metallic Complexes

In 2019, Qin et al. designed and synthesized a new series of Organoplatinum (II) complexes with Quinoline–Coumarin analogues as anticancer agents. These compounds exhibited anticancer activity toward A549/DPP (Cisplatin-resistance of lung adenocarcinoma in humans) and HeLa (cervical cancerous cells). From all

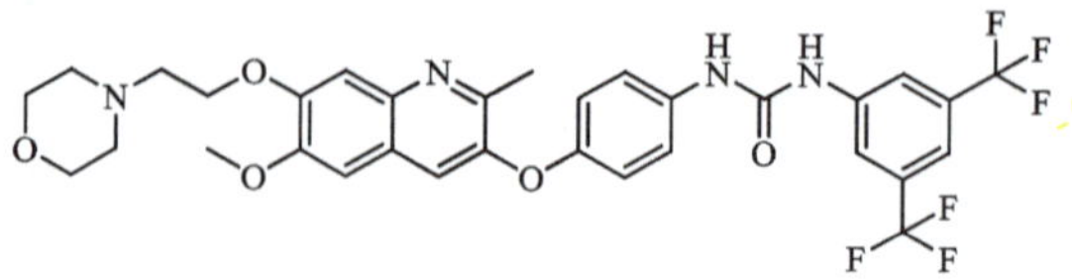

Compound 37

Anticancer activity against 53 cell lines: TGI = 1.18 -12.80

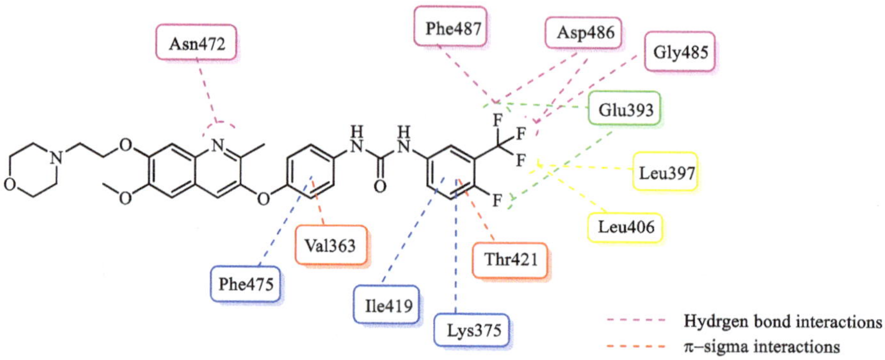

Compound 38

C-RAF kinase inhibition: $IC_{50} = 0.067\ \mu M$

Fig. 32 Quinoline derivatives as C-RAF kinase inhibitors

the synthesized compounds, **compounds 40 and 41** were the most potent anticancer agent with IC_{50} values of 0.1 ± 0.05 μM (A549/DPP), 0.15 ± 0.09 μM (HeLa), and 0.25 ± 0.11 μM (A549/DPP), 0.32 ± 0.14 μM (HeLa), respectively. Moreover, **compound 40** and **41** showed a green colored luminescence, signifying an attack to mitochondrial membrane. **Compound 40** initiated mitochondria conciliate programmed cell death on A549/DPP (Cisplatin-resistance of lung adenocarcinoma in humans) cells **more than compound 41**. SAR study revealed that substitution of 20-quinolyl-6,8-dichloro-hydroxy at C-3 position of coumarin exhibit potential antitumor effect. In vivo study suggests that **compound 40** exhibits significant antitumor activity in treated 21 days later (Fig. 34) (Qin et al. 2019).

In 2021, Shen et al. synthesized three Cu(II) complexes of quinoline derivatives and evaluated them for their chemodynamic anticancer activity against SK-OV-3 cells through ER stress and mitochondrial-mediated apoptosis. Among these, **compound 42** exhibited most effective anticancer activity against SK-OC-3 cell line with the IC_{50} value of 5.27 ± 0.59 μM and against other cell lines T24 (IC_{50} = 5.32 μM), HepG2 (IC_{50} = 14.41 μM), MGC80–3 (IC_{50} = 14.36 μM), WI-38 (IC_{50} = 15.67 μM) (Fig. 35) (Shen et al. 2021).

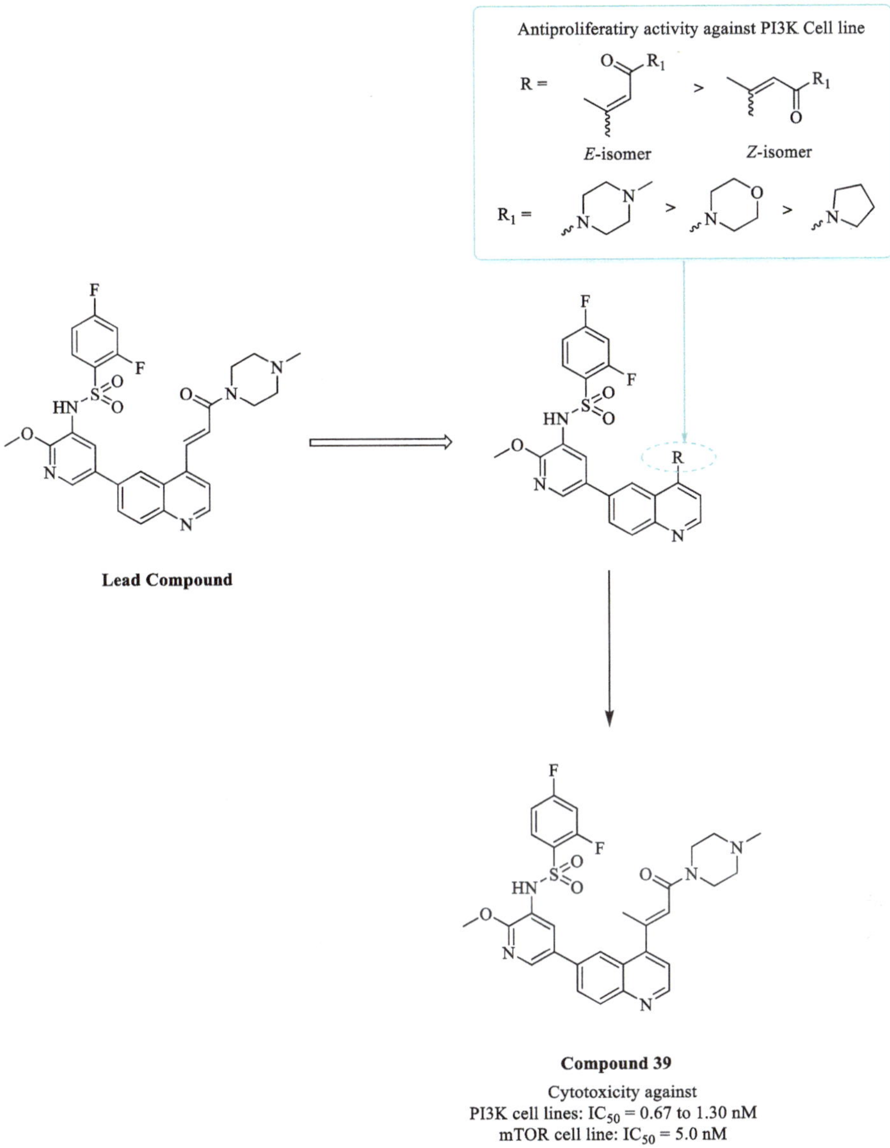

Fig. 33 β-methyl-4-acrylamido quinoline derivatives as PI3K/mTOR dual inhibitors

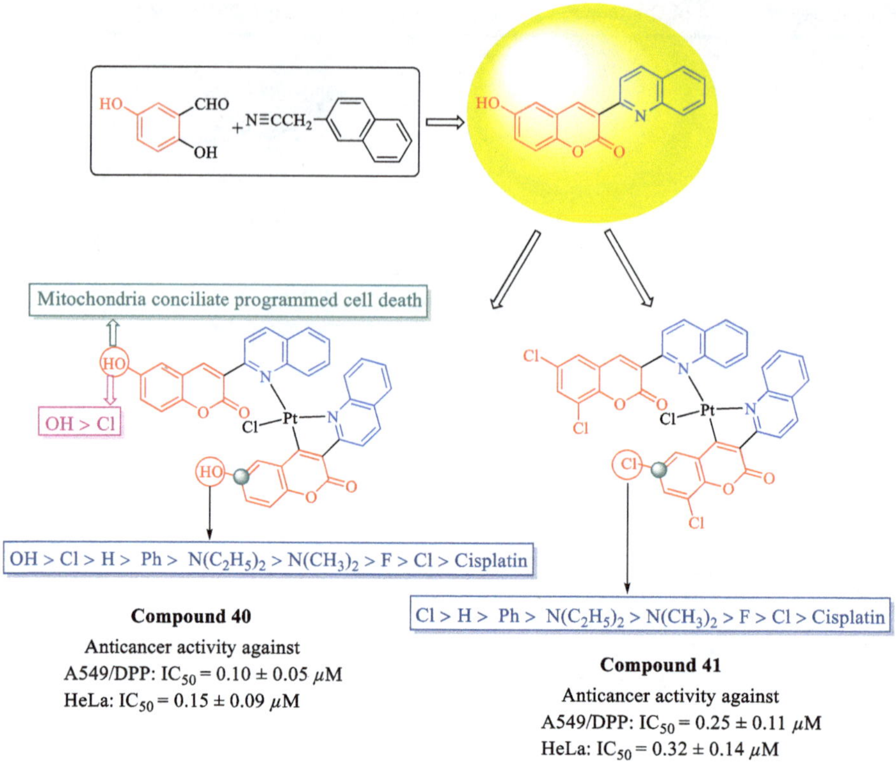

Fig. 34 Organoplatinum (II) complexes with Quinoline–Coumarin analogues as anticancer agents

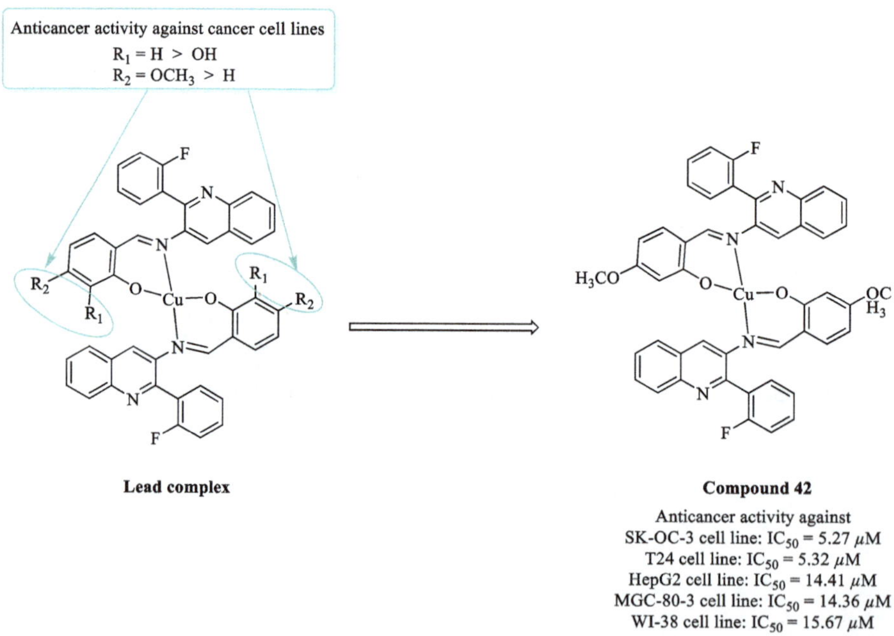

Fig. 35 Cu(II) complexes of quinoline derivatives as anticancer agents

3 Conclusion

Cancer is an uncontrolled cell growth with capabilities to spread and infect nearby tissues and body parts and its current treatment has high toxicity and low efficacy. Moreover, there is an increased rate of emergence of cancer cases due to sedentary lifestyle, global warming, bad eating habits, etc., which has led to increased demand of new molecules that have low toxicity profile and have high efficiency. Therefore, in pursuit of new molecules scientists came across quinoline (C_9H_7N, 129.16 Da), a privileged scaffold that has been associated with multiple biological activities like antiviral, antibacterial, antimalarial, antifungal, antitubercular, antileishmanial, anti-inflammatory, anti-HIV, and anticancer. This multifarious profile helped quinoline to gain the attention of researchers to develop new anticancer moieties by sequential modification of the substituents attached to it. Among all designed and synthesized quinoline compounds, **compound 7** ($IC_{50} = 0.4 \pm 0.04$ nM) against A549 cells, **compound 19** ($IC_{50} = 0.67$ to 1.30 nM) against PI3K cell lines, **compound 22** ($IC_{50} = 0.87$ nM) against PI3Kδ displayed higher potency for antiproliferatory activity after in vitro screening and ligand–receptor interactions. These top three drug molecules proved to be excellent candidates against various cancerous cells. Hence, overall study concluded that quinoline moiety could act as a hot lead for designing of safer and highly potent molecules for the treatment of cancer.

Acknowledgments This work was supported by the research funds under Indian Council of Medical Research (ICMR: BMI/11(04)/2022 and, Council of Scientific and Industrial Research (CSIR: 02(0319)17/EMRII). The contents of this article are solely the responsibility of the authors. The authors are very thankful to Guru Nanak Dev University, Amritsar, India for providing various basic facilities to complete the work.

Conflict of Interests All authors declare that they have no conflict of interest. No writing assistance was utilized in the production of this manuscript.

References

Almansour AI, Arumugam N, Suresh Kumar R, Mahalingam SM, Sau S, Bianchini G, Menéndez JC, Altaf M, Ghabbour HA (2017) Design, synthesis and antiproliferative activity of decarbonyl luotonin analogues. Eur J Med Chem 138:932–941. https://doi.org/10.1016/J.EJMECH.2017.07.027

Alonso C, Fuertes M, Martín-Encinas E, Selas A, Rubiales G, Tesauro C, Knudssen BK, Palacios F (2018) Novel topoisomerase I inhibitors. Syntheses and biological evaluation of phosphorus substituted quinoline derivates with antiproliferative activity. Eur J Med Chem 149:225–237. https://doi.org/10.1016/J.EJMECH.2018.02.058

Antoni F, Bause M, Scholler M, Bauer S, Stark SA, Jackson SM, Manolaridis I, Locher KP, König B, Buschauer A, Bernhardt G (2020) Tariquidar-related triazoles as potent, selective and stable inhibitors of ABCG2 (BCRP). Eur J Med Chem 191:112133. https://doi.org/10.1016/J.EJMECH.2020.112133

Chen C, Hou X, Wang G, Pan W, Yang X, Zhang Y, Fang H (2017) Design, synthesis and biological evaluation of quinoline derivatives as HDAC class I inhibitors. Eur J Med Chem 133: 11–23. https://doi.org/10.1016/J.EJMECH.2017.03.064

Cheung WY, Le LW, Zimmermann C (2009) Symptom clusters in patients with advanced cancers. Support Care Cancer 17:1223–1230. https://doi.org/10.1007/s00520-009-0577-7

Crespo I, Giménez-Dejoz J, Porté S, Cousido-Siah A, Mitschler A, Podjarny A, Pratsinis H, Kletsas D, Parés X, Ruiz FX, Metwally K, Farrés J (2018) Design, synthesis, structure-activity relationships and X-ray structural studies of novel 1-oxopyrimido[4,5-c]quinoline-2-acetic acid derivatives as selective and potent inhibitors of human aldose reductase. Eur J Med Chem 152: 160–174. https://doi.org/10.1016/J.EJMECH.2018.04.015

Ge R, Zhao Q, Xie Z, Lu L, Guo Q, Li Z, Zhao L (2016) Synthesis and biological evaluation of 6-fluoro-3-phenyl-7-piperazinyl quinolone derivatives as potential topoisomerase I inhibitors. Eur J Med Chem 122:465–474. https://doi.org/10.1016/J.EJMECH.2016.06.054

Hauguel C, Ducellier S, Provot O, Ibrahim N, Lamaa D, Balcerowiak C, Letribot B, Nascimento M, Blanchard V, Askenatzis L, Levaique H, Bignon J, Baschieri F, Bauvais C, Bollot G, Renko D, Deroussent A, Prost B, Laisne MC, Michallet S, Lafanechère L, Papot S, Montagnac G, Tran C, Alami M, Apcher S, Hamze A (2022) Design, synthesis and biological evaluation of quinoline-2-carbonitrile-based hydroxamic acids as dual tubulin polymerization and histone deacetylases inhibitors. Eur J Med Chem 240:114573. https://doi.org/10.1016/J.EJMECH.2022.114573

He R, Xu B, Ping L, Lv X (2021) Structural optimization towards promising β-methyl-4-acrylamido quinoline derivatives as PI3K/mTOR dual inhibitors for anti-cancer therapy: the in vitro and in vivo biological evaluation. Eur J Med Chem 214:113249. https://doi.org/10.1016/J.EJMECH.2021.113249

Jitender Dev G, Poornachandra Y, Ratnakar Reddy K, Naresh Kumar R, Ravikumar N, Krishna Swaroop D, Ranjithreddy P, Shravan Kumar G, Nanubolu JB, Ganesh Kumar C, Narsaiah B (2017) Synthesis of novel pyrazolo[3,4-b]quinolinyl acetamide analogs, their evaluation for antimicrobial and anticancer activities, validation by molecular modeling and CoMFA analysis. Eur J Med Chem 130:223–239. https://doi.org/10.1016/J.EJMECH.2017.02.052

John SKP, George S, Primrose JN, Fozard JBJ (2011) Symptoms and signs in patients with colorectal cancer. Color Dis 13:17–25. https://doi.org/10.1111/j.1463-1318.2010.02221.x

Joshi PV, Sayed AA, RaviKumar A, Puranik VG, Zinjarde SS (2017) 4-phenyl quinoline derivatives as potential serotonin receptor ligands with antiproliferative activity. Eur J Med Chem 136:246–258. https://doi.org/10.1016/J.EJMECH.2017.05.002

Khelifi I, Naret T, Renko D, Hamze A, Bernadat G, Bignon J, Lenoir C, Dubois J, Brion JD, Provot O, Alami M (2017) Design, synthesis and anticancer properties of IsoCombretaQuinolines as potent tubulin assembly inhibitors. Eur J Med Chem 127:1025–1034. https://doi.org/10.1016/J.EJMECH.2016.11.012

Khelifi I, Naret T, Hamze A, Bignon J, Levaique H, Garcia Alvarez MC, Dubois J, Provot O, Alami M (2019) N,N-bis-heteroaryl methylamines: potent anti-mitotic and highly cytotoxic agents. Eur J Med Chem 168:176–188. https://doi.org/10.1016/J.EJMECH.2019.02.038

Krstulović L, Stolić I, Jukić M, Opačak-Bernardi T, Starčević K, Bajić M, Glavaš-Obrovac L (2017) New quinoline-arylamidine hybrids: synthesis, DNA/RNA binding and antitumor activity. Eur J Med Chem 137:196–210. https://doi.org/10.1016/J.EJMECH.2017.05.054

Kwak SH, Shin S, Lee JH, Shim JK, Kim M, Lee SD, Lee A, Bae J, Park JH, Abdelrahman A, Müller CE, Cho SK, Kang SG, Bae MA, Yang JY, Ko H, Goddard WA, Kim YC (2018) Synthesis and structure-activity relationships of quinolinone and quinoline-based P2X7 receptor antagonists and their anti-sphere formation activities in glioblastoma cells. Eur J Med Chem 151:462–481. https://doi.org/10.1016/J.EJMECH.2018.03.023

Kwon S, Lee Y, Jung Y, Kim JH, Baek B, Lim B, Lee J, Kim I, Lee J (2018) Mitochondria-targeting indolizino[3,2-c]quinolines as novel class of photosensitizers for photodynamic anticancer activity. Eur J Med Chem 148:116–127. https://doi.org/10.1016/J.EJMECH.2018.02.016

Lee HY, Chang CY, Su CJ, Huang HL, Mehndiratta S, Chao YH, Hsu CM, Kumar S, Sung TY, Huang YZ, Li YH, Yang CR, Liou JP (2016) 2-(Phenylsulfonyl)quinoline N-hydroxyacrylamides as potent anticancer agents inhibiting histone deacetylase. Eur J Med Chem 122:92–101. https://doi.org/10.1016/J.EJMECH.2016.06.023

Li W, Shuai W, Sun H, Xu F, Bi Y, Xu J, Ma C, Yao H, Zhu Z, Xu S (2019) Design, synthesis and biological evaluation of quinoline-indole derivatives as anti-tubulin agents targeting the colchicine binding site. Eur J Med Chem 163:428–442. https://doi.org/10.1016/J.EJMECH.2018.11.070

Liu M, Hou Y, Yin W, Zhou S, Qian P, Guo Z, Xu L, Zhao Y (2016a) Discovery of a novel 6,7-disubstituted-4-(2-fluorophenoxy)quinolines bearing 1,2,3-triazole-4-carboxamide moiety as potent c-Met kinase inhibitors. Eur J Med Chem 119:96–108. https://doi.org/10.1016/J.EJMECH.2016.04.035

Liu J, Nie M, Wang Y, Hu J, Zhang F, Gao Y, Liu Y, Gong P (2016b) Design, synthesis and structure-activity relationships of novel 4-phenoxyquinoline derivatives containing 1,2,4-triazolone moiety as c-Met kinase inhibitors. Eur J Med Chem 123:431–446. https://doi.org/10.1016/J.EJMECH.2016.07.059

Ma CC, Zhang CM, Tang LQ, Liu ZP (2018) Discovery of novel quinazolinone derivatives as high potent and selective PI3Kδ and PI3Kδ/γ inhibitors. Eur J Med Chem 151:9–17. https://doi.org/10.1016/J.EJMECH.2018.03.068

Nippu BN, Sandeep Kumar Jain R, Rahman A, Kumaraswamy HM, Satyanarayan ND (2022) Design and synthesis of novel tetrazolo quinoline bridged isatin derivatives as potential anticancer leads against MIA PaCa-2 human pancreatic cancer cell line. J Mol Struct 1263:133103. https://doi.org/10.1016/J.MOLSTRUC.2022.133103

Omidkhah N, Hadizadeh F, Abnous K, Ghodsi R (2022) Synthesis, structure activity relationship and biological evaluation of a novel series of quinoline–based benzamide derivatives as anticancer agents and histone deacetylase (HDAC) inhibitors. J Mol Struct 1267:133599. https://doi.org/10.1016/J.MOLSTRUC.2022.133599

Palluotto F, Sosic A, Pinato O, Zoidis G, Catto M, Sissi C, Gatto B, Carotti A (2016) Quinolino[3,4-b]quinoxalines and pyridazino[4,3-c]quinoline derivatives: synthesis, inhibition of topoisomerase IIα, G-quadruplex binding and cytotoxic properties. Eur J Med Chem 123:704–717. https://doi.org/10.1016/J.EJMECH.2016.07.063

Perin N, Nhili R, Cindrić M, Bertoša B, Vušak D, Martin-Kleiner I, Laine W, Karminski-Zamola G, Kralj M, David-Cordonnier MH, Hranjec M (2016) Amino substituted benzimidazo[1,2-a]quinolines: Antiproliferative potency, 3D QSAR study and DNA binding properties. Eur J Med Chem 122:530–545. https://doi.org/10.1016/J.EJMECH.2016.07.007

Qin QP, Wang ZF, Huang XL, Tan MX, Zou BQ, Liang H (2019) Strong in vitro and vivo cytotoxicity of novel organoplatinum(II) complexes with quinoline-coumarin derivatives. Eur J Med Chem 184:111751. https://doi.org/10.1016/J.EJMECH.2019.111751

Shaikh SKJ, Kamble RR, Somagond SM, Devarajegowda HC, Dixit SR, Joshi SD (2017) Tetrazolylmethyl quinolines: design, docking studies, synthesis, anticancer and antifungal analyses. Eur J Med Chem 128:258–273. https://doi.org/10.1016/J.EJMECH.2017.01.043

Shen WY, Jia CP, Mo AN, Liang H, Chen ZF (2021) Chemodynamic therapy agents cu (II) complexes of quinoline derivatives induced ER stress and mitochondria-mediated apoptosis in SK-OV-3 cells. Eur J Med Chem 223:113636. https://doi.org/10.1016/J.EJMECH.2021.113636

Shobeiri N, Rashedi M, Mosaffa F, Zarghi A, Ghandadi M, Ghasemi A, Ghodsi R (2016) Synthesis and biological evaluation of quinoline analogues of flavones as potential anticancer agents and tubulin polymerization inhibitors. Eur J Med Chem 114:14–23. https://doi.org/10.1016/J.EJMECH.2016.02.069

Soliman MHA, Ali IAI, El-Sakka SSA, Mohamed OESAB (2022) Novel quinoline derivatives as antitumor agents against HepG2 cells: synthesis, characterization, in silico, in vitro and docking studies. J Mol Struct 1254:132325. https://doi.org/10.1016/J.MOLSTRUC.2021.132325

Teng Y, Li X, Ren S, Cheng Y, Xi K, Shen H, Ma W, Luo G, Xiang H (2020) Discovery of novel quinazoline derivatives as potent PI3Kδ inhibitors with high selectivity. Eur J Med Chem 208: 112865. https://doi.org/10.1016/J.EJMECH.2020.112865

Zaraei SO, Al-Ach NN, Anbar HS, El-Gamal R, Tarazi H, Tokatly RT, Kalla RR, Munther MA, Wahba MM, Alshihabi AM, Shehata MK, Sbenati RM, Shahin AI, El-Awady R, Al-Tel TH, El-Gamal MI (2022) Design and synthesis of new quinoline derivatives as selective C-RAF kinase inhibitors with potent anticancer activity. Eur J Med Chem 238:114434. https://doi.org/10.1016/J.EJMECH.2022.114434

Zhang J, Lv X, Ma X, Hu Y (2017) Discovery of a series of N-(5-(quinolin-6-yl)pyridin-3-yl) benzenesulfonamides as PI3K/mTOR dual inhibitors. Eur J Med Chem 127:509–520. https://doi.org/10.1016/J.EJMECH.2017.01.016

Zhang L, Zhao J, Zhang B, Lu T, Chen Y (2018) Discovery of [1,2,4]triazolo[3,4-b][1,3,4] thiadiazole derivatives as novel, potent and selective c-met kinase inhibitors: synthesis, SAR study, and biological activity. Eur J Med Chem 150:809–816. https://doi.org/10.1016/J.EJMECH.2018.03.049

Zhou Y, Yan W, Cao D, Shao M, Li D, Wang F, Yang Z, Chen Y, He L, Wang T, Shen M, Chen L (2017) Design, synthesis and biological evaluation of 4-anilinoquinoline derivatives as novel potent tubulin depolymerization agents. Eur J Med Chem 138:1114–1125. https://doi.org/10.1016/J.EJMECH.2017.07.040

Antitumor Immunotherapy: Effect of COVID-19 in Cancer Patients

Irina Zh. Shubina, Irina O. Chikileva, and Nikolay Yu. Sokolov

Abstract

Alteration of the immune status leading to impaired immune responses is associated with a more severe course of infectious diseases, including COVID-19. Cancer patients often experience immunosuppression as a result of treatment; therefore, they are at a greater risk of severe COVID-19 and related mortality, as well as the development of serious complications of viral infection. In addition, the malignant disease can cause immunodeficiency, especially in patients with advanced cancer. The review discusses the reported data of the immunological parameters and therapy effectiveness in cancer and non-cancer patients with COVID-19.

A comprehensive search for relevant literature in PubMed (Medline), Embase, Web of Science, Scopus and ClinicalTrials.gov was used to identify the appropriate studies up to June 2022. Various combinations of keywords were used, such as immunity, COVID-19, cancer, immune checkpoint inhibitors (ICI), antitumor immunotherapy, meta-analysis, etc.

The review describes the outcomes of the immunotherapy in cancer patients with SARS-CoV-2 infection, the mechanism of action of immune checkpoint inhibitors (ICI), the immune responses to the coronavirus infection, and the assumption that antitumor therapy with immune checkpoint inhibitors can induce immune competence in patients infected with SARS-CoV-2.

However, to date, only limited studies can clearly demonstrate the protective effect of ICI against SARS-CoV-2 infection. Expanded experimental and clinical

I. Z. Shubina (✉) · I. O. Chikileva
N.N. Blokhin National Medical Research Center of Oncology, Ministry of Health of Russia, Moscow, Russia
e-mail: irinashubina@mail.ru

N. Y. Sokolov
Botkin Hospital, Moscow, Russia

Interdisciplinary Cancer Research, https://doi.org/10.1007/16833_2022_100
Published online: 17 December 2022

studies are required to determine the role of antitumor immunotherapy in the development of COVID-19 in cancer patients.

Keywords

Antitumor immunotherapy · Cancer · COVID-19 · Immune checkpoint inhibitors · Immunity

Abbreviations

CCL2	Chemokine C-C motif ligand 2
CI	Confidence interval
COVID	Coronavirus disease
CTL	Cytotoxic T lymphocytes
DC	Dendritic cells
G-CSF	Granulocyte colony-stimulating factor
ICI	Immune checkpoint inhibitors
IFN	Interferon
IL	Interleukin
IP-10	Interferon gamma-induced protein 10
MCP-1	Monocyte chemoattractant protein 1
MERS-CoV	Middle East respiratory syndrome-related coronavirus
MHC	Major histocompatibility complex
MIP-1A	Macrophage inflammatory proteins 1a
NET	Neutrophil extracellular traps
NK	Natural killer
OR	Odds ratio
PD-1	Programmed cell death protein 1
PD-L1	Ligand for PD-1
RT-PCR	Polymerase chain reaction with reverse transcription
SARS-CoV	Severe acute respiratory syndrome coronavirus
Th	T-helper cells
TNF	Tumor necrosis factor

1 Introduction

A vast number of data about the most severe coronavirus human infections such as MERS-CoV, SARS-CoV and SARS-CoV-2, which have been accumulated over the last decades, demonstrated that multifunctional reactions of CD4+ and CD8+ T cells play a crucial role (Razavi et al. 2021) in the immune response to the viral attack, which are, probably, amplified by the early production of IgM and IgA, and subsequently, IgG.

Although it seems evident that T lymphocyte reactions can provide an effective and long-term defense against SARS-CoV-2, the role of humoral immunity is still unclear.

The analysis of multiple data has led to paradoxical conclusions that the mortality associated with COVID-19 mainly results from the dysregulated immune response to the virus including the "cytokine storm" with overproduction of pro- and anti-inflammatory cytokines, chemokines, pro-apoptotic and other secreted factors (IL-1, IL-2, IL-6, IL-7, IL-8, IL-10, IL-17, IFN-γ, TNF-α, IP-10, MCP-1, G-CSF MIP-1A, CCL2, etc.) (Sun et al. 2020; Vlachakis et al. 2020), but not from the virus replication affecting different organs (Melenotte et al. 2020).

An appropriate interaction of the two parts of the immune system, innate and adaptive immunity, is necessary for the effective immune response to the penetration of the pathogen into the human body. Innate immunity serves as the body's first line of defense acting in a rapid and non-specific way. Along with the innate immune responses, adaptive immune competent cells are activated and transmit antigen-specific signals to T cells, which subsequently differentiate into effector T cells secreting pro- or anti-inflammatory cytokines, and B cells, which differentiate into plasma cells producing specific antibodies. The innate immunity responds to antigens in a non-specific way. The adaptive immunity includes virus-specific CD4+ T cells, CD8+ T cells and antibodies (produced by B cells). Besides, T- and B-memory cells make it possible to store information for a rapid specific immune response upon repeated contact with the antigen (Fig. 1).

Effectors of the innate immunity represent the first line of the antimicrobial defense. Phagocytes such as neutrophils and macrophages capture and destroy viral particles, bacteria, etc. Besides, neutrophils secrete antimicrobial reactive oxygen species and produce neutrophil extracellular traps (NET) that create a

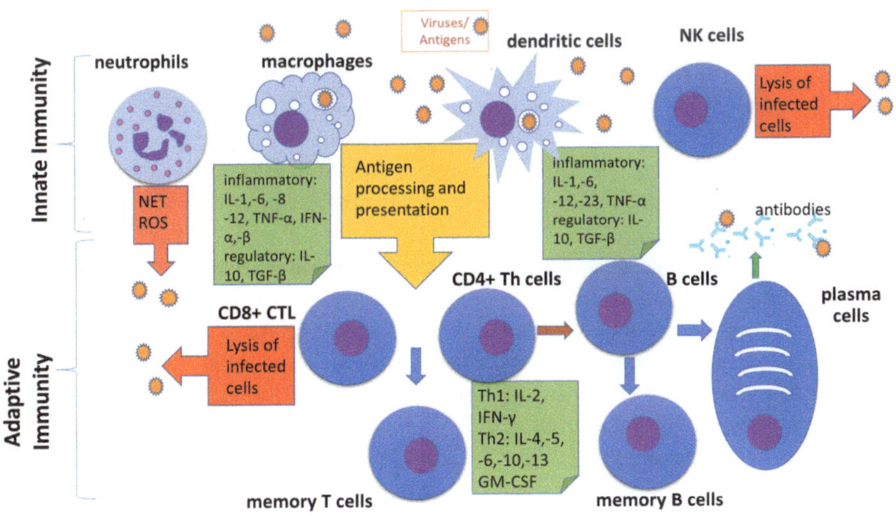

Fig. 1 Major components of the innate and adaptive immune response to the viral infection

specific area with high local concentration of antimicrobial agents. Macrophages and dendritic cells (DC) process pathogenic antigens and present processed antigenic peptides within MHC-I and MHC-II (major histocompatibility complex) molecules to cytotoxic T lymphocytes (CTL) and T-helper (Th) cells, respectively. Thus, they provide innate and adaptive immunity interaction. In addition, DCs and macrophages produce various cytokines and regulate the activated type of the immune response. Natural killer (NK) cells and CTLs recognize and lyse infected cells. However, NK cells respond at an early phase of the immune response since NKs have innate receptors to recognize self or non-self (or infected) cells. Specific CTL functions require priming by antigen-presenting cells such as DCs and macrophages. Th cells produce different cytokines that regulate immune response and promote B-cell differentiation into antibody-producing plasma cells. Antibodies neutralize antigens and may induce antibody-dependent cytotoxicity against antibody-bound infected cells. After infection cessation, effector T and B cells produce adaptive immune memory cells protecting the organism against future pathogen challenges.

The innate immune response develops rapidly within a few hours after the infection has affected the organism. Innate immune reactions detain the replication and spread of the virus, while simultaneously triggering the adaptive immune reactions. The adaptive immune response develops slower due to the essential process of selection and proliferation of virus-specific cells arising from the large pools of naive B and T cells specific to various molecular structures and peptide sequences. Following viral antigen priming, an appropriate adaptive immune response, which involves a sufficient number of the effector cells aimed to fight the infection, develops within approximately 6–10 days.

Adaptive immune response plays an important role in the COVID-19 pathogenesis (Kiselevskiy et al. 2020). In general, the innate immune response after the contact with SARS-CoV-2 develops efficiently within an adequate period that results in an asymptomatic infection (approximately 40% of SARS-CoV-2 infections are asymptomatic) or a clinically "mild" disease ("mild course of the disease" is a clinical definition of COVID-19, meaning that hospitalization is not required), since T-cell reactions and antibody production arise rapidly enough to provide successful control of the infection (Fig. 2). Therefore, an appropriate number of T cells and antibodies are associated with the effective resolution of "mild" cases with COVID-19 (Sette and Crotty 2021).

Considering the general course of COVID-19, the innate immunity can delay the development of the disease for some time, which is enough to activate the adaptive cellular and humoral immune response. Due to this mechanism, the infection often proceeds in an asymptomatic or a mild form, i.e., which requires no hospitalization. (1) Adequate immune response to viral infection starts rapidly with the innate effectors (NK cells, neutrophils, interferons (IFNs)) and is completed by T cells and virus-neutralizing antibodies resulting in the efficient viral clearance. (2) Severe viral infection may result from delayed innate immune response and deficient T cell response.

Basically, virus-specific CD4+ T cells, CD8+ T cells and B-cell produced antibodies represent major components of acute adaptive immunity against viral

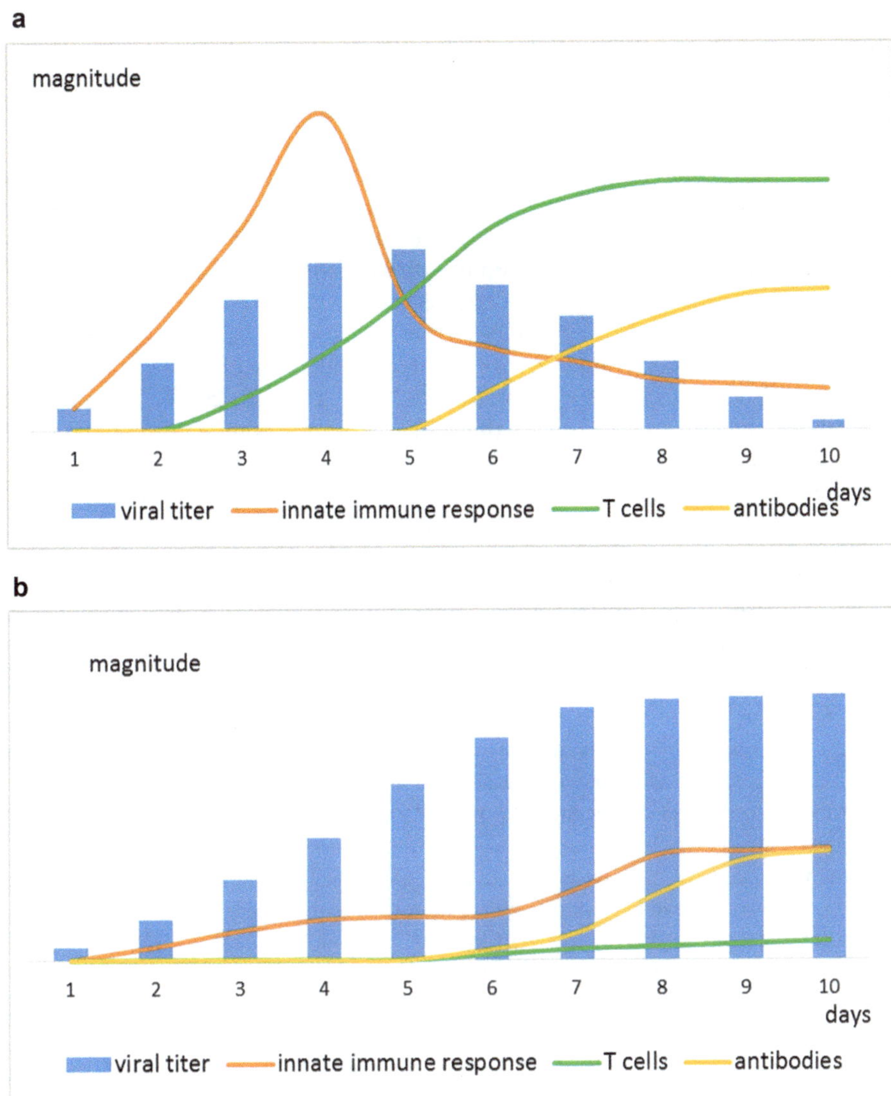

Fig. 2 (**a**, **b**) Schematic presentation of the time periods for the immune response to the viral infection

infection. NK cells, macrophages and neutrophils compose cellular basis for the innate immune response. Recently, some studies have revealed a special role of neutrophil extracellular traps (NET) in the innate defense against pathogens (Brinkmann et al. 2004). These extracellular net-like structures, produced by neutrophils and composed of DNA fibers, histones, enzymes, peptide granules, etc., are characterized by marked immunogenic, trombogenic and toxic functions. Moreover, the reports demonstrated NET involvement in tumor progression and metastatic processes (Masucci et al. 2020), though some evidence was found that NET might have an antitumor function as well (Saffarzadeh et al. 2012).

Alteration of the immune status leading to impaired immune responses is associated with a more severe course of infectious diseases, including COVID-19. Cancer patients often experience immunosuppression as a result of treatment; therefore, they are at a greater risk of severe COVID-19 and related mortality, as well as the development of serious complications of viral infection. In addition, the malignant disease can cause immunodeficiency, especially in patients with advanced cancer. So far, a number of studies have shown that COVID-19 increases complications and the overall risk of death in patients with different types of neoplasms (Dai et al. 2020; Rogado et al. 2020; Zhang et al. 2020). Thus, Dai M et al. found that cancer patients were three times more susceptible to an unfavorable outcome associated with COVID-19 compared to the general population, that was a consequence of the depressed immunity caused both by the malignant process and by the ongoing antitumor therapy (Dai et al. 2020). The researchers analyzed the data of 105 oncological and 536 age-comparable non-oncological patients with COVID-19. Patients with cancer had a relatively higher mortality rate, a higher rate of hospitalization into the intensive care unit, a higher probability of treatment with invasive mechanical lung ventilation and an increased risk of developing critical symptoms associated with COVID-19 compared with those of non-oncological patients (Dai et al. 2020). Patients with hematological diseases, including leukemia, lymphoma and myeloma, had the highest mortality rate; patients with lung cancer and esophageal cancer were also reported to have a high mortality rate, though somewhat lower than the patients with hematoblastoses (Riches 2021; Kuderer et al. 2020a, b; Khoury et al. 2022, Rubinstein et al. 2022). In addition, patients with stage IV metastatic cancer and COVID-19 had an overall higher risk of death, hospitalization in the intensive care unit, the development of severe conditions and treatment with artificial lung ventilation (Dai et al. 2020).

Numerous retrospective studies showed that different antitumor therapies have different effects on the course and outcome of COVID-19 (Dai et al. 2020; Kuderer et al. 2020a, b; Khoury et al. 2022; Yeoh et al. 2020; Mohseni Afshar 2022).

Another important consideration refers to the age-related criteria, since the vast majority of cancer patients are the elderly, and the old age was noted as an additional risk factor (Lunski et al. 2021). In particular, a retrospective study of confirmed COVID-19 outcomes compared 312 cancer patients and 4833 volunteers without cancer. The results showed that patients with oncological diseases had an increased mortality rate if they had SARS-CoV-2 infection when compared to the patients without cancer. The results showed that patients with different cancer types exacerbated by SARS-CoV-2 infection had an increased mortality rate compared to that of patients with COVID-19 but without cancer. Moreover, the authors noted that cancer patients aged 65 years and older with concomitant diseases had the greatest risk of death. In addition, the mortality rates were associated with recent antitumor therapy and the tumor, nodus, metastasis (TNM) stage of the disease (Lunski et al. 2021).

2 Immunological Parameters in Cancer Patients and Non-cancer Patients with COVID-19

A number of studies involving patients with COVID-19 evaluated alterations of immunological parameters that had enhanced plasma levels in patients with severe COVID-19, such as chemokine ligand 2 (CCL2), IFNγ, IFNγ-inducible protein 10, Granulocyte colony-stimulating factor (G-CSF), chemokine C-C motif ligand 3 (CCL3), IL-1β, IL-2, IL-6, IL-7, IL-8, IL-10, IL-17 and TNF-α (Mehta et al. 2020; Huang et al. 2020). Other studies analyzed the T-cell populations including CD4+ T cells, Th17 cells and cytotoxic CD8+ T cells producing TNF-α, HLA-DR (Human Leukocyte Antigen—DR isotype)-positive CD8+ T cells and Treg/CD8 ratio (Thibaudin et al. 2020). Thibaudin and co-authors found that cancer patients suffering from SARS-CoV-2 infection had CD4+ T-cell lymphopenia, accumulation of IFNγ+ TNFα+ CD8+ T and Th17 cells, and inversion of the CD4/CD8 ratio.

Tian J et al. showed that the mean levels of pro-inflammatory cytokines were as following: TNF-α—8.7 and 6.9 pg/ml, $p = 0.004$ in cancer ($n = 89$) and non-cancer ($n = 336$) patients, respectively; IL-6—12.8 and 4.9 pg/ml, $p < 0.0001$, in cancer ($n = 138$) and non-cancer ($n = 350$) patients, respectively; IL-2R—615 and 535 U/ml, $p = 0.012$, in cancer ($n = 79$) and non-cancer ($n = 340$) patients, respectively. In addition, infection-related biomarkers were higher in cancer patients, in particular, mean pro-calcitonin levels were 0.3 and 0.1 ng/ml, $p = 0.0041$, in cancer ($n = 161$) and non-cancer ($n = 251$) patients, respectively; C-reactive protein level was 46.4 and 40.7 mg/l, $p = 0.047$ in cancer ($n = 91$) and non-cancer ($n = 246$) patients, respectively (Tian et al. 2020). Moreover, patients with cancer had a significant decrease in the lymphocyte number, including CD4+ T cells: 370.0 and 625.5 cells/μl, $p < 0.0001$, in cancer ($n = 37$) and non-cancer patients ($n = 82$) and CD8+ T cells: 206.0 and 305.0 cells/μl, $p < 0.0081$, in cancer ($n = 43$) and non-cancer ($n = 82$) patients, respectively. This may be a risk factor for cancer patients, making them more vulnerable to SARS-CoV-2 infection.

Likewise, Diao B et al. reported that the number of T cells was significantly reduced and functionally depleted in patients with COVID-19 (Diao et al. 2020).

The number of CD8+ and CD4+ T cells negatively correlated with the survival of patients with COVID-19. Besides, the increased expression of programmed cell death protein 1 (PD-1), T-cell immunoglobulin and mucin-containing domain 3 (Tim-3) were registered on a large number of CD8+ and CD4+T cells. Increased expression of PD-L1, a transmembrane protein that is a ligand for PD-1, was observed on some tumor cells. PD-L1 binding to PD-1 induces the subsequent transmission of PD-1 receptor signals to T cells, which inhibits their proliferation and cytotoxic functions (McDermott and Atkins 2013). Some authors suggest that due to such mechanism of action of the PD-1 and PD-L1 signaling pathway, cancer patients with high PD-L1 expression may become more susceptible to pathogens such as SARS-COV-2 (Thakkar 2021).

3 Antibody-Dependent Immune Response to SARS-CoV-2 in Cancer Patients in Comparative Studies

The study of Marra A et al. compared the serum levels of antibodies against the SARS-CoV-2 antigen (assessment of the seroconversion level) in cancer patients and medical personnel with confirmed or clinically justified COVID-19 (Marra et al. 2021). The study enrolled 166 people including 61 (36.7%) cancer patients and 105 (63.3%) medical personnel. In general, 86 participants (51.8%) were diagnosed SARS-CoV-2 by RT-PCR (polymerase chain reaction with reverse transcription) of a nasopharyngeal smear, and 60 (36.2%) had a clinical suspicion of COVID-19. The average time from the onset of symptoms (for cases not tested by RT-PCR) or confirmation of RT-PCR to the analysis of serum antibodies was 17 days (interquartile range 26). The population with confirmed RT-PCR included 83.8% of cases positive for IgG. No differences in the qualitative positive assessment of IgG was registered between cancer patients and medical personnel (87.9% and 80.5%, respectively; $p = 0.39$). The authors believe that a positive result for SARS-CoV-2 PCR test on nasopharyngeal material in the absence of clinical evidence requires additional research (Marra et al. 2021).

Another study provided a similar comparison of the antibodies serum levels in cancer patients and health care workers (Yazaki et al. 2021). Similar to the above-mentioned study, the authors reported that the level of serum antibodies to SARS-CoV-2 did not differ between the two cohorts of participants. However, the results showed that systemic therapy, including chemotherapy and immune checkpoint inhibitors, can affect the immune response to SARS-CoV-2. Thus, the levels of N-IgG and S-IgG antibodies in cancer patients were significantly lower than in medical personnel. Besides, N-IgG levels were significantly lower in cancer patients who received chemotherapy than in those who did not receive it.

Humoral immune response to SARS-CoV-2 in patients with cancer was evaluated in a single-center retrospective study, which included adult patients with SARS-CoV-2 hospitalized from March 15 to June 17, 2020 (Esperança-Martins et al. 2021). The antibodies to SARS-CoV-2 receptor binding domain, or spike protein IgM, IgG, and IgA were quantified in patient serum samples. The aims of the study were to assess the level of humoral immune response to SARS-CoV-2; to compare this level in patients with different malignancies, cancer stages and therapies; to clarify the relationship between the humoral response and the clinical outcome of treatment in cancer patients; to compare the level of antibody-dependent response in cancer or non-cancer patients infected with SARS-CoV-2. A total of 72 patients with SARS-CoV-2 were enrolled in the study (19 cancer patients, 53 non-cancer individuals). About 90% of the data of the non-cancer cohort showed a persistent serological reaction. Whereas only 57.9% of cancer patients developed a marked response and 42.1% of patients had a minor response. Fourteen-day chemotherapy before the registered positive result was the only statistically confirmed factor associated with minor serological reactions in patients with cancer.

No significant differences in clinical results were observed between patients with marked and minor immune reactions. The titers of all IgG, IgM, IgA and total antibodies were significantly lower in patients with cancer compared to those without cancer. Previous chemotherapy may be associated with mild serological reactions in patients with cancer. Although cancer patients have a weaker antibody-dependent response to SARS-CoV-2 compared to patients without cancer, most cancer patients developed an appropriate humoral immune response (Esperança-Martins et al. 2021).

Thakkar A et al. reported the results of a retrospective cohort study of patients with cancer tested for IgG to SARS-CoV-2 (Thakkar et al. 2021). Totally 261 cancer patients had the test and the results showed a high level of seroconversion (92%). However, different therapies affected the seroconversion level, such as the following: significantly lower seroconversion was observed in patients with hematological malignancies (82%), in patients receiving anti-CD20 therapy (59%) and stem cell transplantation (60%). It is noteworthy that 17 patients receiving immunotherapy, including 16 individuals who received monoclonal antibodies against PD-1/PD-L1, developed IgG to SARS-CoV-2 (100% seroconversion). The results of the same test for the detection of IgG to SARS-CoV-2 in the general population showed that the level of seroconversion was 90–100% (Bryan et al. 2020; Chew et al. 2020). Indeed, the seroconversion level achieved 91% in a randomly selected cohort of 1,008 patients with SARS-CoV-2 positive PCR which was almost identical to the general seroconversion level in the analyzed cohort of cancer patients (Thakkar et al. 2021).

The researchers of a small study (Qin et al. 2021) performed single-cell RNA sequencing of the peripheral blood samples of three healthy donors, four patients with COVID-19 and four patients with COVID-19 and advanced gynecological cancer before and after antitumor treatment. All patients with acute COVID-19 infection were cured from the infection. Interestingly, molecular profile of the peripheral blood in patients with gynecological cancer were similar to those of patients with COVID-19, which might imply that patients with gynecological cancer recovering from COVID-19 had no serious immunological alterations, and they could develop immunological memory like patients with COVID-19 without cancer. Moreover, chemotherapy in these patients mainly caused neutropenia, having little effect on the proportion and functional phenotype of T and B cells, as well as on the clonal expansion of T cells. The study results showed that anti-PD-L1 therapy significantly increased the cytotoxicity of NK cells and T cells and promoted clonal expansion of T cells in these patients. The authors suggested that T cells could protect patients from re-infection with SARS-CoV-2, while anti-PD-L1 therapy could enhance the antiviral function of T cells (Qin et al. 2021). The assumption about the positive effect of immunotherapy with immune checkpoint inhibitors is based on the blockade mechanism of action (Fig. 3).

Binding PD-1 to PD-L1 may inhibit lytic CTL reactions against tumor or virally infected cells, which is associated with T-cell anergy that results from T-cell receptor interactions with antigen MHC-I peptide complexes. Blockade of either PD-1 or PD-L1 by specific monoclonal antibodies disrupts their functions and leads to CTL efficient lysis of virally infected or tumor cells.

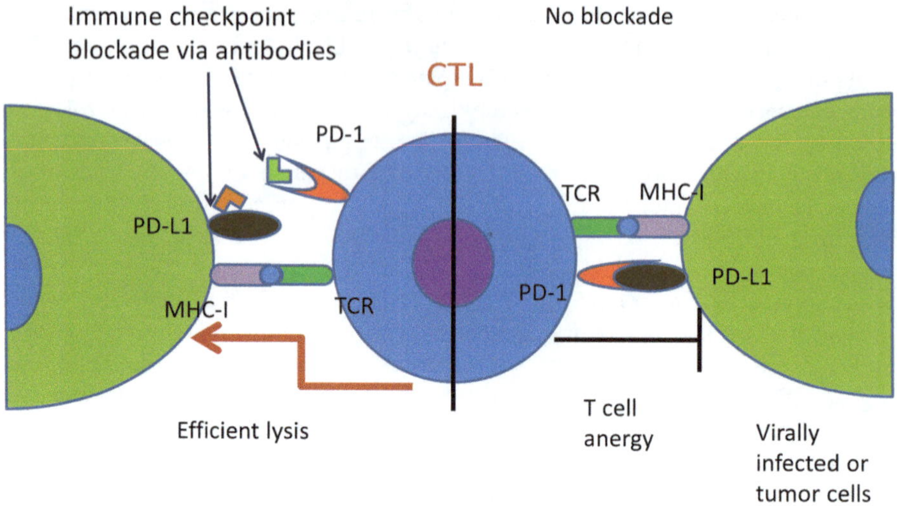

Fig. 3 Proposed mechanism of immune checkpoint blockade

4 Antitumor Immunotherapy and Immune Response to SARS-CoV-2

The patients with severe SARS-CoV-2 infection had significantly more increased number of non-functional CD8+ T cells than patients with moderate symptoms. Nevertheless, the functional activity of CD8+ T cells can be restored by the blockade of PD-1 and CTLA-4, thereby increasing antigen-specific reactions and antiviral activity against SARS-CoV-2 (Zheng 2020).

In addition, in vivo studies have demonstrated rapid stimulation of PD-1 expression after activation of CD8+ T cells in patients with infection of lymphocytic choriomeningitis virus. At an early stage of acute disease, blockade of PD-1 pathway by antibodies against PD-L1 or against PD-1 promotes activation of the response by CD8+ T cells specific to the virus due to accelerated elimination of the infectious factors (Ahn et al. 2018). However, there are still a limited number of studies confirming the positive effect of immunotherapy on the outcome of anti-COVID-19 treatment.

Da Costa CM et al. reported the results of the pembrolizumab-based therapy of a patient with Merkel cell carcinoma who suffered from a severe SARS-CoV-2 infection and respiratory distress syndrome complicated by acute kidney injury, which led to his hospitalization in the intensive care unit. The patient was discharged three months later after a long recovery (Da Costa et al. 2020). Two other papers described the cases of melanoma patients receiving anti-PD-1 therapy who were completely cured of COVID-19 after showing mild symptoms of infection (Di Giacomo et al. 2020).

The study describing in detail the comparative results of the immune checkpoint inhibitor therapy in cancer patients with COVID-19 showed that anti-PD-1 therapy of patients with lung cancer was not associated with an increased risk of developing a severe course of COVID-19 in 41 of 69 patients and, apparently, did not have any impact on the severity of COVID-19 in patients with lung cancer (Luo et al. 2020).

The analysis of the TERAVOLT database that presented 147 patients with malignancies of thoracic localization showed no connection between antitumor treatment including chemotherapy, tyrosine kinase inhibitors, combined chemotherapy and immune checkpoint inhibitors or ICI as monotherapy, and death caused by COVID-19 (Garassino et al. 2020).

Dai M. et al. analyzed 105 cancer patients who underwent immunotherapy and reported that only a small number of them had a severe form of COVID-19 and the disease-associated mortality (Dai et al. 2020).

A comprehensive prospective study CAPTURE was designed to monitor the immune response of a tumor to SARS-CoV-2. One of the objectives was to evaluate the antiviral response to COVID-19 in patients with different cancer types. The authors found that in patients with a number of cancer types the immune response was severely disrupted, and additional infections were registered more often (Au et al. 2020).

The largest study of cancer patients with COVID-19 has recently been finalized and reported in Lancet. The results from the COVID-19 and Cancer Consortium (CCC19) database of more than 900 patients with current or previous cancer were studied and thoroughly analyzed (Kuderer et al. 2020a, b). Less than 4% of patients received any treatment including immunotherapy (such as ICI, allogeneic hematopoietic stem cell transplantation or adoptive cell therapy). Out of 928 examined patients, 38 were diagnosed with melanoma (Kuderer et al. 2020a, b). In particular, the prognostic factors reliably associated with a two-fold increase of a 30-day risk of death were the old age and male sex (odds ratio (OR): 1.63 (confidence interval (CI): 1.07–2.48). The authors made a conclusion that an increased mortality rate of patients with cancer and COVID-19 was associated with both general and cancer-related risk factors, though neither cancer type nor the type of antitumor therapy was associated with the increased mortality rate (Kuderer et al. 2020a, b). Nevertheless, the researchers did not present any analysis of the relationship between different treatment methods (e.g., immunotherapy, chemotherapy) and the incidence of COVID-19.

An Italian study (Isgrò et al. 2021) analyzed the levels of IgM and/or IgG associated with SARS-CoV-2 in three different cohorts: cancer patients receiving innovative ICI immunotherapy, cancer patients undergoing standard chemotherapy (CT), and healthcare workers. Out of 287 patients 9 patients (3.1%) with ICI therapy had IgM and/or IgG-positive test results, which was significantly lower compared to Ig-positive patients receiving CT (39 Ig-positive of 598 patients, i.e., 6.5%) ($p = 0.04$). No statistically significant difference was registered between the group of patients with ICI therapy and healthcare workers: a positive result for IgM and/or IgG was noted in 48 out of 1,050 healthcare workers (4.6%). The authors performed a statistical analysis using a regression logistic model that included the correlation of sex, cancer stage and the treatment effect on seropositivity. The researchers found that ICI immunotherapy was the only protective factor significantly ($p = 0.03$) associated with seropositivity (OR: 0.41; 95% CI 0.18–0.91). Thus, according to the preliminary data, the authors suggested that ICI therapy was a protective factor against SARS-CoV-2 infection (Isgrò et al. 2021).

A prospective study of ICI therapy (Yatim et al. 2021) enrolled 292 patients with melanoma, half of whom received ICI therapy, while 15 patients had COVID-19 in the acute phase or at the stage of recovery. Transcriptomic, proteomic and cellular profiles were evaluated in the patients with COVID-19. The results revealed no association between the ICI therapy and a severe form of COVID-19. The immunotherapy did not affect the induction of inflammatory reactions and enhanced production of INF type I. The data of extended phenotyping showed an increase in the number of effector CD8+ memory T cells, increased activation of T cells and impaired induction of plasmablasts in patients with COVID-19 receiving ICI. Assessment of specific adaptive immunity in recovering patients revealed higher rates of antigen-specific T-cell responses to the spike (S), nucleoprotein (N) and membrane (M) antigens and similar induction of spike-specific antibodies. The study results demonstrated that ICI immunotherapy of patients with COVID-19 enhances T-cell immunity with no aggravation of the inflammation processes.

A significant part of patients who recovered from COVID-19 had symptoms associated with COVID-19 even several months later after being discharged from the hospital. Loretelli C et al. reported a detailed analysis of the immunological characteristics of patients who recovered from COVID-19 (Loretelli et al. 2021). The number of T cells in the observed patients was reduced, while the proportion of PD-1+ T cells increased as compared to the healthy donors of the control group. Plasma levels of IL-1ß, IL-1RA and IL-8 were also elevated in patients who recovered from COVID-19. The altered immunophenotype was represented by a low T-cell response ex vivo to both non-specific and specific stimulation, which implied T-cell dysfunction, including a weak reaction to SARS-CoV-2 antigens. Besides, the analysis also registered altered levels of plasma-soluble PD-L1 protein, as well as methylation of the PD-1 promoter and PD-1-targeted miR-15-5p in CD8+ T cells, that showed an abnormal function of the immune check points PD-1/PD-L1 signaling pathway. Interestingly, the blockade of PD-1 ex vivo practically resulted in the normalization of the immunophenotype and restoration of T-cell functions and the immune disorders after COVID-19. Moreover, the results showed an increased T-cell-mediated response to SARS-CoV-2 peptides. In addition, the neutralization test demonstrated that PD-1 blockade did not alter the T-cell potential to neutralize the SARS-CoV-2 spike pseudotyped lentivirus infection. The authors made a conclusion that inhibition of immune checkpoints restored COVID-19-related immune disorders and stimulated the immune reactions against SARS-CoV-2 (Loretelli et al. 2021). The evidence for the reversibility of CD8+ T-cell exhaustion after ICI treatment was also discussed in a comprehensive review of the effector mechanism of action associated with the antitumor immunotherapy (Budimir et al. 2022).

The authors of a special review performed a thorough analysis of the effect of anti-PD-1 therapy on the course of COVID-19 (Awadasseid et al. 2021) and made a conclusion that ICI immunotherapy with anti-PD-1, anti-PD-L1 and/or anti-CTLA-4 agents did not increase the risk of SARS-CoV-2 infection.

5 Conclusion

A number of various retrospective and prospective studies were completed or started to assess the impact of COVID-19 on the effectiveness of treatment and the status of cancer patients after the rapid spread of SARS-CoV-2 infection.

The reported data showed that the infection mostly affected patients receiving chemotherapy, patients with hematological malignancies, lung cancer, metastatic cancer and patients with different stages of advanced cancer. The elderly age over 65 years was confirmed as a statistically significant risk factor.

The authors of various studies discussed the data of the mechanism of action of ICI immunotherapy and the immune responses to the coronavirus infection and assumed that ICI could induce immune response in patients infected with SARS-CoV-2. However, to date, only limited studies can clearly demonstrate the protective effect of ICI against SARS-CoV-2 infection.

Nevertheless, the published data show that ICI antitumor therapy does not seem to increase mortality or morbidity of patients with cancer and SARS-CoV-2 infection. Such treatment is usually safe for cancer patients with COVID-19 from the practical point of view and taking into account the mechanism of ICI action.

Expanded experimental and clinical studies are required to determine the particular role of antitumor immunotherapy in the development of COVID-19 in cancer patients.

Disclosure of Interests All authors declare they have no conflict of interest.

Funding This study had no special funding.

References

Ahn E, Araki K, Hashimoto M, Li W, Riley JL, Cheung J et al (2018) Role of PD-1 during effector CD8 T cell differentiation. Proc Natl Acad Sci U S A 115(18):4749–4754. https://doi.org/10.1073/pnas.1718217115

Au L, Boos LA, Swerdlow A, Byrne F, Shepherd STC, Fendler A et al (2020) Cancer, COVID-19, and antiviral immunity: the CAPTURE study. Cell 183(1):4–10. https://doi.org/10.1016/j.cell.2020.09.005

Awadasseid A, Yin Q, Wu Y, Zhang W (2021) Potential protective role of the anti-PD-1 blockade against SARS-CoV-2 infection. Biomed Pharmacother 142:111957. https://doi.org/10.1016/j.biopha.2021.111957

Brinkmann V, Reichard U, Goosmann C, Fauler B, Uhlemann Y, Weiss DS et al (2004) Neutrophil extracellular traps kill bacteria. Science 303:1532–1535. https://doi.org/10.1126/science.1092385

Bryan A, Pepper G, Wener MH, Fink SL, Morishima C, Chaudhary A et al (2020) Performance characteristics of the Abbott Architect SARS-CoV-2 IgG assay and seroprevalence in Boise. Idaho J Clin Microbiol 58(8):e00941–e00920. https://doi.org/10.1128/JCM.00941-20

Budimir N, Thomas GD, Dolina JS, Salek-Ardakani S (2022) Reversing T-cell exhaustion in cancer: lessons learned from PD-1/PD-L1 immune checkpoint blockade. Cancer Immunol Res 10(2):146–153. https://doi.org/10.1158/2326-6066.CIR-21-0515

Chew KL, Tan SS, Saw S, Pajarillaga A, Zaine S, Khoo C et al (2020) Clinical evaluation of serological IgG antibody response on the Abbott architect for established SARS-CoV-2 infection. Clin Microbiol Infect 26(9):1256.e9–1256.e11. https://doi.org/10.1016/j.cmi.2020.05.036

Da Costa CM, de Souza ZS, Real Salgues AC, Harada G, Marino Rodrigues Ayres PP, Vieira Nunes DB, Katz A, Munhoz RR (2020) COVID-19 in a patient with advanced Merkel cell carcinoma receiving immunotherapy. Immunotherapy 12(15):1133–1138. https://doi.org/10.2217/imt-2020-0193

Dai M, Liu D, Liu M, Zhou F, Li G, Chen Z et al (2020) Patients with cancer appear more vulnerable to SARS-CoV-2: a multicenter study during the COVID-19 outbreak. Cancer Discov 10:783–791. https://doi.org/10.1158/2159-8290.CD-20-0422

Di Giacomo AM, Gambale E, Monterisi S, Valente M, Maio M (2020) SARS-COV-2 infection in patients with cancer undergoing checkpoint blockade: clinical course and outcome. Eur J Cancer 133:1–3. https://doi.org/10.1016/j.ejca.2020.04.026

Diao B, Wang C, Tan Y, Chen X, Liu Y, Ning L (2020) Reduction and functional exhaustion of T cells in patients with coronavirus disease 2019 (COVID-19). Front Immunol 11:827. https://doi.org/10.3389/fimmu.2020.00827

Esperança-Martins M, Gonçalves L, Soares-Pinho I, Gomes A, Serrano M, Blankenhaus B et al (2021) Humoral immune response of SARS-CoV-2-infected patients with cancer: influencing factors and mechanisms. Oncologist. https://doi.org/10.1002/onco.13828

Garassino MC, Whisenant JG, Huang LC, Trama A, Torri V, Agustoni F et al (2020) COVID-19 in patients with thoracic malignancies (TERAVOLT): first results of an international, registry-based, cohort study. Lancet Oncol 21(7):914–922. https://doi.org/10.1016/S1470-2045(20)30314-4

Huang C, Wang Y, Li X, Ren L, Zhao J, Hu Y et al (2020) Clinical features of patients infected with 2019 novel coronavirus in Wuhan, China. Lancet 395(10223):497–506. https://doi.org/10.1016/S0140-6736(20)30183-5

Isgrò MA, Vitale MG, Celentano E, Nocerino F, Porciello G, Curvietto M et al (2021) Immunotherapy may protect cancer patients from SARS-CoV-2 infection: a single-center retrospective analysis. J Transl Med 19(1):132. https://doi.org/10.1186/s12967-021-02798-2

Khoury E, Nevitt S, Madsen WR, Turtle L, Davies G, Palmieri C (2022) Differences in outcomes and factors associated with mortality among patients with SARS-CoV-2 infection and cancer compared with those without cancer. A systematic review and meta-analysis. JAMA Network Open. https://doi.org/10.1001/jamanetworkopen.2022.10880

Kiselevskiy M, Shubina I, Chikileva I, Sitdikova S, Samoylenko I, Anisimova N et al (2020) Immune pathogenesis of COVID-19 intoxication: storm or silence? Pharmaceuticals (Basel) 13(8):166. https://doi.org/10.3390/ph13080166

Kuderer NM, Choueiri TK, Shah DP, Shyr Y, Rubinstein SM, Rivera DR et al (2020a) Clinical impact of COVID-19 on patients with cancer (CCC19): a cohort study. Lancet 395:1907–1918. https://doi.org/10.1016/S0140-6736(20)31187-9

Kuderer NM, Choueiri TK, Shah DP, Shyr Y, Rubinstein SM, Rivera DR et al (2020b) Clinical impact of COVID-19 on patients with cancer (CCC19): a cohort study [published correction appears in Lancet. 2020. 396(10253):758]. Lancet 395(10241):1907–1918. https://doi.org/10.1016/S0140-6736(20)31187-9

Loretelli C, Abdelsalam A, D'Addio F, Ben Nasr M, Assi E, Usuelli V et al (2021) PD-1 blockade counteracts post-COVID-19 immune abnormalities and stimulates the anti-SARS-CoV-2 immune response. JCI Insight 6(24):e146701. https://doi.org/10.1172/jci.insight.146701

Lunski MJ, Burton J, Tawagi K, Maslov D, Simenson V, Barr D et al (2021) Multivariate mortality analyses in COVID-19: Comparing patients with cancer and patients without cancer in Louisiana. Cancer 127(2):266–274. https://doi.org/10.1002/cncr.33243

Luo J, Rizvi H, Egger JV, Preeshagul IR, Wolchok JD, Hellmann MD (2020) Impact of PD-1 blockade on severity of COVID-19 in patients with lung cancers. Cancer Discov 10(8): 1121–1128. https://doi.org/10.1158/2159-8290.CD-20-0596

Marra A, Generali D, Zagami P, Cervoni V, Gandini S, Venturini S et al (2021) Seroconversion in patients with cancer and oncology health care workers infected by SARS-CoV-2. Ann Oncol 32(1):113–119. https://doi.org/10.1016/j.annonc.2020.10.473

Masucci MT, Minopoli M, Del Vecchio S, Carriero MV (2020) The emerging role of neutrophil extracellular traps (NETs) in tumor progression and metastasis. Front Immunol 11:1749. https://doi.org/10.3389/fimmu.2020.01749

McDermott DF, Atkins MB (2013) PD-1 as a potential target in cancer therapy. Cancer Med 2(5): 662–673. https://doi.org/10.1002/cam4.106

Mehta P, McAuley DF, Brown M, Sanchez E, Tattersall RS, Manson JJ et al (2020) COVID-19: consider cytokine storm syndromes and immunosuppression. Lancet 395(10229):1033–1034. https://doi.org/10.1016/S0140-6736(20)30628-0

Melenotte C, Silvin A, Goubet AG, Lahmar I, Dubuisson A, Zumla A et al (2020) Immune responses during COVID-19 infection. Oncoimmunology 9(1):1807836. https://doi.org/10.1080/2162402X.2020.1807836

Mohseni Afshar Z, Hosseinzadeh R, Barary M, Ebrahimpour S, Alijanpour A, Sayad B et al (2022) Challenges posed by COVID-19 in cancer patients: a narrative review. Cancer Med 11(4): 1119–1135. https://doi.org/10.1002/cam4.4519

Qin T, Guo E, Lu F, Fu Y, Liu S, Xiao R et al (2021) Impact of chemotherapy and immunotherapy on the composition and function of immune cells in COVID-19 convalescent with gynecological tumors. Aging (Albany NY) 13(23):24943–24962. https://doi.org/10.18632/aging.203739

Razavi A, Hamblin MR, Rezaei N (2021) COVID-19 in patients with cancer: risks and precautions. Am J Emerg Med 48:357–360. https://doi.org/10.1016/j.ajem.2021.01.067

Riches JC (2021) Impact of COVID-19 in patients with lymphoid malignancies. World J Virol 10(3):97–110. https://doi.org/10.5501/wjv.v10.i3.97

Rogado J, Pangua C, Serrano-Montero G, Obispo B, Marino AM, Pérez-Pérez M et al (2020) Covid-19 and lung cancer: a greater fatality rate? Lung Cancer 146:19–22. https://doi.org/10.1016/j.lungcan.2020.05.034

Rubinstein SM, Bhutani D, Lynch RC, Hsu CY, Shyr Y, Advani S et al (2022) Patients recently treated for B-lymphoid malignancies show increased risk of severe COVID-19. Blood Cancer Discov 3:181–193. https://doi.org/10.1158/2643-3230.BCD-22-0013

Saffarzadeh M, Juenemann C, Queisser MA, Lochnit G, Barreto G, Galuska SP et al (2012) Neutrophil extracellular traps directly induce epithelial and endothelial cell death: a predominant role of histones. PLoS One. https://doi.org/10.1371/journal.pone.0032366

Sette A, Crotty S (2021) Adaptive immunity to SARS-CoV-2 and COVID-19. Cell 184(4): 861–880. https://doi.org/10.1016/j.cell.2021.01.007

Sun X, Wang T, Cai D, Hu Z, Chen J, Liao H, Zhi L, Wei H, Zhang Z, Qiu Y, Wang J, Wang A (2020) Cytokine storm intervention in the early stages of COVID-19 pneumonia. Cytokine Growth Factor Rev 53:38–42. https://doi.org/10.1016/j.cytogfr.2020.04.002

Thakkar A, Pradhan K, Jindal S, Cui Z, Rockwell B, Shah AP et al (2021) Patterns of seroconversion for SARS-CoV2-IgG in patients with malignant disease and association with anticancer therapy. Nat Cancer 2(4):392–399. https://doi.org/10.1038/s43018-021-00191-y

Thibaudin M, Fumet JD, Bon M, Hampe L, Limagne E, Ghiringhelli F (2020) Immunological features of coronavirus disease 2019 in patients with cancer. Eur J Cancer 139:70–80. https://doi.org/10.1016/j.ejca.2020.08.013

Tian J, Yuan X, Xiao J, Zhong Q, Yang C, Liu B et al (2020) Clinical characteristics and risk factors associated with COVID-19 disease severity in patients with cancer in Wuhan, China: a multicentre, retrospective, cohort study. Lancet Oncol 21(7):893–903. https://doi.org/10.1016/S1470-2045(20)30309-0

Vlachakis PK, Tentolouris A, Tousoulis D, Tentolouris N (2020) Current data on the cardiovascular effects of COVID-19. Hellenic J Cardiol 61(1):46–48. https://doi.org/10.1016/j.hjc.2020.04.001

Yatim N, Boussier J, Tetu P, Smith N, Bruel T, Charbit B et al (2021) Immune checkpoint inhibitors increase T cell immunity during SARS-CoV-2 infection. Sci Adv 7(34):eabg4081. https://doi.org/10.1126/sciadv.abg4081

Yazaki S, Yoshida T, Kojima Y, Yagishita S, Nakahama H, Okinaka K et al (2021) Difference in SARS-CoV-2 antibody status between patients with cancer and health care workers during the COVID-19 pandemic in Japan. JAMA Oncol 7(8):1141–1148. https://doi.org/10.1001/jamaoncol.2021.2159

Yeoh CB, Lee KJ, Rieth EF, Mapes R, Tchoudovskaia AV, Fischer GW et al (2020) COVID-19 in the cancer patient. Anesth Analg 131(1):16–23. https://doi.org/10.1213/ANE.0000000000004884

Zhang L, Zhu F, Xie L, Wang C, Wang J, Chen R et al (2020) Clinical characteristics of COVID-19-infected cancer patients: a retrospective case study in three hospitals within Wuhan, China. Ann Oncol 31:894–901. https://doi.org/10.1016/j.annonc.2020.03.296

Zheng HY, Zhang M, Yang CX, Zhang N, Wang XC, Yang XP et al (2020) Elevated exhaustion levels and reduced functional diversity of T cells in peripheral blood may predict severe progression in COVID-19 patients. Cell Mol Immunol 17(5):541–543. https://doi.org/10.1038/s41423-020-0401-3

The Use of Immunotherapy in Cancer Patients with Autoimmune Diseases

Chung-Shien Lee and Nagashree Seetharamu

Abstract

Immune checkpoint inhibitor (ICI) therapy has revolutionized the way cancer is treated. ICIs have provided prolonged and sustained responses for various tumor types. Through stimulating the immune system, patients with autoimmune disorders (AIDs) were often excluded for clinical trials. The aim of this chapter is to discuss the use of ICIs in patients with AIDs. Evidence for using various types of ICIs [cytotoxic T-lymphocyte-associated protein 4 (CTLA-4), programmed cell death receptor 1 (PD-1) inhibitor, and programmed cell death ligand 1 (PD-L1) inhibitors] in patients with AID disorders are limited. Various studies have investigated the use of ICIs in this patient population. Most studies demonstrate that ICIs can be safely used in these patients with comparable efficacy to patients without AIDs. Immune-related adverse events (irAEs) have been shown to be higher than the general population in some studies, but can be managed. Patients with a history of AIDs can be treated with ICIs, but should be closely monitored for irAEs.

Keywords

Autoimmune disorders · Cytotoxic T-lymphocyte-associated protein 4 · Immune checkpoint inhibitor · Programmed cell death receptor 1

C.-S. Lee (✉)
Department of Clinical Health Professions, St. John's University, Queens, NY, USA

Division of Medical Oncology and Hematology, Northwell Health Cancer Institute, Lake Success, NY, USA
e-mail: leec3@stjohns.edu

N. Seetharamu
Division of Medical Oncology and Hematology, Northwell Health Cancer Institute, Lake Success, NY, USA

Interdisciplinary Cancer Research, https://doi.org/10.1007/16833_2022_63
Published online: 19 November 2022

1 Introduction

Immune checkpoint inhibitor (ICI) therapy, commonly referred to as immunotherapy, has changed the way cancer is treated. Since its initial approval a decade ago, ICIs have demonstrated benefit in various tumor types, improving progression-free survival (PFS) and overall survival (OS) and becoming standard of care (Onitilo and Wittig 2020; Xiong et al. 2021; Rini et al. 2019; Chaudhuri et al. 2021; Golshani and Zhang 2020; Hodi et al. 2010; Eggermont et al. 2018; Larkin et al. 2015; Schachter et al. 2017; Hamid et al. 2019; Robert et al. 2015; Ascierto et al. 2017; Larkin et al. 2019; Ribas et al. 2015; Weber et al. 2015; Langer et al. 2016; Mok et al. 2019; Gandhi et al. 2018; Socinski et al. 2018, 2021; Nishio et al. 2021; Jotte et al. 2020; Horn et al. 2018; Paz-Ares et al. 2018). The estimated percentage of patients with cancer who were eligible for ICIs in 2018 was 44%, and that number has certainly increased and will continue to increase with immunotherapy moving into neoadjuvant and adjuvant space for a variety of cancers (Haslam and Prasad 2019; Lee and Brady 2021; O'Donnell et al. 2019; Kang et al. 2021; Yi et al. 2019; Emens et al. 2017). Currently approved ICIs include cytotoxic T-lymphocyte-associated protein 4 (CTLA-4), programmed cell death receptor 1 (PD-1), and programmed cell death ligand 1 (PD-L1) inhibitors. There are currently eight approved ICIs and several in development. As patients are now living longer due to immunotherapy, the chances of them developing serious toxicity, specifically immune-related adverse event (irAE), are also increasing (Kichloo et al. 2021). In this review, we will focus on checkpoint inhibitor therapy in patients with preexisting autoimmune disorders (AIDs). Patients with AID have an increased risk of developing cancer due to a multitude of reasons (Cappelli and Shah 2020; Schairer et al. 2018; Song et al. 2019; Giat et al. 2017). Patients with AID who develop cancer also pose a challenge for treatment in several different ways. Use of conventional chemotherapy is challenging in these patients due to their already immunosuppressed state, decreased response to treatment, and flare-up of AID (Giat et al. 2017; Richard-Eaglin and Smallheer 2018; Valencia et al. 2019; Elandt and Aletaha 2011). ICI treatment in patients with AID is even more challenging due to overlapping features or AID and ICI toxicity (Rakshit and Molina 2020; He et al. 2017). Some studies have shown that the efficacy of immunotherapy in patients with AID is similar if not superior to those who do not have this preexisting comorbidity (Tang et al. 2021; Tison et al. 2019; Schmerling et al. 2021). However, most of the clinical trials exclude patients with active AID, and hence, majority of the data available is from real-world series, metanalyses, and retrospective case series. The reason for exclusion of these patients is the concern that the occurrence of immune-related adverse events is higher in patients with AID than in general population (Rakshit and Molina 2020, He et al. 2017).

In order to understand the complex interactions between the immune system, autoimmune conditions, and checkpoint inhibitors, we need to focus on the mechanism of action of these agents and the pathogenesis of autoimmune disorders. In the next few paragraphs, we provide a simplified overview of these topics.

2 Pathogenesis of AID

AID encompasses a conglomeration of clinical conditions that result from dysregulated immune system and pathogenic inflammatory responses (Luan et al. 2017; Anaya 2012; Wahren-Herlenius and Dörner 2013). These conditions can present with auto toxic effects involving a single or multiple organs, including the skin, gastrointestinal tract, endocrine glands, kidney, skeletal system, and cranial nervous system. The homeostasis between autoimmunity, which probably exists to some extent in all individuals at a physiological level and immunotolerance, is essential for a healthy immune system (Rosenblum et al. 2015). AID is an extreme manifestation along the same spectrum, usually referring to pathogenic clinical or subclinical autoimmunity directed against one or multiple organ systems (Perl 2012). Although we still do not have a complete understanding of the mechanisms involved, both T- and B-cell lymphocytic subsets seem to be dysregulated to varying extent in most patients with AID (Rosenblum et al. 2015). Unlike individuals with a healthy immune system, people with AID have inappropriate immunotolerance mechanisms, such as anergy and activation-induced cellular apoptosis, unleashing self-destructive lymphocytes upon encounter with autoantigens (Maniati et al. 2010).

Several etiopathologic factors that have been implicated in AID include genetic predisposition, environmental influence, hormonal defects, and quantitative and/or qualitative aberrations of immunoregulatory function (Rosenblum et al. 2015; Taneja 2019; Jörg et al. 2016; Moulton 2018; Benagiano et al. 2019; Cojocaru et al. 2010). These factors lead to abnormal inflammatory response through a series of genetic, epigenetic, cellular, molecular, and microenvironmental changes. Additionally, an imbalance between pro- and anti-inflammatory cytokines and chemokines, abnormal handling of autoantigens, and antigen presentation further perpetrates the autoimmune process (Anaya 2012; Wahren-Herlenius and Dörner 2013; Perl 2012). The vicious cycle thus created negatively impacts the fragile balance between regulatory immune cells such as Tregs and inflammatory cells such as Th17, orchestrated by key regulators of the immune system (e.g., dendritic cell subsets), which can lead to the imbalance between regulatory (e.g., Tregs) and pro-inflammatory cells (e.g., Th17 cells), resulting in a full-blown AID (Knochelmann et al. 2018; Nistala and Wedderburn 2009; Afzali et al. 2007). Abnormal levels of cytokines, such as interleukins (IL), tumor necrosis factor (TNF), cytotoxic T-lymphocyte-associated antigen 4 (CTLA-4), and interferon-γ are commonly noted in AID and have been utilized as therapeutic targets in the recent times (Knochelmann et al. 2018, Nistala and Wedderburn 2009, Afzali et al. 2007).

3 AID and Development of Cancer

Full-blown AID, as mentioned previously, is a pro-inflammatory state with low circulating Tregs. Advanced cancer, on the other hand, is usually associated with high Tregs (Knochelmann et al. 2018). This may make it seem like AID and cancer are immunological opposites, but the low and high Treg states are not binary measures but rather a continuum that will allow immunological overlap between the two conditions. Moreover, the processes that lead to AID and cancer are extremely complex with many overlapping pro- and anti-inflammatory processes that may help explain the association (Cappelli and Shah 2020; Fierabracci and Pellegrino 2016; Kumar et al. 2018; Zarnavalou et al. 2016). Some examples are explained here.

CD8+ T cells are extremely important in mounting innate immunity against cancer (Dolina et al. 2021). One of the first steps in cancer immunity is recognition of major histocompatibility complex (MHC)-1 peptides on cancer cells and subsequent destruction through release of cytolytic enzymes and activation of apoptotic pathways. Tregs, which are typically present in abundance in advanced cancer, suppress CD8+ T cells and other effector T cells, such as Th17, and serve as pro-cancer cells (Nistala and Wedderburn 2009; Takeuchi and Nishikawa 2016). They also hinder development and proliferation of memory T cells. In addition to T cells, there is a growing literature on the pro-cancer role played by tumor-associated neutrophils (TAN) and tumor-associated macrophages (TAM) in response to cytokines such as TGFβ (Wu and Zhang 2020; Galdiero et al. 2018; Keeley et al. 2019). To confuse the picture further, both TAN and TAM can have pro-inflammatory or anti-inflammatory roles depending on the circumstance and the signals they are subject to. Another factor in tumor microenvironment that has been shown to influence cancer progression through complex mechanisms is reactive oxygen species (ROS) (Wigner et al. 2021). The interplay between CD4+ and CD8+ cells and MHC-1 and MHC-II expression on tumor cells also dictate cancer containment or progression (Taneja 2019; Richardson et al. 2021; Marty et al. 2018; Dhatchinamoorthy et al. 2021). Aberrant processes involving all these pathways are hallmark of AID and are possibly responsible for increased incidence of cancer in patients with AID. In addition, autoantibodies in patients with AID that bind anti-tumor antigen will promote carcinogenesis.

The non-so-uncommon occurrence of autoimmune paraneoplastic syndromes is yet another example that ties up AID and cancer (Pelosof and Gerber 2010). Paraneoplastic AID can have phenotypic similarities to known AID syndromes systemic lupus erythematosus (SLE), dermatomyositis, and Sjogren's disease. Treating the underlying cancer is an integral part of AID management suggesting a direct relationship between the two conditions. Treatment of AID with immunosuppressive agents increases the risk of cancer due to nonspecific inhibition of CD8+ T cells, Th1 cells, and other cells that have anti-tumor effects (Vial and Descotes 2003).

4 Mechanism of Action of CTLA-4 Inhibitors

CTLA-4 or CD152 play a very important role in immunotolerance. It is constitutively expressed on Tregs, but its expression can be induced on other T-cell subsets as well, in response to T-cell activation (Rowshanravan et al. 2018). The molecule is present in intracellular vesicles in most T cells and gets transiently expressed upon activation after which is rapidly dissipated through endocytosis (Qureshi et al. 2012).

However, in response to T-cell receptor (TCR) activation, there is upregulation of CTLA-4 on T cells, which in turn engages with antigens on antigen-presenting cells (APC) and gets stabilized in the immunologic synapse (Qureshi et al. 2012). CTLA-4 suppresses cell response by competing with the co-stimulatory receptor CD28. CTLA-4 engages with ligands CD80 and CD86 on APC with much higher affinity than CD28 and reduces immune response to self- and tumor antigens through a multitude of mechanisms (Rowshanravan et al. 2018). One obvious mechanism is immune suppression through competitive inhibition of the immunostimulatory receptor, CD28. CTLA-4 seems to also remove CD80 and CD86 from the cell surfaces of antigen-presenting cells through a process called trans-endocytosis (Soskic et al. 2014). Aberration in the CTLA-4 gene has been shown to result in AID in humans, and overactive CTLA-4 activity has been associated with decreased immune responses to infection and cancer (Lo and Abdel-Motal 2017). By blocking CTLA-4, antibodies such as ipilimumab and tremelimumab reverse the negative influence of CTLA-4 on immune response and result in tumor death (Ascierto et al. 2011). In fact, ipilimumab which was the first immune checkpoint inhibitor that was approved for cancer treatment continues to be an important cancer therapeutic agent today but used mostly in conjunction with PD-1 inhibitors for dual blockade (Mansh 2011; Saung et al. 2021).

5 Mechanism of Programmed Cell Death Receptor 1 (PD-1) and Its Ligand PD-L1 Inhibitors

PD-1, also called CD279, is a receptor that shares similar allelic structure to CD28 and is a key player in the inhibitory immune signaling process and a master regulator of adaptive immune responses (Sullivan et al. 2017; Han et al. 2020). In many species including humans, the receptor is constitutively expressed on some T cells such as follicular helper T cells; most T cells in circulation do not express PD-1 (Simon and Labarriere 2018; Kumagai et al. 2020). Their expression can however be induced by T-cell receptor (TCR) activation or stimulation from cytokines such as interleukins and transforming growth factor. PD-1 can also be expressed on other immune-modulatory cells such as dendritic cells and B cells. PD-1 engages with two specific ligands, PD-L1 (CD274) and PD-L2 (CD273), which are variably expressed on cancer cells, antigen-presenting cells, and some lymphoid cells. Interferon (IFN)-γ stimulates up-regulation of both PD-L1 and PD-L2 (Furuse et al. 2020; Latchman et al. 2001). Engagement of PD-1 with one of its receptors results in phosphorylation of its tyrosine residues which in turn kicks off an intracellular signaling cascade leading up to inactivation of pro-stimulatory molecules such as CD28 and reduced cytokine production. Therefore, the essential player involved in immune homeostasis, PD-1, is only activated upon T-cell activation (Riley 2009). Mice deficient in the receptor develop autoimmune diseases both spontaneously and upon additional insults such as infection. Humans with genetic polymorphisms in the PD-1 locus are also prone to develop autoimmune conditions (Dong et al. 2016; Hashemi et al. 2019). On the contrary in cancer, increased engagement of PD-1 with its ligands, specifically PD-L1, inhibits anti-tumor immune responses and is implicated in cancers (Qin et al. 2019). Antibodies that block PD-1 or PD-L1 can effectively disrupt this engagement and reactivate immune responses (Sullivan 2017). PD-L1 overexpression on tumor cells is associated with poor prognosis but has also shown to predict response to PD-1 and PD-L1 inhibition, but it is important to note that PD-L1 expression on cancer cells can be heterogenous and the expression levels have not been consistently shown to be of predictive value in several types of tumors (Davis and Patel 2019).

6 ICI Therapy and Autoimmune Disorders: Theoretical Considerations

ICIs have not only caused a major paradigm shift in cancer therapeutics but also created a new class of side effect profile, collectively termed as immune-related adverse events (irAEs) (Emens et al. 2017). ICIs work through tilting the balance from immunotolerance to immune activation. ICIs are designed to elicit anti-tumor tumor responses due to their targeted activation of immune system, rather than a systemic inflammatory or immune response (Waldman et al. 2020). However, irAEs frequently occur in patients on ICI and can involve any organ system, often causing significant morbidity and sometime resulting in mortality (Emens et al. 2017). The mechanism of irAEs is understandably complex. In some instances, these are related to a flare-up of inflammation mediated by macrophages and can be easily treated with high-dose steroids and other anti-inflammatory agents (Mihic-Probst et al. 2020). In other situations, the side effects may represent a true autoimmune process characterized by typical phenotypic changes and, frequently, antigen-specific auto-antibody detection in peripheral blood (Young et al. 2018). Patients with underlying autoimmune conditions are at increased risk for the second phenomenon, and there are many examples of this reported in literature (Rakshit and Molina 2020). However, patients who do not have any history of underlying AID can also have classic symptoms of various defined AID conditions (Young et al. 2018). While it is possible that ICI might merely be unmasking a subclinical AID, a true de novo initiation of an AID process, perhaps in conjunction with genetic, environmental, or other factors, is also equally plausible. Contrariwise, there is increasing wealth of literature showing that patients with known AID can tolerate and benefit from ICI, without flare-up of their underlying autoimmune process (Rakshit and Molina 2020).

While there are a number of irAEs that can occur with any ICIs, anti-CTLA-4 and anti-PD-1/PD-L1 antibodies display some unique patterns of irAEs, highlighting differences in the mechanisms of action. Anti-CTLA-4 agents are more likely to cause severe irAEs than PD-1/PD-L1 inhibitors. Colitis, vitiligo, and hypophysitis are more common with CTLA-4 agents, whereas pneumonitis and thyroiditis are more common with PD-1/PD-L1 inhibition (Buchbinder and Desai 2016).

The above statements highlight the need for further characterization of ICI mechanisms of action, specifically in relation to AID and irAEs.

6.1 ICI Therapy in Melanoma

Melanoma was the first type of cancer that ICIs showed promise for, and therefore ICIs have been used the longest in this tumor type. Most large randomized phase III controlled trials excluded patients with AID. Evidence of ICIs use in patients with AID are largely retrospective in nature.

Menzies et al. conducted a retrospective study in advanced melanoma patients treated with anti-PD-1 antibodies with either preexisting AIDs or major irAEs with prior ipilimumab. A total of 119 were included with 52 having a preexisting AID and 67 developed a significant irAE with prior ipilimumab. The majority of patient had received pembrolizumab as their anti-PD-1 therapy. The median age of the 52 patients with a preexisting autoimmune disorder was 71 years (range, 23–88), and 44% had not yet received a systemic melanoma therapy. The most common AID seen was rheumatologic (52%) and dermatologic (15%). Thirty-eight percent of patients had a flare of their underlying AID, most (85%) of which were mild. Flares occurred at a median of 38 days (range, 8–161) after the first dose of anti-PD-1 treatment and occurred more often in patients with active symptoms. Interestingly, patients with gastrointestinal, neurological, or respiratory AIDs did not have a flare. The response rate in those who had a flare was similar to those who did not have a flare (35% vs. 31%, $p > 0.05$). IRAEs occurred in 29% of patients, 6% required a dose interruption and 8% discontinued anti-PD-1 therapy (Menzies et al. 2017).

In a similar, smaller German study, Getzmer R et al. conducted a review of 41 patients with metastatic melanoma with either preexisting AIDs or ipilimumab-triggered irAEs. Nineteen had preexisting AIDs, including two of the patients who also had ipilimumab-triggered autoimmune colitis. The median age was 54 years (range, 38–76), and the most common AID was rheumatologic (47%). Forty-two percent of patients experienced a flare of their underlying AID within 3–20 weeks of starting anti-PD-1 treatment, most of which were mild (89%) (Gutzmer et al. 2017). The rates are comparable to the previously mentioned studied in this patient population. In both studies, the flare in AIDs seems to be more common in patients with rheumatologic AIDs (approximately 50%) (Menzies et al. 2017; Gutzmer et al. 2017). Responses to anti-PD-1 treatment in these patients were reported to be 33% and 32%, respectively, which is similar to advanced melanoma patients without preexisting AIDs (Menzies et al. 2017, Gutzmer et al. 2017). Response rates have been reported in the 33–43% range for frontline treatment and 21–32% as second-line treatment (Larkin et al. 2018; Robert et al. 2015; Ribas et al. 2015; Weber et al. 2015.

There have been a few retrospective studies investigating the use of ipilimumab, a cytotoxic T-lymphocyte-associated antigen 4 (CTLA-4) inhibitor in advanced melanoma patients with preexisting AIDs. Two of these studies showed response in the 12–20% range, while another study by Lee et al., with only eight patients, showed a response of 50% (Kähler et al. 2018; Johnson et al. 2016; Lee et al. 2016). Lee et al. demonstrated an AID flare of 75% and irAE of 100%, while the other two demonstrated 27–29% and 29–33%, respectively. The incidence of irAEs in these studies was lower than that previously seen, likely due to the retrospective nature of the studies (Hodi et al. 2010, Schachter et al. 2017, Larkin et al. 2019).

6.2 ICI Therapy in NSCLC

Similar to melanoma, the evidence of using ICIs in patients with AIDs in other tumor types are retrospective in nature. An estimated 14%–25% of patients with lung cancer will also have a concomitant AID (Khan et al. 2016). In a retrospective, multicenter study, 56 patients with advanced NSCLC and a preexisting AID were investigated. Similar to the melanoma studies, the most common AID was rheumatologic (45%). The median age was 67 years (range, 45–90), and the majority (84%) of patients were receiving an ICI for second-line treatment and beyond. Twenty-three percent of patients experienced a flare of their underlying AID and most of the flares were mild. The onset to flare was variable, ranging from 1 to 260 days after start of ICI. Flares were also experienced more in patients with a rheumatologic AID compared with patients with other AIDs (40% vs. 10%, $p = 0.01$). This observation is consistent with ICI use in melanoma patients with AID. Flares were also more common in patients who were symptomatic from their AID at the time of ICI initiation than those who were asymptomatic (50% vs. 18%, $p = 0.04$). Fourteen percent of patients discontinued the ICI, but none because of an AID flare. This rate of discontinuation was slightly higher than discontinuation rates reported in trials. irAEs occurred in 38% of patients, with 11% of them being grade ≥ 3 (Leonardi et al. 2018). The rate of grade ≥ 3 irAEs seems to be comparable to other clinical trials in this patient population (Brahmer et al. 2015; Herbst et al. 2016; Reck et al. 2016; Rittmeyer et al. 2017).

A retrospective Japanese study evaluated advanced NSCLC patients who were treated with either nivolumab or pembrolizumab monotherapy and underwent a serum antinuclear antibody (ANA) test. A total of 83 patients were included with 18 (22%) patients having a positive ANA test and 65 (78%) negative. No patients in this study had symptomatic AID. The incidence of irAEs was similar among the two groups (33.3% vs. 32.3%, respectively). Patients with a higher ANA titer had a higher frequency of developing irAEs. Patients who were ANA positive had a lower objective response rate (ORR), disease control rate, PFS, and OS (27.8%, 55.6%, 2.9 months, 11.6 months, respectively) compared to patients with a negative ANA [29.2%, 64.6%, 3.8 months ($p = 0.03$), 15.8 months ($p = 0.03$), respectively]. However, in patients who had previously received platinum-based chemotherapy, ORR was greater (33.3% vs. 23.5%; $p = 0.48$) and PFS longer (6.9 vs. 5.4 months; $p = 0.49$) in patients with a positive ANA compared to those who were negative, although not statistically significant. This is the only study that has investigated specifically the ANA status with ICIs and suggests that there may be a relationship. Resistance to ICIs in this population may develop earlier in patients with a positive ANA and may limit its efficacy (Yoneshima et al. 2019).

The TAIL study, which was a prospective, phase III, single-arm study, investigated the use of atezolizumab in diverse patient population of locally advanced or metastatic NSCLC patients who had progressed on chemotherapy. A total of 619 patients were enrolled in this study, with 30 (4.9%) patients having a baseline AID. These patients had similar rates of any grade AE (90% vs. 90.7%) and grade ≥ 3 AE (33.3% vs. 35.6%) compared to the overall population. However, rates of treatment-related AE (70% vs. 53.7%), immune-related AE (13.3% vs. 9.6%), and AE leading to discontinuation (16.7% vs. 4.9%) were higher in the AID group. There were moderately increased incidences of respiratory or gastrointestinal AEs. There was one episode of grade 5 pneumonitis. ORR (10% vs. 11.1%), median PFS (2.9 vs. 2.7 months), and median OS (10.1 vs. 11.1 months) were similar compared to the overall population (Ardizzoni et al. 2021).

6.3 ICI Therapy in Urologic Cancers

The use of ICIs in patients with AIDs has also been investigated in urological cancers. The SAUL trial sought to evaluate the real-world use of atezolizumab in patients with locally advanced or metastatic urothelial or non-urothelial carcinoma of the urinary tract, which included 35 patients with AIDs (Sternberg et al. 2019). The most common AID was dermatologic (49%) in this subset and three patients had two AIDs. The median age was 69 years (range, 41–82); approximately three-quarters were male and most of patients were receiving an ICI for second-line treatment and beyond (66%). Four patients (11%) experienced worsening of their AID, with two of the flares not resolved. The onset to flare was variable, ranging from 21 to 358 days after start of ICI. Patients with an AID had a higher incidence of any grade AE (91% vs. 88%), grade ≥ 3 AE (58% vs. 47%), AEs of special interest (46% vs. 30%), and grade ≥ 3 AEs of special interest (14% vs. 6%). Efficacy data was similar in patients with AID and those who did not have an AID (Loriot et al. 2020).

In another retrospective cohort study, patients with advanced renal cell carcinoma (RCC) and urothelial cancer with a history of AID receiving ICI were investigated. A total of 106 patients were evaluated across 10 centers. The median age was 68 years (range, 25–87) and 80% of patients received a PD-1/PD-L1 inhibitor as monotherapy. The most common AIDs were rheumatologic (34%) and dermatologic (30%). Thirty-six percent of patients experienced an AID flare with the median time to flare being 76 days (range, 25–215) in patients with RCC and 33 days (range, 1–368) in patients with urothelial cancer. Seventy-one percent of flares were low grade and occurred in 50% of patient with a rheumatologic AID and 44% of patients with a dermatologic AID. Forty percent and 34% of patients who had a baseline symptomatic and asymptomatic AID experienced flares. Patients who received combination ICI treatment had a higher frequency of flares (52%) compared to ICI monotherapy (32%). Patients receiving immunomodulators at start of ICI were more likely to experience a flare (50% vs. 35%). irAEs occurred in 38% of patients and 13% were grade ≥ 3. The rate of irAEs in this study was higher than those seen in previous phase III trials with RCC or urothelial cancer (Martinez Chanza et al. 2020).

Many other cohort studies have been done with various tumor types (Table 1). A prospective observational study in France investigated patients with cancer who were treated with ICI and had preexisting AIDs in the REISAMIC registry. A of 397 patients were analyzed in the study with 45 patients having preexisting AIDs. In patients with preexisting AID, the median age in this group was 63 years [interquartile range (IQR), 57–71] and 80% had melanoma. The majority of patients (82%) had one preexisting AID and the rest had two concomitant AIDs. Approximately one-quarter of patients experienced an AID flare and 44% of patients experienced an irAE. The rate of irAE was higher in the patients with preexisting AID compared to those who did not (29%). There was no difference in OS among the two groups ($p = 0.38$) (Danlos et al. 2018).

A retrospective, observational study in Italy investigated patients with advanced cancers that were treated with anti-PD-1 agents. A total of 751 patients were included in the study, with 85 patients (11.3%) having preexisting AIDs and 17.6% of those with clinically active AID. The median age was 69 years (range, 24–92) and approximately two-thirds of the cohort were males. The most common tumor types were non-small cell lung cancer (NSCLC) (65.5%), melanoma (21.2%), and kidney cancer (12.5%). Twenty-three percent of patients received the anti-PD-1 agent as first-line therapy. Forty-seven percent of patients had a flare of their underlying AID with the majority (91%) being mild. Interestingly, the overall incidence of irAEs of any grade and severe was similar, 43% and 9%, respectively. Approximately two-thirds of patients with AIDs experienced an irAE, with 9% of them being severe. When compared with patients without AIDs, the incidence of irAEs of any grade was significantly higher (66% vs. 40%, $p < 0.0001$). Patients with inactive and active AIDs were 2.5 and 4.2 times more likely to develop any grade irAEs, respectively. In a univariate and multivariate analysis, female gender and Eastern Cooperative Oncology Group (ECOG) Performance Status (PS) 0–1 were also shown to be significantly related to a greater incidence of irAEs. There was no difference in discontinuation rates between those with preexisting AIDs and those without, 7% vs. 7.2%, respectively (Cortellini et al. 2019).

7 Conclusion

Evidence of treatment with ICIs in patients with AIDs remain limited, but are much needed. Much of the literature (Table 1) suggests that the efficacy of these agents in this population is similar to that of the general population. Although variable among tumor type, ICI agent, and study, irAEs seem to occur at a higher rate in this population than the general population, but does not seem to vary among tumor types (Table 2). This seems to still be manageable, but clinicians should consider the type of AID, whether or not it's active or inactive, and what type of treatment they are receiving when deciding ICIs for these patients.

Table 1 Immune checkpoint inhibitor efficacy in patients with autoimmune disease

Study	Cancer type	n	ICI	Treatment naive	Type of autoimmune disease						ORR	Median PFS (months)	Median OS (months)
					Rheum	Derm	GI	Neuro	Endo	Resp			
Menzies et al.	Melanoma	52	Pembrolizumab (92%) Nivolumab (8%)[a]	44%	52%	15%	12%	10%	8%	4%	33%	6.2 (95% CI, 4.2–8.2)	NR
Gutzmer et al.	Melanoma	19	Pembrolizumab (37%) Nivolumab (63%)	NR	47%	11%	5%	11%	26%	0%	32%	NR	NR
Kahler et al.	Melanoma	41	Ipilimumab	NR	27%	27%	7%	5%	37%	0%	12%	NR	NR
Johnson et al.	Melanoma	30	Ipilimumab	NR	27%	17%	20%	7%	7%	0%	20%	3.0 (95% CI, 2.0–8.3)	12.5 (95% CI, 6.3 to NE)
Lee et al.	Melanoma	8	Ipilimumab		100%	0%	0%	0%	0%	0%	50%	NR	NR
Leonardi et al.	NSCLC	56	Pembrolizumab (18%) Nivolumab (80%) Atezolizumab (2%)	16%	45%	29%	11%	5%	16%	0%	22%	NR	NR
Yoneshima et al.	NSCLC	18	Pembrolizumab (31%) Nivolumab (69%)[a]	19%	ANA positive ONLY						28%	2.9	11.6
Tison et al.	Melanoma (58.9%) NSCLC (35.7%) Urologic (3.6%) MCC (1.8%)	112	Ipilimumab (13%) Pembrolizumab (24%) Nivolumab (56%) Ipilimumab + nivolumab (2.7) Atezolizumab (2.7%) Avelumab (1.8%)[a]	44%	33%	32%	13%	4%	4%	0%	49%	12.9 (95% CI, 6.9–18.8) (melanoma) 11.8 (95% CI, 7.2–16.5) (NSCLC)	Not reached (melanoma) 22.4 (95% CI, 10.3–34.5)
Ardizzoni A et al.	NSCLC	30	Atezolizumab	0%	NR	NR	NR	NR	NR	NR	10%	2.9 (95% CI, 1.4–4.2)	10.1 (95% CI, 6.5–14.1)

(continued)

Table 1 (continued)

Study	Cancer type	n	ICI	Treatment naive	Type of autoimmune disease						ORR	Median PFS (months)	Median OS (months)
					Rheum	Derm	GI	Neuro	Endo	Resp			
Loriot et al.	Urologic	35	Atezolizumab	34%	14%	49%	6%	3%	31%	0%	11%	4.4 (95% CI, 2.2–6.3)	8.2 (95% CI, 6.5–11.7)
Martinez Chanza et al.	RCC (54.6%) Urothelial (45.4%)	106	PD-1/PD-L1i monotherapy (80%) PD-1/PD-L1i + CTLA-4i (9%) PD-1/PD-L1i + VEGFi (10%)	40%	34%	30%	6%	4%	24%	0%	31% (RCC) 40% (UC)	NR	NR
Danlos et al.	Melanoma (80%) NSCLC (13.3%) Others (6.7%)	45	Pembrolizumab (75.6%) Nivolumab (22.2%) Avelumab (2.2%)	0%	13%	62%	0%	6%	17%	0%	38%	NR	NR
Cortellini et al.	NSCLC (65.5%) Melanoma (21.2%) RCC (12.5%) Others (0.8%)[a]	85	Pembrolizumab (24%) Nivolumab (76%)[a]	24%	12%	16%	5%	1%	60%	0%	38%[b] 50%[c]	14.4[b] 6.8[c]	15.7[b] 9.8[c]
Richter et al.	Melanoma (63%) NSCLC (25%) Others (13%)	16	Ipilimumab (31%) Pembrolizumab (31%) Nivolumab (44%)	6%	100%	0%	0%	0%	0%	0%	NR	NR	NR

Kaur et al.	NR	46	PD-1/PD-L1i monotherapy (74%) CTLA-4i monotherapy (26%)	NR	18%	4%	7%	0%	63%	0%	NR	NR	NR
Abu-Sbeih et al.	Melanoma (44%) NSCLC (23%) GI (17%) Urologic (7%) Others (10%)	102	PD-1/PD-L1i monotherapy (83%) CTLA-4i monotherapy (7%) PD-1/PD-L1i + CTLA-4i (10%)	NR	0%	0%	100%	0%	0%	0%	NR	NR	NR
Braga Neto et al.	Melanoma (54%) Others (46%)	13	Ipilimumab (8%) Pembrolizumab (62%) Nivolumab (38%)	NR	0%	0%	100%	0%	0%	0%	NR	NR	NR
Efuni et al.	Melanoma (32%) NSCLC (32%) Others (36%)	22	Ipilimumab (23%) Pembrolizumab (59%) Nivolumab (41%)	NR	100%	0%	0%	0%	0%	0%	NR	NR	NR

ANA antinuclear antibody, *CI* confidence interval, *derm* dermatologic, *endo* endocrine, *GI* gastrointestinal, *MCC* Merkel cell carcinoma, *neuro* neurologic, *NE* not estimable, *NSCLC* non-small cell lung cancer, *RCC* renal cell carcinoma, *resp* respiratory, *rheum* rheumatologic

Rheumatologic AID: rheumatoid arthritis, myositis, systemic lupus erythematosus (SLE), psoriatic arthritis, vasculitis, polymyalgia rheumatica (PMR), scleroderma, Sjogren's syndrome

Dermatologic AID: psoriasis, eczema, erythema nodosum

Gastrointestinal AID: Crohn's disease, ulcerative colitis, celiac disease

Neurologic AID: Guillain-Barré syndrome (GBS), transverse myelitis, multiple sclerosis, chronic inflammatory demyelinating polyneuropathy (CIDP)

Endocrine AID: hypophysitis, hypoadrenalism, thyroiditis and hyper-/hypothyroidism, Graves' disease

[a]Fom total population; [b]clinically inactive AID; [c]clinically active AID

Table 2 Immune checkpoint inhibitor toxicity and flare in patients with autoimmune disease

Study	Autoimmune disease flare	Grade ≥ 3 autoimmune disease flare	Median time to flare, days (range)	irAEs	Grade ≥ 3 irAEs	ICI discontinuation
Menzies et al.	38%	6%	38 (8–161)	29%	10%	8%
Gutzmer et al.	42%	11%	42% within 20 weeks	58%	16%	0%
Kahler et al.	29%	NR	NR	29%	NR	17%
Johnson et al.	27%	NR	17% at 3 weeks	33%	33%	NR
Lee et al.	75%	25%		100%	75%	63%
Leonardi et al.	23%	4%	64 (1–260)	38%	11%	14%
Yoneshima et al.	NR	NR	NR	33%	11%	11%
Tison et al.	47%	13%	NR	42%	16%	21%
Ardizzoni A et al.	NR	NR	NR	13%	NR	17%
Loriot et al.	11%	6%	74 (21–358)	46%	14%	6%
Martinez Chanza et al.	36%	6%	76 (25–215) RCC 33 (1–368) urothelial cancer	38%	11%	13%
Danlos et al.	24%	11%	NR	44%	NR	9%
Cortellini et al.	47%	9%	NR	66%	9%	7%
Richter et al.	6%	0%	NR	38%	25%	38%
Kaur et al.	20%	NR	NR	NR	NR	2%
Abu-Sbeih et al.	36%	17%	NR	NR	NR	32%
Braga Neto et al.	31%	NR	NR	NR	NR	0%
Efuni et al.	55%	NR	30	32%	9%	9%

irAE immune-related adverse events, *NR* not reported, *RCC* renal cell carcinoma

Acknowledgments None.

Compliance with Ethical Standards The authors declare that there is no conflict of interest.

References

Afzali B, Lombardi G, Lechler RI, Lord GM (2007) The role of T helper 17 (Th17) and regulatory T cells (Treg) in human organ transplantation and autoimmune disease. Clin Exp Immunol. https://doi.org/10.1111/j.1365-2249.2007.03356.x

Anaya JM (2012) Common mechanisms of autoimmune diseases (the autoimmune tautology). Autoimmun Rev. https://doi.org/10.1016/j.autrev.2012.02.002

Ardizzoni A, Azevedo S, Rubio-Viqueira B et al (2021) Primary results from TAIL: a global single-arm safety study of atezolizumab monotherapy in a diverse population of patients with previously treated advanced non-small cell lung cancer. J Immunother Cancer 9(3):e001865. https://doi.org/10.1136/jitc-2020-001865

Ascierto PA, Marincola FM, Ribas A (2011) Anti-CTLA4 monoclonal antibodies: the past and the future in clinical application. J Transl Med. https://doi.org/10.1186/1479-5876-9-196

Ascierto PA, Del Vecchio M, Robert C et al (2017) Ipilimumab 10 mg/kg versus ipilimumab 3 mg/kg in patients with unresectable or metastatic melanoma: a randomised, double-blind, multicentre, phase 3 trial. Lancet Oncol 18(5):611–622. https://doi.org/10.1016/S1470-2045(17)30231-0

Benagiano M, Bianchi P, D'Elios MM, Brosens I, Benagiano G (2019) Autoimmune diseases: role of steroid hormones. Best Pract Res Clin Obstet Gynaecol. https://doi.org/10.1016/j.bpobgyn.2019.03.001

Brahmer J, Reckamp KL, Baas P et al (2015) Nivolumab versus docetaxel in advanced squamous-cell non-small-cell lung cancer. N Engl J Med 373(2):123–135. https://doi.org/10.1056/NEJMoa1504627

Buchbinder EI, Desai A (2016) CTLA-4 and PD-1 pathways similarities, differences, and implications of their inhibition. Am J Clin Oncol Cancer Clin Trials. https://doi.org/10.1097/COC.0000000000000239

Cappelli LC, Shah AA (2020) The relationships between cancer and autoimmune rheumatic diseases. Best Pract Res Clin Rheumatol. https://doi.org/10.1016/j.berh.2019.101472

Chaudhuri S, Thomas S, Munster P (2021) Immunotherapy in breast cancer: a clinician's perspective. J Natl Cancer Cent. https://doi.org/10.1016/j.jncc.2021.01.001

Cojocaru M, Cojocaru IM, Silosi I (2010, Apr) Multiple autoimmune syndrome. Maedica (Bucur) 5(2):132–134

Cortellini A, Buti S, Santini D et al (2019) Clinical outcomes of patients with advanced cancer and pre-existing autoimmune diseases treated with anti-programmed Death-1 immunotherapy: a real-world transverse study. Oncologist 24(6):e327–e337. https://doi.org/10.1634/theoncologist.2018-0618

Danlos FX, Voisin AL, Dyevre V et al (2018) Safety and efficacy of anti-programmed death 1 antibodies in patients with cancer and pre-existing autoimmune or inflammatory disease. Eur J Cancer 91:21–29. https://doi.org/10.1016/j.ejca.2017.12.008

Davis AA, Patel VG (2019) The role of PD-L1 expression as a predictive biomarker: an analysis of all US food and drug administration (FDA) approvals of immune checkpoint inhibitors. J Immunother Cancer 7(1). https://doi.org/10.1186/s40425-019-0768-9

Dhatchinamoorthy K, Colbert JD, Rock KL (2021) Cancer immune evasion through loss of MHC class I antigen presentation. Front Immunol. https://doi.org/10.3389/fimmu.2021.636568

Dolina JS, Van Braeckel-Budimir N, Thomas GD, Salek-Ardakani S (2021) CD8+ T cell exhaustion in cancer. Front Immunol. https://doi.org/10.3389/fimmu.2021.715234

Dong W, Gong M, Shi Z, Xiao J, Zhang J, Peng J (2016) Programmed cell death-1 polymorphisms decrease the cancer risk: a meta-analysis involving twelve case-control studies. PLoS One. https://doi.org/10.1371/journal.pone.0152448

Eggermont AMM, Blank CU, Mandala M et al (2018) Adjuvant Pembrolizumab versus placebo in resected stage III melanoma. N Engl J Med 378(19):1789–1801. https://doi.org/10.1056/NEJMoa1802357

Elandt K, Aletaha D (2011) Treating rheumatic patients with a malignancy. Arthritis Res Ther. https://doi.org/10.1186/ar3352

Emens LA, Ascierto PA, Darcy PK et al (2017) Cancer immunotherapy: opportunities and challenges in the rapidly evolving clinical landscape. Eur J Cancer 81:116–129. https://doi.org/10.1016/j.ejca.2017.01.035

Fierabracci A, Pellegrino M (2016) The double role of p53 in cancer and autoimmunity and its potential as therapeutic target. Int J Mol Sci. https://doi.org/10.3390/ijms17121975

Furuse M, Kuwabara H, Ikeda N et al (2020) PD-L1 and PD-L2 expression in the tumor microenvironment including peritumoral tissue in primary central nervous system lymphoma. BMC Cancer. https://doi.org/10.1186/s12885-020-06755-y

Galdiero MR, Marone G, Mantovani A (2018) Cancer inflammation and cytokines. Cold Spring Harb Perspect Biol. https://doi.org/10.1101/cshperspect.a028662

Gandhi L, Rodríguez-Abreu D, Gadgeel S et al (2018) Pembrolizumab plus chemotherapy in metastatic non-small-cell lung cancer. N Engl J Med 378(22):2078–2092. https://doi.org/10.1056/NEJMoa1801005

Giat E, Ehrenfeld M, Shoenfeld Y (2017) Cancer and autoimmune diseases. Autoimmun Rev. https://doi.org/10.1016/j.autrev.2017.07.022

Golshani G, Zhang Y (2020) Advances in immunotherapy for colorectal cancer: a review. Ther Adv Gastroenterol. https://doi.org/10.1177/1756284820917527

Gutzmer R, Koop A, Meier F et al (2017) Programmed cell death protein-1 (PD-1) inhibitor therapy in patients with advanced melanoma and preexisting autoimmunity or ipilimumab-triggered autoimmunity. Eur J Cancer 75:24–32. https://doi.org/10.1016/j.ejca.2016.12.038

Hamid O, Robert C, Daud A et al (2019) Five-year survival outcomes for patients with advanced melanoma treated with pembrolizumab in KEYNOTE-001. Ann Oncol 30(4):582–588. https://doi.org/10.1093/annonc/mdz011

Han Y, Liu D, Li L (2020) PD-1/PD-L1 pathway: current researches in cancer. Am J Cancer Res 10(3):727–742

Hashemi M, Karami S, Sarabandi S et al (2019) Association between PD-1 and PD-l1 polymorphisms and the risk of cancer: a meta-analysis of case-control studies. Cancers (Basel). https://doi.org/10.3390/cancers11081150

Haslam A, Prasad V (2019) Estimation of the percentage of US patients with cancer who are eligible for and respond to checkpoint inhibitor immunotherapy drugs. JAMA Netw Open 2(5):e192535. Published 2019 May 3. https://doi.org/10.1001/jamanetworkopen.2019.2535

He XS, Gershwin ME, Ansari AA (2017) Checkpoint-based immunotherapy for autoimmune diseases – opportunities and challenges. J Autoimmun. https://doi.org/10.1016/j.jaut.2017.02.004

Herbst RS, Baas P, Kim DW et al (2016) Pembrolizumab versus docetaxel for previously treated, PD-L1-positive, advanced non-small-cell lung cancer (KEYNOTE-010): a randomised controlled trial. Lancet 387(10027):1540–1550. https://doi.org/10.1016/S0140-6736(15)01281-7

Hodi FS, O'Day SJ, McDermott DF et al (2010) Improved survival with ipilimumab in patients with metastatic melanoma [published correction appears in N Engl J Med. 2010 Sep 23;363(13):1290]. N Engl J Med 363(8):711–723. https://doi.org/10.1056/NEJMoa1003466

Horn L, Mansfield AS, Szczęsna A et al (2018) First-line Atezolizumab plus chemotherapy in extensive-stage small-cell lung cancer. N Engl J Med 379(23):2220–2229. https://doi.org/10.1056/NEJMoa1809064

Johnson DB, Sullivan RJ, Ott PA et al (2016) Ipilimumab therapy in patients with advanced melanoma and preexisting autoimmune disorders. JAMA Oncol 2(2):234–240. https://doi.org/10.1001/jamaoncol.2015.4368

Jörg S, Grohme DA, Erzler M et al (2016) Environmental factors in autoimmune diseases and their role in multiple sclerosis. Cell Mol Life Sci. https://doi.org/10.1007/s00018-016-2311-1

Jotte R, Cappuzzo F, Vynnychenko I et al (2020) Atezolizumab in combination with carboplatin and nab-paclitaxel in advanced squamous NSCLC (IMpower131): results from a randomized phase III trial. J Thorac Oncol 15(8):1351–1360. https://doi.org/10.1016/j.jtho.2020.03.028

Kähler KC, Eigentler TK, Gesierich A et al (2018) Ipilimumab in metastatic melanoma patients with pre-existing autoimmune disorders. Cancer Immunol Immunother 67(5):825–834. https://doi.org/10.1007/s00262-018-2134-z

Kang J, Zhang C, Zhong WZ (2021) Neoadjuvant immunotherapy for non–small cell lung cancer: state of the art. Cancer Commun. https://doi.org/10.1002/cac2.12153

Keeley T, Costanzo-Garvey DL, Cook LM (2019) Unmasking the many faces of tumor-associated neutrophils and macrophages: considerations for targeting innate immune cells in cancer. Trends Cancer. https://doi.org/10.1016/j.trecan.2019.10.013

Khan SA, Pruitt SL, Xuan L, Gerber DE (2016) Prevalence of autoimmune disease among patients with lung cancer: implications for immunotherapy treatment options. JAMA Oncol 2(11): 1507–1508. https://doi.org/10.1001/jamaoncol.2016.2238

Kichloo A, Albosta M, Dahiya D et al (2021) Systemic adverse effects and toxicities associated with immunotherapy: a review. World J Clin Oncol. https://doi.org/10.5306/wjco.v12.i3.150

Knochelmann HM, Dwyer CJ, Bailey SR et al (2018) When worlds collide: Th17 and Treg cells in cancer and autoimmunity. Cell Mol Immunol. https://doi.org/10.1038/s41423-018-0004-4

Kumagai S, Togashi Y, Kamada T et al (2020) The PD-1 expression balance between effector and regulatory T cells predicts the clinical efficacy of PD-1 blockade therapies. Nat Immunol. https://doi.org/10.1038/s41590-020-0769-3

Kumar N, Chugh H, Tomar R, Tomar V, Singh VK, Chandra R (2018) Exploring the interplay between autoimmunity and cancer to find the target therapeutic hotspots. Artif Cells Nanomed Biotechnol. https://doi.org/10.1080/21691401.2017.1350188

Langer CJ, Gadgeel SM, Borghaei H et al (2016) Carboplatin and pemetrexed with or without pembrolizumab for advanced, non-squamous non-small-cell lung cancer: a randomised, phase 2 cohort of the open-label KEYNOTE-021 study. Lancet Oncol 17(11):1497–1508. https://doi.org/10.1016/S1470-2045(16)30498-3

Larkin J, Chiarion-Sileni V, Gonzalez R et al (2015) Combined Nivolumab and Ipilimumab or monotherapy in untreated melanoma [published correction appears in N Engl J Med. 2018 Nov 29;379(22):2185]. N Engl J Med 373(1):23–34. https://doi.org/10.1056/NEJMoa1504030

Larkin J, Minor D, D'Angelo S, Neyns B, Smylie M, Miller WH Jr, Gutzmer R, Linette G, Chmielowski B, Lao CD, Lorigan P, Grossmann K, Hassel JC, Sznol M, Daud A, Sosman J, Khushalani N, Schadendorf D, Hoeller C, Walker D, Kong G, Horak C, Weber J (2018, Feb 1) Overall survival in patients with advanced melanoma who received nivolumab versus investigator's choice chemotherapy in checkmate 037: a randomized, controlled, open-label phase III trial. J Clin Oncol 36(4):383–390. https://doi.org/10.1200/JCO.2016.71.8023. Epub 2017 Jul 3

Larkin J, Chiarion-Sileni V, Gonzalez R et al (2019) Five-year survival with combined Nivolumab and Ipilimumab in advanced melanoma. N Engl J Med 381(16):1535–1546. https://doi.org/10.1056/NEJMoa1910836

Latchman Y, Wood CR, Chernova T et al (2001) PD-L2 is a second ligand for PD-1 and inhibits T cell activation. Nat Immunol. https://doi.org/10.1038/85330

Lee AY, Brady MS (2021) Neoadjuvant immunotherapy for melanoma. J Surg Oncol. https://doi.org/10.1002/jso.26229

Lee B, Wong A, Kee D et al (2016) The use of ipilimumab in patients with rheumatoid arthritis and metastatic melanoma. Ann Oncol 27(6):1174–1177. https://doi.org/10.1093/annonc/mdw056

Leonardi GC, Gainor JF, Altan M et al (2018) Safety of programmed Death-1 pathway inhibitors among patients with non-small-cell lung cancer and preexisting autoimmune disorders. J Clin Oncol 36(19):1905–1912. https://doi.org/10.1200/JCO.2017.77.0305

Lo B, Abdel-Motal UM (2017) Lessons from CTLA-4 deficiency and checkpoint inhibition. Curr Opin Immunol. https://doi.org/10.1016/j.coi.2017.07.014

Loriot Y, Sternberg CN, Castellano D et al (2020) Safety and efficacy of atezolizumab in patients with autoimmune disease: subgroup analysis of the SAUL study in locally advanced/metastatic urinary tract carcinoma. Eur J Cancer 138:202–211. https://doi.org/10.1016/j.ejca.2020.07.023

Luan M, Shang Z, Teng Y et al (2017) The shared and specific mechanism of four autoimmune diseases. Oncotarget. https://doi.org/10.18632/oncotarget.19383

Maniati E, Rogers NJ, Morley BJ, Rocchi C (2010) Apoptosis in autoimmunity. In: Apoptosis: modern insights into disease from molecules to man. https://doi.org/10.1201/9781439845431

Mansh M (2011) Ipilimumab and cancer immunotherapy: a new hope for advanced stage melanoma. Yale J Biol Med 84(4):381–389

Martinez Chanza N, Xie W, Issa M et al (2020) Safety and efficacy of immune checkpoint inhibitors in advanced urological cancers with pre-existing autoimmune disorders: a retrospective international multicenter study. J Immunother Cancer 8(1):e000538. https://doi.org/10.1136/jitc-2020-000538

Marty R, Thompson WK, Salem RM, Zanetti M, Carter H (2018) Evolutionary pressure against MHC Class II binding cancer mutations. Cell. https://doi.org/10.1016/j.cell.2018.08.048

Menzies AM, Johnson DB, Ramanujam S et al (2017) Anti-PD-1 therapy in patients with advanced melanoma and preexisting autoimmune disorders or major toxicity with ipilimumab. Ann Oncol 28(2):368–376. https://doi.org/10.1093/annonc/mdw443

Mihic-Probst D, Reinehr M, Dettwiler S et al (2020) The role of macrophages type 2 and T-regs in immune checkpoint inhibitor related adverse events. Immunobiology. https://doi.org/10.1016/j.imbio.2020.152009

Mok TSK, Wu YL, Kudaba I et al (2019) Pembrolizumab versus chemotherapy for previously untreated, PD-L1-expressing, locally advanced or metastatic non-small-cell lung cancer (KEYNOTE-042): a randomised, open-label, controlled, phase 3 trial. Lancet 393(10183): 1819–1830. https://doi.org/10.1016/S0140-6736(18)32409-7

Moulton VR (2018) Sex hormones in acquired immunity and autoimmune disease. Front Immunol. https://doi.org/10.3389/fimmu.2018.02279

Nishio M, Barlesi F, West H et al (2021) Atezolizumab plus chemotherapy for first-line treatment of nonsquamous NSCLC: results from the randomized phase 3 IMpower132 trial. J Thorac Oncol 16(4):653–664. https://doi.org/10.1016/j.jtho.2020.11.025

Nistala K, Wedderburn LR (2009) Th17 and regulatory T cells: rebalancing pro- and anti-inflammatory forces in autoimmune arthritis. Rheumatology. https://doi.org/10.1093/rheumatology/kep028

O'Donnell JS, Hoefsmit EP, Smyth MJ, Blank CU, Teng MWL (2019) The promise of neoadjuvant immunotherapy and surgery for cancer treatment. Clin Cancer Res. https://doi.org/10.1158/1078-0432.CCR-18-2641

Onitilo AA, Wittig JA (2020) Principles of immunotherapy in melanoma. Surg Clin North Am. https://doi.org/10.1016/j.suc.2019.09.009

Paz-Ares L, Luft A, Vicente D et al (2018) Pembrolizumab plus chemotherapy for squamous non-small-cell lung cancer. N Engl J Med 379(21):2040–2051. https://doi.org/10.1056/NEJMoa1810865

Pelosof LC, Gerber DE (2010) Paraneoplastic syndromes: an approach to diagnosis and treatment. Mayo Clin Proc. https://doi.org/10.4065/mcp.2010.0099

Perl A (2012) Pathogenesis and spectrum of autoimmunity. Methods Mol Biol. https://doi.org/10.1007/978-1-60761-720-4_1

Qin W, Hu L, Zhang X et al (2019) The diverse function of PD-1/PD-L pathway beyond cancer. Front Immunol. https://doi.org/10.3389/fimmu.2019.02298

Qureshi OS, Kaur S, Hou TZ et al (2012) Constitutive clathrin-mediated endocytosis of CTLA-4 persists during T cell activation. J Biol Chem. https://doi.org/10.1074/jbc.M111.304329

Rakshit S, Molina JR (2020) Immunotherapy in patients with autoimmune disease. J Thorac Dis. https://doi.org/10.21037/jtd-2019-cptn-10

Reck M, Rodríguez-Abreu D, Robinson AG et al (2016) Pembrolizumab versus chemotherapy for PD-L1-positive non-small-cell lung cancer. N Engl J Med 375(19):1823–1833. https://doi.org/10.1056/NEJMoa1606774

Ribas A, Puzanov I, Dummer R et al (2015) Pembrolizumab versus investigator-choice chemotherapy for ipilimumab-refractory melanoma (KEYNOTE-002): a randomised, controlled, phase 2 trial. Lancet Oncol 16(8):908–918. https://doi.org/10.1016/S1470-2045(15)00083-2

Richard-Eaglin A, Smallheer BA (2018) Immunosuppressive/Autoimmune Disorders. Nurs Clin North Am. https://doi.org/10.1016/j.cnur.2018.04.002

Richardson JR, Schöllhorn A, Gouttefangeas C, Schuhmacher J (2021) CD4+ T cells: multitasking cells in the duty of cancer immunotherapy. Cancers (Basel). https://doi.org/10.3390/cancers13040596

Riley JL (2009) PD-1 signaling in primary T cells. Immunol Rev. https://doi.org/10.1111/j.1600-065X.2009.00767.x

Rini BI, Battle D, Figlin RA et al (2019) The society for immunotherapy of cancer consensus statement on immunotherapy for the treatment of advanced renal cell carcinoma (RCC). J Immunother Cancer. https://doi.org/10.1186/s40425-019-0813-8

Rittmeyer A, Barlesi F, Waterkamp D et al (2017) Atezolizumab versus docetaxel in patients with previously treated non-small-cell lung cancer (OAK): a phase 3, open-label, multicentre randomised controlled trial [published correction appears in Lancet. 2017 Apr 8;389(10077): e5]. Lancet 389(10066):255–265. https://doi.org/10.1016/S0140-6736(16)32517-X

Robert C, Long GV, Brady B et al (2015) Nivolumab in previously untreated melanoma without BRAF mutation. N Engl J Med 372(4):320–330. https://doi.org/10.1056/NEJMoa1412082

Rosenblum MD, Remedios KA, Abbas AK (2015) Mechanisms of human autoimmunity. J Clin Invest. https://doi.org/10.1172/JCI78088

Rowshanravan B, Halliday N, Sansom DM (2018) CTLA-4: a moving target in immunotherapy. Blood. https://doi.org/10.1182/blood-2017-06-741033

Saung MT, Pelosof L, Casak S et al (2021) FDA approval summary: Nivolumab plus Ipilimumab for the treatment of patients with hepatocellular carcinoma previously treated with Sorafenib. Oncologist. https://doi.org/10.1002/onco.13819

Schachter J, Ribas A, Long GV et al (2017) Pembrolizumab versus ipilimumab for advanced melanoma: final overall survival results of a multicentre, randomised, open-label phase 3 study (KEYNOTE-006). Lancet 390(10105):1853–1862. https://doi.org/10.1016/S0140-6736(17)31601-X

Schairer C, Pfeiffer RM, Gadalla SM (2018) Autoimmune diseases and breast cancer risk by tumor hormone-receptor status among elderly women. Int J Cancer. https://doi.org/10.1002/ijc.31148

Schmerling RA, Buzaid AC, Haddad CK et al (2021) Immune manifestations with checkpoint inhibitors in a single Brazilian center: experience and literature review. Futur Sci OA. https://doi.org/10.2144/fsoa-2020-0129

Simon S, Labarriere N (2018) PD-1 expression on tumor-specific T cells: friend or foe for immunotherapy? Onco Targets Ther. https://doi.org/10.1080/2162402X.2017.1364828

Socinski MA, Jotte RM, Cappuzzo F et al (2018) Atezolizumab for first-line treatment of metastatic nonsquamous NSCLC. N Engl J Med 378(24):2288–2301. https://doi.org/10.1056/NEJMoa1716948

Socinski MA, Nishio M, Jotte RM et al (2021) IMpower150 final overall survival analyses for Atezolizumab plus bevacizumab and chemotherapy in first-line metastatic nonsquamous NSCLC. J Thorac Oncol 16(11):1909–1924. https://doi.org/10.1016/j.jtho.2021.07.009

Song M, Latorre G, Ivanovic-Zuvic D, Camargo MC, Rabkin CS (2019) Autoimmune diseases and gastric cancer risk: a systematic review and meta-analysis. Cancer Res Treat. https://doi.org/10.4143/crt.2019.151

Soskic B, Qureshi OS, Hou T, Sansom DM (2014) A transendocytosis perspective on the CD28/CTLA-4 pathway. Adv Immunol. https://doi.org/10.1016/B978-0-12-800147-9.00004-2

Sternberg CN, Loriot Y, James N et al (2019) Primary results from SAUL, a multinational single-arm safety study of Atezolizumab therapy for locally advanced or metastatic urothelial or nonurothelial carcinoma of the urinary tract. Eur Urol 76(1):73–81. https://doi.org/10.1016/j.eururo.2019.03.015

Sullivan K, Preeshagul I, Budman D, Seetharamu N (2017) Immune checkpoint inhibitors in lung cancer: an update. Future Oncol 13(11). https://doi.org/10.2217/fon-2017-0044

Takeuchi Y, Nishikawa H (2016) Roles of regulatory T cells in cancer immunity. Int Immunol. https://doi.org/10.1093/intimm/dxw025

Taneja V (2019) Genetic predisposition to autoimmune diseases conferred by the major histocompatibility complex: utility of animal models. In: The autoimmune diseases. https://doi.org/10.1016/B978-0-12-812102-3.00026-9

Tang H, Zhou J, Bai C (2021) The efficacy and safety of immune checkpoint inhibitors in patients with cancer and preexisting autoimmune disease. Front Oncol. https://doi.org/10.3389/fonc.2021.625872
Tison A, Quéré G, Misery L et al (2019) Safety and efficacy of immune checkpoint inhibitors in patients with cancer and preexisting autoimmune disease: a nationwide, multicenter cohort study. Arthritis Rheumatol. https://doi.org/10.1002/art.41068
Valencia JC, Egbukichi N, Erwin-Cohen RA (2019) Autoimmunity and cancer, the paradox comorbidities challenging therapy in the context of preexisting autoimmunity. J Interf Cytokine Res. https://doi.org/10.1089/jir.2018.0060
Vial T, Descotes J (2003) Immunosuppressive drugs and cancer. Toxicology. https://doi.org/10.1016/S0300-483X(02)00612-1
Wahren-Herlenius M, Dörner T (2013) Immunopathogenic mechanisms of systemic autoimmune disease. Lancet. https://doi.org/10.1016/S0140-6736(13)60954-X
Waldman AD, Fritz JM, Lenardo MJ (2020) A guide to cancer immunotherapy: from T cell basic science to clinical practice. Nat Rev Immunol. https://doi.org/10.1038/s41577-020-0306-5
Weber JS, D'Angelo SP, Minor D et al (2015) Nivolumab versus chemotherapy in patients with advanced melanoma who progressed after anti-CTLA-4 treatment (CheckMate 037): a randomised, controlled, open-label, phase 3 trial. Lancet Oncol 16(4):375–384. https://doi.org/10.1016/S1470-2045(15)70076-8
Wigner P, Grębowski R, Bijak M, Saluk-Bijak J, Szemraj J (2021) The interplay between oxidative stress, inflammation and angiogenesis in bladder cancer development. Int J Mol Sci. https://doi.org/10.3390/ijms22094483
Wu L, Zhang XHF (2020) Tumor-associated neutrophils and macrophages—Heterogenous but not chaotic. Front Immunol. https://doi.org/10.3389/fimmu.2020.553967
Xiong W, Zhao Y, Du H, Guo X (2021) Current status of immune checkpoint inhibitor immunotherapy for lung cancer. Front Oncol. https://doi.org/10.3389/fonc.2021.704336
Yi C, He Y, Xia H, Zhang H, Zhang P (2019) Review and perspective on adjuvant and neoadjuvant immunotherapies in NSCLC. Onco Targets Ther. https://doi.org/10.2147/OTT.S218321
Yoneshima Y, Tanaka K, Shiraishi Y et al (2019) Safety and efficacy of PD-1 inhibitors in non-small cell lung cancer patients positive for antinuclear antibodies. Lung Cancer 130:5–9. https://doi.org/10.1016/j.lungcan.2019.01.014
Young A, Quandt Z, Bluestone JA (2018) The balancing act between cancer immunity and autoimmunity in response to immunotherapy. Cancer Immunol Res. https://doi.org/10.1158/2326-6066.CIR-18-0487
Zarnavalou C, Guri K, Anagnostopoulou FA (2016) Autoimmune diseases and correlation with malignancies. Rev Clin Pharmacol Pharmacokinet Int Ed 30(1):23–29

The Effects of Low-Dose Non-ionizing and Ionizing Radiation on Wound Healing and Cancer

Raahilah Zahir Essa, Ming Tsuey Chew, David A. Bradley, Suat-Cheng Peh, and Sin-Yeang Teow

Abstract

Radiation therapy is a vital integrated part of modern comprehensive cancer management. Aside from the typical use of radiotherapy in treatment of cancer, low-dose radiation (LDR), typically <100 mGy, shows the capacity to improve wound healing by promoting fibroblast-to-myofibroblast differentiation, matrix deposition, keratinocyte proliferation and angiogenesis. Moreover, animal studies have shown LDR attenuates systemic acute inflammatory response by regulating inflammatory cytokines, thus alleviating damage associating with chronic diabetic and burn wounds. Wounds can be classified as open or closed. Open wounds, such as cuts, burns or ulcers, can arise from external factors such as accidents, surgery and trauma or internal factors, such as diabetes mellitus, whereas closed wounds may occur due to blunt force trauma. Additionally, wounds can be either acute or chronic, depending on their healing capacity. These disruptions of the skin's structural and functional integrity go through four distinct phases to achieve complete wound healing, namely, haemostasis, inflammation, cellular migration and proliferation and remodelling. Photobiomodulation and low-dose ionizing

R. Z. Essa · S.-C. Peh · S.-Y. Teow (✉)
Department of Medical Sciences, School of Medical and Life Sciences, Sunway University, Subang Jaya, Malaysia
e-mail: ronaldt@sunway.edu.my

M. T. Chew (✉)
Centre for Applied Physics and Radiation Technologies, Sunway University, Subang Jaya, Malaysia
e-mail: mtchew@sunway.edu.my

D. A. Bradley
Centre for Applied Physics and Radiation Technologies, Sunway University, Subang Jaya, Malaysia

Department of Physics, University of Surrey, Guildford, UK

Interdisciplinary Cancer Research, https://doi.org/10.1007/16833_2022_60
Published online: 25 November 2022

radiation have been studied for their effects on the cellular and molecular processes involved in wound healing. Similarly, both methods of low-dose radiation treatment have also been examined for their cancer therapy-associated adverse effects. In this paper, the molecular and cellular effects of low-dose radiation on wound healing and cancer cells are discussed. Additionally, the protective effects of low-dose radiation against conventional cancer treatments such as high-dose radiation and chemotherapy are also discussed.

Keywords

Cancer · Low-dose radiation · Tissue repair · Wound healing

1 Radiation Therapy

1.1 The History and Current Applications of Ionizing and Non-ionizing Radiation

Non-ionizing radiation (non-IR) is typically characterized as being of relatively low energies (a few eV and less). Within the electromagnetic spectrum, ionizing radiations are considered to be those of energies greater than ultraviolet radiation, sufficiently energetic to displace electrons from their binding to the atom. In addition to ultraviolet radiation, non-IR radiations also include radio waves, microwaves, infrared radiation and visible light. Non-IR has been described by the US Occupational Safety and Health Administration as energy waves composed of oscillating electric and magnetic fields travelling at the speed of light (Non-Ionizing Radiation n.d). While the energy carried by non-IR is too low to displace electrons from the binding they have to the atom, accordingly being insufficient to cause ionization of the atomic media with which interactions occur, it is sufficient to cause excitation to higher atomic orbitals. The biological effects triggered by non-IR occur via photochemical and thermal effects (Daddysman and Fecko 2011; Omer 2021). Heliotherapy, or the use of sunlight for its beneficial properties, can be traced back to ancient Egypt and India (Grzybowski et al. 2016). As early as 1968, Mester et al. experimentally demonstrated the wound healing properties of laser light at low doses, coining the effect as "biostimulation", now more commonly referred to as photobiomodulation (PBM) (Mester et al. 1968).

Ionizing radiation (IR), conventionally used as a prime modality in the treatment of cancer, interacts with tissue by removing electrons from atoms and molecules that make up living tissue. The outcomes of treatment with IR occur through either direct or indirect damage. Direct damage occurs via breaks in the deoxyribonucleic acid (DNA), resulting in single-strand breaks and double-strand breaks (DSBs), which can be fatal to the cells. Indirect damage, on the other hand, primarily occurs as a result of increased reactive oxygen species (ROS) formation (Chew et al. 2021). Three types of ionizing radiation (IR) can be used in external radiation therapy: photon, electron and proton radiation. Photon beams, such as x-rays and γ-rays, are high energy beams now most typically delivered from linear accelerators, the beams being directed to go through the target site, affecting both the tumour and the surrounding cellular and tissue structures. Photon-based radiation is the most common form of radiation therapy that is utilized in the field of radiation oncology, inclusive of both curative and palliative care. Despite improvements in photon-based radiation therapy in regard to both planning and delivery, including intensity or volumetric modulated radiation therapy, the particular physical properties of photons such as high energy and distribution patterns form a major limitation of this treatment plan including potentially high risks of adverse effects, including radiation toxicity to surrounding tissues (Allison et al. 2013). Unlike photon beams, which pass through and exit the body, electron beams have lower penetrative potential and are used to treat tumours on the skin, lymph nodes or other locations with close surface proximity (Gianfaldoni et al. 2017). The interactions with tissue give rise to highly tortuous paths that limit depth penetration such that electron radiation displays a rapid dose fall-off beyond the target tissue, resulting in both high target-specific radiation exposure and lower risk of toxicity and resultant complications in surrounding normal tissue (O'Shea et al. 2008). The negatively charged electron radiation is again typically delivered using linear accelerators (electron linacs), less versatile access being provided by radionuclide sources emitting beta (electron) particles. Another form of particulate IR (electrons are referred to as light particles or low energy transfer radiation) is heavy ions, as, for example, the protons that are increasingly becoming available for radiation therapy, utilizing synchrotrons or cyclotrons to deliver the positively charged particles to deep tissue. Unlike photon radiation, the heavy ion particles do not give rise to a high pattern of radiation scattering to surrounding tissue. Due to high cost, this form of radiation therapy is currently less common compared to the use of photon and electron radiation (Allison et al. 2013; Weber et al. 2006). A notable difference between the more commonly used photon and electron radiations and proton therapy concerns the dose distribution. In particular, for proton irradiation a distinct therapeutic advantage is obtained for deeper-seated tumours. The dose distribution of protons is defined by initial relatively low-dose deposition within the superficial tissues that preface more deep-seated tumours, maximal dose deposition then being obtained in what is referred to as a Bragg peak. Subsequently, beyond the tumour, very steep dose fall-off is obtained, saving tissue at greater depths (Moreno et al. 2019). Other heavy ions such as carbon are less well developed, typically due to the high costs involved (Martins 2018).

Some of the earliest uses of treatment with x-ray radiation can be traced back to the early twentieth century, with reports stating that IR was being used for the treatment of pathologies of the skin, including eczema, psoriasis, lupus vulgaris and mycosis fungoides (Freund 1904; Grzybowski and Pietrzak 2012). On the other hand, recent advancements in radiation therapy against cancer have included the use of intensity-modulated radiation therapy (IMRT), which delivers high doses of photon beams in multiple radiation fields. Additionally, the development of IMRT has allowed delivery of site-specific high-dose radiation with a steep dose fall-off in the non-target regions. This has resulted in decreased radiation-induced toxicities in the surrounding tissue compared to conventional radiation therapy (Pirzkall et al. 2000). While current 3D-IMRT can be used to accurately identify tumour volume, the 2D conventional radiotherapy used prior to the development of 3D techniques was highly reliant on identification of bony landmarks (Purdy 2008). Arguably the most effective anti-tumour therapy, radiation therapy is included in the management of 60–70% of cancer patients (Baumann et al. 2016). However, other than cancer, clinical studies using radiation therapy have also been carried out for benign diseases such as inflammation and infections. For example, low-dose radiotherapy (LDR) has been approved for the treatment of painful degenerative skeletal disorders including enthesopathies and arthrosis (Ott et al. 2015). In addition to degenerative skeletal disorders, groups in Germany have been at the forefront of radiotherapeutics for hyperproliferative and functional diseases (Kriz et al. 2018).

1.2 Low-Dose Ionizing Radiation

The linear no-threshold (LNT) model of radiation describes the risks of radiation at even low doses, implying that there is no threshold dose of radiation below which there is no risk of damaging biological effects, including the development of cancer. However, there is a natural amount of IR that is always present, also known as background radiation. It can originate from both natural and man-made sources and has not been associated with an increased risk of cancer (Sacks et al. 2016; Siegel et al. 2017; Chen et al. 2007). Natural sources of low-dose ionizing radiation (LDIR) include cosmic radiation, as well as radioactive elements in soil and stones, which may be used as building material. In fact, removal of background radiation has shown damaging effects in various model organisms such as bacteria (Castillo et al. 2015, 2021). On the other hand, deliberate LDR exposure primarily occurs due to diagnostic techniques such as x-rays and computed tomography (Radiation in Everyday Life 2014). Total doses of IR less than 0.1 Gy, or 100 mGy, and dose rates of 0.1 Gy/min are commonly denoted as low-dose and low dose-rate radiation, respectively (Biological mechanisms of radiation actions at low doses 2012).

Exposure to high-dose IR (>100 mGy) has been extensively studied and linked to an increase in the number of mutations. However, the linear relationship between radiation dosage and number of mutations is primarily described for high doses of radiation (Sykes et al. 2006). On top of that, despite its detrimental effects at high doses, numerous studies have identified the beneficial effects of radiation at low doses as well. The beneficial effects of low-dose x-rays on acute infections were first observed by Beattie (1921), who showed that exposure to x-ray radiation for diagnostic purposes triggered healing and subsequent alleviation of symptoms and resolution of infections such as otitis media and mastoiditis (Calabrese and Dhawan 2013). Additionally, a majority of the clinical studies highlighted that the dose required to achieve symptom alleviation in acute infection was within 15–20% of the skin erythema dose (starting at 2 Gy with more serious long-term effects arising at 10–15 Gy) (Calabrese and Dhawan 2013; Rehani and Srimahachota 2011). These potential beneficial effects at low doses are modelled in the hormetic model of radiation – which states that beneficial effects will be seen up to threshold level of radiation (<100 mGy), above which detrimental effects are conferred. In addition to the direct effects of LDIR, one of the major non-targeted effects of LDIR occurs as result of an adaptive response in which physiological responses at the time of a primary exposure or "priming" dose provide improved protective effects against the damaging effects induced by subsequent treatment with higher doses (Chew et al. 2021; Guéguen et al. 2019). The adaptive responses are only observed at low doses and are overpowered by damaging effects at higher doses (Feinendegen et al. 2007). They occur after an initial delay and involve changes in existing cellular and molecular cascades, including cellular proliferation and DNA damage repair responses (Feinendegen et al. 2009).

1.3 Photobiomodulation with Low-Dose Non-ionizing Radiation

Photobiomodulation (PBM) using low levels of non-ionizing light waves has also shown potential beneficial effects, including in the improvement of acute, chronic and burn wound healing (Anders et al. 2015). PBM, previously known as low-level laser therapy (LLLT), is a painless and non-invasive technique that utilizes lasers and light-emitting diodes to deliver low levels of non-IR that falls within the range of 0.44–50 J/cm^2 (de Freitas and Hamblin 2016). The biological basis behind PBM lies in the absorption of light energy by photo-acceptor biomolecules, also known as chromophores, both within the mitochondria and other compartments, primarily thought to be cytochrome-c oxidase (Cox) and intracellular water (Passarella and Karu 2014). These photo-acceptor molecules absorb light at red and near-infrared wavelengths, causing them to enter an excited state and trigger a downstream cascade of biochemical reactions resulting in increased mitochondrial respiration and altered redox properties, triggering changes in transcription factors, which then induce protein synthesis (Karu 1999; Chen et al. 2011). Proteins activated in PBM include growth factors and anti-inflammatory cytokines that are involved in downstream effects of irradiation exposure, such as proliferation, differentiation and migration (Hamblin 2017).

Cox is an electron transport chain terminal enzyme involved in catalysing the transfer of four protons from cytochrome c to molecular oxygen. This process is also responsible for the generation of an electrochemical gradient by providing sufficient energy to transport proton across the inner mitochondrial membrane, from the mitochondrial matrix to the intermembrane space, thus driving the activity of ATP synthase (Wikstrom 1977; Sharma et al. 2017). This enzyme consists of 13 peptides and 4 redox-active metal centres and has been previously reported to play a major role as a photo-acceptor of wavelengths ranging from 380 to 880 nm, which represent monochromatic visible light to near-infrared wavelengths (Kadenbach and Hüttemann 2015; Karu 1999). The primary reaction triggered by the absorption of energy by Cox includes the dissociation of inhibitory nitric oxide (NO), which is involved in the regulation of Cox activity. In addition to NO dissociation, the conformation changes that occur in the Cox molecules and heat-activated ion channels in response to transient increase in temperature following energy absorption are also believed to play an essential role in the initiation of downstream biochemical reactions (Karu 2014; Hamblin 2017). However, Sommer (2019) suggests that the absorption of energy by interfacial water layers may also be involved in the molecular effects of PBM. The two key parameters include light-induced volume expansion and viscosity reduction. Sommer et al. (2020) also suggests that in accordance with the hormetic model, the minimal dose required to achieve beneficial effects is dependent on the energy needed to reduce interfacial water layer viscosity. Additionally, the maximum dose at which these beneficial effects are observed is dependent on the interaction with Cox – either through the direct absorption of photons by Cox or indirectly through reactive oxygen species (ROS) generation.

Herein, the molecular and cellular effects of LDR on wound healing and cancer cells are discussed. Additionally, the protective effects of low-dose radiation against conventional cancer treatments such as high-dose radiation and chemotherapy are also examined.

2 Wound Healing

2.1 Types of Wounds

The skin, the largest organ of the body, serves as a protective barrier against external stimuli. In addition to its protective function, the intact epidermal barrier also provides sensory reception and performs the homeostatic functions of temperature regulation, moisture retention, mineral absorption and hormone synthesis. The skin consists of three major layers: the epidermis, dermis and subcutis (Fig. 1a). The epidermis is a layer of stratified squamous epithelial cells that make up the outer layer of the skin. Majority of these epithelial cells are keratin-producing keratinocytes which undergo progressive differentiation from a basal layer to the surface layer, resulting in the formation of four and five layers in thin and thick skin, respectively (Fig. 1b). The dermis houses fibroblasts, myofibroblasts and immune cells, as well as collagen, elastic fibres and proteoglycans produced by fibroblast cells – all of which play a significant role in maintaining the structural and functional integrity of the skin. Additionally, the dermis also provides nutrients to the epidermal layer of the skin through the basement membrane, as the latter lacks a vascular network. Lastly, the subcutaneous layer, also known as the hypodermis, consists primarily of adipose tissue. The primary function of this layer is to provide structural support and insulation for the skin.

Wounds can be classified as either open wounds or closed wounds. Open wounds may be induced intentionally, such as surgical incisions, or may occur accidentally through physical trauma. Closed wounds, on the other hand, are often triggered by blunt force trauma; they do not result in tissue exposure and are associated with internal bleeding or damage. Alternatively, wounds can be classified based on their ability to heal (Irfan-Maqsood 2018). Acute wounds are the most common type of

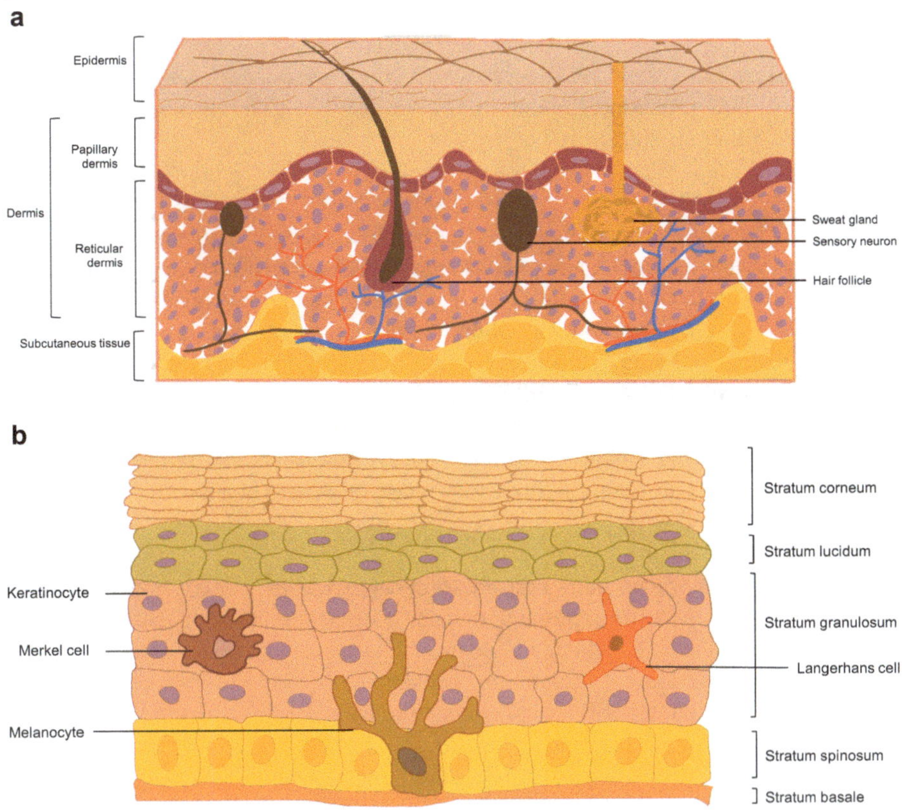

Fig. 1 Layers of the skin (**a**) and cells that make up the epidermis (**b**)

wound and encompass open wounds that undergo an organized wound healing process, whereas chronic wounds are characterized by the lack of tissue volume and integrity, as well as long healing periods lasting a minimum of 3 months (Martin and Nunan 2015). These types of wounds are also associated with pain and persistent inflammation and are usually accompanied by infections. Most common chronic wounds include ulcers such as diabetic foot ulcers, venous ulcers and pressure ulcers, as well as burns and infectious wounds (Frykberg and Banks 2015). In addition to poor quality of life due to pain, chronic wound recurrence occurs in 60–70% of patients and is a significant cause of morbidity in affected individuals (Ottawa 2013).

Damage to the integrity of the skin barrier results in loss of structural and functional capacity of the skin in close proximity to the wound. Additionally, open wounds increase risk of infection by providing a route of entry for external pathogens. The process of wound healing is an intricate cascade of biochemical processes that restore the skin's structural and functional integrity.

2.2 Phases of Wound Healing

Wound healing is a systematic process which constitutes of four sequential phases: haemostasis, inflammation, cellular migration and proliferation and remodelling (Fig. 2) (Velnar et al. 2009).

2.2.1 Haemostasis

Haemostasis, a vascular response which stops blood flow, is triggered immediately after injury. Vasoconstriction and platelet aggregation are triggered to prevent exsanguination through the open wound. Platelets are activated in response to exposure to collagen as a result of wound formation. Activation of platelets causes release of clotting factors including fibronectin, fibrin, vitronectin and thrombospondin, resulting in the formation of an insoluble clot (Velnar et al. 2009). In addition to preventing blood loss, platelet plugs also provide a structural scaffold for incoming immune cells and a barrier against pathogen entry. The formation of the platelet plug also initiates the downstream inflammatory phase of wound healing.

2.2.2 Inflammation

Inflammation is the innate body defence to injury. After the formation of a wound, damaged and necrotic cells expressing damage-associated molecular patterns can be recognised by neutrophils, which are the first immune cells to be recruited to the site of injury. The downstream activation of immune cells found in the skin, including mast, Langerhans and dendritic cells, will then release chemokines and cytokines for the recruitment of circulating leukocytes (Martin and Leibovich 2005). Both cellular debris and pathogens are phagocytized by immune cells.

2.2.3 Proliferation and Cellular Migration

The coordination of wound closure occurs during the proliferative phase (formation of new tissue). The four major cell types that undergo activation and proliferation during this phase of wound healing include endothelial cells, fibroblasts,

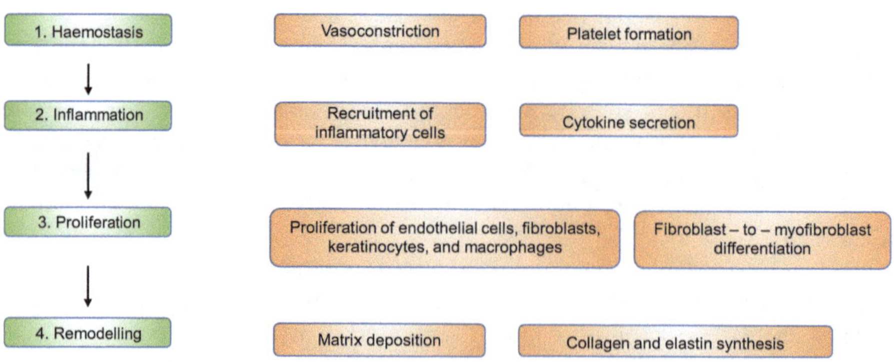

Fig. 2 Four stages of wound healing: haemostasis, inflammation, proliferation and matrix remodelling

keratinocytes and macrophages (Gonzalez et al. 2016). In addition to proliferation, keratinocytes are activated to become more migratory and invasive through an epithelial to partial mesenchymal phenotypic transition. Due to the reformation of the epithelial layer by migratory keratinocytes, this process is also known as re-epithelialization. In addition to re-epithelialization by keratinocytes, matrix deposition and wound contraction are carried out by pro-fibrotic fibroblasts and differentiated myofibroblasts, respectively (Li et al. 2007). The release of matrix deposition and hypoxia-inducible factors further drives migration and recruitment of endothelial cells and macrophages to the site of injury to induce and aid in the process of angiogenesis, respectively (Kalebic et al. 1983; Du Cheyne et al. 2020).

2.2.4 Remodelling

Matrix remodelling takes place throughout the wound healing process and is only completed long after closure of the wound through the formation of collagen-rich scar tissue (Li et al. 2007). After the formation of a wound, fibroblasts are recruited to the site of injury, where they proliferate and form granulation tissue through the production of collagen and other extracellular matrix components (Grinnell 1994). While a majority (80%) of uninjured human skin is composed of type I collagen, during the process of wound healing, epithelial mechanical strength is increased by the replacement of type I collagen with type III collagen during granulation (Witte and Barbul 1997). Another key protein produced during the process of wound healing is elastin – conferring elasticity to the healed epithelial barrier (Duca et al. 2004).

3 Low-Dose Ionizing Radiation and Wound Healing

3.1 Effects of Low-Dose Ionizing Radiation on Open Wound Healing

High doses of IR have been known to cause damaging biological effects, primarily through direct ionization of biomolecules such as DNA DSBs. These DNA lesions may pose a serious threat to genomic stability via mutations and mitotic failure if not repaired correctly, whereas unrepaired DNA lesions may lead to cell death through apoptosis, necrosis and cellular senescence. Indirect effects of IR occur through ionisation of water molecules resulting in water radiolysis and downstream production of harmful radicals such as ROS and $ONOO^-$. On the other hand, due to the beneficial effects of LDIR, one of the potential uses includes improvement of wound healing, as shown in Table 1. Table 1 displays the effects of γ, electron beam and x-ray radiation in different biological models.

The effects of LDIR on fibroblasts were examined by Truong et al. (2018), who showed that while exposure to low-dose x-ray radiation did not induce any observable differences in cell morphology, it did enhance fibroblast proliferation, showing a higher cell number than control cells by day 3 post-treatment. Yim et al. (2017a) demonstrated similar effects of γ-radiation on fibroblast proliferation. The results

Table 1 Results of ionising γ-radiation, x-ray radiation and electron beam radiation on wound healing

Author	Radiation modality	Treatment regimen	Model studied	Findings	Pathways and processes of wound healing
Open wound healing					
Truong et al. (2018)	X-ray	0.55 mGy (550 μGy/h)	3 T3 mouse fibroblast cells	Low-dose x-ray triggers an initial lag in cell cycle progression, followed by significant increase in cell proliferation	Increased proliferation, protein expression, population of cells in the G0/G1 phase of the cell cycle No change in cell morphology and collagen formation function
Yim et al. (2017a)	^{137}Cs γ	0.05, 0.1, 0.2, 0.5, 1, 2 and 4 Gy (1.03 Gy/min)	Normal human lung fibroblasts (MRC-5), normal human dermal fibroblasts (NHDF)	Low-dose γ-radiation induces stimulatory/homeostatic repair responses, whereas high-dose γ-radiation induces higher levels of DNA damage with low repair responses	50 mGy: Increased DNA damage repair responses 2 Gy: Induced DNA damage with strand breaks and reduced cell viability
Yim et al. (2017b)	^{137}Cs γ	0.05, 0.1, 0.2, 0.5, 1, 2 and 4 Gy (1.03 Gy/min)	Normal human lung fibroblasts (MRC-5), normal human dermal fibroblasts (NHDF)	At doses >0.1 Gy and < 2 Gy, increased DNA damage repair responses	50 mGy: Increase in DNA damage repair responses > 100 mGy: Induced DNA damage with strand breaks and reduced cell proliferation
Cho et al. (2017)	^{137}Cs γ	10 and 50 mGy with 3 Gy as negative control	Human mesenchymal stem cells (hMSCs)	Low-dose γ-radiation induces stimulatory/homeostatic repair responses, whereas high-dose γ-radiation induces higher levels of DNA damage with low repair responses	10 mGy: Increased hMSCs viability (by 8% compared to non-irradiated cells) 2 × 10 mGy: Enhanced hMSCs proliferation, maintained stemness and viability 3 Gy: Induced DNA strand breaks, damage, and senescence

Jabbari et al. (2017)	Comparison of electron beam and γ	8 MeV (300 MU/min) electron beam and 0.75 Gy (0.52 Gy/min) γ-radiation	72 healthy Sprague Dawley rats	γ-Rays sped up and promoted wound healing Electron beam radiation inhibited wound healing	γ-Radiation: Increased re-epithelialization and angiogenesis. Increased early fibroblast, neutrophil and macrophage population. Higher tensile strength in healed wounds Electron beam: Delayed increase in fibroblast and macrophage population, slower wound healing with lower tensile strength
Schäffer et al. (2002)	Electron beam	12 and 25 Gy	30 healthy Sprague Dawley rats	Electron beam radiation reduces wound healing capacity	Decrease NO synthesis and collagen formation Increase in pro-inflammatory cytokines
Almeida et al. (2007)	Electron beam	6 MeV	84 healthy Wistar rats	Electron beam radiation caused significant delay in wound healing	Decreased tissue organization, tissue formation Decreased formation, alignment, and density of collagen fibres
Chronic wound healing					
Marques et al. (2020)	X-ray	120–720 mGy	16 rectal cancer patients	X-ray radiation improved wound angiogenesis	Upregulation of pro-angiogenic genes with decrease in pro-inflammatory cytokines
Thanik et al. (2010)	X-ray	5 mGy (10 Gy/min)	50 healthy wild-type FVB mice and 18 tie2/LacZ transgenic mice	X-ray radiation improved wound angiogenesis	Upregulation of pro-angiogenic cytokines

(continued)

Table 1 (continued)

Author	Radiation modality	Treatment regimen	Model studied	Findings	Pathways and processes of wound healing
Mathias et al. (2015)	^{60}Co γ	0.025, 0.05, 0.1, 0.5 and 2 Gy at low-dose rate (1 mGy/min) and high-dose rate (150 mGy/min)	ApoE$^{-/-}$ mice		High- and low-dose rate induced similar effects, and results were more dependent on dose 25 mGy: Increased collagen deposition ≤ 2 Gy: Increased angiogenesis 16 Gy: Damage to capillaries, decreased in micro-vessel density
Gridley et al. (2009)	^{57}Co γ	10, 50 and 100 mGy (02 mGy/min)	192 healthy C57BL/6 mice	Low-dose radiation had more significant effects on decreasing splenic lymphocytes	10 mGy: Long-term decrease in T, B and NK cell population

suggest that while fibroblast proliferation was significantly decreased at high doses 2 Gy, treatment with LDIR at 50 mGy did not show this inhibitory effect.

Treatment of human mesenchymal stem cells (hMSCs) with LDR at 10 mGy of γ-radiation has been shown to improve viability, increase proliferation and enhance the maintenance of stem cell phenotype in mesenchymal stem cells (Cho et al. 2017). Mesenchymal stem cells play an integral role in wound healing, including regulation of immune and inflammatory process, as well as secretion of molecules involved in the regulation of cell survival, proliferation and migration (Maxson et al. 2012). These findings suggest that one of the mechanisms by which γ-radiation may enhance wound healing is through the induction of mesenchymal stem cell activity. One of the major contributors to the wound healing capacity of stem cells is epigenetic regulation, such as histone modification. Kang et al. (2020) demonstrated that histone H3 hypomethylation was an important epigenetic pathway involved in wound healing, and treatment of wounded mice with hypomethylation inhibitors resulted in delayed wound healing. Specifically, only the processes of epithelial cell differentiation and angiogenesis were dependent on this pathway, and inhibition of hypomethylation showed no effect on epithelial cell proliferation and fibroblast recruitment. Numerous studies report exposure to high-dose radiation causes DNA hypomethylation-related genomic instability in various tissues and organs, suggesting the damaging effects of HDR may be as a result of increased genomic instability (Pogribny et al. 2005; Loree et al. 2006).

For comparison, Jabbari et al. (2017) treated full-size incisions in male rats with 52 cGy/min of γ-radiation using a cobalt-60 source and 8 MeV of electron beam radiation. The results of this study demonstrated that despite the same initial wound healing process observed in untreated rats and rats treated with either electron beam or γ-radiation, the wound healing process was significantly enhanced 7 days post-treatment with γ-radiation (75 cGy). While all three groups displayed the initial stages of tissue regeneration on day 3 post-wounding, by day 7, only the γ-radiated group displayed complete wound angiogenesis and significant re-epithelialization. Additionally, the γ-radiated group also displayed significantly increased fibroblast, macrophage and neutrophil populations, providing insight into the biochemical responses to LDR that improve wound healing potential. While γ-radiation enhanced wound healing, rats treated with low-dose electron radiation (8 MeV) demonstrated a delay in both granulation and wound healing (Jabbari et al. 2017). Similar inhibition of wound healing after treatment with electron radiation was reported by Schäffer et al. (2002). While the results did not report any significant changes in inflammatory cell infiltrate, significant decrease in NO synthesis was indicated by a decrease in nitrite and nitrate accumulation and decrease in inducible NOS protein expression, which plays an important role in collagen formation and wound contraction. Additionally, treatment with electron radiation resulted in increased TNF-α and INF-γ, along with a decrease in collagen deposition by fibroblasts, all of which have been identified as important factors in the wound healing process. Therefore, the authors suggested that changes in cellular composition and activity after electron irradiation may play a key role in impaired wound healing. The inhibitory effects of electron beam radiation were corroborated by Almeida et al. (2007), who examined tissue morphology in rat wounds treated with low-dose electron beam radiation (6 MeV with a single dose of 1 Gy). The results of this study showed delayed collagen formation in the irradiated groups compared to control groups; the latter also showed better alignment of collagen fibres. Additionally, delayed granulation was seen in tissues irradiated with electron beams both immediately and 3 days post-wounding, suggesting that treatment with low-dose electron beam radiation induced tissue-damaging effects that resulted in impaired wound healing. Together, the results of these studies suggest that gamma radiation at low doses has stimulatory effects on wound healing, while inhibitory effects may be triggered by electron beam radiation at low doses.

3.2 Effects of Low-Dose Ionizing Radiation on Diabetic Ulcer Healing

Angiogenesis impairment is a major contributor to chronic non-healing wounds, including diabetic ulcers and wounds. Decrease in angiogenic growth factors, including VEGF, FGF and TGF-β, has been associated with both type 1 and type 2 diabetes (Rivard et al. 1999; Nyengaard and Rasch 1993). Marques et al. (2020) demonstrated LDIR-enhanced increase in angiogenesis in individuals treated with 0.12–0.72 Gy of x-ray. These results corroborate the findings of Thanik et al. (2010), who demonstrated in vivo increase in angiogenic cytokines SDF-1 and VEGF 2–7 days after cutaneous treatment with 5 Gy of x-ray radiation. The angiogenic effects of LDIR suggest that this method of treatment may potentially have beneficial effects on improving non-healing chronic wounds. The authors also reported LDIR induced increase in MMP-9 activity that is associated with an increase in hematopoietic progenitor cells, thus suggesting the increase in post-radiation angiogenesis. Cellular migration and matrix deposition, the third and fourth phases of wound healing, can also be modulated via LDIR treatment. Inhibition of Sp1, a major MMP-9 inhibitor, via the upregulation of a miRNA-129 and miRNA-335 demonstrated improved wound healing through improved activity of keratinocyte migratory activity and fibroblast deposition of collagen matrix (Wang et al. 2018). These results suggest that the pathways involved in LDIR-enhanced wound healing may involve increase in angiogenesis – which has been identified as a primary driver of non-healing wounds in diabetic patients – rather than keratinocyte proliferation (Waltenberger et al. 2000).

Another major factor leading to infections and non-healing wounds in diabetic patients is deficient immune responses (Loots et al. 1998). Marques et al. (2020) also reported that treatment with x-ray radiation (0.18–0.72 Gy) downregulated IL-8 gene expression. Pro-inflammatory cytokines, such as IL-8, have been associated with exacerbated immune responses in wounds, resulting in delayed wound healing (Lan et al. 2013). Mathias et al. (2015) compared the systemic effects of low (50 mGy) and high (2 Gy) dose γ-radiation, reporting distinct anti- and pro-inflammatory effects of the treatments, respectively. Gridley et al. (2009) reported a decrease in T cells, B cells and NK cells, the three major leukocytes involved in inflammatory

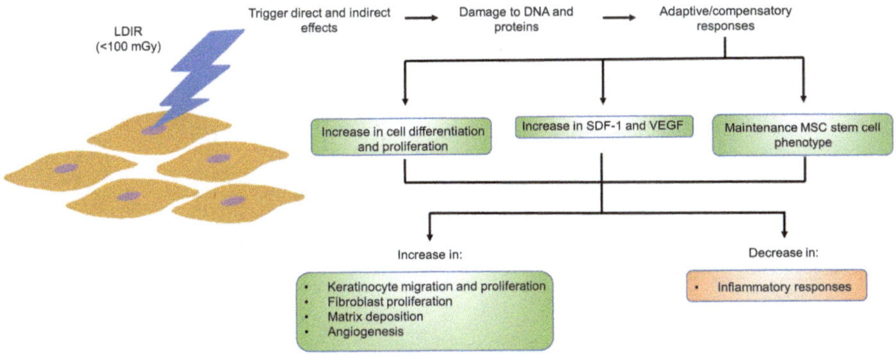

Fig. 3 Mechanisms and pathways involved in low-dose ionizing radiation-enhanced wound healing

responses after treatment of mice with low doses (10 mGy) of γ-radiation. A similar heterogenous decrease in splenic immune cell population was reported in murine models exposed to LDIR (Bogdándi et al. 2010). These results indicate that LDIR modulation of chronic and diabetic wound involves the downregulation of pro-inflammatory genes.

The effects of LDIR on open and chronic diabetic healing are summarised in Fig. 3 and Table 1.

4 Photobiomodulation and Wound Healing

4.1 Effects of Photobiomodulation on Open Wound Healing

The modalities of PBM discussed include diode, aluminium-gallium-indium-phosphide (AlGaAnP), helium-neon (HeNE) and far-infrared lasers, as well as LED and non-coherent light. While the effects of PBM on wound healing are dependent on wavelength and dose, they do not seem to be influenced by radiation modality, as shown by the improvement of wound healing using various laser sources, as well as non-laser light sources as summarised in Table 2.

One of the major cells involved in the process of wound healing is fibroblasts, which undergo a fibroblast-to-myofibroblast differentiation process triggered by injury. These differentiated cells exhibit a highly contractile phenotype and are responsible for the production of numerous extracellular proteins (Li and Wang 2011). Enhanced differentiation of fibroblasts to myofibroblasts after the exposure of cutaneous wounds to a laser diode emitting at a wavelength of 670 nm with an output of 9 mW was reported by Medrado et al. (2003). Similarly, Hawkins and Abrahamse (2005) reported PBM-enhanced wound healing in vitro when exposed to He-Ne laser at a wavelength of 632.8 nm with a single dose of 2.5 J/cm^2. The enhanced

Table 2 Results of non-ionising light and laser radiation on wound healing

Author	Radiation modality	Treatment regimen	Model studied	Findings	Remarks
Open wound healing					
Medrado et al. (2003)	Diode laser	670 nm at 4 and 8 J/cm^2	72 healthy Wistar rats	4 J/cm^2 showed most positive effects on wound healing	4 J/cm^2: More significant decrease in wound size, oedema and leukocyte count, increase in fibroblast and vascular proliferation
Hawkins and Abrahamse (2005)	He-Ne laser	632.8 nm at 0.5, 2.5, 5 and 10 J/cm^2	Human skin fibroblast monolayer culture	2.5 J/cm^2 induced optimal wound healing capacity of fibroblast cells	2.5 J/cm^2 induced improved cell viability, proliferation and fibroblast migration
Demidova-Rice et al. (2007)	Non-coherent light, He-Ne laser and monochromator-coupled-xenon light	635 nm non-coherent light at 1, 2, 10 and 50 J/cm^2	105 healthy BALB/c mice	1 J/cm^2 of 820 nm laser improved wound healing most significantly	All doses <50 J/cm^2 of 635 nm laser improved wound healing
		632.8 nm of he-ne laser at 1 and 2 J/cm^2			50 J/cm^2 of 635 nm light inhibited wound healing
		635, 670, 72 and 820 nm of monochromator-coupled-xenon lamp light at 1 J/cm^2			At 1 J/cm^2, only 820 and 635 nm enhanced wound healing
Toyokawa et al. (2003)	Far infrared laser	900–1,200 nm	110 healthy Sprague Dawley rats	Treatment induced improved wound healing	Wound healing was associated with increased TGF-β1-expressing fibroblast migration and collagen regeneration

Arany et al. (2007)	Far infrared laser	904 nm	Serum-free conditioned medium from transformed human lung adenocarcinoma (A549) and fibrosarcoma (HT1080) and non-transformed mink lung epithelial (CCL64) cells 30 human patients following tooth extraction	Irradiation induced priming effect by activating TGF-β1 both in vitro and in vivo	In vitro: Increased latent TGF-β1 and TGF-β3 activation and made them more sensitive to activation when exposed to subsequent challenges In vivo: Increased TGF-β1 activation and inflammatory infiltrate
Wagner et al. (2016)	InGaAIp laser	660 nm at 4 and 20 J/cm^2	48 healthy Wistar rats	Low dose (4 J/cm^2) had higher stimulatory effects on ulcer healing	Both doses induced significant increase in angiogenesis and IL-1β and decrease in TNF-α, but the effects were more pronounced for 4 J/cm^2
Chronic wound healing					
Schindl et al. (1999)	Diode laser	670 nm at 30 J/cm^2	1 diabetic foot ulcer patient	Laser improved complete ulcer healing	Treatment showed normalized C-reactive protein and fibrinogen levels with complete wound closure and no side effects
Kaviani et al. (2011)	Laser	685 nm at 10 J/cm^2 (in addition to conventional therapy)	23 diabetic foot ulcer patients	Laser improved chronic diabetic foot ulcer healing	Decrease in ulcer size and mean time taken for complete healing, with increased likelihood of complete healing

(continued)

Table 2 (continued)

Author	Radiation modality	Treatment regimen	Model studied	Findings	Remarks
Peplow et al. (2011)	Laser	660 nm of 4.7–6.3 J/cm^2 at 25, 50 and 100 mW	42 diabetic mice	Irradiation improved wound healing in diabetic mice	All power outputs at constant dose and wavelength improved healing of excisional splinted wounds via re-epithelialization, granulation tissue formation and collagen formation
Fujimura et al. (2013)	Diode laser	805 nm	Human gingival tissue samples, and Ca9-22 and SCC-25 human oral squamous epithelial carcinoma cells	Laser treatment promotes wound healing	Increased expression of anti-inflammatory mRNA Del-1, ICAM-1, and epithelial cell migration and proliferation, and decrease in pro-inflammatory IL-6 and IL-8
Lau et al. (2015)	Diode laser	808 nm of 5 J/cm^2 at 0.1, 0.2 and 0.3 W/cm^2	120 diabetic Sprague Dawley rats	Low dose (0.1 and 0.2 W/cm^2) of laser therapy enhanced wound healing, while high dose inhibited the process	All doses: Increased early inflammation, vascularization, re-epithelialization and granulation tissue formation Low-power density: faster wound contraction via granulation tissue formation and collagen synthesis High-power density: Delayed wound contraction and increased scab formation

Feitosa et al. (2015)	Laser	632.8 nm at 4 J/cm^2	16 diabetic ulcer patients	Irradiation improved chronic wound healing with analgesic effects	Decrease in wound size and pain
Amini et al. (2019)	Laser	890 nm at 0.2 J/cm^2	90 diabetic Wistar rats	Irradiation induces wound injury repair in diabetic models	Immune modulation via decrease in macrophage and neutrophil population, as well as increase in fibroblast population, angiogenesis and wound healing-associated factors SDF-1α and bFGF expression

wound healing was attributed to improved cellular viability, proliferation and migration of fibroblasts without a significant increase in DNA damage.

In addition to diode and He-Ne lasers, Demidova-Rice et al. (2007) compared the effects of low and high doses of 635, 670, 720 and 820 nm wavelengths delivered from coherent laser sources and non-coherent light sources. The results of this study demonstrated a PBM-induced increase in fibroblast-to-myofibroblast transition. Specifically, between days 1 and 9 post-wounding, control mice showed a 20% increase in wound size, which is characteristic of wound expansion prior to contraction. On the other hand, mice that were treated with 635 nm (non-coherent red light) at a dose of 2 J/cm^2 and a fluence rate of 80 mW/cm^2 30 min post-wounding did not display expansion of the wound – instead they showed direct progression of wound healing into the contraction phase (wound size decreased by 5%). Additionally, the authors also demonstrated that the stimulatory effects of PBM on wound healing were observed at doses 1, 2 and 10 J/cm^2, whereas increasing the dose to 50 J/cm^2 had inhibitory effects, and wound healing was significantly slower than the control group. These results support the hormesis model. Together these studies suggest myofibroblast-dependent wound contraction may be a major target of PBM-enhanced wound healing.

A key molecule involved in PBM-enhanced wound healing is latent transforming growth factor beta-1 (TGF-β1) complex, which is activated by low-dose near-infrared lasers (630–1000 nm) (Ruh et al. 2018; Arany et al. 2007; Zein et al. 2018). Administration of exogenous transforming growth factor beta-1 (TGF-β1) has shown similar effects on wound healing as PBM, including improved migratory ability of keratinocytes, as well as synthesis of collagen and deposition of extracellular matrix by fibroblasts and resultant wound contraction (Finnson et al. 2013; Tamm et al. 1996). Besides collagen generation and fibroblast proliferation, TGF-β growth factors have also been associated with the modulation of other wound healing processes such as inflammation, angiogenesis and deposition of extracellular matrix (Roberts et al. 1986; Nall et al. 1996). Additionally, chronic wounds with loss of wound healing ability have also been associated with decreased TGF-β1 expression, highlighting their essential role in the healing process (Pastar et al. 2010). Due to the similarities in cellular responses to exogenous TGF-β1 administration and low-level lasers, it has been hypothesized that TGF-β1 activation may be a major molecular mechanism involved in PBM-enhanced wound healing.

Toyokawa et al. (2003) demonstrated PBM-enhanced wound healing in rat models, as well as increase in the migration of TGF-β1-expressing fibroblasts, and collagen regeneration in the group treated with far-infrared wavelengths compared to the control group. Similarly, Arany et al. (2007) showed that exposure of serum representative of the early wound environment to low-power laser radiation resulted in the specific activation of latent TGF-β1. In vitro treatment of serum with near-infrared (904 nm) wavelengths also demonstrated a priming effect, increasing the ability of latent TGF-β1 to become activated by other methods, including heat, chemical and protease exposure. In addition to in vitro assays, the authors demonstrated similar results in human models, highlighting that treatment of post-tooth extraction oral wounds with LLLT resulted in TGF-β1 activation, thus confirming that the role of fibroblasts in PBM-enhanced wound healing is dependent on TGF-β1 activation.

Inflammatory responses are essential for wound healing and are involved in the release of chemokines and cytokines during the early stages of the wound healing process to enable infiltration of the site of injury with inflammatory cells. These inflammatory cells ensure removal of debris and pathogens, thus providing protection against infection and allowing for the process of wound healing to progress into the next stage. Mast cells, an important immune cell in wound healing, are responsible for the production of numerous growth factors such as epidermal and keratinocyte growth factors which stimulate the maturation of cells involved in the re-epithelialization phase (Ud-Din et al. 2020). El Sayed and Dyson (1996) reported a correlation between LLLT exposure and mast cell degranulation and proliferative growth suggesting that mast cell degranulation may be an important molecular mechanism involved in PBM-enhanced wound healing.

Additionally, increased levels of IL-β1 have also been associated with an increase in micro-vessel density. This formation of new blood vessels is an important process for the proliferative phase of wound healing where formation of new cells requires replacement of damaged blood vessels for an adequate supply of oxygen and nutrients (Wagner et al. 2016; Carmi et al. 2009). Wagner et al. (2016) showed that treatment of oral wound ulcers with 4 and 20 J/cm2 of 660 nm of laser irradiation caused an immediate increase in tissue IL-β1 level during the early stages of wound healing. Their results suggest that the increase in IL-β1 seen after treatment with PBM could trigger an increase in endothelial cell-activating factors, thus conferring a pro-angiogenic effect. They also reported a decrease in TNF-α, a pro-inflammatory cytokine which has been linked to exacerbated immune responses and delayed healing of acute wounds. This decrease was observed at all stages of the wound healing post-treatment with a dose of 4 J/cm^2. While excess levels of TNF-α have been linked with the development of chronic wounds, it is also associated with angiogenesis, driving the deposition of extracellular matrix, as well as the differentiation of fibroblasts to myofibroblasts in wound healing (Baum and Duffy 2011; Xu et al. 2016). In addition to increases in IL-β1 levels and angiogenesis, Wagner et al. (2016) also reported more pronounced decrease in TNF-α levels after treatment with 4 J/cm^2 compared to treatment with 20 J/cm^2, suggesting that the lower doses had a more significant stimulatory effect on wound healing which is consistent with the hormetic model.

4.2 Effects of Photobiomodulation on Diabetic Ulcer Healing

Schindl et al. (1999) observed the efficacy of low-intensity laser irradiation on a patient with diabetic neuropathic foot ulcer. The results of this study showed complete healing of the ulcers after being treated with 30 J/cm^2 of 670 nm diode laser at an intensity of 60 mW/cm^2 for 16 sessions. The findings of this case report were corroborated by Kaviani et al. (2011) in a randomized clinical trial demonstrating enhanced diabetic foot ulcer wound healing in patients who received additional treatment with low-level laser therapy at a wavelength of 685 nm and dose of 10 J/cm^2. Similarly, mice with splinted ulcers that are representative of diabetic wounds with delayed healing were treated with 660 nm of continuous laser waves at outputs of 25, 50 and 100 mW and a dose of 2.0 J/day. The results showed that the mice treated with PBM showed almost complete re-epithelialization and formation of granulation tissue, both of which were delayed in the control group (Peplow et al. 2011). The control group exhibiting moderate-to-intense inflammatory responses compared to the irradiated groups' minimal presence of both inflammatory responses and exudate suggested that PBM-enhanced wound healing of diabetic ulcers occurs as a result of a decrease in inflammatory responses.

PBM-enhanced wound contraction, a parameter used to describe percentage of wound closure, has also been linked to the increase in angiogenesis (Lau et al. 2015). Lau et al. (2015) reported the effects of 0.1 and 0.2 W/cm^2 of 808 nm infrared radiation which improved wound healing of diabetic mice. Treatment with these two doses induced increase in epithelial cells, connective tissue and blood vessels, whereas treatment with 0.3 W/cm^2 demonstrated inhibitory effects on wound healing, corroborating the hormetic model of radiation. Feitosa et al. (2015) reported a significant decrease in wound size and pain in diabetic foot ulcer patients treated with a wavelength of 632.8 nm and dose of 4 J/cm^2.

The positive effects of PBM low doses of light on diabetic wound healing are the reduced functions of macrophages and neutrophils, as well as significant reductions in the anti-inflammatory responses (Fujimura et al. 2013; Fekrazad et al. 2015). Treatment of diabetic rat model demonstrated PBM-associated decrease in neutrophils and macrophages, as well as increase in fibroblasts and angiogenesis when treated with 0.2 J/cm^2 of 890 nm radiation. The study also reported a contradiction to the normal process of wound healing: where genes such as stromal cell-derived factor-1α (SDF-1α) and basic fibroblast growth factor (bFGF) show diminished expression, exposure to PBM showed an increase in the expression of these genes (Amini et al. 2019). The major functions of bFGF linked to wound healing include acting as a growth factor for fibroblasts and chemoattractant for various cell types, including vascular endothelial cells (Chakrabarti et al. 2021). Moreover, SDF-1α also acts as a chemoattractant for the recruitment of mesenchymal stem cells and is involved in the activation of growth factors, such as bFGF and vascular endothelial growth factor (Xu et al. 2013). Delayed wound healing has been observed in bFGF knockout model organisms and diabetic models with observable decreases in bFGF levels (Ortega et al. 1998; Shi et al. 2013). Similarly, progression of acute wounds to chronic diabetic wounds has been associated with decreased angiogenesis as a result of decreased SDF-1α expression (Gallagher et al. 2007; Bermudez et al. 2011). Amini et al.'s (2019) findings suggest that PBM-enhanced wound healing could involve the alteration in the expression SDF-1α and bFGF, as well as in the immune response modulation. The effects of PBM on open and chronic diabetic wound healing are summarised in Fig. 4 and Table 2.

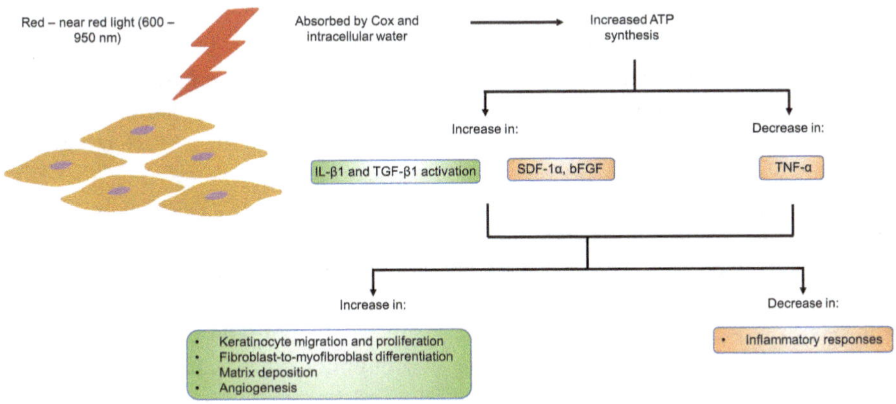

Fig. 4 Mechanisms and pathways involved in low-dose photobiomodulation-enhanced wound healing

5 Low-Dose Radiation and Cancer

5.1 Effects of Low-Dose Ionizing Radiation on Cancer

Unlike high doses of IR, which have a high risk of stochastic effects (such as cancer) due to their harmful ionizing ability, the effects conferred by LDIR stimulate beneficial responses in normal cells and selective anti-cancer effects in tumour cells (Khan and Wang 2022). The primary hormetic responses triggered by LDIR include promotion of cell survival and proliferation and DNA repair responses. The unrepaired or incorrectly repaired DNA damage induced by high doses of IR leads to genomic instability, cell cycle disruption and often eventual downstream carcinogenic effects (Khan and Wang 2022; Lee et al. 2007; Iliakis et al. 2003). One well-known direct effect of IR exposure is the formation of DNA DSBs, which initiate a measurable downstream phosphorylation of histone 2A at serine 139 to produce γ-H2AX (Rogakou et al. 1999). Ulyanenko et al. (2019) examined the effects of both chronic (0.1 mGy/min) and acute (30 mGy/min) low doses of γ-radiation exposure. Their results highlighted a two- to tenfold lower number of repair foci and DSBs when exposed to the chronic low-dose-rate IR (0.1 mGy/min) compared to acute radiation (30 mGy/min). Similarly, Yim et al. (2017a, b) demonstrated disruption of normal fibroblast proliferation as a result of mis-repaired DNA damage and genomic instability when exposed to higher doses of γ-radiation (2 Gy). On the other hand, treatment of the normal fibroblasts with LDIR (0.05 Gy) did not trigger genomic instability, nor did it reduce fibroblast viability and proliferation. Their study demonstrated the different molecular effects of high and low doses of γ-radiation. LDIR initiated an early increase in phospho-NF-κb (Ser536) and phospho-P70S6K (Ser418), suggesting a modulation of the inflammatory responses to initiate repairable DNA damage. Conversely, at high dose there was an increase in PP53 and P53, suggesting this treatment may have triggered higher levels of irreparable or incorrectly repaired DNA damage, resulting in cell cycle arrest. While LDIR confers beneficial effects to normal cells, high doses of IR are associated with cellular and molecular damage resulting in an increased risk of tumorigenesis. These results are agreeable with the hormetic model, highlighting the distinct effects of IR at high and low doses.

The immuno-modulation capacity of LDIR may contribute selectively to anti-cancer effects. While the anti-inflammatory activity of LDIR has been described in Sect. 3, exposure to LDIR has also been observed to increase certain immune functions. Kojima et al. (2002) demonstrated increased cytotoxic function of natural killer (NK) cells following exposure to 0.5 Gy of γ-radiation. The anti-cancer activity conferred by increased immune functions was highlighted by Cheda et al. (2004), who demonstrated that exposure to 100 mGy of x-ray radiation reduced pulmonary tumour metastasis via activation of NK-1 cytotoxic activity. Liu et al. (2010) demonstrated that total body exposure of 1.25 Gy γ-radiation resulted in a selective decrease in T-regulatory cell population in addition to decreasing tumour burden and increasing survival. Together, these results suggest that the anti-cancer effects of LDIR enhanced distinct and selective immune functions (Yang et al. 2016).

The protective effects of LDIR exposure on surrounding normal tissue could provide a potential addition to the conventional radiotherapy treatment plan to reduce high-dose radiation-induced adverse effects. Liang et al. (2016) demonstrated that treatment with low-dose x-ray radiation (25–50 mGy) conferred selective protective effects. Normal human embryonic stem cells displayed an increase in cell proliferation dependent on c-Raf/MAPK/MEK/ERK and PI3K/PDK-1/AKT pathways, whereas apoptotic cell death was triggered in cancer cells. Hauptmann et al. (2016) also demonstrated unique responses of protein levels to 40, 100 and 140 mGy of IR radiation, suggesting different doses of radiation may induce characteristic molecular responses. In fact, the authors demonstrated a significant priming effect of LDIR exposure when cells were treated with 40 mGy prior to being challenged with 100 mGy. There was an increase in protein modulation such as in lamin and vinculin that are associated with maintenance of genomic stability and cell function, respectively (Gonzalez-Suarez and Gonzalo 2010; Wang et al. 2012). These results suggest that pre-treatment with LDIR may confer an adaptive response including enhanced proliferation and stability in normal cells without interfering with the anti-tumour activity of cancer therapies (Jiang et al. 2008; Liang et al. 2011). However, it is important to note that exposure to LDIR may promote tumour invasion and metastasis, inducing similar stimulatory effects on the endothelial cell function within tumours as well as normal cells (Sofia Vala et al. 2010).

5.2 Photobiomodulation for the Management of Adverse Effects of Cancer Treatment

The side effects associated with conventional radiation cancer treatment, such as inflammatory and compensatory responses that are able to break in the protective barriers and play major roles, include fibrosis, mucositis in head and neck cancer patients, pneumonitis in lung cancer patients and radiation-induced dermatitis in most cancer patients. For example, in HNC patients, almost all treated with radiation and approximately 20–40% of patients treated with chemotherapy experience oral mucositis. This inflammatory complication of conventional treatment is driven by ROS formation, NF-κb activation, increased inflammatory responses and alterations in the micro-vessel density and extracellular matrix (Epstein et al. 2012; Trotti et al. 2003; Blijlevens et al. 2016). However, the protective effects of low levels of non-IR are primarily attributed to the adaptive responses triggered by an initial low priming dose that provides sufficient stress to trigger repair responses without causing significant long-term damage to the tissue. This provides an improved protective effect against subsequent treatment with stress-inducing stressors. Therefore, PBM can potentially be used as a prophylactic measure to mitigate the damaging effects induced by other more significant causes of biological stress conventional radiotherapy and chemotherapy.

Pre-treatment of HNC patients with LLLT has been associated with reduced risk, duration and severity of cancer therapy-induced oral mucositis (Bensadoun et al. 1999; Abramoff et al. 2008; Kuhn et al. 2009; Bjordal et al. 2011). Besides analgesic effects, PBM may also have prophylactic effects. Oberoi et al. (2014) reported the consistent findings on the addition of LLLT to HNC treatment regimen were reduction in the pain, severity duration and prevalence of oral mucositis. More specifically, Rizzi et al. (2006) demonstrated that LLLT inhibited trauma-induced NF-κb activation, suggesting this may be a potential target of LLLT. Decrease in severity of oral mucositis following treatment with LLLT was associated with decrease in pro-inflammatory cytokines IL-1β and TNF-α (Oton-Leite et al. 2015). Taken together, these findings suggest that the suppression of immune responses plays a key role in the prophylactic effects of PBM against cancer therapy-induced adverse inflammatory responses. In response to the strong association between oral mucositis and head and neck cancer treatment, Bensadoun (2018) proposes a dose of 2–3 J/cm^2 at wavelengths of 633–685 or 780–830 nm, energy intensity of 10–150 mW and frequency of two to three times a week to achieve the optimal results for management of mucositis.

Radiation targeted to tumour sites in close proximity to lymphatic structures such as HNC and breast cancer has adverse effects such as lymphedema, giving rise to chronic inflammatory exacerbations and eventual fibrosis (Lee and Rockson 2018). Deng et al. (2021) examined the effects of LLLT on head and neck lymphedema severity in HNC patients. They reported a significant reduction in the number and severity of lymphedema sites, its severity and occurrence of fibrosis in patients treated with LLLT. Omar et al. (2012) showed similar management of lymphedema in breast cancer patients treated with PBM. Treatment of mice with tail lymphedema with a wavelength of 904 nm, irradiance of 25 mW/cm^2 and dose of 1.5 J/cm^2 showed reduction in lymphedema via lymphatic vessel regeneration (Jang et al. 2016). These findings suggest that the reduction of post-treatment lymphedema severity in cancer patients treated with LLLT could occur via the decrease in inflammatory processes and in the increase in lymph-angiogenesis (Fig. 5).

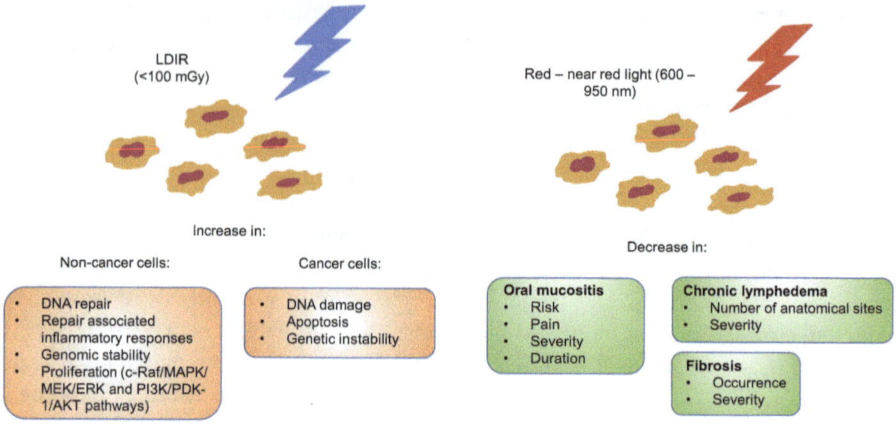

Fig. 5 Mechanisms and pathways involved in treatment of cancer cells with low-dose photobiomodulation and ionizing radiation

6 Discussion and Limitations

Despite the reported beneficial molecular and cellular effects of PBM and LDIR, there is contradictory information between preclinical experimental studies. This could be related to the different model used, as well as the difference in irradiation parameters. In wound healing, radiation intensity and exposure time are known independent factors that could influence the outcome of the LDIR treatment. It has been highlighted that specific combinations of these variables are also required to achieve the desired acceleration of the wound healing process. Lanzafame et al. (2007) showed that exposure to near-infrared light for a shorter length of time ranging from 125 to 625 s in combination with irradiation intensity ranging from 8 to 40 mW resulted in increased wound healing capacity. On the other hand, increasing exposure time and decreasing dose intensity were reported to have inhibitory effects on wound healing, despite obtaining the same total dose administered. Similarly, even though spot diameter plays a significant role in the amount of radiation that is delivered, this has not been reported. This may result in the inconsistent findings of the same methods that were replicated by different authors (Zein et al. 2018). The differences in results between studies highlight the importance for all parameters to be specified for better replicability.

Aside from the controllable factors, the effects of LDR also differ greatly between models. In vitro experimental studies lack replicability as they do could not precisely reflect the complex local cellular environment, cell-to-cell interaction and other host responses inherent to a clinical setting. Additionally, mostly murine models are used in in vivo experimental studies, and the major difference between murine models and human patients is the difference in skin. As loose skin mammals, the wound healing process in rat models proceeds primarily through wound contraction. On the other hand, humans have fixed skin, and the main method of healing involves re-epithelialization and formation of granulation tissue (Grada et al. 2018). Lastly there are limited studies that examine the effects of LDIR on wound healing. Therefore, this paper provides insight into the potential impact of LDIR on the cellular and molecular processes involved in wound healing.

7 Conclusion

There is a potential application of PBM and LDIR as a non-invasive and painless alternative treatment to expedite wound healing. These type of treatments for wound healing may potentially prevent diabetic amputations for the diabetic, reduce the requirement of strong analgesics for critical and severe wound pains and help minimize cancer radiotherapy-associated pain, thus improving the patient quality of life. Low doses of x-ray and γ-radiation (< 100 mGy) can improve wound healing in both open acute and chronic wounds by acting on various stages of the wound healing process. Among the cells affected by LDIR are fibroblasts, keratinocytes, hMSCs and endothelial cells. Post-radiation increase in proliferation and migration in all these cells is accompanied by improved collagen synthesis function of fibroblasts. Additionally, treatment with LDIR was associated with a decrease in pro-inflammatory cytokines and an increase in anti-inflammatory and pro-angiogenic cytokines, giving insight into the molecular targets of LDIR. However, even though x-ray and γ-radiation improved wound healing and reduced time taken for complete wound healing to occur, low doses of electron radiation showed inhibitory effects on wound healing. This inhibitory effect is associated with increased pro-inflammatory cytokines, decreased anti-inflammatory cytokines and collagen deposition.

References

Abramoff MM, Lopes NN, Lopes LA, Dib LL, Guilherme A, Caran EM, Barreto AD, Lee ML, Petrilli AS (2008) Low-level laser therapy in the prevention and treatment of chemotherapy-induced oral mucositis in young patients. Photomed Laser Surg 26(4):393–400. https://doi.org/10.1089/pho.2007.2144

Allison RR, Sibata C, Patel R (2013) Future radiation therapy: photons, protons and particles. Future Oncol 9(4):93–504. https://doi.org/10.2217/fon.13.13

Almeida SMD, Cruz ADD, Ferreira RI, Vizioli MR, Bóscolo FN (2007) Effect of low-dose electron radiation on rat skin wound healing. Braz Dent J 18(3):208–214. https://doi.org/10.1590/S0103-64402007000300006

Amini A, Soleimani H, Abdollhifar MA, Moradi A, Ghoreishi SK, Chien S, Bayat M (2019) Stereological and gene expression examinations on the combined effects of photobiomodulation and curcumin on wound healing in type one diabetic rats. J Cell Biochem 120:17994–18004. https://doi.org/10.1002/jcb.29102

Anders JJ, Lanzafame RJ, Arany PR (2015) Low-level light/laser therapy versus photobiomodulation therapy. Photomed Laser Surg 33:183–184. https://doi.org/10.1089/pho.2015.9848

Arany PR, Nayak RS, Hallikerimath S, Limaye AM, Kale AD, Kondaiah P (2007) Activation of latent TGF-β1 by low-power laser in vitro correlates with increased TGF-β1 levels in laser-enhanced oral wound healing. Wound Repair Regen 15:866–874. https://doi.org/10.1111/j.1524-475X.2007.00306.x

Baum J, Duffy HS (2011) Fibroblasts and myofibroblasts: what are we talking about? J Cardiovasc Pharmacol 57:376–379. https://doi.org/10.1097/FJC.0b013e3182116e39

Baumann M, Krause M, Overgaard J, Debus J, Bentzen SM, Daartz J, Richter C, Zips D, Bortfeld T (2016) Radiation oncology in the era of precision medicine. Nat Rev Cancer 16:234–249. https://doi.org/10.1038/nrc.2016.18

Beattie R (1921) Treatment of subacute and chronic otitis media with use of X-ray. J Mich State Med Soc 20:449–451

Bensadoun R-J (2018) Photobiomodulation or low-level laser therapy in the management of cancer therapy-induced mucositis, dermatitis and lymphedema. Curr Opin Oncol 30(4):226–232. https://doi.org/10.1097/CCO.0000000000000452

Bensadoun RJ, Franquin JC, Ciais G, Darcourt V, Schubert MM, Viot M, Dejou J, Tardieu C, Benezery K, Nguyen TD, Laudoyer Y (1999) Low-energy he/ne laser in the prevention of radiation-induced mucositis. Support Care Cancer 7(4):244–252. https://doi.org/10.1007/s005200050256

Bermudez DM, Xu J, Herdrich BJ, Radu A, Mitchell ME, Liechty KW (2011) Inhibition of stromal cell-derived factor-1α further impairs diabetic wound healing. J Vasc Surg 53(3):774–784. https://doi.org/10.1016/j.jvs.2010.10.056

Biological mechanisms of radiation actions at low doses (2012) United Nations Scientific Committee on the Effects of Atomic Radiation. United Nations, New York

Bjordal JM, Bensadoun R-J, Tunèr J, Frigo L, Gjerde K, Lopes-Martins RAB (2011) A systematic review with meta-analysis of the effect of low-level laser therapy (LLLT) in cancer therapy-induced oral mucositis. Support Care Cancer 19:1069–1077. https://doi.org/10.1007/s00520-011-1202-0

Blijlevens N, Schwenkglenks M, Bacon P, D'Addio A, Einsele H, Maertens J, Niederwieser D, Rabitsch W, Roosaar A, Ruutu T, Schouten H, Stone R, Vokurka S, Quinn B, McCann S (2016) Prospective oral mucositis audit: oral mucositis in patients receiving high-dose melphalan or BEAM conditioning chemotherapy—European Blood and Marrow Transplantation Mucositis Advisory Group. J Clin Oncol 26(9):1519–1525. https://doi.org/10.1200/JCO.2007.13.6028

Bogdándi EN, Balogh A, Felgyinszki N, Szatmári T, Persa E, Hildebrandt G, Sáfrány G, Lumniczky K (2010) Effects of low-dose radiation on the immune system of mice after total-body irradiation. Radiat Res 174(4):480–489. https://doi.org/10.1667/RR2160.1

Calabrese EJ, Dhawan G (2013) Historical use of x-rays: treatment of inner ear infections and prevention of deafness. Hum Exp Toxicol 33(5):542–553. https://doi.org/10.1177/0960327113493303

Carmi Y, Voronov E, Dotan S, Lahat N, Rahat MA, Fogel M, Huszar M, White MR, Dinarello CA, Apte RN (2009) The role of macrophage-derived IL-1 in induction and maintenance of angiogenesis. J Immunol 183(7):4705–4714. https://doi.org/10.4049/jimmunol.0901511

Castillo H, Schoderbek D, Dulal S, Escobar G, Wood J, Nelson R, Smith G (2015) Stress induction in the bacteria Shewanella oneidensis and Deinococcus radiodurans in response to below-background ionizing radiation. Int J Radiat Biol 91(9):749–756. https://doi.org/10.3109/09553002.2015.1062571

Castillo H, Li X, Smith GB (2021) Deinococcus radiodurans UWO298 dependence on background radiation for optimal growth. Front Genet 12:644292. https://doi.org/10.3389/fgene.2021.644292

Chakrabarti S, Mazumder B, Rajkonwar J, Pathak MP, Patowary P, Chattopadhyay P (2021) bFGF and collagen matrix hydrogel attenuates burn wound inflammation through activation of ERK and TRK pathway. Sci Rep 11(1). https://doi.org/10.1038/2Fs41598-021-82888-9

Cheda A, Wrembel-Wargocka J, Lisiak E, Nowosielska EM, Marciniak M, Janiak MK (2004) Single low doses of X rays inhibit the development of experimental tumor metastases and trigger the activities of NK cells in mice. Radiat Res 161(3):335–340. https://doi.org/10.1667/RR3123

Chen WL, Luan YC, Shieh MC, Chen ST, Kung HT, Soong KL, Yeh YC, Chou TS, Mong SH, Wu JT, Sun CP, Deng WP, Wu MF, Shen ML (2007) Effects of cobalt-60 exposure on health of Taiwan residents suggest new approach needed in radiation protection. Abstracts of the Pacific Basin Nuclear Conference 5(1):63–67. https://doi.org/10.2203/2Fdose-response.06-105.Chen

Chen ACH, Arany PR, Huang Y-Y, Tomkinson EM, Sharma SK, Kharkwal GB, Saleem T, Mooney D, Yull FE, Blackwell TS, Hamblin MR (2011) Low-level laser therapy activates NF-kB via generation of reactive oxygen species in mouse embryonic fibroblasts. PLoS One 6(7):e22453. https://doi.org/10.1371/journal.pone.0022453

Chew MT, Daar E, Khandaker MU, Jones B, Nisbet A, Bradley DA (2021) Low radiation dose to treat pneumonia and other inflammations. Br J Radiol 94(1124):20201265. https://doi.org/10.1259/bjr.20201265

Cho W, Kim ES, Kang CM, Ji Y-H, Kim J-I, Park SJ, Son Y, Kim C-H (2017) Low-dose ionizing γ-radiation promotes proliferation of human mesenchymal stem cells and maintains their stem cell characteristics. Tissue Eng Regen Med 14:421–432. https://doi.org/10.1007/s13770-017-0045-2

Daddysman MK, Fecko CJ (2011) DNA multiphoton absorption generates localized damage for studying repair dynamics in live cells. Biophys J 101(9):2294–2303. https://doi.org/10.1016/j.bpj.2011.09.031

De Freitas LF, Hamblin MR (2016) Proposed mechanisms of photobiomodulation or low-level light therapy. IEEE J Sel Top Quantum Electron 22(3):348–364. https://doi.org/10.1109/JSTQE.2016.2561201

Demidova-Rice TN, Salomatina EV, Yaroslavsky AN, Herman IM, Hamblin MR (2007) Low-level light stimulates excisional wound healing in mice. Lasers Surg Med 39(9):706–715. https://doi.org/10.1002/lsm.20549

Deng J, Lukens JN, Swisher-McClure S, Cohn JC, Spinelli BA, Quinn RJ, Chittams J, McMenamin E, Lin A (2021) Photobiomodulation therapy in head and neck cancer-related lymphedema: a pilot feasibility study. Integr Cancer Ther 20. https://doi.org/10.1177/15347354211037938

Du Cheyne C, Tay H, De Spiegelaere W (2020) The complex TIE between macrophages and angiogenesis. Anat Histol Embryol 49(5):585–596. https://doi.org/10.1111/ahe.12518

Duca L, Floquet N, Alix AJP, Haye B, Debelle L (2004) Elastin as a matrikine. Crit Rev Oncol 49(3):235–244. https://doi.org/10.1016/j.critrevonc.2003.09.007

Epstein JB, Thariat J, Bensadoun R-J, Barasch A, Murphy BA, Kolnick L, Popplewell L, Maghami E (2012) Oral complications of cancer and cancer therapy: from cancer treatment to survivorship. CA Cancer J Clin 62(6):400–422. https://doi.org/10.3322/caac.21157

Feinendegen LE, Pollycove M, Neumann RD (2007) Whole-body responses to low-level radiation exposure: new concepts in mammalian radiobiology. Exp Hematol 35(4):37–46. https://doi.org/10.1016/j.exphem.2007.01.011

Feinendegen LE, Pollycove M, Neumann RD (2009) Low-dose cancer risk modeling must recognize up-regulation of protection. Dose-Response 8(2):798–805. https://doi.org/10.2203/2Fdose-response.09-035.Feinendegen

Feitosa MCP, de Carvalho AFM, Feitosa VC, Coelho IM, de Oliveira RA, Arisawa EÂL (2015) Effects of the low-level laser therapy (LLLT) in the process of healing diabetic foot ulcers. Acta Cir Bras 30(12):852–857. https://doi.org/10.1590/S0102-865020150120000010

Fekrazad R, Mirmoezzi A, Kalhori KAM, Arany P (2015) The effect of red, green and blue lasers on healing of oral wounds in diabetic rats. J Photochem Photobiol B Biol 148:242–245. https://doi.org/10.1016/j.jphotobiol.2015.04.018

Finnson KW, Arany PR, Philip A (2013) Transforming growth factor beta Signaling in cutaneous wound healing: lessons learned from animal studies. Adv Wound Caref 2(5):225–237. https://doi.org/10.1089/wound.2012.0419

Freund L (1904) Elements of general radio-therapy for practitioners. Rebman Company, New York

Frykberg RG, Banks J (2015) Challenges in the treatment of chronic wounds. Adv Wound Caref 4(9):560–582. https://doi.org/10.1089/wound.2015.0635

Fujimura T, Mitani A, Fukuda M, Mogi M, Osawa K, Takahashi S, Aino M, Iwamura Y, Miyajima S, Yamamoto H, Noguchi T (2013) Irradiation with a low-level diode laser induces the developmental endothelial locus-1 gene and reduces proinflammatory cytokines in epithelial cells. Lasers Med Sci 29:987–994. https://doi.org/10.1007/s10103-013-1439-6

Gallagher KA, Liu Z-J, Xiao M, Chen H, Goldstein LJ, Buerk DG, Nedeau A, Thom SR, Velazquez OC (2007) Diabetic impairments in NO-mediated endothelial progenitor cell mobilization and homing are reversed by hyperoxia and SDF-1 alpha. J Clin Investig 117(5):1249–1259. https://doi.org/10.1172/JCI29710

Gianfaldoni S, Gianfaldoni R, Wollina U, Lotti J, Tchernev G, Lotti T (2017) An overview on radiotherapy: from its history to its current applications in dermatology. Open Access Maced J Med Sci 5(4):521. https://doi.org/10.3889/oamjms.2017.122

Gonzalez ACDO, Costa TF, Andrade ZDA, Medrado ARAP (2016) Wound healing – a literature review. An Bras Dermatol 91(5):614–620. https://doi.org/10.1590/abd1806-4841.20164741

Gonzalez-Suarez I, Gonzalo S (2010) Nurturing the genome: A-type lamins preserve genomic stability. Nucleus 1(2):129–135. https://doi.org/10.4161/nucl.1.2.10797

Grada A, Mervis J, Falanga V (2018) Research techniques made simple: animal models of wound healing. J Invest Dermatol 138(10):2095–2105.e2091. https://doi.org/10.1016/j.jid.2018.08.005

Gridley DS, Rizvi A, Luo-Owen X, Makinde AY, Pecaut MJ (2009) Low dose, low dose rate photon radiation modifies leukocyte distribution and gene expression in CD4+ T cells. J Radiat Res 50(2):139–150. https://doi.org/10.1269/jrr.08095

Grinnell F (1994) Mini-review on the cellular mechanisms of disease fibroblasts, myofibroblasts, and wound contraction. J Cell Biol 124(4):401–404. https://doi.org/10.1083/jcb.124.4.401

Grzybowski A, Pietrzak K (2012) From patient to discoverer-Niels Ryberg Finsen (1860–1904)-the founder of phototherapy in dermatology. Clin Dermatol 30(4):451–455. https://doi.org/10.1016/j.clindermatol.2011.11.019

Grzybowski A, Sak J, Pawlikowski J (2016) A brief report on the history of phototherapy. Clin Dermatol 34(5):532–537. https://doi.org/10.1016/j.clindermatol.2016.05.002

Guéguen Y, Bontemps A, Ebrahimian TG (2019) Adaptive responses to low doses of radiation or chemicals: their cellular and molecular mechanisms. Cell Mol Life Sci 76:1255–1273. https://doi.org/10.1007/s00018-018-2987-5

Hamblin MR (2017) Mechanisms and mitochondrial redox signaling in photobiomodulation. Photochem Photobiol 94(2):199–212. https://doi.org/10.1111/php.12864

Hauptmann M, Haghdoost S, Gomolka M, Sarioglu H, Ueffing M, Dietz A, Kulka U, Unger K, Babini G, Harms-Ringdahl M, Ottolenghi A, Hornhardt S (2016) Differential response and priming dose effect on the proteome of human fibroblast and stem cells induced by exposure to low doses of ionizing radiation. Radiat Res 185(3):299–312. https://doi.org/10.1667/RR14226.1

Hawkins D, Abrahamse H (2005) Biological effects of helium-neon laser irradiation on normal and wounded human skin fibroblasts. Photomed Laser Surg 23(3):251–259. https://doi.org/10.1089/pho.2005.23.251

Iliakis G, Wang YA, Guan J, Wang H (2003) DNA damage checkpoint control in cells exposed to ionizing radiation. Oncogene 37:5834–5847. https://doi.org/10.1038/sj.onc.1206682

Irfan-Maqsood M (2018) Classification of wounds: know before research and clinical practice. Genes Cells 4:1–4. https://doi.org/10.15562/gnc.61

Jabbari N, Farjah GH, Ghadimi B, Zanjani H, Heshmatian B (2017) Acceleration of skin wound healing by low-dose indirect ionizing radiation in male rats. Kaohsiung J Med Sci 33(8): 385–393. https://doi.org/10.1016/j.kjms.2017.05.013

Jang DH, Song DH, Chang EJ, Jeon JY (2016) Anti-inflammatory and lymphangiogenetic effects of low-level laser therapy on lymphedema in an experimental mouse tail model. Lasers Med Sci 31(2):289–296. https://doi.org/10.1007/s10103-015-1854-y

Jiang H, Li W, Li X, Cai L, Wang G (2008) Low-dose radiation induces adaptive response in normal cells, but not in tumor cells: in vitro and in vivo studies. J Radiat Res 49(3):219–230. https://doi.org/10.1269/jrr.07072

Kadenbach B, Hüttemann M (2015) The subunit composition and function of mammalian cytochrome c oxidase. Mitochondrion 24:64–76. https://doi.org/10.1016/j.mito.2015.07.002

Kalebic T, Garbisa S, Glaser B, Liotta LA (1983) Basement membrane collagen: degradation by migrating endothelial cells. Science 221(4607):281–283. https://doi.org/10.1126/science.6190230

Kang S, Long K, Wang S, Sada A, Tumbar T (2020) Histone H3 K4/9/27 trimethylation levels affect wound healing and stem cell dynamics in adult skin. Stem Cell Rep 14(1):34–48. https://doi.org/10.1016/j.stemcr.2019.11.007

Karu T (1999) Primary and secondary mechanisms of action of visible to near-IR radiation on cells. J Photochem Photobiol B Biol 49(1):1–17. https://doi.org/10.1016/S1011-1344(98)00219-X

Karu TI (2014) Cellular and molecular mechanisms of photobiomodulation (low-power laser therapy). IEEE J Sel Top Quantum Electron 20(2):143–148. https://doi.org/10.1109/JSTQE.2013.2273411

Kaviani A, Djavid GE, Ataie-Fashtami L, Fateh M, Ghodsi M, Salami M, Zand N, Kashef N, Larijani B (2011) A randomized clinical trial on the effect of low-level laser therapy on chronic diabetic foot wound healing: a preliminary report. Photomed Laser Surg 29(2):109–114. https://doi.org/10.1089/pho.2009.2680

Khan MG, Wang Y (2022) Advances in the current understanding of how low-dose radiation affects the cell cycle. Cell 11(3):356. https://doi.org/10.3390/2Fcells11030356

Kojima S, Ishida H, Takahashi M, Yamaoka K (2002) Elevation of glutathione induced by low-dose gamma rays and its involvement in increased natural killer activity. Radiat Res 157(3):275–280. https://doi.org/10.1667/0033-7587(2002)157[0275:eogibl]2.0.co;2

Kriz J, Seegenschmiedt HM, Bartels A, Micke O, Muecke R, Schaefer U, Haverkamp U, Eich HT (2018) Updated strategies in the treatment of benign diseases—a patterns of care study of the German cooperative group on benign diseases. Adv Radiat Oncol 3(3):240–244. https://doi.org/10.1016/j.adro.2018.02.008

Kuhn A, Porto FA, Miraglia P, Brunetto AL (2009) Low-level infrared laser therapy in chemotherapy-induced oral mucositis: a randomized placebo-controlled trial in children. J Pediat Hematol Oncol 31(1):33–37. https://doi.org/10.1097/MPH.0b013e318192cb8e

Lan CC, Wu CS, Huang SM, Wu IH, Chen GS (2013) High-glucose environment enhanced oxidative stress and increased interleukin-8 secretion from keratinocytes: new insights into impaired diabetic wound healing. Diabetes 62(7):2530–2538. https://doi.org/10.2337/2Fdb12-1714

Lanzafame RJ, Stadler I, Kurtz AF, Connelly R, Timothy PA, Brondon P, Olson D (2007) Reciprocity of exposure time and irradiance on energy density during photoradiation on wound healing in a murine pressure ulcer model. Lasers Surg Med 39(6):534–542. https://doi.org/10.1002/lsm.20519

Lau P, Bidin N, Krishnan G, AnaybBaleg SM, Sum MBM, Bakhtiar H, Nassir Z, Hamid A (2015) Photobiostimulation effect on diabetic wound at different power density of near infrared laser. J Photochem Photobiol B Biol 151:201–207. https://doi.org/10.1016/j.jphotobiol.2015.08.009

Lee B-B, Rockson SG (2018) Lymphedema: a concise compendium of theory and practice. Springer, Cham

Lee JH, Kim SY, Kil IS, Park J-W (2007) Regulation of ionizing radiation-induced apoptosis by mitochondrial NADPH+-dependent isocitrate dehydrogenase. J Biol Chem 282(18):13385–13394. https://doi.org/10.1074/jbc.M700303200

Li B, Wang JHC (2011) Fibroblasts and myofibroblasts in wound healing: force generation and measurement. J Tissue Viability 20(4):108–120. https://doi.org/10.1016/j.jtv.2009.11.004

Li J, Chen J, Kirsner R (2007) Pathophysiology of acute wound healing. Clin Dermatol 25(1):9–18. https://doi.org/10.1016/j.clindermatol.2006.09.007

Liang X, So YH, Cui J, Ma K, Xu X, Zhao Y, Cai L, Li W (2011) The low-dose ionizing radiation stimulates cell proliferation via activation of the MAPK/ERK pathway in rat cultured mesenchymal stem cells. J Radiat Res 52(3):380–386. https://doi.org/10.1269/jrr.10121

Liang X, Gu J, Yu D, Wang G, Zhou L, Zhang X, Zhao Y, Chen X, Zheng S, Liu Q, Cai L, Cui J, Li W (2016) Low-dose radiation induces cell proliferation in human embryonic lung fibroblasts but not in lung cancer cells. Dose-Response 14(1):1559325815622174. https://doi.org/10.1177/1559325815622174

Liu R, Xiong S, Zhang L, Chu Y (2010) Enhancement of antitumor immunity by low-dose total body irradiation is associated with selectively decreasing the proportion and number of T regulatory cells. Cell Mol Immunol 7(2):157–162. https://doi.org/10.1038%2Fcmi.2009.117

Loots MAM, Lamme EN, Zeegelaar J, Mekkes JR, Bos JD, Middelkoop E (1998) Differences in cellular infiltrate and extracellular matrix of chronic diabetic and venous ulcers versus acute wounds. J Invest Dermatol 111(5):850–857. https://doi.org/10.1046/j.1523-1747.1998.00381.x

Loree J, Koturbash I, Kutanzi K, Baker M, Pogribny I, Kovalchuk O (2006) Radiation-induced molecular changes in rat mammary tissue: possible implications for radiation-induced carcinogenesis. Int J Radiat Biol 82(11):805–815. https://doi.org/10.1080/09553000600960027

Martins PN (2018) A brief history about radiotherapy. Int J Latest Res Eng Technol 4(2):8–11. https://doi.org/10.5281/zenodo.3824294

Martin P, Leibovich SJ (2005) Inflammatory cells during wound repair: the good, the bad and the ugly. Trends Cell Biol 15(11):599–607. https://doi.org/10.1016/j.tcb.2005.09.002

Martin P, Nunan R (2015) Cellular and molecular mechanisms of repair in acute and chronic wound healing. Br J Dermatol 173(2):320–378. https://doi.org/10.1111/bjd.13954

Marques FG, Poli E, Malaquias J, Carvalho T, Portêlo A, Ramires A, Aldeia F, Ribeiro RM, Vitorino E, Diegues I, Costa L, Coutinho J, Pina F, Mareel M, Constantino Rosa Santos S (2020) Low doses of ionizing radiation activate endothelial cells and induce angiogenesis in peritumoral tissues. Radiother Oncol 151:322–327. https://doi.org/10.1016/j.radonc.2020.06.038

Mathias D, Mitchel REJ, Barclay M, Wyatt H, Bugden M, Priest ND, Whitman SC, Scholz M, Hildebrandt G, Kamprad M, Glasow A (2015) Low-dose irradiation affects expression of inflammatory markers in the heart of ApoE −/− mice. PLoS One 10(3):e0119661. https://doi.org/10.1371/journal.pone.0119661

Maxson S, Lopez EA, Yoo D, Danilkovitch-Miagkova A, Leroux MA (2012) Concise review: role of mesenchymal stem cells in wound repair. Stem Cells Transl Med 1(2):142–149. https://doi.org/10.5966/sctm.2011-0018

Medrado ARAP, Pugliese LS, Reis SRA, Andrade ZA (2003) Influence of low level laser therapy on wound healing and its biological action upon myofibroblasts. Lasers Surg Med 32(3):239–244. https://doi.org/10.1002/lsm.10126

Mester E, Szende B, Gärtner P (1968) The effect of laser beams on the growth of hair in mice. Radiobiol Radiother (Berl) 9(5):621–626

Moreno AC, Frank SJ, Garden AS, Rosenthal DI, Fuller CD, Gunn GB, Reddy JP, Morrison WH, Williamson TD, Holliday EB, Phan J, Blanchard P (2019) Intensity modulated proton therapy (IMPT) – the future of IMRT for head and neck cancer. Oral Oncol 88:66–74. https://doi.org/10.1016/j.oraloncology.2018.11.015

Nall AV, Brownlee RE, Peyton Colvin C, Schultz G, Fein D, Cassisi NJ, Nguyen T, Kalra A, Nall G, Head G, Plastic Surgery F (1996) Transforming growth factor β1 improves wound healing and random flap survival in normal and irradiated rats. Arch Otolaryngol Head Neck Surg 122:171–177. https://doi.org/10.1001/archotol.1996.01890140057011

Non-Ionizing Radiation (n.d.) United States occupational safety and health administration. https://www.osha.gov/non-ionizing-radiation

Nyengaard JR, Rasch R (1993) The impact of experimental diabetes mellitus in rats on glomerular capillary number and sizes. Diabetologia 36(3):189–194. https://doi.org/10.1007/bf00399948

Omer H (2021) Radiobiological effects and medical applications of non-ionizing radiation. Saudi J Biol Sci 28(10):5585–5592. https://doi.org/10.1016/j.sjbs.2021.05.071

O'Shea TP, Foley MJ, Rajasekar D, Downes PA, van der Putten W, Moore M, Shearer A (2008) Electron beam therapy at extended source-to-surface distance: a Monte Carlo investigation. J Appl Clin Med Phys 9(4):57–67. https://doi.org/10.1120/2Fjacmp.v9i4.2811

Oberoi S, Zamperlini-Netto G, Beyene J, Treister NS, Sung L (2014) Effect of prophylactic low level laser therapy on oral mucositis: a systematic review and meta-analysis. PLoS One 9(9): e107418. https://doi.org/10.1371/journal.pone.0107418

Omar MT, Shaheen AA, Zafar H (2012) A systematic review of the effect of low-level laser therapy in the management of breast cancer-related lymphedema. Support Care Cancer 20(11): 2977–2984. https://doi.org/10.1007/s00520-012-1546-0

Ortega S, Ittmann M, Tsang Stephen H, Ehrlich M, Basilico C (1998) Neuronal defects and delayed wound healing in mice lacking fibroblast growth factor 2. Proc Natl Acad Sci 95(10): 5672–5677. https://doi.org/10.1073/pnas.95.10.5672

Oton-Leite AF, Silva GB, Morais MO, Silva TA, Leles CR, Valadares MC, Pinezi JC, Batista AC, Mendonça EF (2015) Effect of low-level laser therapy on chemoradiotherapy-induced oral mucositis and salivary inflammatory mediators in head and neck cancer patients. Laser Surg Med 47(4):296–305. https://doi.org/10.1002/lsm.22349

Ott OJ, Niewald M, Weitmann H-D, Jacob I, Adamietz IA, Schaefer U, Keilholz L, Heyd R, Muecke R, German Cooperative Group on Radiotherapy for Benign Diseases (2015) DEGRO guidelines for the radiotherapy of non-malignant disorders. Strahlenther Onkol 191:1–6. https://doi.org/10.1007/s00066-014-0757-3

Ottawa (2013) Optimal care of chronic, non-healing, lower extremity wounds: a review of clinical evidence and guidelines. Canadian Agency for Drugs and Technologies in Health, Ottawa

Passarella S, Karu T (2014) Absorption of monochromatic and narrow band radiation in the visible and near IR by both mitochondrial and non-mitochondrial photoacceptors results in photobiomodulation. J Photochem Photobiol B Biol 140:344–358. https://doi.org/10.1016/j.jphotobiol.2014.07.021

Pastar I, Stojadinovic O, Krzyzanowska A, Barrientos S, Stuelten C, Zimmerman K, Blumenberg M, Brem H, Tomic-Canic M (2010) Attenuation of the transforming growth factor beta-signaling pathway in chronic venous ulcers. Mol Med 16(3–4):92–101. https://doi.org/10.2119/molmed.2009.00149

Peplow PV, Chung TY, Ryan B, Baxter GD (2011) Laser photobiostimulation of wound healing: reciprocity of irradiance and exposure time on energy density for splinted wounds in diabetic mice. Lasers Surg Med 43(8):843–850. https://doi.org/10.1002/lsm.21094

Pirzkall A, Lohr F, Höss A, Wannenmacher M, Debus J, Carol M (2000) Comparison of intensity-modulated radiotherapy with conventional conformal radiotherapy for complex-shaped tumors. Int J Radiat Oncol Biol Phys 48(5):1371–1380. https://doi.org/10.1016/S0360-3016(00)00772-0

Pogribny I, Koturbash I, Tryndyak V, Hudson D, Stevenson SML, Sedelnikova O, Bonner W, Kovalchuk O (2005) Fractionated low-dose radiation exposure leads to accumulation of DNA damage and profound alterations in DNA and histone methylation in the murine thymus. Mol Cancer Res 3(10):553–561. https://doi.org/10.1158/1541-7786.MCR-05-0074

Purdy JA (2008) Dose to normal tissues outside the radiation therapy patient's treated volume: a review of different radiation therapy techniques. Health Phys 95(5):666–676. https://doi.org/10.1097/01.HP.0000326342.47348.06

Radiation in Everyday Life (2014) International Atomic Energy Agency. https://www.iaea.org/Publications/Factsheets/English/radlife

Rehani MM, Srimahachota S (2011) Skin injuries in interventional procedures. Radiat Prot Dosim 147(1–2):8–12. https://doi.org/10.1093/rpd/ncr257

Rivard A, Silver M, Chen D, Kearney M, Magner M, Annex B, Peters K, Isner JM (1999) Rescue of diabetes-related impairment of angiogenesis by intramuscular gene therapy with adeno-VEGF. Am J Pathol 154(2):355–363. https://doi.org/10.1016/S0002-9440(10)65282-0

Rizzi CF, Mauriz JL, Freitas Corrêa DS, Moreira AJ, Zettler CG, Filippin LI, Marroni NP, González-Gallego J (2006) Effects of low-level laser therapy (LLLT) on the nuclear factor (NF)-κB signaling pathway in traumatized muscle. Lasers Surg Med 38(7):704–713. https://doi.org/10.1002/lsm.20371

Roberts AB, Sporn MB, Assoian RK, Smith JM, Roche NS, Wakefield LM, Heine UI, Liotta LA, Falanga V, Kehrl JH et al (1986) Transforming growth factor type beta: rapid induction of fibrosis and angiogenesis in vivo and stimulation of collagen formation in vitro. Proc Natl Acad Sci 83(12):4167–4171. https://doi.org/10.1073/pnas.83.12.4167

Rogakou EP, Boon C, Redon C, Bonner WM (1999) Megabase chromatin domains involved in DNA double-strand breaks in vivo. J Cell Biol 146(5):905–916. https://doi.org/10.1083/jcb.146.5.905

Ruh AC, Frigo L, Cavalcanti MFXB, Svidnicki P, Vicari VN, Lopes-Martins RAB, Leal Junior ECP, De Isla N, Diomede F, Trubiani O, Favero GM (2018) Laser photobiomodulation in pressure ulcer healing of human diabetic patients: gene expression analysis of inflammatory biochemical markers. Lasers Med Sci 33(1):165–171. https://doi.org/10.1007/s10103-017-2384-6

Sacks B, Meyerson G, Siegel JA (2016) Epidemiology without biology: false paradigms, unfounded assumptions, and specious statistics in radiation science (with commentaries by Inge Schmitz-Feuerhake and Christopher Busby and a reply by the authors). Biol Theory 11:69–101. https://doi.org/10.1007/s13752-016-0244-4

Sayed E, Dyson M (1996) Effect of laser pulse repetition rate and pulse duration on mast cell number and degranulation. Lasers Surg Med 19(4):433–435. https://doi.org/10.1002/(SICI)1096-9101(1996)19:4<3C433::AID-LSM8>3E3.0.CO;2-T

Schäffer M, Weimer W, Wider S, Stülten C, Bongartz M, Budach W, Becker HD (2002) Differential expression of inflammatory mediatiators in radiation-impaired wound healing. J Surg Res 107(1):93–100. https://doi.org/10.1006/jsre.2002.6494

Schindl A, Schindl M, Pernerstorfer-Schön H, Kerschan K, Knobler R, Schindl L (1999) Diabetic neuropathic foot ulcer: successful treatment by low-intensity laser therapy. Dermatology (Basel) 198:314–316. https://doi.org/10.1159/000018140

Sharma V, Jambrina Pablo G, Kaukonen M, Rosta E, Rich Peter R (2017) Insights into functions of the H channel of cytochrome c oxidase from atomistic molecular dynamics simulations. Proc Natl Acad Sci 114(48):E10339–E10348. https://doi.org/10.1073/pnas.1708628114

Shi H-X, Lin C, Lin B-B, Wang Z-G, Zhang H-Y, Wu F-Z, Cheng Y, Xiang L-J, Guo D-J, Luo X, Zhang G-Y, Fu X-B, Bellusci S, Li X-K, Xiao J (2013) The anti-scar effects of basic fibroblast growth factor on the wound repair in vitro and in vivo. PLoS One 8(4):e59966. https://doi.org/10.1371/journal.pone.0059966

Siegel JA, Pennington CW, Sacks B (2017) Subjecting radiologic imaging to the linear no-threshold hypothesis: a non sequitur of non-trivial proportion. J Nucl Med 58(1):1–6. https://doi.org/10.2967/jnumed.116.180182

Sofia Vala I, Martins LR, Imaizumi N, Nunes RJ, Rino J, Kuonen F, Carvalho LM, Rüegg C, Grillo IM, Barata JT, Mareel M, Santos SCR (2010) Low doses of ionizing radiation promote tumor growth and metastasis by enhancing angiogenesis. PLoS One 5(6):e11222. https://doi.org/10.1371/journal.pone.0011222

Sommer AP (2019) Mitochondrial cytochrome c oxidase is not the primary acceptor for near infrared light-it is mitochondrial bound water: the principles of low-level light therapy. Ann Transl Med 7(S13):10.21037/atm.2019.01.43

Sommer AP, Schemmer P, Pavláth AE, Försterling H-D, Mester ÁR, Trelles MA (2020) Quantum biology in low level light therapy: death of a dogma. Ann Transl Med 8(7):440. https://doi.org/10.21037/atm.2020.03.159

Sykes PJ, Day TK, Swinburne SJ, Lane JM, Morley AA, Hooker AM, Bhat M (2006) In vivo mutagenic effect of very low dose radiation. Dose-Response 4(4):309–316. https://doi.org/10.2203/dose-response.06-004.Sykes

Tamm ER, Siegner A, Baur A, Lütjen-Drecoll E (1996) Transforming growth factor-β1 induces α-smooth muscle-actin expression in cultured human and monkey trabecular meshwork. Exp Eye Res 62(4):389–398. https://doi.org/10.1006/exer.1996.0044

Thanik VD, Chang CC, Lerman OZ, Greives MR, Le H, Warren SM, Schneider RJ, Formenti SC, Saadeh PB, Levine JP (2010) Cutaneous low-dose radiation increases tissue vascularity through upregulation of angiogenic and vasculogenic pathways. J Vasc Res 47:472–480. https://doi.org/10.1159/000313875

Toyokawa H, Matsui Y, Uhara J, Tsuchiya H, Teshima S, Nakanishi H, Kwon AH, Azuma Y, Nagaoka T, Ogawa T, Kamiyama Y (2003) Promotive effects of far-infrared ray on full-thickness skin wound healing in rats. Exp Biol Med 228(6):724–729. https://doi.org/10.1177/153537020322800612

Trotti A, Bellm LA, Epstein JB, Frame D, Fuchs HJ, Gwede CK, Komaroff E, Nalysnyk L, Zilberberg MD (2003) Mucositis incidence, severity and associated outcomes in patients with head and neck cancer receiving radiotherapy with or without chemotherapy: a systematic literature review. Radiother Oncol 66(3):253–262. https://doi.org/10.1016/S0167-8140(02)00404-8

Truong K, Bradley S, Baginski B, Wilson JR, Medlin D, Zheng L, Wilson RK, Rusin M, Takacs E, Dean D (2018) The effect of well-characterized, very low-dose x-ray radiation on fibroblasts. PLoS One 13(1):e0190330. https://doi.org/10.1371/journal.pone.0190330

Ud-Din S, Wilgus TA, Bayat A (2020) Mast cells in skin scarring: a review of animal and human research. Front Immunol 11:552205. https://doi.org/10.3389/fimmu.2020.552205

Ulyanenko S, Pustovalova M, Koryakin S, Beketov E, Lychagin A, Ulyanenko L, Kaprin A, Grekhova A, Ozerova AM, Ozerov IV, Vorobyeva N, Shegay P, Ivanov S, Leonov S, Klokov D, Osipov AN (2019) Formation of γH2AX and pATM foci in human mesenchymal stem cells exposed to low dose-rate gamma-radiation. Int J Mol Sci 20(11):2645. https://doi.org/10.3390/ijms20112645

Velnar T, Bailey T, Smrkolj V (2009) The wound healing process: an overview of the cellular and molecular mechanisms. J Int Med 37(5):1528–1542. https://doi.org/10.1177/147323000903700531

Wagner VP, Curra M, Webber LP, Nör C, Matte U, Meurer L, Martins MD (2016) Photobiomodulation regulates cytokine release and new blood vessel formation during oral wound healing in rats. Lasers Med Sci 31:665–671. https://doi.org/10.1007/s10103-016-1904-0

Waltenberger J, Lange J, Kranz A (2000) Vascular endothelial growth factor-A-induced chemotaxis of monocytes is attenuated in patients with diabetes mellitus. Circulation 102:185–190. https://doi.org/10.1161/01.CIR.102.2.185

Wang Y, Kuramitsu Y, Ueno T, Suzuki N, Yoshino S, Iizuka N, Zhang X, Akada J, Oka M, Nakamura K (2012) Proteomic differential display identifies upregulated vinculin as a possible biomarker of pancreatic cancer. Oncol Rep 28(5):1845–1850. https://doi.org/10.3892/or.2012.2004

Wang W, Yang C, Wang XY, Zhou LY, Lao GJ, Liu D, Wang C, Hu MD, Zeng TT, Yan L, Ren M (2018) MicroRNA-129 and -335 promote diabetic wound healing by inhibiting Sp1-mediated MMP-9 expression. Diabetes 67(8):1627–1638. https://doi.org/10.2337/db17-1238

Weber DC, Ares C, Lomax AJ, Kurtz JM (2006) Radiation therapy planning with photons and protons for early and advanced breast cancer: an overview. Radiat Oncol 1(1):1–11. https://doi.org/10.1186/1748-717X-1-22

Wikstrom MKF (1977) Proton pump coupled to cytochrome c oxidase in mitochondria. Nature 266: 271–273. https://doi.org/10.1038/266271a0

Witte MB, Barbul A (1997) General principles of wound healing. Surg Clin North Am 77(3): 509–528. https://doi.org/10.1016/S0039-6109(05)70566-1

Xu X, Zhu F, Zhang M, Zeng D, Luo D, Liu G, Cui W, Wang S, Guo W, Xing W, Liang H (2013) Stromal cell-derived factor-1 enhances wound healing through recruiting bone marrow-derived mesenchymal stem cells to the wound area and promoting neovascularization. Cells Tissues Organs 197(2):103–113. https://doi.org/10.1159/000342921

Xu F, Liu C, Zhou D, Zhang L (2016) TGF-β/SMAD pathway and its regulation in hepatic fibrosis. J Histochem Cytochem 64(3):157–167. https://doi.org/10.1369/0022155415627681

Yang G, Li W, Jiang H, Liang X, Zhao Y, Yu D, Zhou L, Wang G, Tian H, Han F, Cai L (2016) Low-dose radiation may be a novel approach to enhance the effectiveness of cancer therapeutics. Int J Cancer 139(10):2157–2168

Yim JH, Yun JM, Kim JY, Lee IK, Nam SY, Kim CS (2017a) Phosphoprotein profiles of candidate markers for early cellular responses to low-dose γ-radiation in normal human fibroblast cells. J Radiat Res 58(3):329–340. https://doi.org/10.1093/jrr/rrw126

Yim JH, Yun JM, Kim JY, Nam SY, Kim CS (2017b) Estimation of low-dose radiation-responsive proteins in the absence of genomic instability in normal human fibroblast cells. Int J Radiat Biol 93(11):1197–1206. https://doi.org/10.1080/09553002.2017.1350302

Zein R, Selting W, Hamblin MR (2018) Review of light parameters and photobiomodulation efficacy: dive into complexity. J Biomed Opt 23(12):1–17. https://doi.org/10.1117/1.jbo.23.12.120901

How Is Cancer Under the Sea? Hyperbaric Oxygen Therapy in Cancer

Amene Saghazadeh and Nima Rezaei

Abstract

Hyperbaric oxygen therapy (HBOT) provides patients with breathing pure oxygen under higher-than-normal air pressure. Applications of HBOT mainly occur in the management settings for the treatment of radiation-related complications. To date, lymphedema, proctitis and cystitis, and osteoradionecrosis of the jaw have been the most common conditions for using HBOT in post-radiation therapy of breast, prostate, and head and neck cancer. While case reports, case series, and retrospective cohorts produced HBOT-favoring results, the current literature suffers from a paucity of clinical trials, preventing any recommendation against thinking of HBOT for all. However, clinical trials are ongoing and might change the future picture of this field. In addition, the interdisciplinary research can approach further by relating the physics of HBOT and cancer biomechanics and scheduling standard protocols of HBOT for cancer.

A. Saghazadeh
Research Center for Immunodeficiencies, Children's Medical Center, Tehran University of Medical Sciences, Tehran, Iran

Integrated Science Association (ISA), Universal Scientific Education and Research Network (USERN), Tehran, Iran

N. Rezaei (✉)
Research Center for Immunodeficiencies, Children's Medical Center, Tehran University of Medical Sciences, Tehran, Iran

Department of Immunology, School of Medicine, Tehran University of Medical Sciences, Tehran, Iran

Systematic Review and Meta-Analysis Expert Group (SRMEG), Universal Scientific Education and Research Network (USERN), Stockholm, Sweden
e-mail: rezaei_nima@tums.ac.ir

Interdisciplinary Cancer Research, https://doi.org/10.1007/16833_2022_120
Published online: 25 January 2023

Keywords

Cancer · HBOT · Hyperbaric oxygen therapy

1 Introduction

Hyperbaric oxygen therapy (HBOT) serves as an adjuvant in cancer, which is usually used for alleviating late toxic events following radiation therapy; however, it could apply to increase the efficacy of cancer treatments. HBOT effects are observable on both mental and physical health as well as on both general and cancer-specific signs and symptoms. The present chapter reviews studies investigating the effects of HBOT on patients with different types of cancer.

2 Breast Cancer

2.1 Cohort/Pilot

A relatively large-scale, retrospective cohort study, including about 1000 patients with breast cancer, showed a significant improvement in life quality, pain, and breast symptoms with HBOT, which was delivered for 20 or more sessions to all patients (Batenburg et al. 2021). In further analyses, it was possible to see that HBOT is more likely to fail in active smokers and those for whom HBOT was introduced in shorter intervals between HBOT and radiotherapy.

In a prospective pilot study (Koo et al. 2020), ten patients with breast cancer underwent complex decongestive therapy (CDT) with or without HBOT (ten sessions over 2 weeks) for lymphedema. The CDT plus HBOT group was comparable for all bioelectrical impedance spectroscopy-related parameters as well as for most LYMQOL[1] domains, e.g., quality of life, appearance, symptoms, and mood, except for function, whose improvement seems to be significantly superior to that for the CDT group.

Another prospective study recorded pre-post HBOT measurements for 57 patients with LRTI and lymphedema (Teguh et al. 2016). Patients received a mean of 47 HBOT sessions. They self-reported improvements in arm/shoulder pain, arm/hand swelling, arm motility, and pain, swelling, oversensitivity, and skin issues in the cancer-involved breast by about 43%, 26%, 43%, 64%, 58%, 54%, and 41%.

In a non-randomized trial (Gothard et al. 2004) of 21 patients with breast cancer and chronic lymphedema, who underwent a six-week course of HBOT (30 sessions), descriptive statistics 1 year after HBOT included a reduction in arm volume of about 20% of evaluable patients, an improved clearance of nano colloidal technetium

[1]LYMQOL is used for lymphedema-related quality of life measurement.

(99mTc) for about half of evaluable patients, an enhanced shoulder range of motion for about one-third of evaluable patients, an improved feeling about the arm softness for more than 60% of evaluable patients, and a reduction in radiation-induced breast induration in more than half of evaluable patients. However, patients self-reported no significantly higher levels of life quality after HBOT than before HBOT.

Of ten patients with breast cancer and lymphedema, who participated in a pilot project, eight were responders (Teas et al. 2004). They showed a greater than 30% decrease in hand lymphedema and maintained this effect by the last follow-up, which occurred more than 1 year after HBOT was completed. Such an effect was not evident for lymphedema volume. In addition, vascular endothelial growth factor (VEGF) C, which is lymph angiogenesis-specific VEGF, began to increase when HBOT was completed.

Another pilot project (Heys et al. 2006) comprised two groups of patients: one receiving the chemotherapy alone and the other chemotherapy plus a ten-session HBOT. The important point is that the former intervention was tolerable for all patients (17/17), but the latter was not (11/15). Compared to the chemotherapy group, the HBOT group was improved in the extravascular extracellular space of the tumor, as represented in a reduction in VE in MRI. Patients, however, benefited comparably from the two interventions for all other clinical and pathological outcomes.

2.2 Case Report

Two case reports are available; both provide evidence about the HBOT-containing therapeutic protocols. One was a 29-year woman diagnosed with breast cancer of stage IV, BIRADS[2] V, and metastasis to abdomen, liver, and lymph nodes (İyikesici et al. 2017), and the other was a 45-year woman with triple-negative breast cancer complicated with brain necrosis and edema following radiation therapy, which was resistant to therapy with corticosteroids and mannitol (Xing et al. 2019). The former underwent multidisciplinary care made up of chemotherapy, hyperthermia, ketogenic diet, and HBOT, and the latter received Endostar, an angiogenesis inhibitor, plus HBOT. Both were recovered: for the former, pathological response was affirmed, and for the latter, the disappearance of brain necrosis in magnetic resonance imaging (MRI).

2.3 Case Series

In a series (Spruijt and van den Berg 2020), 67 patients with breast cancer and LRTI underwent HBOT for 26–60 sessions (mean: 44). The study assessed LENT-SOMA[3] scores in four points of time: 1, before HBOT, 2, immediately after

[2] Breast Imaging-Reporting and Data System

[3] Late Effects Normal Tissue Task Force-Subjective, Objective, Management, Analytic

HBOT, 3, 3 months after HBOT completion, and 4, 12 months after HBOT completion. Compared to before HBOT, 81% of patients exhibited improvement of one or greater scores in LENT-SOMA at the second time point. Also, such an improvement occurred in 43% of patients at the second time point compared to the first time point. Totally, this improvement was evident for 85% (57 out of 67) of patients at the final point of measurement, i.e., 12 months after HBOT, compared to the first time point, i.e., before HBOT. Patients showed improvement in fibrosis more than in pain more than in the edema subscale (75% vs. 66% vs. 43%). Shoulder motility, which was limited in abduction and anteflexion, increased by 70 and 35°, respectively. Univariate analyses marked different factors as significantly being related to the three subscales of LENT-SOMA, e.g., pain, fibrosis, and edema, as well as to the visual analog scale of pain. These factors included axillary lymph nodes, HBOT occasions, pre-HBOT score, chemotherapy, age, body mass index, and the interval between radiotherapy and HBOT. Multivariate analyses revealed significant correlations only for the pre-HBOT score with LENT-SOMA pain, LENT-SOMA edema, and visual analog scale of pain, and also for smoking with LENT-SOMA fibrosis.

2.4 Clinical Trial

Fifty-eight patients with breast cancer and lymphedema were randomized to receive the standard of care (n = 20) or 30 HBOT sessions (n = 38) (Gothard et al. 2010). Patients who underwent HBOT were not superior in any objective measurements of change in edema volume in ipsilateral and contralateral arms and self-reported assessments.

2.5 Adverse Effects

Among HBOT-related adverse events, myopia and barotrauma most commonly occurred, with estimated incidences of 50% and 18% (Batenburg et al. 2021). The majority of these events appeared to be mild, with moderate-to-severe events occurring in less than 5% of patients.

The series (Spruijt and van den Berg 2020) reported transient vision problems as the most common side effect of HBOT, occurring in more than 80% of patients with a six-month persistence rate of 6%. Increased fatigue (69%) was also prevalent. In addition to persistent vision symptoms, patients were referred to specialists for trouble equalizing ear pressure, which was recorded for 8% of patients.

3 Prostate Cancer

3.1 Cohort/Pilot

A longitudinal study (Nakada et al. 2012) followed 38 patients who underwent HBOT (mean number of sessions; 62) in the context of prostate cancer radiation-induced cystitis over an average of approximately 12 years. In addition to providing data on the baseline and the end of follow-up, the study included measurements of objective and self-reported outcomes at several time points, such as 2 years, 4 years, and 7 years after HBOT. The objective response rate peaked earlier than the subjective response rate, which occurred two and 4 years after HBOT and was between 79% and 95%. Although the response rate for both sets of outcomes, i.e., objective and subjective, slightly began to decline 7 years after HBOT and ranged from 72% to 82%, it was not significant, and patients continued to benefit from the treatment effect until the end of the follow-up duration. More than 70% experienced recurrence-free living, and those who did not have access to this experience had received higher radiation dosages and had started HBOT later relative to the occurrence of cystitis.

In a retrospective cohort study of 27 patients with proctitis who received a mean of 36 HBOT sessions, overall, 67% of patients enjoyed a partial-to-complete recovery, and the remaining did neither improve nor worsen (Dall'Era et al. 2006). Particularly, the majority of patients (75%) experienced pain alleviation, about half of patients could get away from the feeling of urgency, and about 30% documented fewer bleeding episodes.

Elsewhere, 16 patients with proctitis, cystitis, or both completed a median of 26 HBOT occasions (Mayer et al. 2001). All patients with proctitis and 75% of patients with cystitis had stopped bleeding.

3.2 Case Report

There has been reported a case with prostate cancer who developed an abscess and then rectal perforation following external beam radiation therapy (EBRT) (Kashihara et al. 2020). The abscess surrounded the place where the hydrogel spacer, which was located in order to decrease EBRT-related tissue injury. HBOT, in addition to antibiotics, could successfully recover the patient's condition.

The second report (Nakabayashi et al. 2006) is related to a 55-year-old man who presented with tenesmus and severe rectal pain after radiation therapy. Endoscopy revealed an anorectal ulcer. The delivery of one-month HBOT led to the complete response and ulcer resolution.

3.3 Case Series

The study (Kitta et al. 2000) presents four cases of chronic proctitis following radiation therapy. No details over the duration/session number of HBOT were provided. However, overall, patients appeared to improve mucosal appearance and rectal bleeding.

Ten patients complicated with hemorrhagic cystitis received a median of 30 HBOT sessions at a median of 52 months after radiotherapy completion and 11 months after the occurrence of hematuria (Degener et al. 2012). At a median follow-up of 3 years after HBOT, eight patients remained completely recovered from hematuria and reported no serious side effects.

Among 257 patients with proctitis, cystitis, or both in this retrospective cohort study (Fuentes-Raspall et al. 2012), 14 with grade II bladder/rectal toxicity were candidates for HBOT. No details on HBOT protocol are included in the study. However, the authors reported no significant improvement in ten subjects, persistent symptoms in one subject, and recovery in three subjects.

3.4 In Vivo

Four studies randomized SCID mice to investigate the effect of HBOT (Kalns et al. 1998; Chong et al. 2004; Tang et al. 2009a, b). Three of which compared HBOT with normobaric air, and one compared the delivery of chemotherapy drugs under HBOT or normobaric conditions. Cell lines for prostate cancer included LNCaP, PC-3, and Cap. These trials showed no significant effect of HBOT on tumor volume, microvessel density, tumor invasion, and the expression of markers related to cell proliferation, differentiation, and apoptosis, including Ki-67, p53, and p27. Furthermore, the use of HBOT lessened the growth rate of DU-145 cells and enhanced the sensitivity of prostate cancer cell lines to chemotherapy drugs, such as Taxol and Doxorubicin.

In addition, one observational study of the LNCap-injected SCID mice model pointed out HBOT-promoting new DNA synthesis (Kalns and Piepmeier 1999). This effect was dependent upon the pressure under which HBOT was delivered: 44% of cells displayed the new DNA synthesis under the zero-atmosphere pressure, which was increased to 65% of cells under the six-atmosphere pressure. Interestingly, the new DNA caused cells to arrest in the G2/M phase, implying that HBOT might operationalize a cell division-inhibiting mechanism.

4 Head and Neck Cancer

4.1 Cohort/Pilot

A total of 33 patients underwent a 30-session course of HBOT for the treatment of post-radiation osteoradionecrosis (ORN) of the jaw (Gupta et al. 2013). In general, more than 80% benefited from HBOT, with the majority achieving marked-to-complete healing (66%). In particular, the most improved outcomes were mouth dryness and pain (71% and 70%), followed by the ability to speak (41%).

A pilot project was made up of 80 patients candidate for HBOT for the management of ORN-related complications, mainly dry mouth (86%) and salivary gland hypofunction (56%) (Forner et al. 2011). HBOT, including 30 sessions, was effective in reducing both of these complications. Of note, more than half of those with salivary gland hypofunction responded to HBOT, of which again about half could experience normal salivary function.

Also, a prospectively designed study followed patients with oral and oropharyngeal cancer for one to 2 years after HBOT was completed for radiotherapy-induced ORN management (Gerlach et al. 2008). This study obtained similar results as mentioned above, i.e., higher saliva production and higher ability to swallow, as well as a better taste perception.

In a retrospective study (Slotman et al. 2011), 43 patients received surgery with or without post-operative HBOT. Those who received the HBOT-containing therapy showed a reduction in blood loss (700 ml vs. 1000 ml), with experiencing few major adverse events (17% vs. 63%) compared to those who underwent standard surgery. However, the two groups were not different in recurrence rate and cancer-related death.

4.2 Clinical Trial

Several randomized trials have published interim and final reports on the effect of HBOT in the short and long term.

In a trial (Teguh et al. 2009), 19 patients were randomized into two groups to receive or not receive HBOT (eight and 11 patients) and were followed up for 1.5 years after the intervention was completed. Patients who underwent HBOT showed an increased ability to swallow and eat in public while experiencing a reduction in dry mouth and sticky saliva, as well as pain alleviation. Another randomized trial (Schoen et al. 2007) published in the 2000s compared the effect of HBOT and antibiotics on implant survival. Patients who underwent HBOT after implantation had no superiority over those who received antibiotics in the proportion of well-maintained implants (about 85% vs. 94%) and life quality and satisfaction.

A group of trials was published before 2000 (Sealy et al. 1974, 1986; Henk et al. 1977; Henk and Smith 1977; Sealy and Cridland 1984; Henk 1986; Denham et al. 1987). These trials considered hyperbaric oxygen a means under which other interventions, such as radiotherapy and chemotherapy, were applicable and intended to see whether or not the effectiveness of cancer therapies delivered under hyperbaric oxygen differs from those under normal air. In general, the findings are positive for these few published trials, with reports of improved survival and local disease control rate and reduced need for surgery. The findings for one trial are not provided (Denham et al. 1987).

4.3 Systematic Review

A systematic review (Sultan et al. 2017) is available that investigated the effect of HBOT on ORN prevention and treatment. This review considered only qualified studies eligible and accordingly included three studies in the prevention setting and four studies in the management setting (Marx et al. 1985; Vudiniabola et al. 1999; Maier et al. 2000; David et al. 2001; Sulaiman et al. 2003; Annane et al. 2004; D'Souza et al. 2014). ORN occurrence in the prevention setting was up to 5% with HBOT and between 2% and 30% with the control intervention or antibiotics therapy. In the management setting, HBOT was comparable to surgery or placebo; however, one trial showed a reduction in complete healing with HBOT compared to medical/surgical treatment (14% vs. 20–28%). The multidisciplinary review team was against recommending HBOT for all patients, while the consideration of individual cases, including those who do not respond to medical/surgical therapies or those high-risk patients who cannot undergo such therapies, might be well.

5 Esophagus Cancer

A clinical trial investigated whether or not HBOT increases the efficacy of 125I particle-integrated esophageal covered stent (Zhang et al. 2021). There were two groups of patients: one received a 125I particle-integrated esophageal covered stent without HBOT, and the other received 125I particle-integrated esophageal covered stent plus HBOT. The latter group exhibited a significantly better efficacy soon after the treatment started and maintained it over the long term, with an estimated total efficacy rate of 80.7% vs. 63.1%.

6 Gastric Cancer

6.1 Case Series

In the breast cancer section, a case with metastatic breast cancer was reported who had undergone a combined therapeutic and supportive protocol, comprising a ketogenic diet, hyperthermia, HBOT, and chemotherapy. The same author did a similar job for patients with gastric adenocarcinoma ($n = 24$), stage III-IV; all of them, except for two, responded to the therapy protocol without presenting any serious adverse events (Iyikesici 2020a, b). Patients were followed for an average of 2 years, during which overall survival and progression-free survival were close to each other, and about 3 years for all evaluable patients.

6.2 In Vitro

In vitro studies investigated the effect of HBOT alone or combined with melatonin on the same gastric cancer cell line, SGC7901 (Qi et al. 2017; Wei et al. 2018). When combined with melatonin, HBOT appeared to contribute to melatonin-induced tumor-suppressing effects by increasing the cell sensitivity to respond to melatonin and inducing the expression or activation of apoptosis-promoting molecules, such as p53, caspase 3, and LC3. By contrast, when introduced alone, HBOT caused cell proliferation.

7 Pancreatic Cancer

Like metastatic breast cancer and gastric cancer, 25 patients received combined therapy with the ketogenic diet, hyperthermia, HBOT, and chemotherapy (Iyikesici 2020a, b). The average follow-up was about 2 years, with an average overall survival and progression-free survival of about 16 and 13 months.

8 Colorectal Cancer

8.1 Case Report

A patient with rectal cancer was presented with a rectal wound along with superficial mesorectal necrosis following radiotherapy and total mesorectal excision (TME) (Araujo et al. 2011). HBOT could resolve the wound completely.

8.2 In Vivo

In vivo studies of colorectal cancer in CBA mice (Daruwalla and Christophi 2006; Daruwalla et al. 2007) show findings similar to that reported by in vitro studies of gastric cancer cell lines. Accordingly, HBOT alone had no significant effect on liver metastases, apoptosis, and microvasculature; however, there was a transient effect observed on day 13 with regard to a reduction in necrosis and proliferation in the tumor area, which was no longer evident on day 25. When combined with SMA-pirarubicin, HBOT appeared to increase the tumor area-reducing effect of SMA-prirarubicin.

9 Pelvic Cancer

Patients with pelvic cancer commonly develop late radiation tissue injury (LRTI), which will cause pain, affect life quality, and interfere with daily functioning. In a simple pre-post study (Velure et al. 2022), HBOT could boost life quality while alleviating pain, bowel and bladder symptoms, sleep problems, and fatigue. Of note, patients exhibited this significant effect immediately after receiving HBOT and continued to benefit in the long term, i.e., 6 months after completing HBOT.

A case (76 years) with vaginal recurrence of cervical cancer developed necrosis of the external urethral orifice 21 months after receiving high-dose radiation therapy (Arakaki et al. 2021). Two cycles of HBOT could remove necrosis and contribute to normal mucosa formation.

10 Lung Cancer

10.1 In Vivo

In vivo, HBOT showed a growth-suppressing effect on tumor cells (A549 model for non-small cell lung cancer, NSCLC) in the severe combined immunodeficiency (SCID) mice (Chen et al. 2021). The suppression appeared to be increased with time and accompanied by different molecular events, including the decreased level of p53 and increased level of caspase 3, along with the observation of apoptotic cells. In another study using the same NSCLC cell line and the introduction of cobalt chloride to model hypoxia (Wang et al. 2018), HBOT showed that HBOT might be protective against hypoxia by interfering with LDH-induced cell migration and invasion.

10.2 Cohort/Pilot

Under the combined protocol of ketogenic diet, hyperthermia, HBOT, and chemotherapy, about 61% of patients with metastatic NSCLC ($n = 44$) could achieve an objective response rate; about 16% remained unchanged; about 23% progressed to severe condition (Iyikesici 2019). Overall, patients, on average, survived for about 3.5 years.

In post-lung resection settings, a short-term course of HBOT (median: seven sessions) could help patients rescue from ischemic bronchitis (Endoh et al. 2018). Also, patients who underwent HBOT in pre-operative and post-operative periods showed a reduction in hypoxia-related lipid peroxidation products, implying the protective effect of HBOT against hypoxia (Nikolaeva et al. 1991). Patients who received combined treatment with HBOT and chemotherapy responded to therapy more than those treated with chemotherapy alone (64% vs. 44%) (Ohguri et al. 2009). When used with photodynamic therapy, HBOT improved both patient-reported and objective outcomes, including dyspnea, hemoptysis, and Karnofsky's[4] performance status (Tomaselli et al. 2001).

[4] It is a scale used for assessing the performance of patients with cancer.

11 Conclusion

In the present chapter, given that the results of most clinical trials are unavailable, we searched for all eligible studies published in PubMed. Overall, the relevant studies were mostly small-scale pilot projects or cohort studies, case series, case reports, and to a very lesser extent, randomized clinical trials. In patients with breast cancer, HBOT was mainly applied for treating lymphedema following radiation therapy. Pilot projects and case series mostly reported the favorable effects of HBOT on lymphedema, while the only available randomized trial showed no significant difference between HBOT and standard of care. Brain necrosis and metastatic breast cancer were the other breast cancer-related conditions, and for their treatment, HBOT was considered and led to their recovery in case reports. In patients with prostate cancer, cystitis and proctitis were the main post-radiation conditions considered for HBOT in cohort studies and case series, where HBOT was advantageous to at least a substantial proportion of all patients. The two studies of individual cases reported their experience successfully utilizing HBOT to manage abscess, rectal perforation, and an anorectal junction-located ulcer. A few in vivo studies on prostate cancer cell lines-injected SCID mice ruled out the role of HBOT in tumor progression, which was previously thought, and added that HBOT might sensitize cells, enhancing chemotherapy effectiveness and also cause G2/M phase arrest, contributing to tumor suppression. The major complication following radiation in the context of head and neck cancer is ORN. Cohort and pilot studies favor HBOT in the healing of ORN and improvement in related complications, mainly dry mouth, pain, and salivary gland hypofunction. Also, a randomized study supported these complications' improvement. Post-operative HBOT failed to change the clinical endpoint of recurrence rate and cancer-related death in a retrospective study. Also, a randomized trial found HBOT comparable to antibiotics in maintaining the implants. Before the 2000s, trials used hyperbaric oxygen as a vehicle for chemotherapy/radiotherapy delivery, and all of them published its positive effect in improving survival and disease control. In addition to these cohort and pilot studies and randomized trials, there have been published better-deigned studies, which were reviewed by a multidisciplinary team in 2016, leading to a recommendation against HBOT as a routine intervention for all patients and instead its consideration only in individual cases and conditions. The number of studies available on other cancer types, including gastric cancer, esophagus cancer, colorectal cancer, pancreatic cancer, and NSCLC, was small, calling the need for research throughout the hierarchy of evidence.

The findings reviewed in the present chapter point out HBOT as an effective adjuvant in cancer therapy, with small side effects. Despite this, the most studies available are case reports and observational studies, including case-control and cohort studies, with very few prospectively designed interventional studies. Table 1 provides a list of interventional studies registered with ClinicalTrials.gov. As of October 04, 2022, 29 interventional studies (excluding withdrawn trials) exist. Figures 1 and 2 show the distribution of these few available trials by cancer type, status, sample size, location, and phase. It is, therefore, to consider that:

Table 1 Interventional studies investigating the efficacy of hyperbaric oxygen therapy in patients with cancer registered with clinicaltrials.gov (Date of access: October 04, 2022)

NCT number	Status	Study results	Cancer	Country	Phases	Enrollment
NCT01850563	Completed	Available	CNS cancer	USA	NA	22
NCT01449539	Terminated	Available	Hematologic malignancies	USA	NA	8
NCT02099266	Completed	Available	Hematologic malignancies	USA	NA	15
NCT03916068	Active, not recruiting	NA	Breast cancer	USA	Phase 2	60
NCT04193722	Recruiting	NA	Breast cancer	Netherlands	Phase 3	120
NCT01808625	Terminated	NA	CNS cancer	Israel	NA	2
NCT00077090	Unknown status	NA	Breast cancer	UK	Phase 2	63
NCT00026975	Completed	NA	Head and neck cancer	USA	Phase 2	150
NCT00906269	Unknown status	NA	Urological cancer	USA	Phase 4	100
NCT02575014	Enrolling by invitation	NA	Gastrointestinal cancer	USA	NA	50
NCT01087268	Unknown status	NA	Pelvic cancer	UK	Phase 3	75
NCT01822405	Unknown status	NA	Gastrointestinal cancer	Spain	Phase 2	42
NCT02895724	Unknown status	NA	Breast cancer	Denmark	Phase 2	20
NCT00087815	Unknown status	NA	CNS cancer	USA	NA	30
NCT00006460	Unknown status	NA	CNS cancer	USA	Phase 1 | Phase 2	5-to-10
NCT00474825	Completed	NA	Head and neck cancer	USA	Phase 1	12
NCT03843671	Not yet recruiting	NA	Head and neck cancer	USA	Phase 2	400
NCT05189496	Recruiting	NA	Cancer	China	NA	380
NCT03398200	Active, not recruiting	NA	Hematologic malignancies	USA	Phase 2	99
NCT04862676	Recruiting	NA	Hematologic malignancies	USA	Early Phase 1	15
NCT03964506	Recruiting	NA	Hematologic malignancies	USA	Early Phase 1	24
NCT03144206	Recruiting	NA	Soft tissue cancers	USA	Phase 4	20
NCT05031949	Recruiting	NA	Gastrointestinal cancer	China	Phase 1	20

NCT02087657	Unknown status	NA	Hematologic malignancies	USA	NA	20
NCT00936052	Unknown status	NA	CNS cancer	USA	Phase 2	20
NCT03411408	Unknown status	NA	CNS cancer	Italy	NA	24
NCT02084927	Unknown status	NA	CNS cancer	Israel	Phase 1	62
NCT02122042	Unknown status	NA	CNS cancer	Israel	Phase 1	62
NCT03739502	Recruiting	NA	Hematologic malignancies	USA	Phase 2	64

NA, not available (for the Study results column) and NA (for the Phases column)

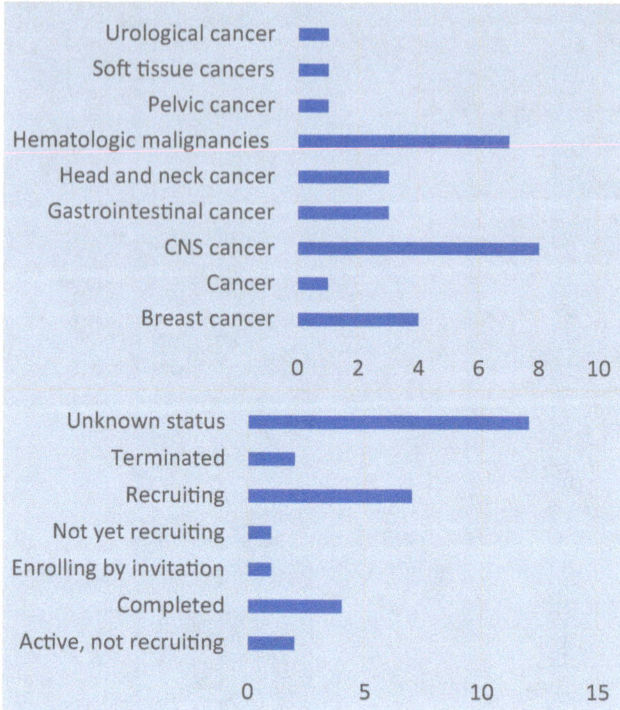

Fig. 1 Interventional studies investigating the efficacy of hyperbaric oxygen therapy in patients with cancer registered with clinicaltrials.gov by cancer type and status

(1) hematologic malignancies and CNS tumors, either primary or secondary (metastatic), are the most-investigated cancer types, followed by breast cancer; (2) USA-related centers are the top-active ones, with being the provider of more than 60 studies, followed by European centers; (3) studies are mostly of phase 1 and 2, with only four studies of phase 3 or 4; (4) studies' sample sizes are small, with only three studies including greater than 100 subjects; and (5) it is possible to understand that the cancer type-based distribution of registered clinical trials, of which only four are completed, is very different from that of the current literature. In our review, head and neck cancers are the most common cancers for which HBOT has been applied to date, followed by breast and prostate cancer. When the ongoing trials' findings become published, we might be able to decide when, who, and how of HBOT in cancer. In the future, larger, high-quality clinical trials are required to assess the effectiveness of HBOT in different settings worldwide.

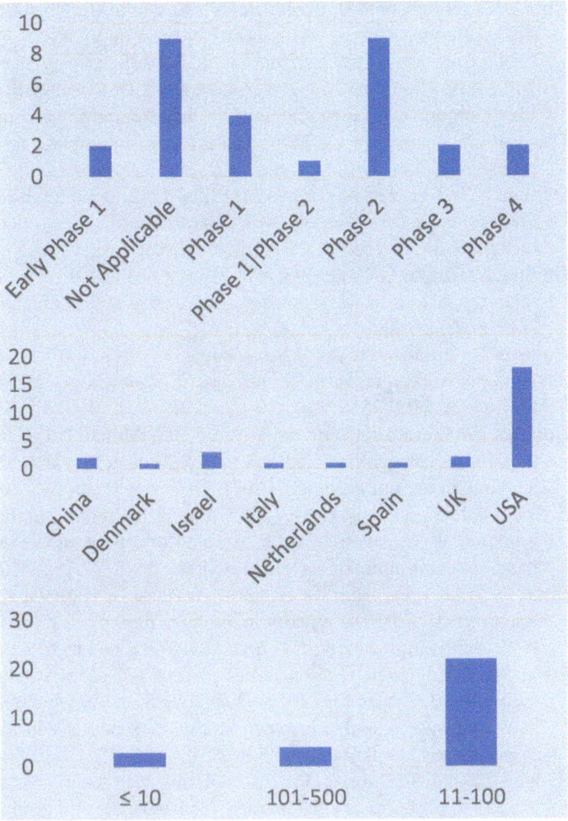

Fig. 2 Interventional studies investigating the efficacy of hyperbaric oxygen therapy in patients with cancer registered with clinicaltrials.gov by phase, location, and sample size

References

Annane D, Depondt J, Aubert P, Villart M, Géhanno P, Gajdos P, Chevret S (2004) Hyperbaric oxygen therapy for radionecrosis of the jaw: a randomized, placebo-controlled, double-blind trial from the ORN96 study group. J Clin Oncol 22:4893–4900

Arakaki Y, Shimoji Y, Nakasone T, Taira Y, Nakamoto T, Kudaka W, Mekaru K, Aoki Y (2021) Hyperbaric oxygen therapy for suburethral vaginal mucosal necrosis after interstitial irradiation for recurrent cervical cancer. Case Rep Obstet Gynecol 2021:1737975

Araujo SE, Bammann RH, Seid VE, Nahas SC, Nahas CS, Cecconello I (2011) Neoadjuvant chemoradiation therapy followed by curative transanal endoscopic microsurgery (TEM) for rectal cancer complicated by major suture dehiscence: avoiding ileostomy through hyperbaric oxygen therapy. Int J Color Dis 26:1359–1361

Batenburg MCT, Maarse W, van der Leij F, Baas IO, Boonstra O, Lansdorp N, Doeksen A, van den Bongard D, Verkooijen HM (2021) The impact of hyperbaric oxygen therapy on late radiation toxicity and quality of life in breast cancer patients. Breast Cancer Res Treat 189:425–433

Chen SY, Tsuneyama K, Yen MH, Lee JT, Chen JL, Huang SM (2021) Hyperbaric oxygen suppressed tumor progression through the improvement of tumor hypoxia and induction of tumor apoptosis in A549-cell-transferred lung cancer. Sci Rep 11:12033

Chong KT, Hampson NB, Bostwick DG, Vessella RL, Corman JM (2004) Hyperbaric oxygen does not accelerate latent in vivo prostate cancer: implications for the treatment of radiation-induced haemorrhagic cystitis. BJU Int 94:1275–1278
Dall'Era MA, Hampson NB, Hsi RA, Madsen B, Corman JM (2006) Hyperbaric oxygen therapy for radiation induced proctopathy in men treated for prostate cancer. J Urol 176:87–90
Daruwalla J, Christophi C (2006) The effect of hyperbaric oxygen therapy on tumour growth in a mouse model of colorectal cancer liver metastases. Eur J Cancer 42:3304–3311
Daruwalla J, Greish K, Nikfarjam M, Millar I, Malcontenti-Wilson C, Iyer AK, Christophi C (2007) Evaluation of the effect of SMA-pirarubicin micelles on colorectal cancer liver metastases and of hyperbaric oxygen in CBA mice. J Drug Target 15:487–495
David LA, Sàndor GKB, Evans AW, Brown DH (2001) Hyperbaric oxygen therapy and mandibular osteoradionecrosis: a retrospective study and analysis of treatment outcomes. J Can Dent Assoc 67:384–385
Degener S, Strelow H, Pohle A, Lazica DA, Windolf J, Zumbé J, Roth S, Brandt AS (2012) Hyperbaric oxygen in the treatment of hemorrhagic radiogenic cystitis after prostate cancer. Urologe A 51:1735–1740
Denham JW, Yeoh EK, Wittwer G, Ward GG, Ahmad AS, Harvey ND (1987) Radiation therapy in hyperbaric oxygen for head and neck cancer at Royal Adelaide Hospital – 1964 to 1980. Int J Radiat Oncol Biol Phys 13:201–208
D'Souza J, Lowe D, Rogers SN (2014) Changing trends and the role of medical management on the outcome of patients treated for osteoradionecrosis of the mandible: experience from a regional head and neck unit. Br J Oral Maxillofac Surg 52:356–362
Endoh M, Oizumi H, Kato H, Suzuki J, Watarai H, Hamada A, Suzuki K, Nakahashi K, Shiono S, Sadahiro M (2018) Hyperbaric oxygen therapy for postoperative ischemic bronchitis after resection of lung cancer. J Thorac Dis 10:6176–6183
Forner L, Hyldegaard O, von Brockdorff AS, Specht L, Andersen E, Jansen EC, Hillerup S, Nauntofte B, Jensen SB (2011) Does hyperbaric oxygen treatment have the potential to increase salivary flow rate and reduce xerostomia in previously irradiated head and neck cancer patients? A pilot study. Oral Oncol 47:546–551
Fuentes-Raspall R, Inoriza JM, Martí-Utzet MJ, Auñón-Sanz C, Garcia-Martin P, Oliu-Isern G (2012) Hyperbaric oxygen therapy for late rectal and bladder toxicity after radiation in prostate cancer patients. A symptom control and quality-of-life study. Clin Oncol (R Coll Radiol) 24: e126
Gerlach NL, Barkhuysen R, Kaanders JH, Janssens GO, Sterk W, Merkx MA (2008) The effect of hyperbaric oxygen therapy on quality of life in oral and oropharyngeal cancer patients treated with radiotherapy. Int J Oral Maxillofac Surg 37:255–259
Gothard L, Stanton A, MacLaren J, Lawrence D, Hall E, Mortimer P, Parkin E, Pritchard J, Risdall J, Sawyer R, Woods M, Yarnold J (2004) Non-randomised phase II trial of hyperbaric oxygen therapy in patients with chronic arm lymphoedema and tissue fibrosis after radiotherapy for early breast cancer. Radiother Oncol 70:217–224
Gothard L, Haviland J, Bryson P, Laden G, Glover M, Harrison S, Woods M, Cook G, Peckitt C, Pearson A, Somaiah N, Stanton A, Mortimer P, Yarnold J (2010) Randomised phase II trial of hyperbaric oxygen therapy in patients with chronic arm lymphoedema after radiotherapy for cancer. Radiother Oncol 97:101–107
Gupta P, Sahni T, Jadhav GK, Manocha S, Aggarwal S, Verma S (2013) A retrospective study of outcomes in subjects of head and neck cancer treated with hyperbaric oxygen therapy for radiation induced osteoradionecrosis of mandible at a tertiary care Centre: an Indian experience. Indian J Otolaryngol Head Neck Surg 65:140–143
Henk JM (1986) Late results of a trial of hyperbaric oxygen and radiotherapy in head and neck cancer: a rationale for hypoxic cell sensitizers? Int J Radiat Oncol Biol Phys 12:1339–1341
Henk JM, Smith CW (1977) Radiotherapy and hyperbaric oxygen in head and neck cancer. Interim report of second clinical trial. Lancet 2:104–105

Henk JM, Kunkler PB, Smith CW (1977) Radiotherapy and hyperbaric oxygen in head and neck cancer. Final report of first controlled clinical trial. Lancet 2:101–103

Heys SD, Smith IC, Ross JA, Gilbert FJ, Brooks J, Semple S, Miller ID, Hutcheon A, Sarkar T, Eremin O (2006) A pilot study with long term follow up of hyperbaric oxygen pretreatment in patients with locally advanced breast cancer undergoing neo-adjuvant chemotherapy. Undersea Hyperb Med 33:33–43

Iyikesici MS (2019) Feasibility study of metabolically supported chemotherapy with weekly carboplatin/paclitaxel combined with ketogenic diet, hyperthermia and hyperbaric oxygen therapy in metastatic non-small cell lung cancer. Int J Hyperth 36:446–455

Iyikesici MS (2020a) Long-term survival outcomes of metabolically supported chemotherapy with gemcitabine-based or FOLFIRINOX regimen combined with ketogenic diet, hyperthermia, and hyperbaric oxygen therapy in metastatic pancreatic cancer. Complement Med Res 27:31–39

Iyikesici MS (2020b) Survival outcomes of metabolically supported chemotherapy combined with ketogenic diet, hyperthermia, and hyperbaric oxygen therapy in advanced gastric cancer. Niger J Clin Pract 23:734–740

İyikesici MS, Slocum AK, Slocum A, Berkarda FB, Kalamian M, Seyfried TN (2017) Efficacy of metabolically supported chemotherapy combined with ketogenic diet, hyperthermia, and hyperbaric oxygen therapy for stage IV triple-negative breast cancer. Cureus 9:e1445

Kalns JE, Piepmeier EH (1999) Exposure to hyperbaric oxygen induces cell cycle perturbation in prostate cancer cells. In Vitro Cell Dev Biol Anim 35:98–101

Kalns J, Krock L, Piepmeier E Jr (1998) The effect of hyperbaric oxygen on growth and chemosensitivity of metastatic prostate cancer. Anticancer Res 18:363–367

Kashihara T, Inaba K, Komiyama M, Nakayama H, Iijima K, Nishioka S, Okamoto H, Kikkawa N, Kubo Y, Shima S, Nakamura S, Takahashi A, Takahashi K, Okuma K, Murakami N, Igaki H, Nakayama Y, Fukunaga A, Matsui Y, Fujimoto H, Itami J (2020) The use of hyperbaric oxygen to treat actinic rectal fistula after SpaceOAR use and radiotherapy for prostate cancer: a case report. BMC Urol 20:196

Kitta T, Shinohara N, Shirato H, Otsuka H, Koyanagi T (2000) The treatment of chronic radiation proctitis with hyperbaric oxygen in patients with prostate cancer. BJU Int 85:372–374

Koo JH, Song SH, Oh HS, Oh SH (2020) Comparison of the short-term effects of hyperbaric oxygen therapy and complex decongestive therapy on breast cancer-related lymphedema: a pilot study. Medicine (Baltimore) 99:e19564

Maier A, Gaggl A, Klemen H, Santler G, Anegg U, Fell B, Kärcher H, Smolle-Jüttner FM, Friehs GB (2000) Review of severe osteoradionecrosis treated by surgery alone or surgery with postoperative hyperbaric oxygenation. Br J Oral Maxillofac Surg 38:173–176

Marx RE, Johnson RP, Kline SN (1985) Prevention of osteoradionecrosis: a randomized prospective clinical trial of hyperbaric oxygen versus penicillin. J Am Dent Assoc 111:49–54

Mayer R, Klemen H, Quehenberger F, Sankin O, Mayer E, Hackl A, Smolle-Juettner FM (2001) Hyperbaric oxygen – an effective tool to treat radiation morbidity in prostate cancer. Radiother Oncol 61:151–156

Nakabayashi M, Beard C, Kelly SM, Carr-Locke DL, Oh WK (2006) Treatment of a radiation-induced rectal ulcer with hyperbaric oxygen therapy in a man with prostate cancer. Urol Oncol 24:503–508

Nakada T, Nakada H, Yoshida Y, Nakashima Y, Banya Y, Fujihira T, Karasawa K (2012) Hyperbaric oxygen therapy for radiation cystitis in patients with prostate cancer: a long-term follow-up study. Urol Int 89:208–214

Nikolaeva EE, Stepanenko EM, Chubukhchiev GB (1991) The effect of hyperbaric oxygenation on the indices of lipid peroxidation in the blood of patients with lung cancer. Anesteziol Reanimatol:67–68

Ohguri T, Imada H, Narisada H, Yahara K, Morioka T, Nakano K, Miyaguni Y, Korogi Y (2009) Systemic chemotherapy using paclitaxel and carboplatin plus regional hyperthermia and hyperbaric oxygen treatment for non-small cell lung cancer with multiple pulmonary metastases: preliminary results. Int J Hyperth 25:160–167

Qi Y, Ruan J, Wang M, Dai Y, Zhou Q, Gui S, Zhang S, Wang Y (2017) Effects of hyperbaric oxygen treatment on gastric cancer cell line SGC7901. Biomed Rep 6:475–479

Schoen PJ, Raghoebar GM, Bouma J, Reintsema H, Vissink A, Sterk W, Roodenburg JL (2007) Rehabilitation of oral function in head and neck cancer patients after radiotherapy with implant-retained dentures: effects of hyperbaric oxygen therapy. Oral Oncol 43:379–388

Sealy R, Cridland S (1984) The treatment of locally advanced head and neck cancer with misonidazole, hyperbaric oxygen and irradiation: an interim report. Int J Radiat Oncol Biol Phys 10:1721–1723

Sealy R, Helman P, Greenstein A, Shepstone B (1974) The treatment of locally advanced cancer of the head and neck with intra-arterial cytotoxics, cobalt, and hyperbaric oxygen therapy. Cancer 34:497–500

Sealy R, Cridland S, Barry L, Norris R (1986) Irradiation with misonidazole and hyperbaric oxygen: final report on a randomized trial in advanced head and neck cancer. Int J Radiat Oncol Biol Phys 12:1343–1346

Slotman GJ, Matthews M, Fahey L, Thom S, Clark J, Hardy K (2011) Operative Nd:YAG laser plus postoperative hyperbaric oxygen reduces surgical morbidity after radical head and neck cancer surgery and complex reconstruction. Undersea Hyperb Med 38:159–165

Spruijt NE, van den Berg R (2020) The effect of hyperbaric oxygen treatment on late radiation tissue injury after breast cancer: a case-series of 67 patients. Diving Hyperb Med 50:206–213

Sulaiman F, Huryn JM, Zlotolow IM (2003) Dental extractions in the irradiated head and neck patient: a retrospective analysis of Memorial Sloan-Kettering Cancer Center protocols, criteria, and end results. J Oral Maxillofac Surg 61:1123–1131

Sultan A, Hanna GJ, Margalit DN, Chau N, Goguen LA, Marty FM, Rabinowits G, Schoenfeld JD, Sonis ST, Thomas T, Tishler RB, Treister NS, Villa A, Woo SB, Haddad R, Mawardi H (2017) The use of hyperbaric oxygen for the prevention and management of osteoradionecrosis of the jaw: a Dana-Farber/Brigham and Women's Cancer Center multidisciplinary guideline. Oncologist 22:343–350

Tang H, Sun Y, Xu C, Zhou T, Gao X, Wang L (2009a) Effects of hyperbaric oxygen therapy on tumor growth in murine model of PC-3 prostate cancer cell line. Urology 73:205–208

Tang H, Zhang ZY, Ge JP, Zhou WQ, Gao JP (2009b) Effects of hyperbaric oxygen on tumor growth in the mouse model of LNCaP prostate cancer cell line. Zhonghua Nan Ke Xue 15:713–716

Teas J, Cunningham JE, Cone L, Jansen K, Raghavan SK, Nitcheva DK, Xie D, Butler WM (2004) Can hyperbaric oxygen therapy reduce breast cancer treatment-related lymphedema? A pilot study. J Women Heal (Larchmt) 13:1008–1018

Teguh DN, Levendag PC, Noever I, Voet P, van der Est H, van Rooij P, Dumans AG, de Boer MF, van der Huls MP, Sterk W, Schmitz PI (2009) Early hyperbaric oxygen therapy for reducing radiotherapy side effects: early results of a randomized trial in oropharyngeal and nasopharyngeal cancer. Int J Radiat Oncol Biol Phys 75:711–716

Teguh DN, Bol Raap R, Struikmans H, Verhoef C, Koppert LB, Koole A, Huang Y, van Hulst RA (2016) Hyperbaric oxygen therapy for late radiation-induced tissue toxicity: prospectively patient-reported outcome measures in breast cancer patients. Radiat Oncol 11:130

Tomaselli F, Maier A, Sankin O, Anegg U, Stranzl U, Pinter H, Kapp K, Smolle-Jüttner FM (2001) Acute effects of combined photodynamic therapy and hyperbaric oxygenation in lung cancer--a clinical pilot study. Lasers Surg Med 28:399–403

Velure GK, Müller B, Hauken MA (2022) Symptom burden and health-related quality of life six months after hyperbaric oxygen therapy in cancer survivors with pelvic radiation injuries. Support Care Cancer 30:5703–5711

Vudiniabola S, Pirone C, Williamson J, Goss AN (1999) Hyperbaric oxygen in the prevention of osteoradionecrosis of the jaws. Aust Dent J 44:243–247

Wang Y, Qi Y, Wei X, Chen S, Jia N, Zhou Q, Zhang S, Gui S, Wang Y (2018) Hyperbaric oxygen rescues lung cancer cells from chemical hypoxia-induced low differentiation and apoptosis resistance. Exp Lung Res 44:417–423

Wei X, Qi Y, Jia N, Zhou Q, Zhang S, Wang Y (2018) Hyperbaric oxygen treatment sensitizes gastric cancer cells to melatonin-induced apoptosis through multiple pathways. J Cell Biochem 119:6723–6731

Xing S, Fan Z, Shi L, Yang Z, Bai Y (2019) Successful treatment of brain radiation necrosis resulting from triple-negative breast cancer with Endostar and short-term hyperbaric oxygen therapy: a case report. Onco Targets Ther 12:2729–2735

Zhang QZ, Li GL, Shang JB, Ren YM, Xie JL (2021) Clinical study of a 125I particle-integrated esophageal covered stent and hyperbaric oxygen in the treatment of advanced esophageal cancer. Rev Esp Enferm Dig 113:576–579

Interventional Oncology Techniques: A Primer for Non-users

Dimitrios K. Filippiadis, Evgenia Efthymiou, Athanasios Gianakis, George Charalampopoulos, and Stavros Spiliopoulos

Abstract

Interventional oncology, along with surgical, medical and radiation oncology, constitutes the four pillars of cancer management. Interventional oncology therapies are image-guided, minimally invasive percutaneous or trans-arterial techniques aiming to provide diagnostic or therapeutic (both curative and palliative) solutions in a plethora of malignant pathologies. Amongst others, these techniques include, but are not limited to, biopsy, ablation, trans-arterial embolization and chemo- or radioembolisation, whilst techniques such as neurolysis and biliary and fluid drainage provide palliative treatment and comfort in cancer patients. The purpose of the current chapter is to focus on the current role of interventional oncology procedures for curative or palliative treatment of a wide variety of cancer pathologies.

Keywords

Ablation · Biopsy · Bone augmentation · Cancer · Embolization

1 Introduction

Modern management of cancer includes a personalized approach combining techniques and therapies from surgical, medical, radiation and interventional oncology. Multidisciplinary meetings as well interdisciplinary discussions play a key role in the management of cancer patients. Interventional oncology techniques include a wide variety of percutaneous and trans-arterial procedures, which are performed

D. K. Filippiadis (✉) · E. Efthymiou · A. Gianakis · G. Charalampopoulos · S. Spiliopoulos
2nd Department of Radiology, University General Hospital "ATTIKON", Medical School, National and Kapodistrian University of Athens, Athens, Greece
e-mail: stavspiliop@med.uoa.gr

Interdisciplinary Cancer Research, https://doi.org/10.1007/16833_2023_175
Published online: 29 July 2023

under image guidance. Characteristic features of these techniques include the minimally invasive character, rendering them tolerable even in co-morbid patients, which is combined with high efficacy and safety as well as morbidity and mortality rates. Percutaneous biopsy contributes to diagnosis and evaluation of molecular and other characteristics governing a neoplastic disease, whilst therapeutic techniques performed either for curative or palliative goals include, but are not limited to, ablation, trans-arterial embolization, chemo- or radioembolisation, neurolysis and biliary and fluid drainage. The purpose of the current chapter is to focus on the current role of interventional oncology procedures for curative or palliative treatment of a wide variety of cancer pathologies.

1.1 Biopsy

The importance of image-guided biopsy in establishing the diagnosis of malignancy, identifying tumour histology and staging the disease is very well recognised (Trumm et al. 2013; O'Shea et al. 2021; Tam et al. 2016). However, the role of image-guided biopsy evolved with the rise of precision medicine and personalisation of cancer care. Nowadays, biopsies provide cellular, molecular and genetic information of tumour tissue, which may play a vital role in determining standard-of-care therapy options, predicting prognosis and enrolment into clinical trials (Trumm et al. 2013; O'Shea et al. 2021; Tam et al. 2016). Furthermore, biopsies performed after the initial diagnosis can detect progression and guide next-line therapy.

Ultrasound (US) and computed tomography (CT) represent the two most frequently used techniques for image-guided biopsies (Trumm et al. 2013; Kim et al. 2017; Copelan et al. 2016). Magnetic resonance (MR) imaging, which was introduced later than US and CT as guidance method for biopsy, is not regarded as a "first line" option and is reserved for cases where the lesions are not clearly visible using the other two imaging techniques. Fluoroscopy with or without cone beam CT can be used mainly in spine or peripheral skeleton biopsies (Tomasian et al. 2020; Meek et al. 2020). The chosen imaging technique for biopsy guidance is usually the technique which can best visualise the target. Further important factors represent operator preference, scanner availability and patients' compatibility.

The two main techniques used to obtain diagnostic tissue are fine-needle aspiration biopsy (FNAB) and core needle biopsy (CNB) (Gupta et al. 2010; Veltri et al. 2017). Fine-needle biopsies are performed with 21- to 25-G needles (smaller diameter). The needle is introduced into the lesion and then moved back and forth several times to collect the samples. The samples collected are rarely suitable for histopathologic analysis. FNAB is a technique more suitable for patients having a known primary tumour. With the use of 12- to 20-G cutting needles, CNB collects cores of tissue suitable for histopathologic diagnosis. Due to better reproducibility of CNB- in comparison to FNA-results and comparable rate of complications, CNB is the technique of choice in most radiological departments with FNA having specific indications (i.e. breast and thyroid lesions). In the case of bone lesions with accessible extraosseous components, a CNB can be performed. When no obvious extraosseous component is present, the use of a drilling-type needle is mandatory. A manual bone drill or a battery-powered drill may be used.

In the case of inadequate previous imaging, new imaging should be performed to narrow the differential diagnosis, choose the most representative lesion or even obviate the need for biopsy if a lesion exhibits radiological characteristics that are, with no doubt, benign. Before planning any image-guided biopsy, the radiologist should check for any conditions that could make the intervention unsafe. Although there are no absolute contraindications for image-guided biopsy, there are relative contraindications which should be carefully evaluated before the start of the intervention. Relative contraindications include (i) coagulopathy that cannot be adequately corrected and might increase the risk of bleeding (especially in deeper located organs, where direct pressure for haemostasis cannot be applied), (ii) hemodynamic instable patients, (iii) lack of a safe pathway from the skin to the target lesion, (iv) uncooperative patient, and (v) pregnancy in case of imaging modalities using ionizing radiation. Most image-guided biopsies can be performed on an outpatient basis under local anaesthesia. However, as mentioned before, the inability of a patient to cooperate represent a contraindication for biopsy. In those cases, conscious sedation or general anaesthesia may be necessary.

The complications of image-guided interventions are divided into two types: generic and organ-specific (Gupta et al. 2010; Veltri et al. 2017; Kennedy et al. 2015). Generic refers to those complications that can affect every biopsied organ. Organ-specific refers to those complications which are associated most with a specific organ. To the generic complications belong haemorrhage, infection, perforation and injury of an adjacent organ. Concerning haemorrhage after image-guided biopsy, it seems important to note the difference between minor and major bleeding. A small, non-enlarging haematoma that is not clinically relevant and does not require further medical attention is something that every interventional radiologist faces once and again. On the other hand, major haemorrhage is defined as bleeding requiring blood transfusion or further intervention. The incidence of major haemorrhage is low and dependent on the vascularity of the biopsied organ, as well as the size of the used needle and ranges from 0.1% to 8.3% in the reported literature. Organ-specific complications are those associated with biopsy of a specific organ. Examples of organ-specific complications are pneumothorax after lung biopsy or accidental puncture of the lung, haematuria after renal or prostate biopsy and haemoptysis after lung biopsy. Although not necessarily rare, these organ-specific complications rarely require therapy.

In the case of an uneventful image-guided biopsy, vital signs of the patients are checked for 1 hour after the intervention of for up to 3 hours in case of high-risk patients. The small puncture wound must be checked for bleeding or swelling, and bathing must be avoided for the first 24 hours. Image-guided biopsy is not only served for the initial diagnosis of cancer but can also aid in staging, therapy planning and detection of tumour recurrence (Fig. 1).

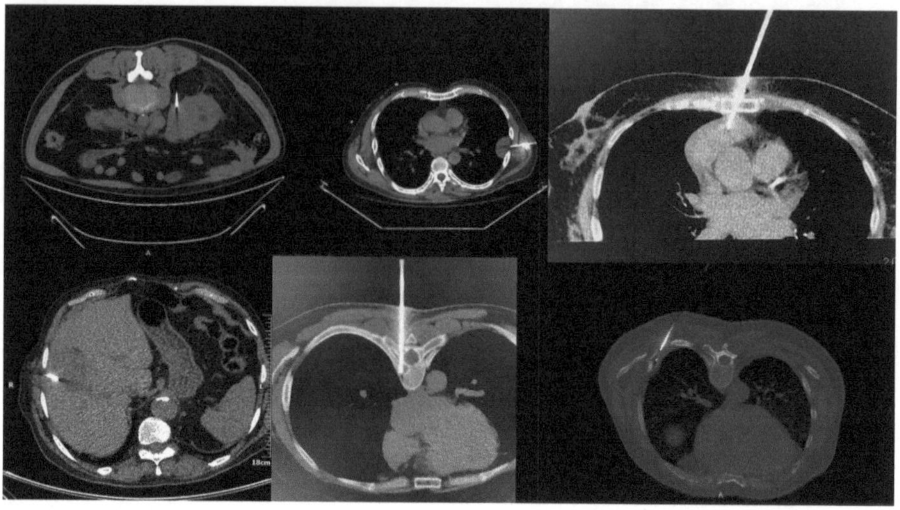

Fig. 1 Computed tomography is the most commonly used image modality used for guidance in percutaneous biopsy. Different examples of percutaneous core biopsies are illustrated, including biopsy cases in renal, pulmonary, mediastinal, liver, spine and thopracic rib tumours

1.2 Ablation

Imaging-guided tumour ablation includes the application of non-energy or energy-based (i.e. thermal and non-thermal) therapies under imaging guidance to treat neoplastic tissue. Ablation therapy belongs to minimally invasive treatments, further categorised according to the type of tissue injury to chemical (e.g. Ethanol) and energy-based ablation (Ahmed et al. 2011).

1.2.1 Chemical Ablation

Chemical ablation includes the usage of a chemical agent such as absolute ethanol causing cellular dehydration, vascular thrombosis and ischemia. Ethanol is the commonest substance used, either as a standalone procedure or in combination with other techniques like TACE and/or radiofrequency ablation. Chemical ablation has been mostly studied in HCC and RCC (Filippiadis et al. 2019a, b; Clark and Soulen 2002). Access is gained to the tumour through a percutaneously placed needle. Iodinated contrast and lidocaine may be injected to demonstrate the extent of diffusion and provide analgesia, respectively. Nowadays, newer thermal ablation techniques have been developed that have replaced chemical ablation, limiting its role in interventional oncology. Chemical ablation is used in cases in which thermal ablation is contraindicated and in lesions sized <3 cm (Saldanha et al. 2010). One major drawback of the method is the unpredictable diffusivity of the agent through the tumour and peritumoural tissues (Saldanha et al. 2010; Filippiadis et al. 2014). Major complications include portal venous thrombosis, hemoperitoneum, haemolysis, peritoneal seeding, liver failure and transient renal insufficiency (Saldanha et al. 2010).

1.2.2 Thermal Ablation

Thermal ablation techniques aim to eliminate neoplastic cells by applying extreme temperatures sufficiently to induce irreversible cellular injury.

Radiofrequency ablation (RF) utilizes a generator to create alternating current, typically between 200 and 1200 Hz. The alternating current agitates ions in the adjacent tissue, thus increasing the tissue temperature (temperatures of 60–100 °C) and resulting in rapid coagulative necrosis of tumour cells and tumour-free margin. Heating is more intense in the centre of the lesions, whereas peripheral areas receive heat by thermal conduction. In general, the goal of thermal ablation is to produce a zone of coagulative necrosis with a 0.5–1.0 cm tumour-free margin (Saldanha et al. 2010). Electrodes can be monopolar or bipolar, and they can have different designs (multitoned expandable, internally cooled, perfused) (Ahmed et al. 2011; Saldanha et al. 2010).

Microwave ablation (MWA) uses also electromagnetic energy functioning at 915 MHz or 2.45 GHz, resulting in frictional heat (temperatures of 60–100 °C) and subsequent protein denaturation and coagulation necrosis. Microwave ablation is less severely affected by heat-sink effect, thus proved attractive for highly vascular lesions (Kurup and Callstrom 2010). Heat sink effect is a phenomenon when the target lesion is in close proximity (within 1 cm) to a large blood vessel (≥3 mm in diameter), the blood has a cooling effect, thereby reducing the ablation zone and therefore limiting the effectiveness of the ablation (Filippiadis et al. 2019a, b; Crocetti et al. 2020). Additional advantages of microwaves include the more homogenous tissue coagulation compared to RF, the absence of ground pads and the fact that multiple antennas can be operated simultaneously (Saldanha et al. 2010).

Cryoablation (CA) utilizes cryoprobes to deliver room temperature-pressurized argon gas, which results in rapid tissue cooling of the target tissue (reaching −100 °C) within a few seconds, alternating with delivering of helium gas, which achieves active thawing (Filippiadis et al. 2014; Kurup and Callstrom 2010). Cell death derives from the sequence of freezing and thawing cycles. Although cryoablation is an expensive and long-lasting procedure compared to the other thermal techniques, it offers the advantage of low peri- and post-procedural pain and the ability to visualise the ice ball formation during the procedure (Filippiadis et al. 2014; Kurup and Callstrom 2010).

High-intensity focused ultrasound (HIFU) is a newer ablative technique in which an extracorporeal ultrasound probe with a piezoelectric transducer is placed on the patient and a focused beam of sound energy is delivered under MR guidance, resulting in temperature elevation (Kurup and Callstrom 2010). Currently, the use of HIFU is limited to small target zones (less than 1 cm) and the need of multiple repeated sessions (Saldanha et al. 2010).

Irreversible electroporation (IRE) is a relatively new, recently introduced technique, using electric field pulses, lasting hundreds of microseconds to cells. The IRE generator produces direct current (25–45 A) electric pulses of high voltage (1500–3000 V), resulting in large volumes of coagulation necrosis (Saldanha et al. 2010).

Ablation therapies have been widely applied in the treatment of malignant lesions, offering great oncological outcomes, comparable to those of surgery and radiotherapy. Nowadays, strong recommendations and international guidelines are available regarding the utility of ablation in different neoplastic tissue (Crocetti et al. 2020; Krokidis et al. 2017; Venturini et al. 2020; Ryan et al. 2022). The role of a multidisciplinary team in the management of the patient is extremely important, since in the majority of the cases, more than one specialty are involved and interdisciplinary discussions are necessary. Following the decision to proceed with ablation therapy, there are many technical parameters that should be taken under consideration.

- The most optimal ablation method should be used in terms of safety and effectiveness. In the majority of cases, there is not a definite answer, as it is a multifactorial decision, depending on the histology of the tumour, patient's characteristics and the preference of the operator.
- An ablation with necrosis of the whole tumour and safety margins of at least 5–10 mm should be the goal for local tumour control.
- Common absolute contraindications for all ablation techniques include lack of a safe access, severe immunosuppression, local or systemic infection, uncorrected coagulopathy and patient refusal to consent.
- General anaesthesia (GA) is a prerequisite for IRE.
- Recent preoperative imaging is required in all the cases.
- Major life-threatening complications are rather rare. Nevertheless, the physician should be aware and plan a step ahead. Post-ablation syndrome occurs from 24 to 48 hours following ablation. Post-ablation syndrome is characterized by low-grade fever, nausea and general weakness following ablation. It is usually self-limited and resolves usually within 1 week.
- Common nomenclature with standardised definitions for oncologic outcomes following ablation and the grading of complications has been well established (Puijk et al. 2021; Filippiadis et al. 2017a, b).

1.3 Liver

Liver lesions are one of the most frequent ablation targets in everyday practice. Ablation therapies including thermal and non-thermal ablation methods constitute attractive options for both primary and secondary liver tumours. Preoperatively, the size and location of the lesion are of great importance, as they affect the prognostic outcome. Overall, a tumoutr sized <3 cm has a good prognostic outcome and a subsequent ablation provides similar results to resection. For larger tumours >3 and <5 cm, a careful planning is needed along with the use of multiple probes. Location of the tumour could also affect the ablation result, especially in cases with close proximity to central bile ducts; in such cases, alternative techniques (e.g. IRE) could be used. For difficult locations, additional techniques, including hydro/gas dissection, could be used, or even the new upcoming robotic and stereotactic systems. For

HCC and liver metastases, ablation margins should be minimum 5–10 mm; several studies highlighted the need for larger ablation margins >10 mm to achieve acceptable oncological outcomes (Crocetti et al. 2020; Gillams et al. 2015). In cases this is not feasible, the limit of 5 mm ablation margin should be maintained (Lin et al. 2021). Specifically for intrahepatic cholangiocarcinoma, margins should be at least 10 mm. Additional general contraindications for liver tumour ablation constitute close proximity <1 cm from the main biliary duct, significant ascites and untreatable/unmanageable coagulopathy (Crocetti et al. 2018, 2020). Prophylactic antibiotic is usually recommended prior to procedure (Crocetti et al. 2020). The choice of imaging guidance used is mainly dependent on physicians' experience and preference. Major complications in liver ablation are rare (2–3%) and mainly include intraperitoneal bleeding, pneumothorax, and hemothorax (Crocetti et al. 2020). Tumour seeding is highly unlikely, especially in cases in which track ablation is performed.

Hepatocellular carcinoma (HCC) is the fifth most common malignancy in the world and the most common primary liver tumour, more often occurring in patients with underlying cirrhosis (Crocetti et al. 2020). Nowadays percutaneous ablation is integrated in the treatment of HCC, and it is strongly recommended by the latest guidelines (Crocetti et al. 2020, 2017; Galle et al. 2018). The Barcelona-Clínic Liver Cancer (BCLC) staging system was based on the results of several cohort studies and randomized controlled trials and categorized HCC to different stages taking under consideration different prognostic factors, aiming to treatment guidance (Llovet et al. 1999). As a result, percutaneous ablation is strongly recommended as an alternative to surgery for:

- Stage 0 (performance status ECOG status 0 and Child-Pugh score A) – very early stage: single liver lesion measuring <2 cm
- Stage A (performance status 0–2 and Child-Pugh score A-C) – early stage: solitary lesion >2 cm or early multifocal disease characterized by up to 3 lesions measuring less than 3 cm

Moreover, percutaneous ablation has emerged a valuable tool for patients anticipating liver transplantation, impeding the progression of the disease (Agopian et al. 2017).

Radiofrequency ablation has been successfully used in patients with cirrhosis and very early and early-stage HCC, with complete response above 95% and with 5 years survival rates in 62–68% of cases (Crocetti et al. 2017; Livraghi et al. 2007). Similarly, MWA has proven a safe and effective technique in the treatment of HCC. Dong et al. (2003) studied 234 patients who underwent microwave ablation for HCCs, demonstrating survival rates of 92.7%, 81.6%, 72.9%, 66.4% and 56.7% at 1, 2, 3, 4 and 5 years following the ablation, with a local recurrence rate of 7%. Multiple studies have shown similar results with different MWA systems, confirming, thus, its efficacy in the treatment of HCC (Ziemlewicz et al. 2015; Iannitti et al. 2007; Lu et al. 2001). Interestingly, promising results have also been published for tumours sized >2 cm. Sun et al. (2015) reported retrospective data of patients with a single medium-sized HCC (mean size, 3.72 ± 0.54 cm) showing overall survival rates of 89%, 74% and 60% and cumulative recurrence-free survival of 51%, 36% and 27% at 1, 2 and 3 years, respectively. Cryoablation has also been used effectively in the treatment of HCC. One of the largest studies evaluating cryoablation and HCC was performed by Yang et al. (2012a, b). The authors enrolled 300 patients with unresectable HCC treated with cryoablation, demonstrating a mean survival time of 45.7, 28.4 and 17.7 months, in increasing order of tumour stage. The same authors proved that size and tumour location were significantly correlated with the risk of recurrence. IRE has recently been introduced in the treatment option of HCC, offering the advantage of approaching and treating lesions in difficult anatomic locations, which are unsuitable for RFA, MWA and SBRT (perihilar and/or perivascular) (Cheung et al. 2013; Cannon et al. 2013).

Several studies comparing different ablation techniques in the treatment of early HCC are available, in the majority demonstrating no significant difference between the distinctive modalities (Shibata et al. 2002; Lu et al. 2005; Vietti Violi et al. 2018; Wu et al. 2015). Additionally, there is growing number of data evaluating the combination of trans-arterial treatments and ablation (Poggi et al. 2013). The combination of necrosis, ischemia and chemotherapeutic agents increases the sensitivity of neoplastic cells to hyperthermia, resulting in synergy with the thermal ablation effect (Poggi et al. 2015; Liu et al. 2011). Despite a plethora of literature on the topic, due to the inhomogeneity in enrolled patient population and treatment protocols, further research to determine optimal methods of combining chemotherapeutic regimens (agent, route of administration, time interval between TACE and ablation or vice versa) with ablation (RF or MW) is needed (Crocetti et al. 2020).

1.3.1 Liver Metastatic Disease

Ablation has successfully been applied in the treatment of secondary hepatic lesions. Indications for ablation of secondary liver tumours include patients unfit for surgery, patients with non-resectable hepatic lesions or as an assist to systemic therapy (Crocetti et al. 2020). Liver ablation of secondary tumours is highly recommended in:

- Lesions sized <3 cm, but with allowance to <5 cm in lesions with easy access
- Number of lesions: <5

Additionally, besides the curative intent, ablation therapies may aim to partially control a long-term disease, thus contributing potentially to overall survival (Crocetti et al. 2020; Van Cutsem et al. 2016; Clavien et al. 2007; Solbiati et al. 2012; Weiser et al. 2013). Moreover, ablation treatments have proven efficient in recurrent cases following hepatectomy (Sofocleous et al. 2011).

RFA has proven highly efficient in the treatment of colorectal liver metastasis sized <3 cm, demonstrating outcomes comparable to surgery (Puijk et al. 2018). Moreover, RFA could prolong the overall survival when combined with chemotherapy in contrast to chemotherapy alone (Ruers et al. 2017). MWA achieves also great results; overall survival for MW ablation ranges between 35–79%, 35–58% and 17–18% at 3-, 4- and 5-year follow up (Puijk et al. 2018). Cryoablation, although used very early in the advent of ablation treatments, has been associated with higher rates of local recurrence and complications and is therefore rarely applied in clinical practice (Seifert and Junginger 2004). On the other hand, IRE is a promising and upcoming technique in the treatment of colorectal metastasis. Two retrospective studies found a 2-year overall survival rates of up to 62% in patients treated with IRE for colorectal liver metastasis and a 2-year progression-free survival of 18–40.5% (Cornelis et al. 2020; Hosein et al. 2014).

It is highly important to take under consideration the biological behavior of the tumour as it seems to affect the postoperative outcome. For colorectal cancer liver metastatic disease, mutation of the *RAS* gene family (*KRAS, NRAS and HRAS*) is one of the relevant prognostic biomarkers for locoregional CLM treatment as mutation in the RAS family (approx. present in 40% of patients) is related to worse prognosis (Lin et al. 2021). In tumours with such biological characteristics, an ablation margin of at least 10 mm is strongly recommended (Calandri et al. 2018).

Besides colorectal metastasis ablation, nowadays, there is ongoing research regarding the application of ablation techniques in metastasis from other primary tumours, exhibiting satisfactory results, mainly from neuroendocrine tumour, breast, sarcoma, thyroid and melanoma (Crocetti et al. 2020; de Baere et al. 2015a, b; Barral et al. 2016; Cazzato et al. 2018; Efthymiou et al. 2023; Filippiadis et al. 2022).

Take home points
Hepatocellular carcinoma Single nodule <2 cm (even in surgical patients) Single or up to 3 nodules >3 cm in non-surgical patients
Colorectal liver metastases Up to 5 metastases <3 cm
For the rest tumours: Multidisciplinary approach
Ablation margins 0.5–1 cm
The size <3 cm and the location of the lesion are important prognostic factors.
For colorectal Mets, check RAS mutation status.

1.3.2 Renal Cell Cancer

Renal cancer ranks seventh in the list of most common malignancies, accounting for 5% and 3% of all female and male adult neoplasm, respectively (Higgins and Hong 2015). Although partial nephrectomy is considered the standard of care, percutaneous ablative techniques have been proven a safe and effective treatment for localized and early diagnosed RCC, with progression-free and overall survival rates comparable to surgical options (Humphrey et al. 2016).

Nowadays, international guidelines advocate the application of percutaneous ablative nephron sparing techniques, including radiofrequency ablation (RFA), cryoablation (CA) and microwave ablation (MWA), as an alternative attractive therapeutic option for the management of localized renal mass with a diameter ≤3 cm, when complete ablation is technically feasible while remaining skeptical for larger tumours (>3 cm), and in T1b renal tumours, due to the increased rates of recurrence (Krokidis et al. 2017; Katsanos et al. 2014; Finelli et al. 2017; Motzer et al. 2017; Campbell et al. 2017; Escudier et al. 2019; Ljungberg et al. 2019). ESMO guidelines support the utility of ablation in patients with small cortical tumours (<3 cm) and age >70 years, high surgical risk, solitary kidney, compromised renal function, hereditary RCC or multiple bilateral tumours (Escudier et al. 2019). The recommendation of EAU is that ablation could be offered to elderly and/or comorbid patients with small renal masses (Ljungberg et al. 2019). Recent evidence demonstrates that larger tumours (>3 cm and T1b) can also be treated successfully with favourable outcomes (Aarts et al. 2020; Guo and Arellano 2020; Efthymiou et al. 2021).

Several technical points may affect the ablation result and should be carefully addressed prior to procedure, starting from the ideal placement of the patient in the surgical bed (prone, decubitus, etc.) to any additional manoeuvres needed in order to avoid vital proximal structures (e.g. bowel), including hydro-dissection and ureteral stent placement (Seager et al. 2021).

The role of several morphometric parameters of the tumour, including the size, the endophytic or exophytic location in the kidney, the proximity with the hilar structures in the procedural outcome, has been assessed, and respective morphological scores have been proposed aiming to predict the peri- and post-procedural result (Kutikov and Uzzo 2009; Gahan et al. 2015; Schmit et al. 2014; Camacho et al. 2015; Reyes et al. 2013; Ierardi et al. 2017).

Complication rate is generally low, and the majority of the procedures are performed as day cases. Commonest complications include haemorrhage (massive bleeding <1%), haematuria (0.5–1%) and thermal injury of the surrounding organs (mostly bowel), urinoma (1–3%) (Krokidis et al. 2017).

In current literature, there is a plethora of studies demonstrating favourable results after thermal ablation of renal cell tumours. Psutka et al. (2013) treated 185 T1 renal cell tumours, with RFA reporting 96.1% 5-year recurrence-free survival and 91.5% disease-free survival for T1a lesions. Georgiades et al. (2013), in a large single-centre series including 134 patients treated with percutaneous CA, reported a 5-year efficacy of 97.0% and 5-year recurrence-free survival of 100%. Similar results have been reported by other authors (Tracy et al. 2010; Zagoria et al. 2011; McDougal et al. 2005; Levinson et al. 2008; Wah et al. 2014; Nielsen et al. 2020; Lim et al. 2020). Microwave ablation, although less studied, has also emerged as a safe and effective alternative treatment in RCCs. Kidney is a highly perfused organ, and this unique physiology results in important implications on efficacy of different ablative techniques due to significant alteration of bio-heat equation because of this perfusion difference. Guo and Arellano (2021) performed CT-guided microwave ablation for T1a renal tumours in 106 patients. At the first follow-up imaging study, complete response was achieved in 101 (95.3%) patients and partial response was achieved in 5 (4.7%) patients; the 1-, 2- and 3-year local progression-free survival rates were 100.0%, 92.8% and 90.6%, respectively, and 3-year overall survival were 99.0%, 97.7%, and 94.6%, respectively. Several series demonstrate comparable results (Aarts et al. 2020; Efthymiou et al. 2021; Hao et al. 2018; Maciolek et al. 2019; Klapperich et al. 2017).

Although partial nephrectomy remains the standard of care in the treatment of RCCs, percutaneous ablation techniques show comparable results for patients that are not suitable or refuse surgery (Katsanos et al. 2014). Talenfeld et al. (2018) evaluated retrospectively T1a lesions treated either with RF-, cryo- or MW ablation reporting similar outcomes with total or partial nephrectomy with less periprocedural complications, reduced 30- and 90-day mortality and lower risk of long-term renal insufficiency. Moreover, a recent retrospective analysis performed on a large patient cohort reported that 3-, 5-, and 9-year survival rates were not statistically significant among thermal ablation, partial and total nephrectomy (Xing et al. 2018). Literature comparing the distinct ablation techniques remains limited. Generally, when compared to radiofrequency, microwave ablation is less affected by perfusion differences and the heat-sink effect, an advantage which renders this technique ideal for the hyper-vascular renal tumours. Recent trials comparing MWA, RFA and cryoablation have demonstrated significantly decreased procedure times in favour of MWA with similar complication rates and renal function changes post-procedure (Zhou and Arellano 2018). Similarly, De Cobelli et al. (2020) compared percutaneous MWA and cryoablation for T1a RCC and showed comparable safety and efficacy between the two modalities. Overall, evidence in literature suggests that there are no significant outcome differences regarding overall complications, metastasis-free rates and cancer-specific survival between thermal ablation techniques. However, there is a lack of big randomized controlled trials (RCT) comparing the different ablation techniques.

Take-home points for RCC ablation
1. Current guidelines advocate the use of ablation techniques in RCCs sized <3 cm.
2. Not clear guidelines yet about larger tumours, although there are promising results in terms of efficiency and safety.
3. Ablation techniques have comparable results to surgery, with lower complication rates and shorter hospital stay.
4. Each ablation technique has advantages – not enough data yet to choose one over the other.

1.3.3 Pulmonary Tumours

Lung cancer is the commonest type of malignancy in both sexes and a leading cause of death worldwide, constituting 19.4% of all cancer deaths (Postmus et al. 2017). In addition, lung remains one of the most frequent sites of metastatic spread (Cornelis et al. 2020). Apart from surgical options and radiation therapy, percutaneous ablation constitutes an additional alternative technique for local treatment of primary or secondary lung lesions (Herold et al. 1996; Welch et al. 2015; Lam et al. 2018).

Both size and location of tumours should be taken under consideration prior to decision-making. Tumour size and the number of the lesions are described in more details below. Extra care should be taken for lesions with a distance <1 cm from hilum, large vessel or main bronchi, oesophagus or trachea and for tumours abutting a vessel or myocardium, as the above locations could be relative contraindications (Venturini et al. 2020). Moreover, in bilateral lesions physicians are advised not to treat in the same session due to the relative risk of bilateral pneumothorax (Venturini et al. 2020). Poor results of spirometry are not an absolute contraindication but should be further discussed.

Striking technical differences in lung ablation comparing to other tissues constitute the lower power (30–40 W) energy used in RFA as well as the triple-freeze protocol during CWA, which is accompanied with lower recurrence and complication rates (Crocetti and Lencioni 2010; Lyons et al. 2018). Moreover, MWA has some advantages over RFA, such as the less severe heat-sink effect and the faster and higher heating, resulting in larger ablation zone, shorter procedural time and more tolerable pain (Venturini et al. 2020). Advantages of cryoablation include good visualization of ice ball during CT and low periprocedural pain, enabling performing procedures under minor sedation. However, a major limitation of cryoablation is the smaller size of the ablation zone, which increases the need for more cryoprobes, thus increasing the risk for complications.

Commonest procedural complications include small pneumothoraxes and pleural effusions occurring in up to 50% of patients, in the vast majority do not require any intervention (Venturini et al. 2020). Rarer and more severe complications included hemorrhage, air embolism, lung abscess formation and bronchopleural fistula.

In primary lung tumours, thermal ablation is indicated (Venturini et al. 2020; Welch et al. 2015; Donington et al. 2012):

- For patients with stage I NSCLC who present contraindications to surgery or stereotactic radiotherapy due to cardiorespiratory comorbidity or insufficient vital lung reserve
- In patients with T1a and T1b NSCLC with lesion sized <2 cm

Regarding ablation techniques, radiofrequency is the modality mostly studied, with two large multi-centre prospective studies including 54 and 42 patients, respectively, with inoperable stage IA NSCLC, showing an overall survival rate of approximately 90% at 1 year, 70% at 2 years and 60% at 3 years (Palussière et al. 2018; Dupuy et al. 2015). Similar results have been reported by other authors (Uhlig et al. 2018). Microwave and cryoablation, although less studied, have proven a safe and effective treatment in primary lung disease (Palussière et al. 2019; Moussa et al. 2019).

Minimally invasive image-guided thermal ablative therapies have emerged as an alternative curative option for the treatment of oligometastatic pulmonary disease. Percutaneous ablation techniques in metastatic lung disease have been mostly assessed in colorectal metastasis and to a lesser extent to metastatic lung cancer, renal cell carcinoma, melanoma, hepatocellular carcinoma and sarcoma. Consensus has not yet been reached regarding the optimal size and number of lesions, but the majority of centres treat patients with five or fewer pulmonary metastases with a diameter <2 cm (Venturini et al. 2020). de Baère (2011) evaluated 566 patients with 1037 metastases and reported overall survival rates of 92.4%, 79.4%, 67.7%, 58.9% and 51.5% in 1-, 2-, 3-, 4- and 5-year follow-up, respectively, whereas the progression-free survival rates were 40.2%, 23.3%, 16.4% and 13.1% at 1, 2,

3 and 4 years, respectively. Similarly, in one of the largest series using MWA, Wolf et al. (2008) reported a 1-year local control rate of 67%, with a mean of 16.2 months to the first local recurrence after microwave ablation in 50 patients with 82 intrapulmonary lesions. Moreover, the initial results published from the ECLIPSE trial (de Baere et al. 2015a, b) investigating the feasibility, safety and local tumour control of cryoablation in pulmonary metastases reported a local tumour control of 96.6% and 94.2% at 6 and 12 months, respectively, whereas the 1-year OS rate was 97.5%. Several authors have shown comparable outcomes (Kurilova et al. 2018; Vogl et al. 2011).

In current literature, there are few studies comparing the different ablation modalities. The Italian multi-centre randomized LUMIRA trial, which compared RFA to MWA for the treatment of primary and secondary lung tumours in a palliative setting, showed that there was not significant difference between the two groups in terms of survival time (Macchi et al. 2017). However, the pain level was significantly lower in MWA group than in RFA group (Guo and Arellano 2021). Das et al. (2019) showed that both cryoablation and microwave were comparably effective, with similar survival benefits in patients with advanced NSCLC (stages IIIb/IV) and small tumours (size less than 3 cm) with cryoablation offering the advantage of reduced intra-procedural pain. On the other hand, a metanalysis by Jiang et al. (2018) showed that radiofrequency and microwave lung ablation were more effective than cryoablation in terms of local progression rate with no significant difference regarding the complication rates. In conclusion, the current literature regarding the application of ablation in primary and secondary lung tumours is limited and more ideally randomized controlled trials are needed.

Take-home points for lung ablation

1. Thermal ablation techniques have proven safe and efficient in the treatment of either primary or secondary lung tumours.
2. *For primary lung cancer:* Stage I NSCLC, unfit for surgery/radiotherapy.
3. *For metastatic disease:* Five or fewer pulmonary metastases with a diameter <2 cm.
4. Better results when lesion size <2 cm and tumour margin recommendation is >1 cm.
5. RFA and MWA present comparable efficacy, but MWA is better tolerated and more suitable for larger tumours.
6. Cryoablation offers the advantage of direct visualization during procedure + lower periprocedural pain but smaller ablation zone.

1.4 Bone

Historically, ablative techniques have been successfully used in the treatment of benign bone lesions, as well as for curative purposes in oligometastatic patients or as a palliative treatment in symptomatic patients suffering from pain and mobility impairment. Although radiation therapy is the standard of care in the treatment of bone malignancies, it is accompanied by several limitations, including the radiosensitivity of the tumor and the upper dose that can be applied. Furthermore, surgical resection of bone lesions is technically challenging, with a high mortality and morbidity rate (Ryan et al. 2022).

In terms of the most optimal ablative modality used, RFA, MWA and CA have been successfully applied in the treatment of bone malignancies (Vaswani et al. 2018; McMenomy et al. 2013; Deschamps et al. 2014). RFA is strongly suggested in osteolytic or mixed osteolytic-osteoblastic lesions, preferably with minimal soft tissue extent (Tomasian and Jennings 2020). Although not absolutely contraindicated, extra care should be given in the case of metallic surgical fixation devices (Ryan et al. 2022). MWA, on the other hand, is indicated for sclerotic lesions, as it is not affected by the high impedance of the sclerotic bone (Prud'homme et al. 2017). CA has proven highly efficient in the treatment of bone lesions, partially due to the ability of direct visualization of the ice ball and the synchronous use of multiple cryoprobes, enabling to treat larger lesions (Ryan et al. 2022).

Additional to general contraindications as in other tissues, the proximity with neural structures should be highlighted since it could potentially consist a contraindication. Techniques to avoid thermal injury to non-target sensitive structures include passive monitoring or active protection (Ryan et al. 2022).

Spinal interventions are often technically challenging due to the close proximity with neural vital structures. Extra care should be taken, as some technical modifications may be needed; ipsilateral lesions of the vertebral body may be entirely ablated with a unipedicular approach, in comparison to more extensive lesions exceeding the sagittal midline of the vertebral body, in which bipedicular approach is recommended (Ryan et al. 2022). Additionally, unstable fractures and metastatic epidural spinal cord compression are the most frequent relative contraindications in spinal treatments.

In some cases, especially in weight-bearing bones, ablation is used in combination with bone consolidation/augmentation techniques, for greater support and stability. Apart from the above techniques, it has been proven that ablation therapies could be successfully combined with embolization and radiotherapy (Pellerin et al. 2014; Kelekis et al. 2017; Ma et al. 2017). Further research is required to investigate the optimal timing and sequence of operative events.

Clinically significant complications are not common (approx. 2.3%), with pathological fracture being the commonest (1.8%). Other rarely encountered complications include infection, skin burn, peripheral sensory or motor neuropathy and haematoma (Cazzato et al. 2020).

Overall, ablation therapies have emerged as an essential tool in today's oncological treatment (Fig. 2). Undoubtedly, further research is required, especially large randomized trials, to establish the role of ablation techniques in various malignancies and to investigate their distinctive characteristics (e.g. RAS), taken under consideration prior to procedure.

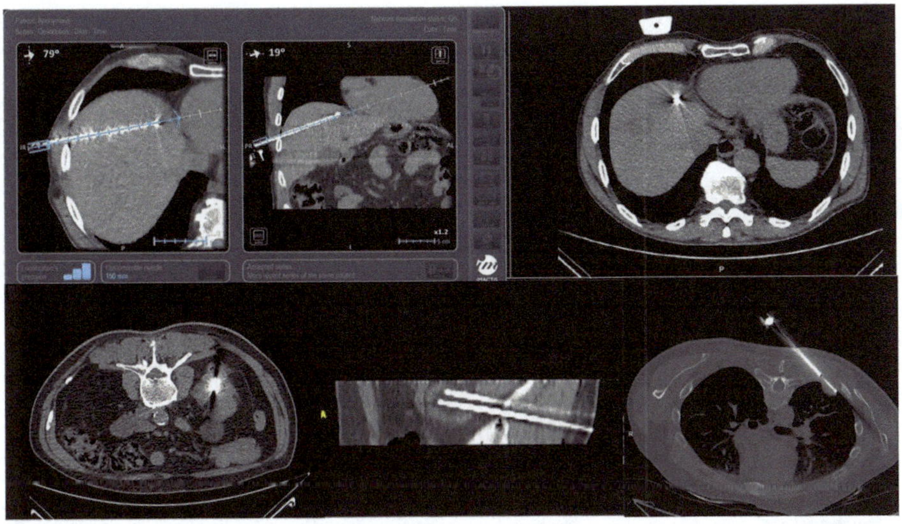

Fig. 2 Percutaneous imaging-guided ablation is a safe and efficacious therapy against cancer; ablation is not limited by tumour histology and, at the same time, preserves the rest physiologic parenchyma of the organ. Different examples of percutaneous ablative therapies are illustrated including liver, renal and thoracic wall tumour ablation

1.5 Locoregional Intraarterial Therapies

1.5.1 General Considerations

Locoregional intra-arterial techniques include embolization therapies such as conventional trans-arterial chemoembolization (cTACE) drug-eluting microparticle trans arterial chemoembolization (DEM-TACE) and selective internal radiation therapy (SIRT). Less popular endovascular treatment options are trans-arterial bland embolization (TAE), hepatic arterial infusion (HAI) and chemo saturation (also known as percutaneous hepatic perfusion; PHP) (Vogel et al. 2023; Hu et al. 2023). Intra-arterial therapies are performed in an angiography suite, under local anaesthesia, using small diameter arterial access (4–5 Fr) via common femoral or radial artery, although brachial artery or distal trans-radial access are also a valid option, according to the patient's anatomical details (Iezzi et al. 2017; van Dam et al. 2019). Following meticulous patient selection, decided during an appropriate oncologic multidisciplinary team meeting, baseline imaging, CT and/or MRI, is the basic pre-procedural step for all intra-arterial therapies. This should always include an arterial phase not only for diagnostic reasons but also for pre-procedural planning, which includes arterial mapping and detailed tumour arterial supply, in order to maximize technical success and minimize procedural time and complications. The usual target vessels of such procedures are the hepatic arteries (HA), but anatomical variation may include mainly the gastric (GA) and the superior mesenteric arteries (SMA).

1.5.2 Trans-arterial Chemoembolization (TACE)

TACE is the delivery of both embolic and chemotherapeutic agents within the tumour using its arterial supply (West and Jin 2015). The concept of TACE is based on the fact that liver tumours are supplied by the hepatic arteries, while the main (approx. 80%) healthy liver blood supply is guaranteed by the portal vein (Mitra and Metcalf 2009). Therefore, TACE decreases the malignant blood supply by administrating embolic material within the tumoural microcirculation but also enables local intra-tumoural delivery of large doses of chemotherapeutic drugs, without the unnecessary risk of systemic exposure (Lencioni et al. 2013) (Fig. 3).

There are two main categories of TACE, discriminated according to the agents used for delivery. cTACE, in which the chemotherapeutic agent is emulsified with Lipiodol, and DEM-TACE, where the agent is loaded on drug eluting microparticles. The latter has the theoretical advantage of deeper penetration and increased selectivity of delivery and longer indwelling time of the chemotherapeutic agent within the neoplastic vascular bed, also resulting in reduced systemic exposure of the drug (Malagari et al. 2014). Both have been widely studied for the management of hepatocellular carcinoma and their efficacy and safety the safety is well established. The most commonly used chemotherapeutic agents for TACE in HCC are doxorubicin and Idarubicin and doses should be adjusted according to liver function (Jogi et al. 2020). TACE can be also proposed as palliative treatment of intrahepatic cholangiocarcinoma (ICC) and metastatic disease in cases of systemic chemotherapeutic failure or in synergy with ablation and systemic therapy schemes (Lencioni et al. 2013; Mosconi et al. 2023; Helmberger et al. 2022; Spiliopoulos et al. 2023). According to the recently amended Barcelona Clinic Liver Cancer (BCLC) recommendations, indications for TACE (both cTACE and DEM-TACE) in HCC include BCLC early stages 0-A when ablation and resection are not indicated (recommendation class IB) and intermediate-stage stage B in the transplant setting (recommendation class IA), aiming to reduce down-staging within the transplant criteria, bridging (tumor growth control if on transplant list), and palliative

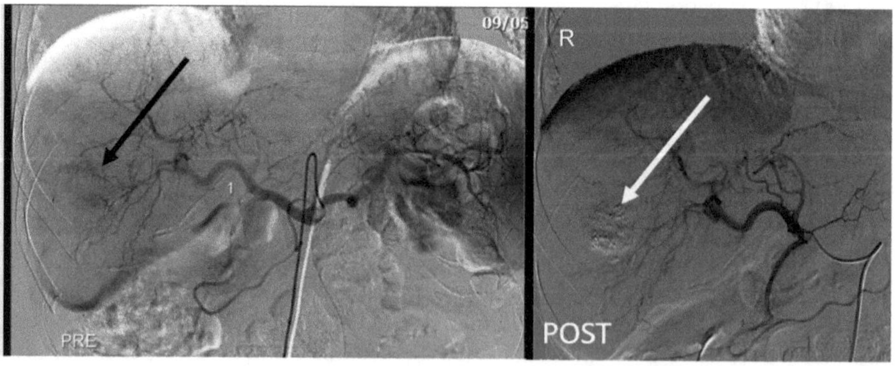

Fig. 3 Trans-arterial chemoembolization in a hypervascular HCC (black arrow). Fluoroscopy image post embolization illustrates coverage of the tumour with lipiodol and lack of vasculature (white arrow)

(improving survival in patients not eligible for transplantation). According to the European Society for Medical Oncology (ESMO) guidelines, TACE is the only guideline-recommended global standard of care for stage B HCC. In ICC, TACE is indicated for patients with surgically unresectable or inoperable liver-only or liver-dominant disease (Lucatelli et al. 2021; Vogel et al. 2018).

In metastatic disease, the ESMO guidelines recommend TACE in cases of colorectal liver metastasis in patients with liver-limited disease when available chemotherapeutic lines have failed. The more frequently used chemotherapeutic agent for colorectal metastasis is irinotecan (Van Cutsem et al. 2016). Further indications for metastatic disease include patients with neuroendocrine tumours (NET) limited to the liver, when systemic therapy fails and NET liver metastasis without surgical resection option (Lucatelli et al. 2021; de Baere et al. 2015a, b). TACE could also be considered in selected cases of non-colorectal, non-NET liver metastasis, such as cancer and melanoma not responding to standard treatments, but the level of evidence is low and data from major studies are scarce (Storozhakova et al. 2020; Tao et al. 2023; Bale et al. 2019). Procedure-related complications of TACE are expected in approximately 10% of the cases and include vascular injury or haemorrhage, non-target arterial thrombosis, ischemia due to non-target embolization, liver failure, peribiliary necrosis, abscess and bilioma. In nearly 30% of the cases, post-embolisation syndrome (PES) is expected, characterized by nausea, vomiting, fever, pain and fatigue. PES is not considered a complication as it is an indicator of sufficient embolic effect and auto-resolves within 2 weeks, necessitating only symptomatic medical treatment. Persisting symptoms should prompt further evaluation (Lucatelli et al. 2021).

According to the literature, TACE results in an overall survival of over 2.5 years in patients with intermediate BCLC stage B (Reig et al. 2022). Regarding the different TACE techniques, in a recent network, metaanalysis of randomized controlled trials, cTACE and DEM-TACE demonstrated similar survival benefit (estimated median survival 18.1 months for cTACE, 20.6 months for DEB-TACE). Notably, bland embolization (TAE) also demonstrated similar survival benefit (estimated median survival 20.8 months), while TACE combined with external radiation or liver ablation achieved the best patient survival (30.1 months TACE plus external radiotherapy, 33.3 months in TACE plus liver ablation) (Katsanos et al. 2017). Less data is available for TACE in metastatic disease. The use of Irinotecan-loaded drug-eluting bead TACE (DEBIRI) has been reported to be safe and provides a median overall survival rate ranging from 16.8 to 25 months (Aliberti et al. 2011; Fiorentini et al. 2012; Martin et al. 2015; Akinwande et al. 2017).

Selective Internal Radiation Therapy (SIRT)

SIRT, also known as radioembolization, is a more recent trans-arterial therapy which uses embolic micron-sized embolic particles as carriers of a radioisotope (Radioshperes, mainly resin or glass microspheres) capable of irradiating the tumour from within. Very high doses of radiation can be selectively administered within hepatic tumours and only a small dose to the surrounding normal liver (Memon et al. 2011). The major difference compared to TACE is the use of irradiation instead of ischemia and chemotherapy, as the radioactive microparticles do not produce a substantial embolic effect (Brown et al. 2023). One of the most common agents used in SIRT is yttrium 90 (Y-90), a near-pure beta emitter, but recently, other agents such as Holmium-166 have been made available in the market (Memon et al. 2011; Pérez-López et al. 2022). Currently available SIRT systems are: SIR-Spheres® resin microspheres (SIRTEX, USA), Therasphere™ glass microspheres (Boston Scientific, USA), and Quiremspheres™ 166Ho microspheres (TERUMO, Japan). Current indications for SIRT include unresectable primary liver cancer (HCC or cholangiocarcinoma) and liver metastases from colorectal and neuroendocrine tumors, but also for other liver-dominant metastases as a salvage therapy. Specifically, it is indicated for HCC across all stages: curative setting in BCLC stage A, for downstaging and bridging in the transplant patient and for palliation in BCLC stages B and C (Vogel et al. 2017). In the latest version of National Comprehensive Cancer Network guidelines, radioembolization is classified with uniform consensus as category 2 A for the treatment of liver-dominant, chemo-refractory colorectal metastasis (CRM) (Benson et al. 2017). Absolute contraindications include severely compromised hepatic function (i.e. ascites, icterus, encephalopathy), poor performance status (ECOG 4 2), active hepatic infection, significant extrahepatic metastases, pregnancy or breast-feeding, life expectancy <3 months, inability to administer microspheres without non-target embolization to the bowel and high lung shunt fraction (LSF) leading to >30-Gy dose to the lungs with a single treatment. Relative contraindications include uncorrectable coagulopathy, severe radiographic contrast medium allergy and renal impairment (> 2.5 mg/dl) not medically addressed, increased bilirubin level and significant ascites, Child–Pugh >B7, high intrahepatic tumour burden (50–70%), and previous external radiotherapy (Padia et al. 2017). Notably, one of the core advantages of SIRT is that as opposed to TACE, it can be safely performed in patients with main portal vein branch thrombosis, due to its mild embolic effect. SIRT is a multi-step procedure which initially requires meticulous clinical evaluation, radiological imaging (contrast-enhanced CT or MRI within 30 days of the procedure for staging and the calculation of the tumour volume, patient selection and dose calculation (dosimetry). Selective digital subtracted intra-arterial angiography of the hepatic vasculature and embolization of arteries such as the gastroduodenal or the right gastric arteries could be necessary as to avoid non-target dissemination of the radio spheres to the gastrointestinal system. Following DSA and embolization, an 99mTc-MAA or 166Ho-microsphere scout dose is administrated via the microcatheter in order to simulate the administration of the radio spheres, and the patient is sent for pretreatment planar scintigraphy or bremsstrahlung single-photon emission computed tomography with integrated computed tomography (SPECT/CT). If gastrointestinal dispersion and/or significant LSF are not noted, the next step, which is the actual administration of the radio spheres, can be performed the same day or within the next 14 days (Weber et al. 2022; Kim et al. 2019). The final step is post-procedural imaging with planar scintigraphy or SPECT/CT to confirm sufficient tumour uptake, acceptable pulmonary absorbed dose and the absence of visceral concentration. The most fearful major complication of SIRT is radiation-induced hepatitis (radiation induced liver disfunction; RILD). It occurs at 4–8 weeks (up to 6 months) and in the majority of the cases is lethal. There is no effective treatment, and it has been reported in up to 4% of the cases, but the true incidence is unknown. Predisposing factors include pre-treatment total serum bilirubin >2.0 mg/ml, low-volume "healthy" liver remnant and bi-lobar single-session treatment. Other complications include radio-induced cholocistitis, biloma, abscess (<2%), peptic ulcer (<5%; due to non-targeted delivery), radiation pneumonitis <1% or pulmonary fibrosis (lung dose <30 Gray each time and και <50 Gray totally), abdominal wall radiation dermatitis and ulceration. It should be noted that high doses in liver segments in proximity to colon and stomach could induce necrosis-abscess and fistula requiring drainage and surgery. Post-embolic syndrome is reported to be 20–55% milder compared to TACE (Padia et al. 2017). Although initial outcomes in patients with unresectable HCC did not demonstrate a net survival benefit of SIRT versus TACE, results from more recent randomized controlled trials indicate that SIRT results in superior time to progression and survival compared to TACE in patients with early or intermediate HCC (Dhondt et al. 2022). In a 2017 network metatanalysis of RCTs the median survival following SIRT was 24.3 months, while SIRT was proven the safest intervention compared to TACE, TAE and external radiotherapy (Katsanos et al. 2017). This has led major centres in a current clinical practice switch to use SIRT as a first-line treatment for HCC independently of BCLC stage (Salem et al. 2018). For intrahepatic cholangiocarcinoma, a metanalysis of 13 studies on TACE (906 patients) and 18 on SIRT (789 patients) indicated a median survival 14.2 and 13.5 months, respectively (95%C.I.: 11.4–16.1) (Mosconi et al. 2021). For colorectal metastasis (CLM), three large RCTs (Sirflox study, Foxfire and Foxfire global) did not demonstrate a significant improvement in overall survival. This has been attributed to the increase in the extrahepatic disease, as an improvement in the overall survival was noted when TARE was combined with systemic chemotherapy as opposed to chemotherapy alone (van Hazel et al. 2016; Wasan et al. 2017). More recently, the EPOCH RCT demonstrated that SIRT using Yttrium-90 glass radio spheres demonstrated a significant improvement of 31% in progression-free survival and 41% in liver progression-free survival when added to systemic chemotherapy for second-line CLM compared to systemic chemotherapy alone (Mulcahy et al. 2021). In a more recent network metaanalysis of seven trials Regorafenib, TAS-102 (trifluridine/tipiracil) and using Y-90 resin SIRT, were found more effective than best supportive care, in third-line treatment of CLM. Moreover, following an analysis of the NHS SIRT program for CLM in the UK, (399 patients; in 10 centres), median overall survival was 7.6 months with only an 8% of grade 3 adverse events. Median progression-free and liver progression-free survival were 3.0 and 3.7 months, respectively. During the follow-up period, 143 patients experienced an adverse event (White et al. 2019). Future major studies for CLM will investigate personalized dosimetry and high doses to ablate segmental disease (SIRT segmentectomy), which are expected to improve survival outcomes (Chiu et al. 2023).

In patients with NET, SIRT has repeatedly shown excellent tumour response rates with significant improvement in survival, but evidence remain very limited. In a retrospective study of 148 patients, a median survival of 70 months was reported

(Kennedy et al. 2008), while a systematic review comparing chemoembolization and radioembolization demonstrated similar response and survival rates (Yang et al. 2012a, b). Therefore, optimal trans-arterial treatment for NET remains to be determined, although SIRT seems to be a reasonable alternative to chemo refractory NET. SIRT outcomes in non-CLM, non-NET metastatic disease, include satisfactory overall survival in patients with breast cancer (median survival 9.8–10.6 months) (Liu et al. 2022), pancreatic cancer (median survival 5.6 months) and melanoma (median survival 14.6 months), with reasonable rates of ≥grade 3 adverse events (2.1–2.5%) (Helmberger et al. 2021; Liu et al. 2022).

1.6 Palliative Care

Interventional oncology techniques have been proven to be highly efficient in the local therapy of various cancerous tumours, in treatment of complications related to the primary tumor or metastases and in providing supportive procedures to improve quality of life of patients with high levels of technical success and excellent safety profiles. The risk of death from cancer has been decreasing continuously the last decades (Siegel et al. 2022) and population size and life expectancy have been increasing (Wang et al. 2020; Vos et al. 2020), so the need for techniques that can provide effective disease control for cancer patients is also increasing.

2 Percutaneous Paliation of Pain

Most cancer patients experience pain, which is of moderate severity at least in most of the cases, and it is difficult to treat (Heptonstall et al. 2023; Scott-Warren and Bhaskar 2014). Cancer pain can result from direct tissue damage (nociceptive pain) or from dysfunction of nerves (neuropathic pain). Cancer pain significantly reduces quality of life, and in 56–82% of cases, management of pain is inadequate (Ripamonti et al. 2012). Percutaneous interventional oncology techniques include nerve blocks, chemical and thermal neurolysis and augmentation techniques in the spine and peripheral skeleton (Filippiadis et al. 2019a, b; Tomasian et al. 2022). Neurolysis is safe and effective and has been used for the palliation of pain of peripheral, cranial, splanchnic and intercostal nerves and also nerve ganglia and plexuses (Tomasian et al. 2022). Percutaneous neurolysis is indicated in advanced stage cancer patients with a life expectancy of 6–12 months (Filippiadis et al. 2019a, b) and improves pain and quality of life in more than half of patients (65–82%), while complication rate is low (Heptonstall et al. 2023). Percutaneous neurolysis has been successfully used for many different types of cancers, including pancreatic, hepatobiliary, adrenal and upper gastrointestinal cancers; retroperitoneal lymph node metastases; neck, facial and breast cancers; and visceral and perineal pelvic cancers (Heptonstall et al. 2023).

Neurolysis can be achieved either by injection of alcohol or phenol (chemical neurolysis) or by thermal means, such as radiofrequency or microwave ablation or cryoablation and high-intensity focused ultrasound (thermal neurolysis) (Filippiadis et al. 2019a, b; Filippiadis et al. 2020; Tomasian et al. 2022). Alcohol causes nerve oedema and sclerosis, while phenol causes protein denaturation due to diffusion of the chemical agent into the vessels of the axon and the perineurium (Koyyalagunta et al. 2016). Alcohol is most used in clinical practice. Thermal ablation causes direct pain fibre damage by placing the probe of the ablation device close to the target nerve, and then heat (up to 60–80 °C) or extreme cold is applied. Prior to thermal neurolysis, pain can be induced by electrical stimulation so the proper location where the probe of the ablation device should be placed can be confirmed (Filippiadis et al. 2017a, b).

For percutaneous neurolysis, CT guidance is mostly used as it outperforms all other imaging techniques in terms of resolution and needle placement and location (Kambadakone et al. 2011), and in daily practice, neurolysis is performed under local anaesthesia and conscious sedation (Filippiadis et al. 2017a, b). Percutaneous neurolysis is a safe procedure with low complications rate (<2%) (Filippiadis et al. 2017a, b). Complications include dysaesthesia, neuritis or neuroma formation, failure to relieve pain and early return of pain (Filippiadis et al. 2019a, b). Other reported complications are cardiovascular compromise, orthostatic hypotension, Horner's syndrome, transient diarrhoea, iatrogenic vascular damage and bleeding, pneumothorax, intestinal perforation and death (Filippiadis et al. 2019a, b). Neurolysis may be repeated to treat early return of pain.

Cancer patients commonly report pain related to bone metastases, or pathological fractures and the spine is the most common site of metastatic disease with painful lesions occurring in 30–70% of patients (Molina et al. 2012) and compression fractures in 21% of patients (Mattie et al. 2021). Spine and peripheral skeleton augmentation techniques are used to relieve pain and include percutaneous cementoplasty and percutaneous fixation with internally cemented screws in the peripheral skeleton and vertebral augmentation, including percutaneous vertebroplasty, balloon kyphoplasty or spinal implants (Heptonstall et al. 2023; Filippiadis et al. 2019a, b). In addition to pain palliation, bone augmentation should also be considered for structural support post chemotherapy or radiotherapy to provide structural stability in necrotic bone that is subject to fracture (Filippiadis et al. 2019a, b). Vertebral augmentation is highly successful (80–100% success rate), and reported complications are <11.5% (Tsoumakidou et al. 2017).

3 Percutaneous Drainage of Fluid Collections

Pleural effusion and ascites are common complications in patients with cancer (Yang et al. 2022; Matsusaki et al. 2022). Pleural effusion occurs either by in situ pleural involvement or by metastatic deposits (Feller-Kopman and Light 2018), and its occurrence in cancer patients is indicative of disseminated or advanced disease (Asciak and Rahman 2018). Ascites frequently occurs in abdominal malignancy and indicates the presence of peritoneal metastases, being a grave prognostic sign (Sangisetty 2012). Pleural effusion and ascites, especially when massive, cause severe discomfort, reduce quality of life and denote a poor prognosis. Percutaneous drainage of pleural or peritoneal fluid collections is a simple and effective procedure offered by interventional radiology and can be safely performed under local anesthesia (Matsusaki et al. 2022; Dariushnia et al. 2020).

In common clinical practice, drainage of pleural effusion or ascites is performed under ultrasound guidance as ultrasonography is highly sensitive and accurate in detecting pleural or ascitic fluid (Soni et al. 2015; Cho et al. 2019). In the case of free pleural effusion, positioning the patient in a more upright posture will facilitate the detection of fluid as, in this position, fluid gravitates to the costophrenic sulcus and can be easily and quickly seen with ultrasound. In the case of ascites, fluid is easily detected along the paracolic gutters and in the pelvis. Fluid detection and aspiration can be facilitated by positioning the patient in decubitus or semi-recumbent positions so the fluid can be shifted towards the dependent parts of the abdominal cavity. If the collection is loculated, it may be more difficult to be detected by ultrasound imaging, and computed tomography can be used in these cases.

The presence of a large amount of fluid collection in the peritoneal cavity or the pleural space causes severe abdominal bloating and respiratory distress in the patient, but it is worth to mention that in immunocompromised patients, even a small amount of effusion can be infected and cause symptoms. The infected fluid collection can be percutaneously drained or aspirated so the obtained sample can be sent for bacterial culture and fluid characterization (Dariushnia et al. 2020).

Various catheters can be used for percutaneous drainage and aspiration of fluid collections, with the reported success rates for aspiration and curative drainage reaching 93–100% and 62–100% accordingly (Dariushnia et al. 2020). Success rates can be improved by tailoring the size of the catheter to the consistency of the fluid collection (Dariushnia et al. 2020). The most commonly used type of catheters are non-tunnelled pigtail catheters, and these catheters can be used for either a Seldinger or trocar technique (Jaffe and Nelson 2016). There are no absolute contraindications, but relative contraindications include significant coagulopathy that cannot be adequately corrected, severely compromised cardiopulmonary function or hemodynamic instability, lack of a safe pathway to the fluid collection, inability of the patient to cooperate and patient refusal of the procedure (Dariushnia et al. 2020). Serious complications arising from percutaneous drainage procedures are generally rare, and the reported rate of all major adverse events is 0–15% (Dariushnia et al. 2020). Complications include bacteremia; superinfection and, rarely, septic shock; bowel or pleural transgression, leading to bowel perforation; peritonitis, pneumothorax or hemothorax; and injury to adjacent organs, such as the liver and spleen, leading to haemorrhage (Dariushnia et al. 2020; Martinez-Zayas et al. 2022), which can be significant in the rare case of intercostal or inferior epigastric vessels injury. Malignant seeding along the catheter track is also possible. Other reported complications are paracentesis-induced circulatory dysfunction after large volume drainage of ascitic fluid and pulmonary oedema after rapid drainage of pleural fluid (Lindsay et al. 2014; Sunderland et al. 2016).

Other catheters that are used in clinical practice are indwelling tunnelled catheters. These catheters have a cuffed segment located within the subcutaneous layer that promotes fibrosis, preventing infection from the skin entry and protecting against catheter dislodgement so they can be used as a long term palliative option. Tunnelled pleural catheters are recommended as first line definitive intervention for management of dyspnea for patients with suspected expandable lung and no previous definitive therapy (Feller-Kopman et al. 2018; Bibby et al. 2018). Tunnelled pleural catheters are not only used as a simple drainage system, but they can also be used for instillation of sclerosants aimed at inducing rapid pleurodesis, with favourable results (Walker et al. 2020). Tunnelled peritoneal catheters are used for refractory or recurrent ascites with symptom relief in most patients, and they are more cost-effective than serial large volume paracenteses in patients with recurrent ascites due to the reduced risk of infection, emergency department visits, and length of hospitalization (Wu et al. 2022; Murray et al. 2022).

Pleuroperitoneal shunts that are tunnelled under the skin from the chest to the abdomen have been used for refractory cases, trapped lung and chylothorax secondary to malignancy, but there is insufficient evidence to support their routine use and require great compliance from the patient and can be associated with significant complications (Leung et al. 2013; Koegelenberg et al. 2018). Peritoneovenous shunting has been used for malignant ascites, but because of the technically difficult procedures and high rates of serious complications with mortality reaching 10–20%, it is not being routinely used in clinical practice (Lindsay et al. 2014; Sangisetty 2012).

Pleurodesis has been the historical choice for prevention of pleural collection recurrence, and talc is widely regarded as the best agent for pleurodesis, but this technique is suitable only if adequate pulmonary re-expansion can be demonstrated before the procedure (Fortin and Tremblay 2015; Addala et al. 2022).

In cancer patients, the occurrence of abscesses is not uncommon. They can be related to the primary cancer or metastases, and they can occur as a post-treatment complication. In most cases, CT guidance is used for percutaneous drainage and treatment with very good results (Dariushnia et al. 2020; Jaffe and Nelson 2016).

4 Percutaneous Management of Malignant Biliary Obstruction

Malignant biliary obstruction is a common complication in cancer patients, and it can be related to either intraluminal (related to presence of cholangiocarcinoma) or extraluminal (related to presence of primary cancers, such as hepatocellular carcinoma, gastric, duodenal, gall bladder or pancreatic cancer, as well as to presence of hepatic metastases or metastatic lymph nodes with subsequent tumour infiltration, extrinsic compression and desmoplastic or inflammatory responses) causes (Das et al. 2021).

If biliary obstruction is not decompressed, liver function impairment or infection are caused and may lead to early mortality in the patient. Percutaneous management of malignant biliary obstruction is a multi-step process including percutaneous transhepatic cholangiography, followed by biliary drainage and stenting.

Percutaneous access is considered an alternative to endoscopic approaches in cases of failure to catheterize the papilla or the obstruction as well as in cases of failure to advance a stent; however, it can be considered the first-choice approach in anatomically challenging situations. Uncorrectable coagulopathy is the only absolute contraindication, whilst presence of ascites, extensive intrahepatic cystic or metastatic disease, multifocal intra-hepatic segmental stenosis, infection at puncture side and low life expectancy are considered relative contraindications for percutaneous management of malignant biliary obstruction (Das et al. 2021).

Pre-procedural imaging evaluation through ultrasound and more preferably computed tomography or magnetic resonance imaging is used to provide invaluable information upon the level of obstruction and the pre-interventional planning including optimal side and access route. Patients are usually instructed to fast for 3–6 hours prior to the procedure depending upon the type of anaesthesia used (sedation or general anaesthesia). Combined ultrasound and fluoroscopy guidance increases safety and efficacy of percutaneous management of malignant biliary obstruction; ultrasound allows for adequate biliary tree visualization and evaluation of potential complications, whilst fluoroscopy can be used for duct navigation and dilatation as well as drainage catheter placement or stenting. In the case of diagnostic dilemmas, biopsy can be performed during the process by means of brush cytology or forceps tissue biopsy. Biliary internal-external drain catheters of 8.5–10 French are more commonly used for drainage whilst self-expandable stents of 7–10 mm are used for biliary stenting; now there no clear evidence supporting superiority of covered over metallic stents. Balloon dilatation of a malignant stricture is not commonly performed due to association with bleeding and thrombus formation. However, if preferred, an 8–10 mm balloon is used prior to metallic stent placement aiming to enhance stent's expansion. Bilateral stenting can be performed in the case of a hilar tumour, obstructing both hepatic ducts if contra-lateral bile ducts are not opacified during percutaneous cholangiography and if jaundice fails to resolve post-unilateral approach. Identical stents should be used in case of bilateral stenting since identical radial forces will avoid compression of one stent from the other.

Complications' rate ranges from 4% to12%, with high experience centres, subsegmental entry and dilated bile ducts being factors related to lower reported rates; the most common complication is haemobilia (10%), whilst bleeding requiring intervention, biliovascular fistulas, infection and sepsis, as well as pneumothorax or peritonitis are encountered less frequently (Das et al. 2021; Liu et al. 2018; Rees et al. 2020). Central biliary access, use of 18Gauge access needles, multiple needle passes, non-dilated biliary tree, liver cirrhosis or renal insufficiency and advanced age and coagulopathy or uptake of anticoagulants are considered risk factors significantly increasing bleeding risk (Devane et al. 2020). Technical success rate of percutaneous trans-hepatic biliary drainage and stenting ranges from 90–100% and 82–100%, respectively, whilst 12-month stent patency is up to 86% (Devane et al. 2020; Uberoi et al. 2012; Weber et al. 2009). Clinical success is determined and evaluated by laboratory tests of hepatic function and cholestasis parameters.

5 Conclusion

Interventional oncology constitutes one of the four pillars for modern cancer management. Image-guided biopsy is an established, safe and effective intervention for patients with suspected or known malignancy. The integration of ablation procedures in given guidelines highlights the significance of interventional oncology and, at the same time, the need for further exploration. Various minimal invasive, image-guided, intra-arterial therapies are currently indicated as loco-regional treatment options of both primary and metastatic liver malignancies. Palliative therapies such as neurolysis and biliary and fluid drainage reduce pain and discomfort in cancer patients.

Conflict of Interest The authors declare that they have no conflict of interest.

Funding This study was not supported by any funding.

References

Aarts BM, Prevoo W, Meier MAJ, Bex A, Beets-Tan RGH, Klompenhouwer EG, Gómez FM (2020) Percutaneous microwave ablation of histologically proven T1 renal cell carcinoma. Cardiovasc Intervent Radiol 43(7):1025–1033. https://doi.org/10.1007/s00270-020-02423-7

Addala DN, Kanellakis NI, Bedawi EO, Dong T, Rahman NM (2022) Malignant pleural effusion: updates in diagnosis, management and current challenges. Front Oncol 12:1053574. https://doi.org/10.3389/fonc.2022.1053574

Agopian VG, Harlander-Locke MP, Ruiz RM, Klintmalm GB, Senguttuvan S, Florman SS, Haydel B, Hoteit M, Levine MH, Lee DD, Taner CB, Verna EC, Halazun KJ, Abdelmessih R, Tevar AD, Humar A, Aucejo F, Chapman WC, Vachharajani N et al (2017) Impact of pretransplant bridging locoregional therapy for patients with hepatocellular carcinoma within Milan criteria undergoing liver transplantation: analysis of 3601 patients from the US Multicenter HCC Transplant Consortium. Ann Surg 266(3):525–535. https://doi.org/10.1097/SLA.0000000000002381

Ahmed M, Brace CL, Lee FT, Goldberg SN (2011) Principles of and advances in percutaneous ablation. Radiology 258(2):351–369. https://doi.org/10.1148/radiol.10081634

Akinwande O, Dendy M, Ludwig JM, Kim HS (2017) Hepatic intra-arterial injection of irinotecan drug eluting beads (DEBIRI) for patients with unresectable colorectal liver metastases: a systematic review. Surg Oncol 26(3):268–275. https://doi.org/10.1016/j.suronc.2017.05.003

Aliberti C, Fiorentini G, Muzzio PC, Pomerri F, Tilli M, Dallara S, Benea G (2011) Trans-arterial chemoembolization of metastatic colorectal carcinoma to the liver adopting DC Bead®, drug-eluting bead loaded with irinotecan: results of a phase II clinical study. Anticancer Res 31(12): 4581–4587

Asciak R, Rahman NM (2018) Malignant pleural effusion. Clin Chest Med 39(1):181–193. https://doi.org/10.1016/j.ccm.2017.11.004

Bale R, Putzer D, Schullian P (2019) Local treatment of breast cancer liver metastasis. Cancers 11(9):1341. https://doi.org/10.3390/cancers11091341

Barral M, Auperin A, Hakime A, Cartier V, Tacher V, Otmezguine Y, Tselikas L, de Baere T, Deschamps F (2016) Percutaneous thermal ablation of breast cancer metastases in oligometastatic patients. Cardiovasc Intervent Radiol 39(6):885–893. https://doi.org/10.1007/s00270-016-1301-x

Benson AB, Venook AP, Cederquist L, Chan E, Chen Y-J, Cooper HS, Deming D, Engstrom PF, Enzinger PC, Fichera A, Grem JL, Grothey A, Hochster HS, Hoffe S, Hunt S, Kamel A, Kirilcuk N, Krishnamurthi S, Messersmith WA et al (2017) Colon cancer, version 1.2017, NCCN clinical practice guidelines in oncology. J Natl Compr Cancer Netw 15(3):370–398. https://doi.org/10.6004/jnccn.2017.0036

Bibby AC, Dorn P, Psallidas I, Porcel JM, Janssen J, Froudarakis M, Subotic D, Astoul P, Licht P, Schmid R, Scherpereel A, Rahman NM, Cardillo G, Maskell NA (2018) ERS/EACTS statement on the management of malignant pleural effusions. Eur Respir J 52(1):1800349. https://doi.org/10.1183/13993003.00349-2018

Brown AM, Kassab I, Massani M, Townsend W, Singal AG, Soydal C, Moreno-Luna L, Roberts LR, Chen VL, Parikh ND (2023) TACE versus TARE for patients with hepatocellular carcinoma: overall and individual patient level meta analysis. Cancer Med 12(3):2590–2599. https://doi.org/10.1002/cam4.5125

Calandri M, Yamashita S, Gazzera C, Fonio P, Veltri A, Bustreo S, Sheth RA, Yevich SM, Vauthey J-N, Odisio BC (2018) Ablation of colorectal liver metastasis: interaction of ablation margins and RAS mutation profiling on local tumour progression-free survival. Eur Radiol 28(7): 2727–2734. https://doi.org/10.1007/s00330-017-5273-2

Camacho JC, Kokabi N, Xing M, Master VA, Pattaras JG, Mittal PK, Kim HS (2015) R.E.N.A.L. (radius, exophytic/endophytic, nearness to collecting system or sinus, anterior/posterior, and location relative to polar lines) nephrometry score predicts early tumor recurrence and complications after percutaneous ablative therapies for renal cell carcinoma: a 5-year experience. J Vasc Interv Radiol 26(5):686–693. https://doi.org/10.1016/j.jvir.2015.01.008

Campbell S, Uzzo RG, Allaf ME, Bass EB, Cadeddu JA, Chang A, Clark PE, Davis BJ, Derweesh IH, Giambarresi L, Gervais DA, Hu SL, Lane BR, Leibovich BC, Pierorazio PM (2017) Renal mass and localized renal cancer: AUA guideline. J Urol 198(3):520–529. https://doi.org/10.1016/j.juro.2017.04.100

Cannon R, Ellis S, Hayes D, Narayanan G, Martin RCG (2013) Safety and early efficacy of irreversible electroporation for hepatic tumors in proximity to vital structures: IRE for hepatic tumors. J Surg Oncol 107(5):544–549. https://doi.org/10.1002/jso.23280

Cazzato RL, Garnon J, Koch G, Shaygi B, Tsoumakidou G, Caudrelier J, Boatta E, Buy X, Palussiere J, Gangi A (2018) Current role of interventional radiology in the management of visceral and bone metastases from thyroid cancer. Gland Surg 7(2):80–88. https://doi.org/10.21037/gs.2017.12.08

Cazzato RL, Palussière J, Auloge P, Rousseau C, Koch G, Dalili D, Buy X, Garnon J, De Marini P, Gangi A (2020) Complications following percutaneous image-guided radiofrequency ablation of bone tumors: a 10-year dual-center experience. Radiology 296(1):227–235. https://doi.org/10.1148/radiol.2020191905

Cheung W, Kavnoudias H, Roberts S, Szkandera B, Kemp W, Thomson KR (2013) Irreversible electroporation for unresectable hepatocellular carcinoma: initial experience and review of safety and outcomes. Technol Cancer Res Treat 12(3):233–241. https://doi.org/10.7785/tcrt.2012.500317

Chiu AM, Savoor R, Gordon AC, Riaz A, Sato KT, Hohlastos E, Salem R, Lewandowski RJ (2023) Yttrium-90 radiation segmentectomy in oligometastatic secondary hepatic malignancies. J Vasc Interv Radiol 34(3):362–368. https://doi.org/10.1016/j.jvir.2022.12.021

Cho J, Jensen TP, Reierson K, Mathews BK, Bhagra A, Franco-Sadud R, Grikis L, Mader M, Dancel R, Lucas BP, Society of Hospital Medicine Point-of-care Ultrasound Task Force, Soni NJ (2019) Recommendations on the use of ultrasound guidance for adult abdominal paracentesis: a position statement of the society of hospital medicine. J Hosp Med 14(1):E7. https://doi.org/10.12788/jhm.3095

Clark TWI, Soulen MC (2002) Chemical ablation of hepatocellular carcinoma. J Vasc Interv Radiol 13(9):S245–S252. https://doi.org/10.1016/S1051-0443(07)61792-8

Clavien P-A, Petrowsky H, DeOliveira ML, Graf R (2007) Strategies for safer liver surgery and partial liver transplantation. N Engl J Med 356(15):1545–1559. https://doi.org/10.1056/NEJMra065156

Collision Trial Group, Puijk RS, Ruarus AH, Vroomen LGPH, van Tilborg AAJM, Scheffer HJ, Nielsen K, de Jong MC, de Vries JJJ, Zonderhuis BM, Eker HH, Kazemier G, Verheul H, van der Meijs BB, van Dam L, Sorgedrager N, Coupé VMH, van den Tol PMP, Meijerink MR (2018) Colorectal liver metastases: surgery versus thermal ablation (COLLISION) – a phase III single-blind prospective randomized controlled trial. BMC Cancer 18(1):821. https://doi.org/10.1186/s12885-018-4716-8

Copelan A, Scola D, Roy A, Nghiem HV (2016) The myriad advantages of ultrasonography in image-guided interventions. Ultrasound Q 32(3):247–257. https://doi.org/10.1097/RUQ.0000000000000188

Cornelis FH, Cindrič H, Kos B, Fujimori M, Petre EN, Miklavčič D, Solomon SB, Srimathveeravalli G (2020) Peri-tumoral metallic implants reduce the efficacy of irreversible electroporation for the ablation of colorectal liver metastases. Cardiovasc Intervent Radiol 43(1):84–93. https://doi.org/10.1007/s00270-019-02300-y

Crocetti L, Lencioni R (2010) Radiofrequency ablation of pulmonary tumors. Eur J Radiol 75(1): 23–27. https://doi.org/10.1016/j.ejrad.2010.04.011

Crocetti L, Bargellini I, Cioni R (2017) Loco-regional treatment of HCC: current status. Clin Radiol 72(8):626–635. https://doi.org/10.1016/j.crad.2017.01.013

Crocetti L, Iezzi R, Goldberg SN, Bilbao JI, Sami A, Akhan O, Giuliante F, Pompili M, Malagari K, Valentini V, Gasbarrini A, Colosimo C, Manfred R (2018) The ten commandments of liver ablation: expert discussion and report from Mediterranean Interventional Oncology (MIOLive) congress 2017. Eur Rev Med Pharmacol Sci 22(12):3896–3904. https://doi.org/10.26355/eurrev_201806_15274

Crocetti L, de Baére T, Pereira PL, Tarantino FP (2020) CIRSE standards of practice on thermal ablation of liver tumours. Cardiovasc Intervent Radiol 43(7):951–962. https://doi.org/10.1007/s00270-020-02471-z

Dariushnia SR, Mitchell JW, Chaudry G, Hogan MJ (2020) Society of Interventional Radiology Quality Improvement Standards for image-guided percutaneous drainage and aspiration of abscesses and fluid collections. J Vasc Interv Radiol 31(4):662–666.e4. https://doi.org/10.1016/j.jvir.2019.12.001

Das S, Huang Y, Li B, Yu X, Xiao R, Yang H (2019) Comparing cryoablation and microwave ablation for the treatment of patients with stage IIIB/IV non-small cell lung cancer. Oncol Lett 19:1031. https://doi.org/10.3892/ol.2019.11149

Das M, van der Leij C, Katoh M, Benten D, Hendriks BMF, Hatzidakis A (2021) CIRSE standards of practice on percutaneous transhepatic cholangiography, biliary drainage and stenting. Cardiovasc Intervent Radiol 44(10):1499–1509. https://doi.org/10.1007/s00270-021-02903-4

de Baère T (2011) Lung tumor radiofrequency ablation: where do we stand? Cardiovasc Intervent Radiol 34(2):241–251. https://doi.org/10.1007/s00270-010-9860-8

de Baere T, Deschamps F, Tselikas L, Ducreux M, Planchard D, Pearson E, Berdelou A, Leboulleux S, Elias D, Baudin E (2015a) GEP-NETS UPDATE: interventional radiology: role in the treatment of liver metastases from GEP-NETs. Eur J Endocrinol 172(4): R151–R166. https://doi.org/10.1530/EJE-14-0630

de Baere T, Tselikas L, Woodrum D, Abtin F, Littrup P, Deschamps F, Suh R, Aoun HD, Callstrom M (2015b) Evaluating cryoablation of metastatic lung tumors in patients—safety and efficacy The ECLIPSE trial—interim analysis at 1 year. J Thorac Oncol 10(10):1468–1474. https://doi.org/10.1097/JTO.0000000000000632

De Cobelli F, Papa M, Panzeri M, Colombo M, Steidler S, Ambrosi A, Cao R, Gusmini S, Marra P, Capitanio U, Bertini R, Venturini M, Losa A, Gaboardi F, Montorsi F, Cardone G (2020) Percutaneous microwave ablation versus cryoablation in the treatment of T1a renal tumors. Cardiovasc Intervent Radiol 43(1):76–83. https://doi.org/10.1007/s00270-019-02313-7

Deschamps F, Farouil G, Ternes N, Gaudin A, Hakime A, Tselikas L, Teriitehau C, Baudin E, Auperin A, de Baere T (2014) Thermal ablation techniques: a curative treatment of bone metastases in selected patients? Eur Radiol 24(8):1971–1980. https://doi.org/10.1007/s00330-014-3202-1

Devane AM, Annam A, Brody L, Gunn AJ, Himes EA, Patel S, Tam AL, Dariushnia SR (2020) Society of Interventional Radiology Quality Improvement Standards for percutaneous cholecystostomy and percutaneous transhepatic biliary interventions. J Vasc Interv Radiol 31(11):1849–1856. https://doi.org/10.1016/j.jvir.2020.07.015

Dhondt E, Lambert B, Hermie L, Huyck L, Vanlangenhove P, Geerts A, Verhelst X, Aerts M, Vanlander A, Berrevoet F, Troisi RI, Van Vlierberghe H, Defreyne L (2022) 90 Y radioembolization versus drug-eluting bead chemoembolization for unresectable hepatocellular carcinoma: results from the TRACE phase II randomized controlled trial. Radiology 303(3): 699–710. https://doi.org/10.1148/radiol.211806

Dong B, Liang P, Yu X, Su L, Yu D, Cheng Z, Zhang J (2003) Percutaneous sonographically guided microwave coagulation therapy for hepatocellular carcinoma: results in 234 patients. Am J Roentgenol 180(6):1547–1555. https://doi.org/10.2214/ajr.180.6.1801547

Donington J, Ferguson M, Mazzone P, Handy J Jr, Schuchert M, Fernando H, Loo B, Lanuti M, de Hoyos A, Detterbeck F, Pennathur A, Howington J, Landreneau R, Silvestri G (2012) American College of Chest Physicians and Society of Thoracic Surgeons consensus statement for evaluation and management for high-risk patients with stage I non-small cell lung cancer. Chest 142(6):1620–1635. https://doi.org/10.1378/chest.12-0790

Dupuy DE, Fernando HC, Hillman S, Ng T, Tan AD, Sharma A, Rilling WS, Hong K, Putnam JB (2015) Radiofrequency ablation of stage IA non-small cell lung cancer in medically inoperable patients: results from the American College of Surgeons Oncology Group Z4033 (Alliance) trial: radiofrequency ablation of stage IA NSCLC. Cancer 121(19):3491–3498. https://doi.org/10.1002/cncr.29507

Efthymiou E, Siatelis A, Liakouras C, Makris G, Chrisofos M, Kelekis A, Brountzos E, Kelekis N, Filippiadis D (2021) Computed tomography-guided percutaneous microwave ablation for renal cell carcinoma: impact of tumor size on the progression survival rates. Diagnostics 11(9):1618. https://doi.org/10.3390/diagnostics11091618

Efthymiou E, Charalampopoulos G, Velonakis G, Grigoriadis S, Kelekis A, Kelekis N, Filippiadis D (2023) Ablative techniques for sarcoma metastatic disease: current role and clinical applications. Medicina 59(3):485. https://doi.org/10.3390/medicina59030485

Escudier B, Porta C, Schmidinger M, Rioux-Leclercq N, Bex A, Khoo V, Grünwald V, Gillessen S, Horwich A (2019) Renal cell carcinoma: ESMO Clinical Practice Guidelines for diagnosis, treatment and follow-up. Ann Oncol 30(5):706–720. https://doi.org/10.1093/annonc/mdz056

Feller-Kopman D, Light R (2018) Pleural disease. N Engl J Med 378(8):740–751. https://doi.org/10.1056/NEJMra1403503

Feller-Kopman DJ, Reddy CB, DeCamp MM, Diekemper RL, Gould MK, Henry T, Iyer NP, Lee YCG, Lewis SZ, Maskell NA, Rahman NM, Sterman DH, Wahidi MM, Balekian AA (2018) Management of malignant pleural effusions. An official ATS/STS/STR clinical practice guideline. Am J Respir Crit Care Med 198(7):839–849. https://doi.org/10.1164/rccm.201807-1415ST

Filippiadis DK, Tutton S, Mazioti A, Kelekis A (2014) Percutaneous image-guided ablation of bone and soft tissue tumours: a review of available techniques and protective measures. Insights Imaging 5(3):339–346. https://doi.org/10.1007/s13244-014-0332-6

Filippiadis DK, Binkert C, Pellerin O, Hoffmann RT, Krajina A, Pereira PL (2017a) CIRSE quality assurance document and standards for classification of complications: the CIRSE classification system. Cardiovasc Intervent Radiol 40(8):1141–1146. https://doi.org/10.1007/s00270-017-1703-4

Filippiadis D, Tutton S, Kelekis A (2017b) Pain management: the rising role of interventional oncology. Diagn Interv Imaging 98(9):627–634. https://doi.org/10.1016/j.diii.2017.06.015

Filippiadis D, Mauri G, Marra P, Charalampopoulos G, Gennaro N, De Cobelli F (2019a) Percutaneous ablation techniques for renal cell carcinoma: current status and future trends. Int J Hyperth 36(2):21–30. https://doi.org/10.1080/02656736.2019.1647352
Filippiadis DK, Cornelis FH, Kelekis A (2019b) Interventional oncologic procedures for pain palliation. Presse Med 48(7–8):e251–e256. https://doi.org/10.1016/j.lpm.2019.06.006
Filippiadis DK, Tselikas L, Bazzocchi A, Efthymiou E, Kelekis A, Yevich S (2020) Percutaneous management of cancer pain. Curr Oncol Rep 22(5):43. https://doi.org/10.1007/s11912-020-00906-x
Filippiadis D, Efthymiou E, Palialexis K, Brountzos E, Kelekis N (2022) Interventional oncology procedures for breast cancer metastatic disease: current role and clinical applications. Diagn Interv Radiol 28(3):249–256. https://doi.org/10.5152/dir.2022.20911
Finelli A, Ismaila N, Bro B, Durack J, Eggener S, Evans A, Gill I, Graham D, Huang W, Jewett MAS, Latcha S, Lowrance W, Rosner M, Shayegan B, Thompson RH, Uzzo R, Russo P (2017) Management of small renal masses: American Society of Clinical Oncology clinical practice guideline. J Clin Oncol 35(6):668–680. https://doi.org/10.1200/JCO.2016.69.9645
Fiorentini G, Aliberti C, Tilli M, Mulazzani L, Graziano F, Giordani P, Mambrini A, Montagnani F, Alessandroni P, Catalano V, Coschiera P (2012) Intra-arterial infusion of irinotecan-loaded drug-eluting beads (DEBIRI) versus intravenous therapy (FOLFIRI) for hepatic metastases from colorectal cancer: final results of a phase III study. Anticancer Res 32(4):1387–1395
Fortin M, Tremblay A (2015) Pleural controversies: indwelling pleural catheter vs. pleurodesis for malignant pleural effusions. J Thorac Dis 7(6):1052–1057. https://doi.org/10.3978/j.issn.2072-1439.2015.01.51
Gahan JC, Richter MD, Seideman CA, Trimmer C, Chan D, Weaver M, Olweny EO, Cadeddu JA (2015) The performance of a modified RENAL nephrometry score in predicting renal mass radiofrequency ablation success. Urology 85(1):125–129. https://doi.org/10.1016/j.urology.2014.08.026
Galle PR, Forner A, Llovet JM, Mazzaferro V, Piscaglia F, Raoul J-L, Schirmacher P, Vilgrain V (2018) EASL clinical practice guidelines: management of hepatocellular carcinoma. J Hepatol 69(1):182–236. https://doi.org/10.1016/j.jhep.2018.03.019
Georgiades C, Rodriguez R, Azene E, Weiss C, Chaux A, Gonzalez-Roibon N, Netto G (2013) Determination of the nonlethal margin inside the visible "ice-ball" during percutaneous cryoablation of renal tissue. Cardiovasc Intervent Radiol 36(3):783–790. https://doi.org/10.1007/s00270-012-0470-5
Gillams A, Goldberg N, Ahmed M, Bale R, Breen D, Callstrom M, Chen MH, Choi BI, de Baere T, Dupuy D, Gangi A, Gervais D, Helmberger T, Jung E-M, Lee F, Lencioni R, Liang P, Livraghi T, Lu D et al (2015) Thermal ablation of colorectal liver metastases: a position paper by an international panel of ablation experts, the interventional oncology sans frontières meeting 2013. Eur Radiol 25(12):3438–3454. https://doi.org/10.1007/s00330-015-3779-z
Guo J, Arellano RS (2020) Percutaneous microwave ablation of stage T1b renal cell carcinoma: short-term assessment of technical feasibility, short-term oncologic outcomes, and safety. J Endourol 34(10):1021–1027. https://doi.org/10.1089/end.2020.0382
Guo J, Arellano RS (2021) Percutaneous microwave ablation of category T1a renal cell carcinoma: intermediate results on safety, technical feasibility, and clinical outcomes of 119 tumors. AJR Am J Roentgenol 216(1):117–124. https://doi.org/10.2214/AJR.20.22818. Epub 2020 Nov 19. PMID: 32603227
Gupta S, Wallace MJ, Cardella JF, Kundu S, Miller DL, Rose SC (2010) Quality improvement guidelines for percutaneous needle biopsy. J Vasc Interv Radiol 21(7):969–975. https://doi.org/10.1016/j.jvir.2010.01.011
Hao G, Hao Y, Cheng Z, Zhang X, Cao F, Yu X, Han Z, Liu F, Mu M, Dou J, Li X, Dupuy DE, Yu J, Liang P (2018) Local tumor progression after ultrasound-guided percutaneous microwave ablation of stage T1a renal cell carcinoma: risk factors analysis of 171 tumors. Int J Hyperth 35(1):62–70. https://doi.org/10.1080/02656736.2018.1475684

Helmberger T, Golfieri R, Pech M, Pfammatter T, Arnold D, Cianni R, Maleux G, Munneke G, Pellerin O, Peynircioglu B, Sangro B, Schaefer N, de Jong N, Bilbao JI, On behalf of the CIRT Steering Committee, Pelage J-P, Manas DM, Kolligs FT, Ezziddin S et al (2021) Clinical application of trans-arterial radioembolization in hepatic malignancies in Europe: first results from the prospective multicentre observational study CIRSE registry for SIR-spheres therapy (CIRT). Cardiovasc Intervent Radiol 44(1):21–35. https://doi.org/10.1007/s00270-020-02642-y

Helmberger T, Lucatelli P, Pereira PL, Gjoreski A, Jovanoska I, Bansaghi Z, Spiliopoulos S, Carchesio F, Arnold D, Baierl A, Zeka B, Kaufmann NC, Taieb J, Iezzi R (2022) Safety, feasibility and technical considerations from a prospective, observational study—CIREL: irinotecan-TACE for CRLM in 152 patients. J Clin Med 11(20):6178. https://doi.org/10.3390/jcm11206178

Heptonstall N, Scott-Warren J, Berman R, Filippiadis D, Bell J (2023) Role of interventional radiology in pain management in oncology patients. Clin Radiol 78(4):245–253. https://doi.org/10.1016/j.crad.2022.05.022

Herold CJ, Bankier AA, Fleischmann D (1996) Lung metastases. Eur Radiol 6(5). https://doi.org/10.1007/BF00187656

Higgins LJ, Hong K (2015) Renal ablation techniques: state of the art. Am J Roentgenol 205(4): 735–741. https://doi.org/10.2214/AJR.15.14752

Hosein PJ, Echenique A, Loaiza-Bonilla A, Froud T, Barbery K, Rocha Lima CM, Yrizarry JM, Narayanan G (2014) Percutaneous irreversible electroporation for the treatment of colorectal cancer liver metastases with a proposal for a new response evaluation system. J Vasc Interv Radiol 25(8):1233–1239.e2. https://doi.org/10.1016/j.jvir.2014.04.007

Hu L, Zheng Y, Lin J, Shi X, Wang A (2023) Does adjuvant hepatic artery infusion chemotherapy improve patient outcomes for hepatocellular carcinoma following liver resection? A meta-analysis. World J Surg Oncol 21(1):121. https://doi.org/10.1186/s12957-023-03000-1

Humphrey PA, Moch H, Cubilla AL, Ulbright TM, Reuter VE (2016) The 2016 WHO classification of tumours of the urinary system and male genital organs—part B: prostate and bladder Tumours. Eur Urol 70(1):106–119. https://doi.org/10.1016/j.eururo.2016.02.028

Iannitti DA, Martin RCG, Simon CJ, Hope WW, Newcomb WL, Mcmasters KM, Dupuy D (2007) Hepatic tumor ablation with clustered microwave antennae: the US phase II trial. HPB 9(2): 120–124. https://doi.org/10.1080/13651820701222677

Ierardi AM, Puliti A, Angileri SA, Petrillo M, Duka E, Floridi C, Lecchi M, Carrafiello G (2017) Microwave ablation of malignant renal tumours: intermediate-term results and usefulness of RENAL and mRENAL scores for predicting outcomes and complications. Med Oncol 34(5):97. https://doi.org/10.1007/s12032-017-0948-8

Iezzi R, Pompili M, Posa A, Annicchiarico E, Garcovich M, Merlino B, Rodolfino E, Di Noia V, Basso M, Cassano A, Barone C, Gasbarrini A, Manfredi R, Colosimo C (2017) Transradial versus transfemoral access for hepatic chemoembolization: intrapatient prospective single-center study. J Vasc Interv Radiol 28(9):1234–1239. https://doi.org/10.1016/j.jvir.2017.06.022

Jaffe TA, Nelson RC (2016) Image-guided percutaneous drainage: a review. Abdom Radiol 41(4): 629–636. https://doi.org/10.1007/s00261-016-0649-3

Jiang B, Mcclure M, Chen T, Chen S (2018) Efficacy and safety of thermal ablation of lung malignancies: a network meta-analysis. Ann Thorac Med 13(4):243. https://doi.org/10.4103/atm.ATM_392_17

Jogi S, Varanai R, Bantu SS, Manne A (2020) Selecting the first line treatment in non-metastatic hepatocellular carcinoma—comparing clinical practice guidelines. Oncol Rev 14(2). https://doi.org/10.4081/oncol.2020.515

Kambadakone A, Thabet A, Gervais DA, Mueller PR, Arellano RS (2011) CT-guided celiac plexus neurolysis: a review of anatomy, indications, technique, and tips for successful treatment. RadioGraphics 31(6):1599–1621. https://doi.org/10.1148/rg.316115526

Katsanos K, Mailli L, Krokidis M, McGrath A, Sabharwal T, Adam A (2014) Systematic review and meta-analysis of thermal ablation versus surgical nephrectomy for small renal tumours. Cardiovasc Intervent Radiol 37(2):427–437. https://doi.org/10.1007/s00270-014-0846-9

Katsanos K, Kitrou P, Spiliopoulos S, Maroulis I, Petsas T, Karnabatidis D (2017) Comparative effectiveness of different transarterial embolization therapies alone or in combination with local ablative or adjuvant systemic treatments for unresectable hepatocellular carcinoma: a network meta-analysis of randomized controlled trials. PLoS One 12(9):e0184597. https://doi.org/10.1371/journal.pone.0184597

Kelekis A, Cornelis F, Tutton S, Filippiadis D (2017) Metastatic osseous pain control: bone ablation and cementoplasty. Semin Interv Radiol 34(04):328–336. https://doi.org/10.1055/s-0037-1608747

Kennedy AS, Dezarn WA, McNeillie P, Coldwell D, Nutting C, Carter D, Murthy R, Rose S, Warner RRP, Liu D, Palmedo H, Overton C, Jones B, Salem R (2008) Radioembolization for unresectable neuroendocrine hepatic metastases using resin 90Y-microspheres: early results in 148 patients. Am J Clin Oncol 31(3):271–279. https://doi.org/10.1097/COC.0b013e31815e4557

Kennedy S, Milovanovic L, Midia M (2015) Major bleeding after percutaneous image-guided biopsies: frequency, predictors, and periprocedural management. Semin Interv Radiol 32(01):026–033. https://doi.org/10.1055/s-0034-1396961

Kim SY, Chung HW, Oh TS, Lee J-S (2017) Practical guidelines for ultrasound-guided Core needle biopsy of soft-tissue lesions: transformation from beginner to specialist. Korean J Radiol 18(2):361. https://doi.org/10.3348/kjr.2017.18.2.361

Kim SP, Cohalan C, Kopek N, Enger SA (2019) A guide to 90Y radioembolization and its dosimetry. Phys Med 68:132–145. https://doi.org/10.1016/j.ejmp.2019.09.236

Klapperich ME, Abel EJ, Ziemlewicz TJ, Best S, Lubner MG, Nakada SY, Hinshaw JL, Brace CL, Lee FT, Wells SA (2017) Effect of tumor complexity and technique on efficacy and complications after percutaneous microwave ablation of stage T1a renal cell carcinoma: a single-center, retrospective study. Radiology 284(1):272–280. https://doi.org/10.1148/radiol.2016160592

Koegelenberg CFN, Shaw JA, Irusen EM, Lee YCG (2018) Contemporary best practice in the management of malignant pleural effusion. Ther Adv Respir Dis 12:175346661878509. https://doi.org/10.1177/1753466618785098

Koyyalagunta D, Engle MP, Yu J, Feng L, Novy DM (2016) The effectiveness of alcohol versus phenol based splanchnic nerve neurolysis for the treatment of intra-abdominal cancer pain. Pain Physician 19(4):281–292

Krokidis ME, Orsi F, Katsanos K, Helmberger T, Adam A (2017) CIRSE guidelines on percutaneous ablation of small renal cell carcinoma. Cardiovasc Intervent Radiol 40(2):177–191. https://doi.org/10.1007/s00270-016-1531-y

Kurilova I, Gonzalez-Aguirre A, Beets-Tan RG, Erinjeri J, Petre EN, Gonen M, Bains M, Kemeny NE, Solomon SB, Sofocleous CT (2018) Microwave ablation in the management of colorectal cancer pulmonary metastases. Cardiovasc Intervent Radiol 41(10):1530–1544. https://doi.org/10.1007/s00270-018-2000-6

Kurup A, Callstrom M (2010) Image-guided percutaneous ablation of bone and soft tissue tumors. Semin Interv Radiol 27(03):276–284. https://doi.org/10.1055/s-0030-1261786

Kutikov A, Uzzo RG (2009) The R.E.N.A.L. Nephrometry score: a comprehensive standardized system for quantitating renal tumor size, location and depth. J Urol 182(3):844–853. https://doi.org/10.1016/j.juro.2009.05.035

Lam A, Yoshida EJ, Bui K, Fernando D, Nelson K, Abi-Jaoudeh N (2018) A National Cancer Database analysis of radiofrequency ablation versus stereotactic body radiotherapy in early-stage non–small cell lung cancer. J Vasc Interv Radiol 29(9):1211–1217.e1. https://doi.org/10.1016/j.jvir.2018.04.029

Lencioni R, Petruzzi P, Crocetti L (2013) Chemoembolization of hepatocellular carcinoma. Semin Interv Radiol 30(01):003–011. https://doi.org/10.1055/s-0033-1333648

Leung L, Hsin M, Lam KC (2013) Management of malignant pleural effusion: options and recommended approaches: management of malignant pleural effusion. Thorac Cancer 4(1):9–13. https://doi.org/10.1111/j.1759-7714.2012.00150.x

Levinson AW, Su L-M, Agarwal D, Sroka M, Jarrett TW, Kavoussi LR, Solomon SB (2008) Long-term oncological and overall outcomes of percutaneous radio frequency ablation in high risk surgical patients with a solitary small renal mass. J Urol 180(2):499–504. https://doi.org/10.1016/j.juro.2008.04.031

Lim E, Kumar S, Seager M, Modi S, Mandal I, Neves JB, Jones S, Tran MGB, Munneke G, Bandula S, Walkden M (2020) Outcomes of renal tumors treated by image-guided percutaneous cryoablation: immediate and 3- and 5-year outcomes at a regional center. Am J Roentgenol 215(1):242–247. https://doi.org/10.2214/AJR.19.22213

Lin Y-M, Paolucci I, Brock KK, Odisio BC (2021) Image-guided ablation for colorectal liver metastasis: principles, current evidence, and the path forward. Cancers 13(16):3926. https://doi.org/10.3390/cancers13163926

Lindsay A, Burton J, Ray C (2014) Paracentesis-induced circulatory dysfunction: a primer for the interventional radiologist. Semin Interv Radiol 31(03):276–278. https://doi.org/10.1055/s-0034-1382799

Liu C, Liang P, Liu F, Wang Y, Li X, Han Z, Liu C (2011) MWA combined with TACE as a combined therapy for unresectable large-sized hepotocellular carcinoma. Int J Hyperth 27(7): 654–662. https://doi.org/10.3109/02656736.2011.605099

Liu Y-S, Lin C-Y, Chuang M-T, Tsai Y-S, Wang C-K, Ou M-C (2018) Success and complications of percutaneous transhepatic biliary drainage are influenced by liver entry segment and level of catheter placement. Abdom Radiol 43(3):713–722. https://doi.org/10.1007/s00261-017-1258-5

Liu C, Tadros G, Smith Q, Martinez L, Jeffries J, Yu Z, Yu Q (2022) Selective internal radiation therapy of metastatic breast cancer to the liver: a meta-analysis. Front Oncol 12:887653. https://doi.org/10.3389/fonc.2022.887653

Livraghi T, Meloni F, Di Stasi M, Rolle E, Solbiati L, Tinelli C, Rossi S (2007) Sustained complete response and complications rates after radiofrequency ablation of very early hepatocellular carcinoma in cirrhosis: is resection still the treatment of choice? Hepatology 47(1):82–89. https://doi.org/10.1002/hep.21933

Ljungberg B, Albiges L, Abu-Ghanem Y, Bensalah K, Dabestani S, Fernández-Pello S, Giles RH, Hofmann F, Hora M, Kuczyk MA, Kuusk T, Lam TB, Marconi L, Merseburger AS, Powles T, Staehler M, Tahbaz R, Volpe A, Bex A (2019) European Association of Urology guidelines on renal cell carcinoma: the 2019 update. Eur Urol 75(5):799–810. https://doi.org/10.1016/j.eururo.2019.02.011

Llovet J, Brú C, Bruix J (1999) Prognosis of hepatocellular carcinoma: the BCLC staging classification. Semin Liver Dis 19(03):329–338. https://doi.org/10.1055/s-2007-1007122

Lu M, Chen J, Xie X, Liu L, Huang X, Liang L, Huang J (2001) Hepatocellular carcinoma: US-guided percutaneous microwave coagulation therapy. Radiology 221(1):167–172. https://doi.org/10.1148/radiol.2211001783

Lu M-D, Xu H-X, Xie X-Y, Yin X-Y, Chen J-W, Kuang M, Xu Z-F, Liu G-J, Zheng Y-L (2005) Percutaneous microwave and radiofrequency ablation for hepatocellular carcinoma: a retrospective comparative study. J Gastroenterol 40(11):1054–1060. https://doi.org/10.1007/s00535-005-1671-3

Lucatelli P, Burrel M, Guiu B, de Rubeis G, van Delden O, Helmberger T (2021) CIRSE standards of practice on hepatic transarterial chemoembolisation. Cardiovasc Intervent Radiol 44(12): 1851–1867. https://doi.org/10.1007/s00270-021-02968-1

Lyons GR, Askin G, Pua BB (2018) Clinical outcomes after pulmonary cryoablation with the use of a triple freeze protocol. J Vasc Interv Radiol 29(5):714–721. https://doi.org/10.1016/j.jvir.2017.12.029

Ma Y, Wallace AN, Waqar SN, Morgensztern D, Madaelil TP, Tomasian A, Jennings JW (2017) Percutaneous image-guided ablation in the treatment of osseous metastases from non-small cell lung cancer. Cardiovasc Intervent Radiol 41:726. https://doi.org/10.1007/s00270-017-1843-6

Macchi M, Belfiore MP, Floridi C, Serra N, Belfiore G, Carmignani L, Grasso RF, Mazza E, Pusceddu C, Brunese L, Carrafiello G (2017) Radiofrequency versus microwave ablation for treatment of the lung tumours: LUMIRA (lung microwave radiofrequency) randomized trial. Med Oncol 34(5):96. https://doi.org/10.1007/s12032-017-0946-x

Maciolek KA, Abel EJ, Posielski NM, Hinshaw JL, Lubner MG, Lee FT, Ziemlewicz TJ, Wells SA (2019) Tumor location does not impact oncologic outcomes for percutaneous microwave ablation of clinical T1a renal cell carcinoma. Eur Radiol 29(11):6319–6329. https://doi.org/10.1007/s00330-019-06121-y

Malagari K, Pomoni M, Moschouris H, Kelekis A, Charokopakis A, Bouma E, Spyridopoulos T, Chatziioannou A, Sotirchos V, Karampelas T, Tamvakopoulos C, Filippiadis D, Karagiannis E, Marinis A, Koskinas J, Kelekis DA (2014) Chemoembolization of hepatocellular carcinoma with hepasphere 30–60 μm. Safety and efficacy study. Cardiovasc Intervent Radiol 37(1): 165–175. https://doi.org/10.1007/s00270-013-0777-x

Martin RCG, Scoggins CR, Schreeder M, Rilling WS, Laing CJ, Tatum CM, Kelly LR, Garcia-Monaco RD, Sharma VR, Crocenzi TS, Strasberg SM (2015) Randomized controlled trial of irinotecan drug-eluting beads with simultaneous FOLFOX and bevacizumab for patients with unresectable colorectal liver-limited metastasis: irinotecan intrahepatic arterial chemotherapy. Cancer 121(20):3649–3658. https://doi.org/10.1002/cncr.29534

Martinez-Zayas G, Molina S, Ost DE (2022) Sensitivity and complications of thoracentesis and thoracoscopy: a meta-analysis. Eur Respir Rev 31(166):220053. https://doi.org/10.1183/16000617.0053-2022

Matsusaki K, Aridome K, Emoto S, Kajiyama H, Takagaki N, Takahashi T, Tsubamoto H, Nagao S, Watanabe A, Shimada H, Kitayama J (2022) Clinical practice guideline for the treatment of malignant ascites: section summary in clinical practice guideline for peritoneal dissemination (2021). Int J Clin Oncol 27(1):1–6. https://doi.org/10.1007/s10147-021-02077-6

Mattie R, Brar N, Tram JT, McCormick ZL, Beall DP, Fox A, Saltychev M (2021) Vertebral augmentation of cancer-related spinal compression fractures: a systematic review and meta-analysis. Spine 46(24):1729–1737. https://doi.org/10.1097/BRS.0000000000004093

McDougal WS, Gervais DA, McGovern FJ, Mueller PR (2005) Long-term followup of patients with renal cell carcinoma treated with radio frequency ablation with curative intent. J Urol 174(1):61–63. https://doi.org/10.1097/01.ju.0000162046.45024.2b

McMenomy BP, Kurup AN, Johnson GB, Carter RE, McWilliams RR, Markovic SN, Atwell TD, Schmit GD, Morris JM, Woodrum DA, Weisbrod AJ, Rose PS, Callstrom MR (2013) Percutaneous cryoablation of musculoskeletal oligometastatic disease for complete remission. J Vasc Interv Radiol 24(2):207–213. https://doi.org/10.1016/j.jvir.2012.10.019

Meek RD, Mills MK, Hanrahan CJ, Beckett BR, Leake RL, Allen H, Williams DD, Tommack M, Schmahmann S, Hansford BG (2020) Pearls and pitfalls for soft-tissue and bone biopsies: a cross-institutional review. RadioGraphics 40(1):266–290. https://doi.org/10.1148/rg.2020190089

Memon K, Lewandowski RJ, Kulik L, Riaz A, Mulcahy MF, Salem R (2011) Radioembolization for primary and metastatic liver cancer. Semin Radiat Oncol 21(4):294–302. https://doi.org/10.1016/j.semradonc.2011.05.004

Mitra V, Metcalf J (2009) Functional anatomy and blood supply of the liver. Anaesth Intensive Care Med 10(7):332–333. https://doi.org/10.1016/j.mpaic.2009.03.012

Molina CA, Gokaslan ZL, Sciubba DM (2012) Diagnosis and management of metastatic cervical spine tumors. Orthop Clin N Am 43(1):75–87. https://doi.org/10.1016/j.ocl.2011.08.004

Mosconi C, Solaini L, Vara G, Brandi N, Cappelli A, Modestino F, Cucchetti A, Golfieri R (2021) Transarterial chemoembolization and radioembolization for unresectable intrahepatic cholangiocarcinoma—a systemic review and meta-analysis. Cardiovasc Intervent Radiol 44(5):728–738. https://doi.org/10.1007/s00270-021-02800-w

Mosconi C, O'Rourke J, Kloeckner R, Sturm L, Golfieri R, Celsa C, Fateen W, Odisio BC, Garanzini EM, Peck-Radosavljevic M, Borghi A, Ma YT, Stoehr F, Bettinger D, Giuffrida P, Aithal GP, Lin Y-M, Spreafico C, Giampalma E et al (2023) Textbook outcome after transarterial chemoembolization for hepatocellular carcinoma. Cardiovasc Intervent Radiol 46(4): 449–459. https://doi.org/10.1007/s00270-023-03375-4

Motzer RJ, Jonasch E, Agarwal N, Bhayani S, Bro WP, Chang SS, Choueiri TK, Costello BA, Derweesh IH, Fishman M, Gallagher TH, Gore JL, Hancock SL, Harrison MR, Kim W, Kyriakopoulos C, LaGrange C, Lam ET, Lau C et al (2017) Kidney cancer, version 2.2017, NCCN clinical practice guidelines in oncology. J Natl Compr Cancer Netw 15(6):804–834. https://doi.org/10.6004/jnccn.2017.0100

Moussa AM, Ziv E, Solomon SB, Camacho JC (2019) Microwave ablation in primary lung malignancies. Semin Interv Radiol 36(04):326–333. https://doi.org/10.1055/s-0039-1700567

Mulcahy MF, Mahvash A, Pracht M, Montazeri AH, Bandula S, Martin RCG, Herrmann K, Brown E, Zuckerman D, Wilson G, Kim T-Y, Weaver A, Ross P, Harris WP, Graham J, Mills J, Yubero Esteban A, Johnson MS, Sofocleous CT et al (2021) Radioembolization with chemotherapy for colorectal liver metastases: a randomized, open-label, international, multicenter, phase III trial. J Clin Oncol 39(35):3897–3907. https://doi.org/10.1200/JCO.21.01839

Murray FR, Gnehm F, Schindler V, Morell B, Gubler C, Kretschmer E-M, Bütikofer S (2022) Permanent tunneled drainage of ascites in palliative patients: timing needs evaluation. J Palliat Med 25(7):1132–1135. https://doi.org/10.1089/jpm.2021.0506

Nielsen TK, Vedel PF, Borgbjerg J, Andersen G, Borre M (2020) Renal cryoablation: five- and 10-year survival outcomes in patients with biopsy-proven renal cell carcinoma. Scand J Urol 54(5):408–412. https://doi.org/10.1080/21681805.2020.1794954

O'Shea A, Tam AL, Kilcoyne A, Flaherty KT, Lee SI (2021) Image-guided biopsy in the age of personalised medicine: strategies for success and safety. Clin Radiol 76(2):154.e1–154.e9. https://doi.org/10.1016/j.crad.2020.08.010

Padia SA, Lewandowski RJ, Johnson GE, Sze DY, Ward TJ, Gaba RC, Baerlocher MO, Gates VL, Riaz A, Brown DB, Siddiqi NH, Walker TG, Silberzweig JE, Mitchell JW, Nikolic B, Salem R (2017) Radioembolization of hepatic malignancies: background, quality improvement guidelines, and future directions. J Vasc Interv Radiol 28(1):1–15. https://doi.org/10.1016/j.jvir.2016.09.024

Palussière J, Chomy F, Savina M, Deschamps F, Gaubert JY, Renault A, Bonnefoy O, Laurent F, Meunier C, Bellera C, Mathoulin-Pelissier S, de Baere T (2018) Radiofrequency ablation of stage IA non–small cell lung cancer in patients ineligible for surgery: results of a prospective multicenter phase II trial. J Cardiothorac Surg 13(1):91. https://doi.org/10.1186/s13019-018-0773-y

Palussière J, Catena V, Lagarde P, Cousin S, Cabart M, Buy X, Chomy F (2019) Primary tumors of the lung: should we consider thermal ablation as a valid therapeutic option? Int J Hyperth 36(2): 46–52. https://doi.org/10.1080/02656736.2019.1647351

Pellerin O, Medioni J, Vulser C, Déan C, Oudard S, Sapoval M (2014) Management of painful pelvic bone metastasis of renal cell carcinoma using embolization, radio-frequency ablation, and cementoplasty: a prospective evaluation of efficacy and safety. Cardiovasc Intervent Radiol 37(3):730–736. https://doi.org/10.1007/s00270-013-0740-x

Pérez-López A, Martín-Sabroso C, Gómez-Lázaro L, Torres-Suárez AI, Aparicio-Blanco J (2022) Embolization therapy with microspheres for the treatment of liver cancer: state-of-the-art of clinical translation. Acta Biomater 149:1–15. https://doi.org/10.1016/j.actbio.2022.07.019

Poggi G, Montagna B, Di Cesare P, Melchiorre F, Riva G. (2013) Combined percutaneous microwave ablation (MWA) and transarterial chemoembolization for hepatocellular carcinoma. J Hepatol 58:S113

Poggi G, Tosoratti N, Montagna B, Picchi C (2015) Microwave ablation of hepatocellular carcinoma. World J Hepatol 7(25):2578–2589. https://doi.org/10.4254/wjh.v7.i25.2578

Postmus PE, Kerr KM, Oudkerk M, Senan S, Waller DA, Vansteenkiste J, Escriu C, Peters S (2017) Early and locally advanced non-small-cell lung cancer (NSCLC): ESMO clinical practice guidelines for diagnosis, treatment and follow-up. Ann Oncol 28:iv1–iv21. https://doi.org/10.1093/annonc/mdx222

Prud'homme C, Nueffer J-P, Runge M, Dubut J, Kastler B, Aubry S (2017) Prospective pilot study of CT-guided microwave ablation in the treatment of osteoid osteomas. Skelet Radiol 46(3): 315–323. https://doi.org/10.1007/s00256-016-2558-5

Psutka SP, Feldman AS, McDougal WS, McGovern FJ, Mueller P, Gervais DA (2013) Long-term oncologic outcomes after radiofrequency ablation for T1 renal cell carcinoma. Eur Urol 63(3): 486–492. https://doi.org/10.1016/j.eururo.2012.08.062

Puijk RS, Ahmed M, Adam A, Arai Y, Arellano R, de Baère T, Bale R, Bellera C, Binkert CA, Brace CL, Breen DJ, Brountzos E, Callstrom MR, Carrafiello G, Chapiro J, de Cobelli F, Coupé VMH, Crocetti L, Denys A et al (2021) Consensus guidelines for the definition of time-to-event end points in image-guided tumor ablation: results of the SIO and DATECAN initiative. Radiology 301(3):533–540. https://doi.org/10.1148/radiol.2021203715

Rees J, Mytton J, Evison F, Mangat KS, Patel P, Trudgill N (2020) The outcomes of biliary drainage by percutaneous transhepatic cholangiography for the palliation of malignant biliary obstruction in England between 2001 and 2014: a retrospective cohort study. BMJ Open 10(1): e033576. https://doi.org/10.1136/bmjopen-2019-033576

Reig M, Forner A, Rimola J, Ferrer-Fàbrega J, Burrel M, Garcia-Criado Á, Kelley RK, Galle PR, Mazzaferro V, Salem R, Sangro B, Singal AG, Vogel A, Fuster J, Ayuso C, Bruix J (2022) BCLC strategy for prognosis prediction and treatment recommendation: the 2022 update. J Hepatol 76(3):681–693. https://doi.org/10.1016/j.jhep.2021.11.018

Reyes J, Canter D, Putnam S, Simhan J, Smaldone MC, Kutikov A, Viterbo R, Chen DYT, Uzzo RG (2013) Thermal ablation of the small renal mass: case selection using the R.E.N.A.L.-Nephrometry Score. Urol Oncol Semin Orig Investig 31(7):1292–1297. https://doi.org/10.1016/j.urolonc.2011.09.006

Ripamonti CI, Santini D, Maranzano E, Berti M, Roila F (2012) Management of cancer pain: ESMO Clinical Practice Guidelines. Ann Oncol 23:vii139–vii154. https://doi.org/10.1093/annonc/mds233

Ruers T, Van Coevorden F, Punt CJA, Pierie J-PEN, Borel-Rinkes I, Ledermann JA, Poston G, Bechstein W, Lentz M-A, Mauer M, Folprecht G, Van Cutsem E, Ducreux M, Nordlinger B (2017) Local treatment of unresectable colorectal liver metastases: results of a randomized phase II trial. J Natl Cancer Inst 109(9). https://doi.org/10.1093/jnci/djx015

Ryan A, Byrne C, Pusceddu C, Buy X, Tsoumakidou G, Filippiadis D (2022) CIRSE standards of practice on thermal ablation of bone tumours. Cardiovasc Intervent Radiol 45(5):591–605. https://doi.org/10.1007/s00270-022-03126-x

Saldanha D, Khiatani V, Carrillo T, Yap F, Bui J, Knuttinen M, Owens C, Gaba R (2010) Current tumor ablation technologies: basic science and device review. Semin Interv Radiol 27(03): 247–254. https://doi.org/10.1055/s-0030-1261782

Salem R, Gabr A, Riaz A, Mora R, Ali R, Abecassis M, Hickey R, Kulik L, Ganger D, Flamm S, Atassi R, Atassi B, Sato K, Benson AB, Mulcahy MF, Abouchaleh N, Asadi AA, Desai K, Thornburg B et al (2018) Institutional decision to adopt Y90 as primary treatment for hepatocellular carcinoma informed by a 1,000-patient 15-year experience. Hepatology 68(4): 1429–1440. https://doi.org/10.1002/hep.29691

Sangisetty SL (2012) Malignant ascites: a review of prognostic factors, pathophysiology and therapeutic measures. World J Gastrointest Surg 4(4):87. https://doi.org/10.4240/wjgs.v4.i4.87

Schmit GD, Schenck LA, Thompson RH, Boorjian SA, Kurup AN, Weisbrod AJ, Kor DJ, Callstrom MR, Atwell TD, Carter RE (2014) Predicting renal cryoablation complications: new risk score based on tumor size and location and patient history. Radiology 272(3): 903–910. https://doi.org/10.1148/radiol.14132548

Scott-Warren J, Bhaskar A (2014) Cancer pain management—part I: general principles. Contin Educ Anaesth Crit Care Pain 14(6):278–284

Seager M, Kumar S, Lim E, Munneke G, Bandula S, Walkden M (2021) Renal cryoablation – a practical guide for interventional radiologists. Br J Radiol 94(1118):20200854. https://doi.org/10.1259/bjr.20200854

Seifert JK, Junginger T (2004) Cryotherapy for liver tumors: current status, perspectives, clinical results, and review of literature. Technol Cancer Res Treat 3(2):151–163. https://doi.org/10.1177/153303460400300208

Shibata T, Iimuro Y, Yamamoto Y, Maetani Y, Ametani F, Itoh K, Konishi J (2002) Small hepatocellular carcinoma: comparison of radio-frequency ablation and percutaneous microwave coagulation therapy. Radiology 223(2):331–337. https://doi.org/10.1148/radiol.2232010775

Siegel RL, Miller KD, Fuchs HE, Jemal A (2022) Cancer statistics, 2022. CA Cancer J Clin 72(1): 7–33. https://doi.org/10.3322/caac.21708

Sofocleous CT, Petre EN, Gonen M, Brown KT, Solomon SB, Covey AM, Alago W, Brody LA, Thornton RH, D'Angelica M, Fong Y, Kemeny NE (2011) CT-guided radiofrequency ablation as a salvage treatment of colorectal cancer hepatic metastases developing after hepatectomy. J Vasc Interv Radiol 22(6):755–761. https://doi.org/10.1016/j.jvir.2011.01.451

Solbiati L, Ahmed M, Cova L, Ierace T, Brioschi M, Goldberg SN (2012) Small liver colorectal metastases treated with percutaneous radiofrequency ablation: local response rate and long-term survival with up to 10-year follow-up. Radiology 265(3):958–968. https://doi.org/10.1148/radiol.12111851

Soni NJ, Franco R, Velez MI, Schnobrich D, Dancel R, Restrepo MI, Mayo PH (2015) Ultrasound in the diagnosis and management of pleural effusions: ultrasound and pleural effusions. J Hosp Med 10(12):811–816. https://doi.org/10.1002/jhm.2434

Spiliopoulos S, Moschovaki-Zeiger O, Sethi A, Festas G, Reppas L, Filippiadis D, Kelekis N (2023) An update on locoregional percutaneous treatment technologies in colorectal cancer liver metastatic disease. Expert Rev Med Devices 20(4):293–302. https://doi.org/10.1080/17434440.2023.2185137

Storozhakova AE, Vladimirova LY, Kit OI, Kolesnikov EN, Snezhko AV, Chernyak MN, Snezhko TA, Samaneva NY, Svetitskaya YV, Kalabanova EA, Kabanov SN, Tishina AV, Teplyakova MA, Lisutin AE (2020) Outcomes of transarterial chemoembolization (TACE) of the liver in patients with metastatic triple-negative breast cancer (TNBC). J Clin Oncol 38(15_suppl): e13107. https://doi.org/10.1200/JCO.2020.38.15_suppl.e13107

Sun AX, Cheng ZL, Wu PP, Sheng YH, Qu XJ, Lu W, Zhao CG, Qian GJ (2015) Clinical outcome of medium-sized hepatocellular carcinoma treated with microwave ablation. World J Gastroenterol 21(10):2997. https://doi.org/10.3748/wjg.v21.i10.2997

Sunderland N, Maweni R, Akunuri S, Karnovitch E (2016) Re-expansion pulmonary oedema: a novel emergency therapeutic option. BMJ Case Rep bcr2016215076. https://doi.org/10.1136/bcr-2016-215076

Talenfeld AD, Gennarelli RL, Elkin EB, Atoria CL, Durack JC, Huang WC, Kwan SW (2018) Percutaneous ablation versus partial and radical nephrectomy for T1a renal cancer: a population-based analysis. Ann Intern Med 169(2):69. https://doi.org/10.7326/M17-0585

Tam AL, Lim HJ, Wistuba II, Tamrazi A, Kuo MD, Ziv E, Wong S, Shih AJ, Webster RJ, Fischer GS, Nagrath S, Davis SE, White SB, Ahrar K (2016) Image-guided biopsy in the era of personalized cancer care: proceedings from the Society of Interventional Radiology Research Consensus Panel. J Vasc Interv Radiol 27(1):8–19. https://doi.org/10.1016/j.jvir.2015.10.019

Tao YX, Li HW, Luo JT, Li Y, Wei WB (2023) Regional chemotherapy for uveal melanoma liver metastases. Int J Ophthalmol 16(2):293–300. https://doi.org/10.18240/ijo.2023.02.18

Tomasian A, Jennings JW (2020) Percutaneous minimally invasive thermal ablation of osseous metastases: evidence-based practice guidelines. Am J Roentgenol 215(2):502–510. https://doi.org/10.2214/AJR.19.22521

Tomasian A, Hillen TJ, Jennings JW (2020) Bone biopsies: what radiologists need to know. Am J Roentgenol 215(3):523–533. https://doi.org/10.2214/AJR.20.22809

Tomasian A, Filippiadis DK, Tutton S, Deschamps F, Cazzato RL, Prologo JD, Kelekis A, Levy J, Gangi A, Garnon J, Jennings JW (2022) Comprehensive palliative musculoskeletal interventional radiology care for patients with cancer. RadioGraphics 42(6):1654–1669. https://doi.org/10.1148/rg.220009

Tracy CR, Raman JD, Donnally C, Trimmer CK, Cadeddu JA (2010) Durable oncologic outcomes after radiofrequency ablation: experience from treating 243 small renal masses over 7.5 years. Cancer 116(13):3135–3142. https://doi.org/10.1002/cncr.25002

Trumm CG, Hoffmann R-T, Thomas C (2013) Biopsy. In: Mahnken AH, Wilhelm KE, Ricke J (eds) CT- and MR-guided interventions in radiology. Springer, Berlin Heidelberg, pp 115–148

Tsoumakidou G, Too CW, Koch G, Caudrelier J, Cazzato RL, Garnon J, Gangi A (2017) CIRSE guidelines on percutaneous vertebral augmentation. Cardiovasc Intervent Radiol 40(3): 331–342. https://doi.org/10.1007/s00270-017-1574-8

Uberoi R, Das N, Moss J, Robertson I (2012) British Society of Interventional Radiology: biliary drainage and stenting registry (BDSR). Cardiovasc Intervent Radiol 35(1):127–138. https://doi.org/10.1007/s00270-011-0103-4

Uhlig J, Ludwig JM, Goldberg SB, Chiang A, Blasberg JD, Kim HS (2018) Survival rates after thermal ablation versus stereotactic radiation therapy for stage 1 non–small cell lung cancer: a National Cancer Database Study. Radiology 289(3):862–870. https://doi.org/10.1148/radiol.2018180979

Van Cutsem E, Cervantes A, Adam R, Sobrero A, Van Krieken JH, Aderka D, Aranda Aguilar E, Bardelli A, Benson A, Bodoky G, Ciardiello F, D'Hoore A, Diaz-Rubio E, Douillard J-Y, Ducreux M, Falcone A, Grothey A, Gruenberger T, Haustermans K et al (2016) ESMO consensus guidelines for the management of patients with metastatic colorectal cancer. Ann Oncol 27(8):1386–1422. https://doi.org/10.1093/annonc/mdw235

van Dam L, Geeraedts T, Bijdevaate D, van Doormaal PJ, The A, Moelker A (2019) Distal radial artery access for noncoronary endovascular treatment is a safe and feasible technique. J Vasc Interv Radiol 30(8):1281–1285. https://doi.org/10.1016/j.jvir.2019.01.011

van Hazel GA, Heinemann V, Sharma NK, Findlay MPN, Ricke J, Peeters M, Perez D, Robinson BA, Strickland AH, Ferguson T, Rodríguez J, Kröning H, Wolf I, Ganju V, Walpole E, Boucher E, Tichler T, Shacham-Shmueli E, Powell A et al (2016) SIRFLOX: randomized phase III trial comparing first-line mFOLFOX6 (plus or minus bevacizumab) versus mFOLFOX6 (plus or minus bevacizumab) plus selective internal radiation therapy in patients with metastatic colorectal cancer. J Clin Oncol 34(15):1723–1731. https://doi.org/10.1200/JCO.2015.66.1181

Vaswani D, Wallace AN, Eiswirth PS, Madaelil TP, Chang RO, Tomasian A, Jennings JW (2018) Radiographic local tumor control and pain palliation of sarcoma metastases within the musculoskeletal system with percutaneous thermal ablation. Cardiovasc Intervent Radiol 41(8): 1223–1232. https://doi.org/10.1007/s00270-018-1932-1

Veltri A, Bargellini I, Giorgi L, Almeida PAMS, Akhan O (2017) CIRSE guidelines on percutaneous needle biopsy (PNB). Cardiovasc Intervent Radiol 40(10):1501–1513. https://doi.org/10.1007/s00270-017-1658-5

Venturini M, Cariati M, Marra P, Masala S, Pereira PL, Carrafiello G (2020) CIRSE standards of practice on thermal ablation of primary and secondary lung tumours. Cardiovasc Intervent Radiol 43(5):667–683. https://doi.org/10.1007/s00270-020-02432-6

Vietti Violi N, Duran R, Guiu B, Cercueil J-P, Aubé C, Digklia A, Pache I, Deltenre P, Knebel J-F, Denys A (2018) Efficacy of microwave ablation versus radiofrequency ablation for the treatment of hepatocellular carcinoma in patients with chronic liver disease: a randomised controlled phase 2 trial. Lancet Gastroenterol Hepatol 3(5):317–325. https://doi.org/10.1016/S2468-1253(18)30029-3

Vogel A, ESMO, Padia SA, Lewandowski RJ, Johnson GE, et al; Society of Interventional Radiology Standards of Practice Committee (2017) Radioembolization of hepatic malignancies: background, quality improvement guidelines, and future directions. J Vasc Interv Radiol 28(1): 1–15

Vogel A, Cervantes A, Chau I, Daniele B, Llovet JM, Meyer T, Nault J-C, Neumann U, Ricke J, Sangro B, Schirmacher P, Verslype C, Zech CJ, Arnold D, Martinelli E (2018) Hepatocellular carcinoma: ESMO Clinical Practice Guidelines for diagnosis, treatment and follow-up. Ann Oncol 29:iv238–iv255. https://doi.org/10.1093/annonc/mdy308

Vogel A, Ochsenreither S, Zager JS, Wacker F, Saborowski A (2023) Chemosaturation for primary and secondary liver malignancies: a comprehensive update of current evidence. Cancer Treat Rev 113:102501. https://doi.org/10.1016/j.ctrv.2022.102501

Vogl TJ, Naguib NNN, Lehnert T, Nour-Eldin N-EA (2011) Radiofrequency, microwave and laser ablation of pulmonary neoplasms: clinical studies and technical considerations—review article. Eur J Radiol 77(2):346–357. https://doi.org/10.1016/j.ejrad.2009.07.034

Vos T, Lim SS, Abbafati C, Abbas KM, Abbasi M, Abbasifard M, Abbasi-Kangevari M, Abbastabar H, Abd-Allah F, Abdelalim A, Abdollahi M, Abdollahpour I, Abolhassani H, Aboyans V, Abrams EM, Abreu LG, Abrigo MRM, Abu-Raddad LJ, Abushouk AI et al (2020) Global burden of 369 diseases and injuries in 204 countries and territories, 1990–2019: a systematic analysis for the Global Burden of Disease Study 2019. Lancet 396(10258):1204–1222. https://doi.org/10.1016/S0140-6736(20)30925-9

Wah TM, Irving HC, Gregory W, Cartledge J, Joyce AD, Selby PJ (2014) Radiofrequency ablation (RFA) of renal cell carcinoma (RCC): experience in 200 tumours: RFA for RCC. BJU Int 113(3):416–428. https://doi.org/10.1111/bju.12349

Walker S, Mercer R, Maskell N, Rahman NM (2020) Malignant pleural effusion management: keeping the flood gates shut. Lancet Respir Med 8(6):609–618. https://doi.org/10.1016/S2213-2600(19)30373-X

Wang H, Abbas KM, Abbasifard M, Abbasi-Kangevari M, Abbastabar H, Abd-Allah F, Abdelalim A, Abolhassani H, Abreu LG, Abrigo MRM, Abushouk AI, Adabi M, Adair T, Adebayo OM, Adedeji IA, Adekanmbi V, Adeoye AM, Adetokunboh OO, Advani SM et al (2020) Global age-sex-specific fertility, mortality, healthy life expectancy (HALE), and population estimates in 204 countries and territories, 1950–2019: a comprehensive demographic analysis for the Global Burden of Disease Study 2019. Lancet 396(10258):1160–1203. https://doi.org/10.1016/S0140-6736(20)30977-6

Wasan HS, Gibbs P, Sharma NK, Taieb J, Heinemann V, Ricke J, Peeters M, Findlay M, Weaver A, Mills J, Wilson C, Adams R, Francis A, Moschandreas J, Virdee PS, Dutton P, Love S, Gebski V, Gray A et al (2017) First-line selective internal radiotherapy plus chemotherapy versus chemotherapy alone in patients with liver metastases from colorectal cancer (FOXFIRE, SIRFLOX, and FOXFIRE-Global): a combined analysis of three multicentre, randomised, phase 3 trials. Lancet Oncol 18(9):1159–1171. https://doi.org/10.1016/S1470-2045(17)30457-6

Weber A, Gaa J, Rosca B, Born P, Neu B, Schmid RM, Prinz C (2009) Complications of percutaneous transhepatic biliary drainage in patients with dilated and nondilated intrahepatic bile ducts. Eur J Radiol 72(3):412–417. https://doi.org/10.1016/j.ejrad.2008.08.012

Weber M, Lam M, Chiesa C, Konijnenberg M, Cremonesi M, Flamen P, Gnesin S, Bodei L, Kracmerova T, Luster M, Garin E, Herrmann K (2022) EANM procedure guideline for the treatment of liver cancer and liver metastases with intra-arterial radioactive compounds. Eur J Nucl Med Mol Imaging 49(5):1682–1699. https://doi.org/10.1007/s00259-021-05600-z

Weiser MR, Jarnagin WR, Saltz LB (2013) Colorectal cancer patients with oligometastatic liver disease: what is the optimal approach? Oncology (Williston Park) 27(11):1074–1078

Welch BT, Brinjikji W, Schmit GD, Callstrom MR, Kurup AN, Cloft HJ, Woodrum DA, Nichols FC, Atwell TD (2015) A national analysis of the complications, cost, and mortality of percutaneous lung ablation. J Vasc Interv Radiol 26(6):787–791. https://doi.org/10.1016/j.jvir.2015.02.019

West H(J), Jin JO (2015) Transarterial chemoembolization. JAMA Oncol 1(8):1178. https://doi.org/10.1001/jamaoncol.2015.3702

White J, Carolan-Rees G, Dale M, Morgan HE, Patrick HE, See TC, Beeton EL, Swinson DEB, Bell JK, Manas DM, Crellin A, Slevin NJ, Sharma RA (2019) Analysis of a national programme for selective internal radiation therapy for colorectal cancer liver metastases. Clin Oncol 31(1): 58–66. https://doi.org/10.1016/j.clon.2018.09.002

Wolf FJ, Grand DJ, Machan JT, DiPetrillo TA, Mayo-Smith WW, Dupuy DE (2008) Microwave ablation of lung malignancies: effectiveness, CT findings, and safety in 50 patients. Radiology 247(3):871–879. https://doi.org/10.1148/radiol.2473070996

Wu S, Hou J, Ding Y, Wu F, Hu Y, Jiang Q, Mao P, Yang Y (2015) Cryoablation versus radiofrequency ablation for hepatic malignancies: a systematic review and literature-based analysis. Medicine 94(49):e2252. https://doi.org/10.1097/MD.0000000000002252

Wu X, Rabei R, Keller EJ, King B, Kothary N, Kohi M, Taylor A, Heller M (2022) Tunneled peritoneal catheter vs repeated paracenteses for recurrent ascites: a cost-effectiveness analysis. Cardiovasc Intervent Radiol 45(7):972–982. https://doi.org/10.1007/s00270-022-03103-4

Xing M, Kokabi N, Zhang D, Ludwig JM, Kim HS (2018) Comparative effectiveness of thermal ablation, surgical resection, and active surveillance for T1a renal cell carcinoma: a surveillance, epidemiology, and end results (SEER)–medicare-linked population study. Radiology 288(1): 81–90. https://doi.org/10.1148/radiol.2018171407

Yang Y, Wang C, Lu Y, Bai W, An L, Qu J, Gao X, Chen Y, Zhou L, Wu Y, Feng Y, Zhang M, Chang X, Lv J (2012a) Outcomes of ultrasound-guided percutaneous argon-helium cryoablation of hepatocellular carcinoma. J Hepatobiliary Pancreat Sci 19(6):674–684. https://doi.org/10.1007/s00534-011-0490-6

Yang TX, Chua TC, Morris DL (2012b) Radioembolization and chemoembolization for unresectable neuroendocrine liver metastases – a systematic review. Surg Oncol 21(4): 299–308. https://doi.org/10.1016/j.suronc.2012.07.001

Yang Y, Du J, Wang Y, Kang H, Zhai K, Shi H (2022) Prognostic impact of pleural effusion in patients with malignancy: a systematic review and meta-analysis. Clin Transl Sci 15(6): 1340–1354. https://doi.org/10.1111/cts.13260

Zagoria RJ, Pettus JA, Rogers M, Werle DM, Childs D, Leyendecker JR (2011) Long-term outcomes after percutaneous radiofrequency ablation for renal cell carcinoma. Urology 77(6): 1393–1397. https://doi.org/10.1016/j.urology.2010.12.077

Zhou W, Arellano RS (2018) Thermal ablation of T1c renal cell carcinoma: a comparative assessment of technical performance, procedural outcome, and safety of microwave ablation, radiofrequency ablation, and cryoablation. J Vasc Interv Radiol 29(7):943–951. https://doi.org/10.1016/j.jvir.2017.12.020

Ziemlewicz TJ, Hinshaw JL, Lubner MG, Brace CL, Alexander ML, Agarwal P, Lee FT (2015) Percutaneous microwave ablation of hepatocellular carcinoma with a gas-cooled system: initial clinical results with 107 tumors. J Vasc Interv Radiol 26(1):62–68. https://doi.org/10.1016/j.jvir.2014.09.012

Future Perspectives of Phytochemicals in Cancer Therapy

Bakiye Goker Bagca and Cigir Biray Avci

Abstract

Cancer is a heterogeneous group of diseases originating from genetic or epigenetic abnormalities of a single cell. It is the second most common cause of death after cardiovascular diseases. To minimize the handicaps such as side effects and drug resistance that occur in chemotherapy, which forms the basis of current treatment methods in cancer treatment, the potential of the use of chemicals obtained from natural sources is currently researched. Although there is a countless research on phytochemicals in conventional treatment applications, the potential of phytochemicals in modern molecular cancer research is reviewed in this chapter. The current works, which include the possible utilization of phytochemicals for eliminating cancer stem cells or in combinational usage with conventional drugs and nanomedicine approaches, were reviewed. It was determined that phytochemicals target cancer stem cells which are the major liable for therapy resistance, relapse, and tumor heterogeneity. It was also determined that phytochemicals improve chemotherapy and radiotherapy treatments in combinational approaches. Moreover, nanoparticle encapsulation or conjugation strategies also enhance the bioavailability of the phytochemicals. It should be kept in mind that phytochemicals, like all other chemicals, can take their place in the modern medical approach after passing many in vitro and in vivo steps including selection of appropriate extraction method and elucidation of molecular mechanism.

B. Goker Bagca
Department of Medical Biology, Faculty of Medicine, Aydin Adnan Menderes University, Aydin, Turkey

C. Biray Avci (✉)
Department of Medical Biology, Faculty of Medicine, Ege University, Izmir, Turkey
e-mail: cigir.biray@ege.edu.tr; cbavci@gmail.com

Interdisciplinary Cancer Research, https://doi.org/10.1007/16833_2022_45
Published online: 29 November 2022

Keywords

Cancer stem cells · Combinational approaches · Nanoparticle · Phytochemical

1 Introduction

Since ancient times, people have sought treatment of all diseases in nature. Therefore, the origins of the usage of plants in therapies are quite old.

Phytochemicals are the common class of chemicals obtained from plants and include alkaloids, organosulfur, phenolic compounds, flavonoids, carbohydrates, lipids, and proteins (Bolling et al. 2011).

Cancer is a heterogeneous group of diseases originating from genetic or epigenetic abnormalities of a single cell. It is the second most common cause of death after cardiovascular diseases (Bray et al. 2018). To minimize the handicaps such as side effects and drug resistance that occur in chemotherapy, which forms the basis of current treatment methods in cancer treatment, the potential of the use of chemicals obtained from natural sources is currently researched.

Since cancer originates from the uncontrolled proliferation of cells, the potential effect on the cell cycle is one of the most frequent topics in phytochemical research. Caffeic acid and its phenethyl ester (CAPE), quercetin, and genistein are among the most frequently evaluated phytochemicals known to cause cell cycle arrest by affecting the cycle-related genes (Angst et al. 2013; Spagnuolo et al. 2015; Dziedzic et al. 2017).

The other conventional strategy is programmed cell death, especially apoptosis, induction by using phytochemicals. Phytochemicals such as caffeic acid, genistein, quercetin, and resveratrol are known to direct different cancer cells to apoptosis by affecting mitochondrial membrane potential, pro-apoptotic and anti-apoptotic members of the Bcl2 family, and caspases (Chang et al. 2010; Yu et al. 2016; Dziedzic et al. 2017; Granato et al. 2017; Hashemzaei et al. 2017; Li et al. 2017b, 2018a; Blanquer-Rossello et al. 2017; Liu et al. 2018; Heo et al. 2018; Wu et al. 2018).

The induction of autophagy, known as type II cell death, is one of the current topics of cancer research. Phytochemicals such as CAPE, genistein, and quercetin have been demonstrated to regulate autophagy in different cancers by controlling AKT/mTOR and AMPK signaling pathways (Yu et al. 2011; Wang et al. 2011).

Although there is a countless research on phytochemicals in conventional treatment applications, the potential of phytochemicals in modern molecular cancer research is reviewed in this chapter.

2 Phytochemicals in Future Cancer Therapy Perspectives

2.1 Cancer Stem Cell Targeting Approach

Cancer stem cells are pivotal factors which play essential role in tumor initiation, metastasis, tumor heterogeneity, chemotherapy and radiotherapy resistance, relapse, and recurrence. They may originate from normal cells, embryonic or adult stem cells, or tumor cells due to abnormal activation of Notch, WNT, Hedgehog stem cell signaling pathways (Clevers 2011). Current cancer therapeutics aim to target cancer stem cells directly.

Inhibition of p38/NFKB pathway by CAPE suppresses cancer stem cell properties (Yang et al. 2013). Carnosol induces apoptosis of glioblastoma stem cells (Giacomelli et al. 2017). Curcumin suppresses liver, breast, bladder, lung, liver cancer stem cell proliferation via regulating PI3K/MTOR, WNT/B-catenin, Hedgehog, NFKB pathways (Mukherjee et al. 2014; Marquardt et al. 2015; Mirza et al. 2017; Zhu et al. 2017; Liang et al. 2017; Wang et al. 2017a, 2018b; Li et al. 2018d). Ellagic acid inhibits breast cancer metastasis via controlling cancer stem cells (Wang et al. 2017b). Epigallocatechin-3-gallate targets colorectal, breast, lung, head and neck stem cells via suppressing WNT and Notch pathways (Stearns and Wang 2011; Goker et al. 2014; Kilic et al. 2014; Jiang et al. 2020). Genistein suppresses stem cell properties of gastric cancer, breast, and prostate cancer (Zhang et al. 2012; Fan et al. 2013; Huang et al. 2014; Yu et al. 2014b). Phenethyl isothiocyanate inhibit colon and breast cancer stem cells both in vitro and in vivo model (Yun et al. 2017; Nguyen et al. 2020; Shin et al. 2021). Quercetin has also antiproliferative and apoptotic effects on human colon, prostate, breast, gastric cancer stem cells, it regulates expression levels of autophagy, resistance, and EMT genes, additively (Atashpour et al. 2015; Shen et al. 2016; Tsai et al. 2016; Wang et al. 2018c; Li et al. 2018b, e; Erdogan et al. 2018). Ursolic acid has antiproliferative effect on human ovarian cancer stem cells by mediating the resistance genes as ABC transporters (Wang et al. 2016b). Sulforaphane targets squamous cancer stem cells (Liu et al. 2017; Fisher et al. 2017). Vanillin suppresses stem-like phenotype of lung cancer cells via Akt pathway (Srinual et al. 2017).

2.2 Combinational Approach

Phytochemicals are natural compounds are accepted that they have less side-effect than conventional chemotherapeutics. Therefore, researches in which phytochemicals are combined with current therapy strategies are popular. Combination studies are also promising about improve chemotherapy and radiotherapy efficiency, overcome therapy resistance.

Allicin is reported that improved effect of conventional chemotherapy agents on hepatocellular carcinoma cell (Zou et al. 2016). It is currently reported that apigenin improves the apoptotic effect of 5-fluorouracil in colon cancer (Yang et al. 2021). Caffeic acid and derivatives also improves cytotoxic and apoptotic effects of chemotherapeutic agents (Tolba et al. 2013; Sirota et al. 2017; Koraneekit et al. 2018). CAPE enhances radiotherapy and chemotherapy effectiveness in breast cancer cells (Motawi et al. 2016a, b; Khoram et al. 2016). It is suggested that catechol improves therapy efficiency in pancreatic cancer (Moon et al. 2021). Capsaicin shows synergistic effect with sorafenib and pirarubicin (Arulmozhi et al. 2013; Mady and Shaker 2017). It also improves effect of radiotherapy in prostate cancer model (Venier et al. 2015). Alpha-carotene improves anticancer activity of taxol on lung cancer (Liu et al. 2015). Curcumin improves anticancer effects of taxols on breast, lung, gastric, prostate, over cancer cells (Liu et al. 2016; Quispe-Soto and Calaf 2016; Ebrahimifar et al. 2017; Banerjee et al. 2017; Lu et al. 2017; Calaf et al. 2018). It enhances antitumor effects of 5-fluorouracil on colon, gastric cancer cells (Kang et al. 2016; Yang et al. 2017; Zhang et al. 2017a). It also supports to overcome chemotherapy resistance in neuroblastoma, glioblastoma, hepatocellular, colon, breast, pancreatic, and bladder cancer cells against different agents including cisplatin (Park et al. 2016; Zhao et al. 2017; Huang et al. 2017; Yoshida et al. 2017; Zou et al. 2018; Abdallah et al. 2018; Namkaew et al. 2018; Su et al. 2018). Curcumin potentiates effects of radiotherapy on colon, renal cancer cells (Kang et al. 2016; Yang et al. 2017). Ellagic acid improves radiotherapy efficiency on breast cancer and hepatocellular carcinoma cells (Wang et al. 2016a; Sanchez-Carranza et al. 2018). It also supports activity of chemotherapeutics in breast and colon cancer (Kao et al. 2012; Shi et al. 2015; Gonzalez-Sarrias et al. 2015). Epigallocatechin-3-gallate enhances chemotherapeutic agents anticancer property in prostate, cervical cancers and it also improves apoptotic effect of ponatinib in chronic myeloid leukemia (Stearns and Wang 2011; Goker et al. 2014; Kilic et al. 2014). Gallic acid enhances chemotherapeutic effects of paclitaxel and cisplatin on over and lung cancer cells via overcoming resistance (Wang et al. 2016a; Sanchez-Carranza et al. 2018). It is currently determined that Glaucocalyxin B, a diterpenoid, enhances chemotherapy effectiveness on over cancers (Zhang et al. 2022). 6-Gingerol improves apoptotic effect of radiotherapy on gastric cancer cells (Venier et al. 2015). 3,3′-Diindolylmethane improves the effectiveness of paclitaxel, erlotinib, docetaxel, taxotere, cisplatin, herceptin, and γ-irradiation (McGuire et al. 2006; Ali et al. 2008; Ichite et al. 2009; Rahman et al. 2009; Ahmad et al. 2011, 2013; Kandala and Srivastava 2012; Jin et al. 2015; Wang et al. 2016c). Phenethyl isothiocyanate sensitizes lung cancer cells to gefitinib induced apoptosis (Hsia et al. 2018). Phenethyl isothiocyanate also improves anticancer activity of taxanes include paclitaxel and docetaxel on breast and prostate cancer cells (Cang et al. 2014). It also increases chemotherapeutic effects of doxorubicin and cisplatin on breast and cervical cancer (Cang et al. 2014; Eisa et al. 2015). Differently, benzyl isothiocyanate sensitizes pancreas cancer cells to radiotherapy (Ohara et al. 2011). Allyl isothiocyanate enhances not only radiotherapy but also chemotherapy efficiency in lung and bladder cancer (Bhattacharya et al. 2013; Tripathi et al. 2015). Lycopene improves chemotherapy effectiveness in prostate cancer cells (Chen et al. 2022). It is recently demonstrated that naringenin improves the effects of temozolomide in glioblastoma (Gautam and Gabrani 2022). Oleuropein induces chemotherapy and radiotherapy efficiency in breast and over cancer (Arulmozhi et al. 2013; Mady and Shaker 2017). Piceatannol decreases IC_{50} dose of gemcitabine in lung cancer and it increases sensitivity of over cancer to cisplatin (Farrand et al. 2013; Xu and Tao 2014). Piperine enhances chemotherapy efficiency in prostate, breast, lung, over, cervical cancers (Li et al. 2011; Makhov et al. 2012; Han et al. 2017). Resveratrol improves anticancer effect of 5-fluorouracil, cisplatin, paclitaxel, docetaxel on colon, lung, liver, prostate cancer cells, respectively (Jiang et al. 2017; Chung et al. 2018; Li et al. 2018c; Lee and Lee 2021). It synergists doxorubicin in breast, and gastric cancers (Chung et al. 2018;

Li et al. 2018c). It also improves effects of radiation and temozolomide on glioma stem cell (Wang et al. 2015; Li et al. 2016). Sulforaphane enhances chemotherapy efficiency in lung, breast, kidney, gastric, prostate, colon cancers (Hussain et al. 2013; Erzinger et al. 2016; Khurana et al. 2016; Wang et al. 2016d, 2018a; Juengel et al. 2016; Kim et al. 2017; Mokhtari et al. 2021). It has also synergistic effect with photodynamic therapy in head and neck cancer cells (Lee et al. 2015). Ursolic acid induces anticancer effects of platin compounds on different cancer types (Wu et al. 2016; Shan et al. 2016; Li et al. 2017a; Zhang et al. 2018).

2.3 Nanoparticle Utilization Approach

Bioavailability is major challenge of clinical phytochemical usage. Nanotechnology helps researches to overcome the problem. Nanoparticles which has >100 nm diameter, are used as nanocarriers and scaffolds for drug delivering (Cesmeli and Biray Avci 2018). Nanoparticle-conjugated drugs are being popular day by day in cancer therapy approaches.

Capsaicin conjugated lipid nanoparticles improves therapeutic response in over cancer cells (Venier et al. 2015). Beta-carotene conjugated with zein, lipid nanoparticles have enhanced anticancer effect on breast cancer. Organic polymer-encapsulated ellagic acid shows increased efficiency in oral cancer cells (Arulmozhi et al. 2013; Mady and Shaker 2017). Gallic acid which encapsulated silver, gold, and polyethylene glycol has enhanced anticancer activity on lung, breast, cervical, and colon cancer cells with inhibition of EMT- related genes (Daduang et al. 2015; Chen et al. 2016; Rosman et al. 2018; Sunil Gowda et al. 2018). Lycopene loaded nanocarriers improves anticancer effectiveness (Zhang et al. 2017b; Jain et al. 2017, 2018). It is currently reported that nimbolide-encapsulated nanoparticles have anticancer effects on pancreatic cancer by targeting stem cells (Singh et al. 2022). Chitosan and polylactic acid-coated nanocarriers improves cytotoxic and apoptotic efficiency of piceatannol on liver, lung and breast cancer cells (Dhanapal and Balaraman Ravindrran 2018). It is currently demonstrated that piperine encapsulated nanoparticles have anticancer effects on breast cancer (Kazmi et al. 2022). It is recently shown that resveratrol encapsulated micels have potential on breast cancer (Gregoriou et al. 2020). The anticancer potential of the Quercetin-loaded nanoparticles on glioblastoma is currently demonstrated (Ersoz et al. 2020). Sulforaphane with gold and polyethyleneglycol nanoparticles as drug delivery systems improve cytotoxic, apoptotic and antitumor activity in breast cancer (Danafar et al. 2017; Soni and Kohli 2018).

Moreover, the use of plant-originated compounds in the synthesis of nanoparticles or drug carriers, called the green strategy, has recently been a popular research topic in cancer research (Takei et al. 2010; Bosio et al. 2012; Chittasupho et al. 2013; Chandran et al. 2013; Yu et al. 2014a; Izadi et al. 2016; Hussien et al. 2018; Namasivayam et al. 2021; Yang et al. 2022).

3 Conclusions

Cancer, which is the second leading cause of death after cardiovascular disease, is a heterogeneous disease group which originates genetic or epigenetic factors. Considering the heterogeneity of cancer types, it is clear that the standard chemotherapy and radiotherapy applications used for cancer treatment should be specialize as targeted.

Since the methods used in cancer treatment are not target- specific, they also cause many side effects by affecting healthy cells. In addition, chemotherapy and/or radiotherapy resistance occurs over time. Cancer stem cells that are not affected the dose administered to the tumor mass are primary responsible for therapy resistance. Cancer stem cells are also responsible for the heterogeneous structure of the cancer mass and the metastasis, which causes most cancer-related deaths. Therefore, aiming to eliminate cancer stem cells is one of the current treatment approaches.

The use of natural products against diseases has been the first method since the first people. Today, many natural products are using as prescription drugs in the treatment of certain diseases.

Since the higher doses of safety compared to conventional agents, phytochemicals have a great potential for cancer therapy, both individual and combine usage with current chemotherapeutics. Studies are underway to explain the molecular action mechanisms, anticancer stem cell potentials of phytochemicals in various types of cancer.

The foremost handicap about use of phytochemicals in cancer models is the bioavailability. To overcome this problem, drug transport systems are used which are products of nanotechnology. In addition, phytochemicals also function as organic scaffolds.

It should be kept in mind that phytochemicals, like all other chemicals, can take their place in the modern medical approach after passing many in vitro and in vivo steps including selection of appropriate extraction method and elucidation of molecular mechanism.

Acknowledgements None.

Data availability Statements All data generated or analyzed during this study are included in this published article.

Compliance with Ethical Standards All authors declared that they have no conflict of interest. This manuscript does not include any human or animal subjects.

References

Abdallah FM, Helmy MW, Katary MA, Ghoneim AI (2018) Synergistic antiproliferative effects of curcumin and celecoxib in hepatocellular carcinoma HepG2 cells. Naunyn Schmiedeberg's Arch Pharmacol. https://doi.org/10.1007/s00210-018-1557-6

Ahmad A, Ali S, Wang Z et al (2011) 3,3′-diindolylmethane enhances taxotere-induced growth inhibition of breast cancer cells through downregulation of FoxM1. Int J Cancer 129:1781–1791. https://doi.org/10.1002/ijc.25839

Ahmad A, Ali S, Ahmed A et al (2013) 3,3′-diindolylmethane enhances the effectiveness of herceptin against HER-2/neu-expressing breast cancer cells. PLoS One 8:e54657. https://doi.org/10.1371/journal.pone.0054657

Ali S, Banerjee S, Ahmad A et al (2008) Apoptosis-inducing effect of erlotinib is potentiated by 3,3′-diindolylmethane in vitro and in vivo using an orthotopic model of pancreatic cancer. Mol Cancer Ther 7:1708–1719. https://doi.org/10.1158/1535-7163.MCT-08-0354

Angst E, Park JL, Moro A et al (2013) The flavonoid quercetin inhibits pancreatic cancer growth in vitro and in vivo. Pancreas. https://doi.org/10.1097/MPA.0b013e318264ccae

Arulmozhi V, Pandian K, Mirunalini S (2013) Ellagic acid encapsulated chitosan nanoparticles for drug delivery system in human oral cancer cell line (KB). Colloids Surf B Biointerfaces 110:313–320. https://doi.org/10.1016/j.colsurfb.2013.03.039

Atashpour S, Fouladdel S, Movahhed TK et al (2015) Quercetin induces cell cycle arrest and apoptosis in CD133(+) cancer stem cells of human colorectal HT29 cancer cell line and enhances anticancer effects of doxorubicin. Iran J Basic Med Sci 18:635–643

Banerjee S, Singh SK, Chowdhury I et al (2017) Combinatorial effect of curcumin with docetaxel modulates apoptotic and cell survival molecules in prostate cancer. Front Biosci (Elite Ed) 9:235–245

Bhattacharya A, Li Y, Shi Y, Zhang Y (2013) Enhanced inhibition of urinary bladder cancer growth and muscle invasion by allyl isothiocyanate and celecoxib in combination. Carcinogenesis 34:2593–2599. https://doi.org/10.1093/carcin/bgt280

Blanquer-Rossello M, Hernandez-Lopez R, Roca P et al (2017) Resveratrol induces mitochondrial respiration and apoptosis in SW620 colon cancer cells. Biochim Biophys Acta Gen Subj 1861: 431–440. https://doi.org/10.1016/j.bbagen.2016.10.009

Bolling BW, Chen CYO, McKay DL, Blumberg JB (2011) Tree nut phytochemicals: composition, antioxidant capacity, bioactivity, impact factors. A systematic review of almonds, brazils, cashews, hazelnuts, macadamias, pecans, pine nuts, pistachios and walnuts. Nutr Res Rev 24(2):244–275

Bosio VE, Machain V, Lopez AG et al (2012) Binding and encapsulation of doxorubicin on smart pectin hydrogels for oral delivery. Appl Biochem Biotechnol 167:1365–1376. https://doi.org/10.1007/s12010-012-9641-8

Bray F, Ferlay J, Soerjomataram I et al (2018) Global cancer statistics 2018: GLOBOCAN estimates of incidence and mortality worldwide for 36 cancers in 185 countries. CA Cancer J Clin. https://doi.org/10.3322/caac.21492

Calaf GM, Ponce-Cusi R, Carrion F (2018) Curcumin and paclitaxel induce cell death in breast cancer cell lines. Oncol Rep 40:2381–2388. https://doi.org/10.3892/or.2018.6603

Cang S, Ma Y, Chiao J-W, Liu D (2014) Phenethyl isothiocyanate and paclitaxel synergistically enhanced apoptosis and alpha-tubulin hyperacetylation in breast cancer cells. Exp Hematol Oncol 3:5. https://doi.org/10.1186/2162-3619-3-5

Cesmeli S, Biray Avci C (2018) Application of titanium dioxide (TiO2) nanoparticles in cancer therapies. J Drug Target:1–13. https://doi.org/10.1080/1061186X.2018.1527338

Chandran S, Praveen G, Snima KS et al (2013) Potential use of drug loaded nano composite pectin scaffolds for the treatment of ovarian cancer. Curr Drug Deliv 10:326–335

Chang W-C, Hsieh C-H, Hsiao M-W et al (2010) Caffeic acid induces apoptosis in human cervical cancer cells through the mitochondrial pathway. Taiwan J Obstet Gynecol 49:419–424. https://doi.org/10.1016/S1028-4559(10)60092-7

Chen Y-J, Lee Y-C, Huang C-H, Chang L-S (2016) Gallic acid-capped gold nanoparticles inhibit EGF-induced MMP-9 expression through suppression of p300 stabilization and NFkappaB/c-Jun activation in breast cancer MDA-MB-231 cells. Toxicol Appl Pharmacol 310:98–107. https://doi.org/10.1016/j.taap.2016.09.007

Chen X, Yang G, Liu M et al (2022) Lycopene enhances the sensitivity of castration-resistant prostate cancer to enzalutamide through the AKT/EZH2/androgen receptor signaling pathway. Biochem Biophys Res Commun 613:53–60. https://doi.org/10.1016/j.bbrc.2022.04.126

Chittasupho C, Jaturanpinyo M, Mangmool S (2013) Pectin nanoparticle enhances cytotoxicity of methotrexate against HepG2 cells. Drug Deliv 20:1–9. https://doi.org/10.3109/10717544.2012.739214

Chung SS, Dutta P, Austin D et al (2018) Combination of resveratrol and 5-flurouracil enhanced anti-telomerase activity and apoptosis by inhibiting STAT3 and Akt signaling pathways in human colorectal cancer cells. Oncotarget 9:32943–32957. https://doi.org/10.18632/oncotarget.25993

Clevers H (2011) The cancer stem cell: premises, promises and challenges. Nat Med 17:313–319. https://doi.org/10.1038/nm.2304

Daduang J, Palasap A, Daduang S et al (2015) Gallic acid enhancement of gold nanoparticle anticancer activity in cervical cancer cells. Asian Pac J Cancer Prev 16:169–174

Danafar H, Sharafi A, Kheiri Manjili H, Andalib S (2017) Sulforaphane delivery using mPEG-PCL co-polymer nanoparticles to breast cancer cells. Pharm Dev Technol 22:642–651. https://doi.org/10.3109/10837450.2016.1146296

Dhanapal J, Balaraman Ravindrran M (2018) Chitosan/poly (lactic acid)-coated piceatannol nanoparticles exert an in vitro apoptosis activity on liver, lung and breast cancer cell lines. Artif Cells Nanomed Biotechnol:1–9. https://doi.org/10.1080/21691401.2017.1422130

Dziedzic A, Kubina R, Kabala-Dzik A, Tanasiewicz M (2017) Induction of cell cycle arrest and apoptotic response of head and neck squamous carcinoma cells (Detroit 562) by caffeic acid and caffeic acid phenethyl ester derivative. Evid Based Complement Alternat Med 2017:6793456. https://doi.org/10.1155/2017/6793456

Ebrahimifar M, Hasanzadegan Roudsari M, Kazemi SM et al (2017) Enhancing effects of curcumin on cytotoxicity of paclitaxel, methotrexate and vincristine in gastric cancer cells. Asian Pac J Cancer Prev 18:65–68. https://doi.org/10.22034/APJCP.2017.18.1.65

Eisa NH, ElSherbiny NM, Shebl AM et al (2015) Phenethyl isothiocyanate potentiates anti-tumour effect of doxorubicin through Akt-dependent pathway. Cell Biochem Funct 33:541–551. https://doi.org/10.1002/cbf.3153

Erdogan S, Turkekul K, Dibirdik I et al (2018) Midkine downregulation increases the efficacy of quercetin on prostate cancer stem cell survival and migration through PI3K/AKT and MAPK/ERK pathway. Biomed Pharmacother 107:793–805. https://doi.org/10.1016/j.biopha.2018.08.061

Ersoz M, Erdemir A, Derman S et al (2020) Quercetin-loaded nanoparticles enhance cytotoxicity and antioxidant activity on C6 glioma cells. Pharm Dev Technol. https://doi.org/10.1080/10837450.2020.1740933

Erzinger MM, Bovet C, Hecht KM et al (2016) Sulforaphane preconditioning sensitizes human colon cancer cells towards the bioreductive anticancer prodrug PR-104A. PLoS One 11:e0150219. https://doi.org/10.1371/journal.pone.0150219

Fan P, Fan S, Wang H et al (2013) Genistein decreases the breast cancer stem-like cell population through hedgehog pathway. Stem Cell Res Ther 4:146. https://doi.org/10.1186/scrt357

Farrand L, Byun S, Kim JY et al (2013) Piceatannol enhances cisplatin sensitivity in ovarian cancer via modulation of p53, X-linked inhibitor of apoptosis protein (XIAP), and mitochondrial fission. J Biol Chem 288:23740–23750. https://doi.org/10.1074/jbc.M113.487686

Fisher ML, Ciavattone N, Grun D et al (2017) Sulforaphane reduces YAP/Np63alpha signaling to reduce cancer stem cell survival and tumor formation. Oncotarget 8:73407–73418. https://doi.org/10.18632/oncotarget.20562

Gautam M, Gabrani R (2022) Combinatorial effect of temozolomide and naringenin in human glioblastoma multiforme cell lines. Nutr Cancer. https://doi.org/10.1080/01635581.2021.1952438

Giacomelli C, Daniele S, Natali L et al (2017) Carnosol controls the human glioblastoma stemness features through the epithelial-mesenchymal transition modulation and the induction of cancer stem cell apoptosis. Sci Rep 7:15174. https://doi.org/10.1038/s41598-017-15360-2

Goker B, Caliskan C, Onur Caglar H et al (2014) Synergistic effect of ponatinib and epigallocatechin-3-gallate induces apoptosis in chronic myeloid leukemia cells through altering expressions of cell cycle regulatory genes. J BUON 19:992–998

Gonzalez-Sarrias A, Tome-Carneiro J, Bellesia A et al (2015) The ellagic acid-derived gut microbiota metabolite, urolithin A, potentiates the anticancer effects of 5-fluorouracil chemotherapy on human colon cancer cells. Food Funct 6:1460–1469. https://doi.org/10.1039/c5fo00120j

Granato M, Rizzello C, Montani MSG et al (2017) Quercetin induces apoptosis and autophagy in primary effusion lymphoma cells by inhibiting PI3K/AKT/mTOR and STAT3 signaling pathways. J Nutr Biochem. https://doi.org/10.1016/j.jnutbio.2016.12.011

Gregoriou Y, Gregoriou G, Yilmaz V et al (2020) Resveratrol loaded polymeric micelles for theranostic targeting of breast cancer cells. Nano. https://doi.org/10.7150/ntno.51955

Han S-Z, Liu H-X, Yang L-Q et al (2017) Piperine (PP) enhanced mitomycin-C (MMC) therapy of human cervical cancer through suppressing Bcl-2 signaling pathway via inactivating STAT3/NF-kappaB. Biomed Pharmacother 96:1403–1410. https://doi.org/10.1016/j.biopha.2017.11.022

Hashemzaei M, Far AD, Yari A et al (2017) Anticancer and apoptosis-inducing effects of quercetin in vitro and in vivo. Oncol Rep. https://doi.org/10.3892/or.2017.5766

Heo J-R, Kim S-M, Hwang K-A et al (2018) Resveratrol induced reactive oxygen species and endoplasmic reticulum stressmediated apoptosis, and cell cycle arrest in the A375SM malignant melanoma cell line. Int J Mol Med 42:1427–1435. https://doi.org/10.3892/ijmm.2018.3732

Hsia T-C, Huang Y-P, Jiang Y-W et al (2018) Phenethyl isothiocyanate induces apoptotic cell death through the mitochondria-dependent pathway in gefitinib-resistant NCI-H460 human lung cancer cells in vitro. Anticancer Res 38:2137–2147. https://doi.org/10.21873/anticanres.12454

Huang W, Wan C, Luo Q et al (2014) Genistein-inhibited cancer stem cell-like properties and reduced chemoresistance of gastric cancer. Int J Mol Sci 15:3432–3443. https://doi.org/10.3390/ijms15033432

Huang Y-F, Zhu D-J, Chen X-W et al (2017) Curcumin enhances the effects of irinotecan on colorectal cancer cells through the generation of reactive oxygen species and activation of the endoplasmic reticulum stress pathway. Oncotarget 8:40264–40275. https://doi.org/10.18632/oncotarget.16828

Hussain A, Mohsin J, Prabhu SA et al (2013) Sulforaphane inhibits growth of human breast cancer cells and augments the therapeutic index of the chemotherapeutic drug, gemcitabine. Asian Pac J Cancer Prev 14:5855–5860

Hussien NA, Isiklan N, Turk M (2018) Pectin-conjugated magnetic graphene oxide nanohybrid as a novel drug carrier for paclitaxel delivery. Artif Cells Nanomed Biotechnol:1–10. https://doi.org/10.1080/21691401.2017.1421211

Ichite N, Chougule MB, Jackson T et al (2009) Enhancement of docetaxel anticancer activity by a novel diindolylmethane compound in human non-small cell lung cancer. Clin Cancer Res 15: 543–552. https://doi.org/10.1158/1078-0432.CCR-08-1558

Izadi Z, Divsalar A, Saboury AA, Sawyer L (2016) Beta-lactoglobulin-pectin nanoparticle-based oral drug delivery system for potential treatment of colon cancer. Chem Biol Drug Des 88:209–216. https://doi.org/10.1111/cbdd.12748

Jain A, Sharma G, Kushwah V et al (2017) Fabrication and functional attributes of lipidic nanoconstructs of lycopene: an innovative endeavour for enhanced cytotoxicity in MCF-7 breast cancer cells. Colloids Surf B Biointerfaces 152:482–491. https://doi.org/10.1016/j.colsurfb.2017.01.050

Jain A, Sharma G, Ghoshal G et al (2018) Lycopene loaded whey protein isolate nanoparticles: an innovative endeavor for enhanced bioavailability of lycopene and anti-cancer activity. Int J Pharm 546:97–105. https://doi.org/10.1016/j.ijpharm.2018.04.061

Jiang Q, Yang M, Qu Z et al (2017) Resveratrol enhances anticancer effects of paclitaxel in HepG2 human liver cancer cells. BMC Complement Altern Med 17:477. https://doi.org/10.1186/s12906-017-1956-0

Jiang P, Xu C, Zhang P et al (2020) Epigallocatechin-3-gallate inhibits self-renewal ability of lung cancer stem-like cells through inhibition of CLOCK. Int J Mol Med. https://doi.org/10.3892/ijmm.2020.4758

Jin H, Park MH, Kim SM (2015) 3,3′-diindolylmethane potentiates paclitaxel-induced antitumor effects on gastric cancer cells through the Akt/FOXM1 signaling cascade. Oncol Rep 33:2031–2036. https://doi.org/10.3892/or.2015.3758

Juengel E, Maxeiner S, Rutz J et al (2016) Sulforaphane inhibits proliferation and invasive activity of everolimus-resistant kidney cancer cells in vitro. Oncotarget 7:85208–85219. https://doi.org/10.18632/oncotarget.13421

Kandala PK, Srivastava SK (2012) Diindolylmethane suppresses ovarian cancer growth and potentiates the effect of cisplatin in tumor mouse model by targeting signal transducer and activator of transcription 3 (STAT3). BMC Med 10:9. https://doi.org/10.1186/1741-7015-10-9

Kang Y, Hu W, Bai E et al (2016) Curcumin sensitizes human gastric cancer cells to 5-fluorouracil through inhibition of the NFkappaB survival-signaling pathway. Onco Targets Ther 9:7373–7384. https://doi.org/10.2147/OTT.S118272

Kao T-Y, Chung Y-C, Hou Y-C et al (2012) Effects of ellagic acid on chemosensitivity to 5-fluorouracil in colorectal carcinoma cells. Anticancer Res 32:4413–4418

Kazmi I, Al-Abbasi FA, Imam SS et al (2022) Formulation of piperine nanoparticles: in vitro breast cancer cell line and in vivo evaluation. Polymers (Basel). https://doi.org/10.3390/polym14071349

Khoram NM, Bigdeli B, Nikoofar A, Goliaei B (2016) Caffeic acid phenethyl ester increases radiosensitivity of estrogen receptor-positive and -negative breast cancer cells by prolonging radiation-induced DNA damage. J Breast Cancer 19:18–25. https://doi.org/10.4048/jbc.2016.19.1.18

Khurana N, Talwar S, Chandra PK et al (2016) Sulforaphane increases the efficacy of anti-androgens by rapidly decreasing androgen receptor levels in prostate cancer cells. Int J Oncol 49:1609–1619. https://doi.org/10.3892/ijo.2016.3641

Kilic U, Sahin K, Tuzcu M et al (2014) Enhancement of cisplatin sensitivity in human cervical cancer: epigallocatechin-3-gallate. Front Nutr 1:28. https://doi.org/10.3389/fnut.2014.00028

Kim S-H, Park H-J, Moon D-O (2017) Sulforaphane sensitizes human breast cancer cells to paclitaxel-induced apoptosis by downregulating the NF-kappaB signaling pathway. Oncol Lett 13:4427–4432. https://doi.org/10.3892/ol.2017.5950

Koraneekit A, Limpaiboon T, Sangka A et al (2018) Synergistic effects of cisplatin-caffeic acid induces apoptosis in human cervical cancer cells via the mitochondrial pathways. Oncol Lett 15:7397–7402. https://doi.org/10.3892/ol.2018.8256

Lee SH, Lee YJ (2021) Synergistic anticancer activity of resveratrol in combination with docetaxel in prostate carcinoma cells. Nutr Res Pract. https://doi.org/10.4162/nrp.2021.15.1.12

Lee SJ, Hwang H-J, Shin J-I et al (2015) Enhancement of cytotoxic effect on human head and neck cancer cells by combination of photodynamic therapy and sulforaphane. Gen Physiol Biophys 34:13–21. https://doi.org/10.4149/gpb_2014025

Li S, Lei Y, Jia Y et al (2011) Piperine, a piperidine alkaloid from Piper nigrum re-sensitizes P-gp, MRP1 and BCRP dependent multidrug resistant cancer cells. Phytomedicine 19:83–87. https://doi.org/10.1016/j.phymed.2011.06.031

Li H, Liu Y, Jiao Y et al (2016) Resveratrol sensitizes glioblastoma-initiating cells to temozolomide by inducing cell apoptosis and promoting differentiation. Oncol Rep 35:343–351. https://doi.org/10.3892/or.2015.4346

Li L, Hou Y, Yu J et al (2017a) Synergism of ursolic acid and cisplatin promotes apoptosis and enhances growth inhibition of cervical cancer cells via suppressing NF-kappaB p65. Oncotarget 8:97416–97427. https://doi.org/10.18632/oncotarget.22133

Li S, Li J, Dai W et al (2017b) Genistein suppresses aerobic glycolysis and induces hepatocellular carcinoma cell death. Br J Cancer. https://doi.org/10.1038/bjc.2017.323

Li L, Qiu R-L, Lin Y et al (2018a) Resveratrol suppresses human cervical carcinoma cell proliferation and elevates apoptosis via the mitochondrial and p53 signaling pathways. Oncol Lett 15:9845–9851. https://doi.org/10.3892/ol.2018.8571

Li S, Zhao Q, Wang B et al (2018b) Quercetin reversed MDR in breast cancer cells through down-regulating P-gp expression and eliminating cancer stem cells mediated by YB-1 nuclear translocation. Phytother Res 32:1530–1536. https://doi.org/10.1002/ptr.6081

Li W, Shi Y, Wang R et al (2018c) Resveratrol promotes the sensitivity of small-cell lung cancer H446 cells to cisplatin by regulating intrinsic apoptosis. Int J Oncol 53:2123–2130. https://doi.org/10.3892/ijo.2018.4533

Li X, Wang X, Xie C et al (2018d) Sonic hedgehog and Wnt/beta-catenin pathways mediate curcumin inhibition of breast cancer stem cells. Anti-Cancer Drugs 29:208–215. https://doi.org/10.1097/CAD.0000000000000584

Li X, Zhou N, Wang J et al (2018e) Quercetin suppresses breast cancer stem cells (CD44(+)/CD24(−)) by inhibiting the PI3K/Akt/mTOR-signaling pathway. Life Sci 196:56–62. https://doi.org/10.1016/j.lfs.2018.01.014

Liang Z, Lu L, Mao J et al (2017) Curcumin reversed chronic tobacco smoke exposure induced urocystic EMT and acquisition of cancer stem cells properties via Wnt/beta-catenin. Cell Death Dis 8:e3066. https://doi.org/10.1038/cddis.2017.452

Liu Y-Z, Yang C-M, Chen J-Y et al (2015) Alpha-carotene inhibits metastasis in Lewis lung carcinoma in vitro, and suppresses lung metastasis and tumor growth in combination with taxol in tumor xenografted C57BL/6 mice. J Nutr Biochem 26:607–615. https://doi.org/10.1016/j.jnutbio.2014.12.012

Liu Z, Zhu Y-Y, Li Z-Y, Ning S-Q (2016) Evaluation of the efficacy of paclitaxel with curcumin combination in ovarian cancer cells. Oncol Lett 12:3944–3948. https://doi.org/10.3892/ol.2016.5192

Liu C-M, Peng C-Y, Liao Y-W et al (2017) Sulforaphane targets cancer stemness and tumor initiating properties in oral squamous cell carcinomas via miR-200c induction. J Formos Med Assoc 116:41–48. https://doi.org/10.1016/j.jfma.2016.01.004

Liu G-L, Han N-Z, Liu S-S (2018) Caffeic acid phenethyl ester inhibits the progression of ovarian cancer by regulating NF-?B signaling. Biomed Pharmacother 99:825–831. https://doi.org/10.1016/j.biopha.2018.01.129

Lu Y, Wang J, Liu L et al (2017) Curcumin increases the sensitivity of paclitaxel-resistant NSCLC cells to paclitaxel through microRNA-30c-mediated MTA1 reduction. Tumour Biol 39:1010428317698353. https://doi.org/10.1177/1010428317698353

Mady FM, Shaker MA (2017) Enhanced anticancer activity and oral bioavailability of ellagic acid through encapsulation in biodegradable polymeric nanoparticles. Int J Nanomedicine 12:7405–7417. https://doi.org/10.2147/IJN.S147740

Makhov P, Golovine K, Canter D et al (2012) Co-administration of piperine and docetaxel results in improved anti-tumor efficacy via inhibition of CYP3A4 activity. Prostate 72:661–667. https://doi.org/10.1002/pros.21469

Marquardt JU, Gomez-Quiroz L, Arreguin Camacho LO et al (2015) Curcumin effectively inhibits oncogenic NF-kappaB signaling and restrains stemness features in liver cancer. J Hepatol 63:661–669. https://doi.org/10.1016/j.jhep.2015.04.018

McGuire KP, Ngoubilly N, Neavyn M, Lanza-Jacoby S (2006) 3,3′-diindolylmethane and paclitaxel act synergistically to promote apoptosis in HER2/Neu human breast cancer cells. J Surg Res 132:208–213. https://doi.org/10.1016/j.jss.2006.02.008

Mirza S, Vasaiya A, Vora H et al (2017) Curcumin targets circulating cancer stem cells by inhibiting self-renewal efficacy in non-small cell lung carcinoma. Anti Cancer Agents Med Chem 17:859–864. https://doi.org/10.2174/1871520616666160923102549

Mokhtari RB, Qorri B, Baluch N et al (2021) Next-generation multimodality of nutrigenomic cancer therapy: sulforaphane in combination with acetazolamide actively target bronchial carcinoid cancer in disabling the PI3K/Akt/mTOR survival pathway and inducing apoptosis. Oncotarget. https://doi.org/10.18632/oncotarget.28011

Moon JY, Ediriweera MK, Ryu JY et al (2021) Catechol enhances chemo- and radio-sensitivity by targeting AMPK/hippo signaling in pancreatic cancer cells. Oncol Rep. https://doi.org/10.3892/or.2021.7924

Motawi TK, Abdelazim SA, Darwish HA et al (2016a) Modulation of tamoxifen cytotoxicity by caffeic acid phenethyl ester in MCF-7 breast cancer cells. Oxidative Med Cell Longev 2016: 3017108. https://doi.org/10.1155/2016/3017108

Motawi TK, Abdelazim SA, Darwish HA et al (2016b) Could caffeic acid phenethyl ester expand the antitumor effect of tamoxifen in breast carcinoma? Nutr Cancer 68:435–445. https://doi.org/10.1080/01635581.2016.1153669

Mukherjee S, Mazumdar M, Chakraborty S et al (2014) Curcumin inhibits breast cancer stem cell migration by amplifying the E-cadherin/beta-catenin negative feedback loop. Stem Cell Res Ther 5:116. https://doi.org/10.1186/scrt506

Namasivayam SKR, Venkatachalam G, Bharani RSA et al (2021) Molecular intervention of colon cancer and inflammation manifestation by tannin capped biocompatible controlled sized gold nanoparticles from Terminalia bellirica: a green strategy for pharmacological drug formulation based on nanotechnology principles. 3 Biotech. https://doi.org/10.1007/s13205-021-02944-z

Namkaew J, Jaroonwitchawan T, Rujanapun N et al (2018) Combined effects of curcumin and doxorubicin on cell death and cell migration of SH-SY5Y human neuroblastoma cells. In Vitro Cell Dev Biol Anim. https://doi.org/10.1007/s11626-018-0288-9

Nguyen YTK, Moon JY, Ediriweera MK, Cho SK (2020) Phenethyl isothiocyanate suppresses stemness in the chemo-and radio-resistant triple-negative breast cancer cell line MDA-MB-231/IR via downregulation of metadherin. Cancers (Basel). https://doi.org/10.3390/cancers12020268

Ohara M, Kimura S, Tanaka A et al (2011) Benzyl isothiocyanate sensitizes human pancreatic cancer cells to radiation by inducing apoptosis. Int J Mol Med 28:1043–1047. https://doi.org/10.3892/ijmm.2011.770

Park BH, Lim JE, Jeon HG et al (2016) Curcumin potentiates antitumor activity of cisplatin in bladder cancer cell lines via ROS-mediated activation of ERK1/2. Oncotarget 7:63870–63886. https://doi.org/10.18632/oncotarget.11563

Quispe-Soto ET, Calaf GM (2016) Effect of curcumin and paclitaxel on breast carcinogenesis. Int J Oncol 49:2569–2577. https://doi.org/10.3892/ijo.2016.3741

Rahman KMW, Banerjee S, Ali S et al (2009) 3,3′-diindolylmethane enhances taxotere-induced apoptosis in hormone-refractory prostate cancer cells through survivin down-regulation. Cancer Res 69:4468–4475. https://doi.org/10.1158/0008-5472.CAN-08-4423

Rosman R, Saifullah B, Maniam S et al (2018) Improved anticancer effect of magnetite nanocomposite formulation of GALLIC acid (Fe(3)O(4)-PEG-GA) against lung, breast and colon cancer cells. Nanomater (Basel, Switzerland) 8. https://doi.org/10.3390/nano8020083

Sanchez-Carranza JN, Diaz JF, Redondo-Horcajo M et al (2018) Gallic acid sensitizes paclitaxel-resistant human ovarian carcinoma cells through an increase in reactive oxygen species and subsequent downregulation of ERK activation. Oncol Rep 39:3007–3014. https://doi.org/10.3892/or.2018.6382

Shan J, Xuan Y, Zhang Q et al (2016) Ursolic acid synergistically enhances the therapeutic effects of oxaliplatin in colorectal cancer. Protein Cell 7:571–585. https://doi.org/10.1007/s13238-016-0295-0

Shen X, Si Y, Wang Z et al (2016) Quercetin inhibits the growth of human gastric cancer stem cells by inducing mitochondrial-dependent apoptosis through the inhibition of PI3K/Akt signaling. Int J Mol Med 38:619–626. https://doi.org/10.3892/ijmm.2016.2625

Shi L, Gao X, Li X et al (2015) Ellagic acid enhances the efficacy of PI3K inhibitor GDC-0941 in breast cancer cells. Curr Mol Med 15:478–486

Shin JM, Lim E, Cho YS, Nho CW (2021) Cancer-preventive effect of phenethyl isothiocyanate through tumor microenvironment regulation in a colorectal cancer stem cell xenograft model. Phytomedicine. https://doi.org/10.1016/j.phymed.2021.153493

Singh D, Mohapatra P, Kumar S et al (2022) Nimbolide-encapsulated PLGA nanoparticles induces mesenchymal-to-epithelial transition by dual inhibition of AKT and mTOR in pancreatic cancer stem cells. Toxicol Vitr. https://doi.org/10.1016/j.tiv.2021.105293

Sirota R, Gibson D, Kohen R (2017) The timing of caffeic acid treatment with cisplatin determines sensitization or resistance of ovarian carcinoma cell lines. Redox Biol 11:170–175. https://doi.org/10.1016/j.redox.2016.12.006

Soni K, Kohli K (2018) Sulforaphane decorated gold nanoparticle for anti-cancer activity: in vitro and in vivo studies. Pharm Dev Technol:1–37. https://doi.org/10.1080/10837450.2018.1507038

Spagnuolo C, Russo GL, Orhan IE et al (2015) Genistein and cancer: current status, challenges, and future directions. Adv Nutr 6:408–419. https://doi.org/10.3945/an.114.008052

Srinual S, Chanvorachote P, Pongrakhananon V (2017) Suppression of cancer stem-like phenotypes in NCI-H460 lung cancer cells by vanillin through an Akt-dependent pathway. Int J Oncol 50:1341–1351. https://doi.org/10.3892/ijo.2017.3879

Stearns ME, Wang M (2011) Synergistic effects of the green tea extract epigallocatechin-3-gallate and taxane in eradication of malignant human prostate tumors. Transl Oncol 4:147–156

Su P, Yang Y, Wang G et al (2018) Curcumin attenuates resistance to irinotecan via induction of apoptosis of cancer stem cells in chemoresistant colon cancer cells. Int J Oncol 53:1343–1353. https://doi.org/10.3892/ijo.2018.4461

Sunil Gowda SN, Rajasowmiya S, Vadivel V et al (2018) Gallic acid-coated sliver nanoparticle alters the expression of radiation-induced epithelial-mesenchymal transition in non-small lung cancer cells. Toxicol In Vitro 52:170–177. https://doi.org/10.1016/j.tiv.2018.06.015

Takei T, Sato M, Ijima H, Kawakami K (2010) In situ gellable oxidized citrus pectin for localized delivery of anticancer drugs and prevention of homotypic cancer cell aggregation. Biomacromolecules 11:3525–3530. https://doi.org/10.1021/bm1010068

Tolba MF, Esmat A, Al-Abd AM et al (2013) Caffeic acid phenethyl ester synergistically enhances docetaxel and paclitaxel cytotoxicity in prostate cancer cells. IUBMB Life 65:716–729. https://doi.org/10.1002/iub.1188

Tripathi K, Hussein UK, Anupalli R et al (2015) Allyl isothiocyanate induces replication-associated DNA damage response in NSCLC cells and sensitizes to ionizing radiation. Oncotarget 6:5237–5252. https://doi.org/10.18632/oncotarget.3026

Tsai P-H, Cheng C-H, Lin C-Y et al (2016) Dietary flavonoids luteolin and quercetin suppressed cancer stem cell properties and metastatic potential of isolated prostate cancer cells. Anticancer Res 36:6367–6380. https://doi.org/10.21873/anticanres.11234

Venier NA, Colquhoun AJ, Sasaki H et al (2015) Capsaicin: a novel radio-sensitizing agent for prostate cancer. Prostate 75:113–125. https://doi.org/10.1002/pros.22896

Wang K, Liu R, Li J et al (2011) Quercetin induces protective autophagy in gastric cancer cells: involvement of Akt-mTOR- and hypoxia-induced factor 1alpha-mediated signaling. Autophagy 7:966–978

Wang L, Long L, Wang W, Liang Z (2015) Resveratrol, a potential radiation sensitizer for glioma stem cells both in vitro and in vivo. J Pharmacol Sci 129:216–225. https://doi.org/10.1016/j.jphs.2015.11.001

Wang R, Ma L, Weng D et al (2016a) Gallic acid induces apoptosis and enhances the anticancer effects of cisplatin in human small cell lung cancer H446 cell line via the ROS-dependent mitochondrial apoptotic pathway. Oncol Rep 35:3075–3083. https://doi.org/10.3892/or.2016.4690

Wang W-J, Sui H, Qi C et al (2016b) Ursolic acid inhibits proliferation and reverses drug resistance of ovarian cancer stem cells by downregulating ABCG2 through suppressing the expression of hypoxia-inducible factor-1alpha in vitro. Oncol Rep 36:428–440. https://doi.org/10.3892/or.2016.4813

Wang W, Lv M, Wang Y, Zhang J (2016c) Development of novel application of 3,3′-diindolylmethane: sensitizing multidrug resistance human breast cancer cells to gamma-irradiation. Pharm Biol 54:3164–3168. https://doi.org/10.1080/13880209.2016.1192198

Wang X, Li Y, Dai Y et al (2016d) Sulforaphane improves chemotherapy efficacy by targeting cancer stem cell-like properties via the miR-124/IL-6R/STAT3 axis. Sci Rep 6:36796. https://doi.org/10.1038/srep36796

Wang D, Kong X, Li Y et al (2017a) Curcumin inhibits bladder cancer stem cells by suppressing Sonic Hedgehog pathway. Biochem Biophys Res Commun 493:521–527. https://doi.org/10.1016/j.bbrc.2017.08.158
Wang N, Wang Q, Tang H et al (2017b) Direct inhibition of ACTN4 by ellagic acid limits breast cancer metastasis via regulation of beta-catenin stabilization in cancer stem cells. J Exp Clin Cancer Res 36:172. https://doi.org/10.1186/s13046-017-0635-9
Wang F, Wang W, Li J et al (2018a) Sulforaphane reverses gefitinib tolerance in human lung cancer cells via modulation of sonic hedgehog signaling. Oncol Lett 15:109–114. https://doi.org/10.3892/ol.2017.7293
Wang J, Wang C, Bu G (2018b) Curcumin inhibits the growth of liver cancer stem cells through the phosphatidylinositol 3-kinase/protein kinase B/mammalian target of rapamycin signaling pathway. Exp Ther Med 15:3650–3658. https://doi.org/10.3892/etm.2018.5805
Wang R, Yang L, Li S et al (2018c) Quercetin inhibits breast cancer stem cells via downregulation of aldehyde dehydrogenase 1A1 (ALDH1A1), chemokine receptor type 4 (CXCR4), mucin 1 (MUC1), and epithelial cell adhesion molecule (EpCAM). Med Sci Monit 24:412–420
Wu S, Zhang T, Du J (2016) Ursolic acid sensitizes cisplatin-resistant HepG2/DDP cells to cisplatin via inhibiting Nrf2/ARE pathway. Drug Des Devel Ther 10:3471–3481. https://doi.org/10.2147/DDDT.S110505
Wu X, Xu Y, Zhu B et al (2018) Resveratrol induces apoptosis in SGC-7901 gastric cancer cells. Oncol Lett 16:2949–2956. https://doi.org/10.3892/ol.2018.9045
Xu B, Tao Z-Z (2014) Piceatannol enhances the antitumor efficacy of gemcitabine in human A549 non-small cell lung cancer cells. Oncol Res 22:213–217. https://doi.org/10.3727/096504015X14386062091398
Yang Y, Li Y, Wang K et al (2013) P38/NF-kappaB/snail pathway is involved in caffeic acid-induced inhibition of cancer stem cells-like properties and migratory capacity in malignant human keratinocyte. PLoS One 8:e58915. https://doi.org/10.1371/journal.pone.0058915
Yang H, Huang S, Wei Y et al (2017) Curcumin enhances the anticancer effect of 5-fluorouracil against gastric cancer through down-regulation of COX-2 and NF- kappaB signaling pathways. J Cancer 8:3697–3706. https://doi.org/10.7150/jca.20196
Yang C, Song J, Hwang S et al (2021) Apigenin enhances apoptosis induction by 5-fluorouracil through regulation of thymidylate synthase in colorectal cancer cells. Redox Biol. https://doi.org/10.1016/j.redox.2021.102144
Yang CM, Chu TH, Tsai KW et al (2022) Phytochemically derived zingerone nanoparticles inhibit cell proliferation, invasion and metastasis in human oral squamous cell carcinoma. Biomedicines. https://doi.org/10.3390/biomedicines10020320
Yoshida K, Toden S, Ravindranathan P et al (2017) Curcumin sensitizes pancreatic cancer cells to gemcitabine by attenuating PRC2 subunit EZH2, and the lncRNA PVT1 expression. Carcinogenesis 38:1036–1046. https://doi.org/10.1093/carcin/bgx065
Yu S-H, Kao Y-T, Wu J-Y et al (2011) Inhibition of AMPK-associated autophagy enhances caffeic acid phenethyl ester-induced cell death in C6 glioma cells. Planta Med 77:907–914. https://doi.org/10.1055/s-0030-1250682
Yu C-Y, Wang Y-M, Li N-M et al (2014a) In vitro and in vivo evaluation of pectin-based nanoparticles for hepatocellular carcinoma drug chemotherapy. Mol Pharm 11:638–644. https://doi.org/10.1021/mp400412c
Yu D, Shin H-S, Lee YS et al (2014b) Genistein attenuates cancer stem cell characteristics in gastric cancer through the downregulation of Gli1. Oncol Rep 31:673–678. https://doi.org/10.3892/or.2013.2893
Yu X-D, Yang J-L, Zhang W-L, Liu D-X (2016) Resveratrol inhibits oral squamous cell carcinoma through induction of apoptosis and G2/M phase cell cycle arrest. Tumour Biol 37:2871–2877. https://doi.org/10.1007/s13277-015-3793-4
Yun JH, Kim K-A, Yoo G et al (2017) Phenethyl isothiocyanate suppresses cancer stem cell properties in vitro and in a xenograft model. Phytomedicine 30:42–49. https://doi.org/10.1016/j.phymed.2017.01.015

Zhang L, Li L, Jiao M et al (2012) Genistein inhibits the stemness properties of prostate cancer cells through targeting Hedgehog-Gli1 pathway. Cancer Lett 323:48–57. https://doi.org/10.1016/j.canlet.2012.03.037

Zhang P, Lai Z-L, Chen H-F et al (2017a) Curcumin synergizes with 5-fluorouracil by impairing AMPK/ULK1-dependent autophagy, AKT activity and enhancing apoptosis in colon cancer cells with tumor growth inhibition in xenograft mice. J Exp Clin Cancer Res 36:190. https://doi.org/10.1186/s13046-017-0661-7

Zhang X-F, Huang F-H, Zhang G-L et al (2017b) Novel biomolecule lycopene-reduced graphene oxide-silver nanoparticle enhances apoptotic potential of trichostatin A in human ovarian cancer cells (SKOV3). Int J Nanomedicine 12:7551–7575. https://doi.org/10.2147/IJN.S144161

Zhang Y, Huang L, Shi H et al (2018) Ursolic acid enhances the therapeutic effects of oxaliplatin in colorectal cancer by inhibition of drug resistance. Cancer Sci 109:94–102. https://doi.org/10.1111/cas.13425

Zhang T, Xu C, Zheng P et al (2022) Glaucocalyxin B attenuates ovarian cancer cell growth and cisplatin resistance in vitro via activating oxidative stress. Oxidative Med Cell Longev. https://doi.org/10.1155/2022/6324292

Zhao J, Zhu J, Lv X et al (2017) Curcumin potentiates the potent antitumor activity of ACNU against glioblastoma by suppressing the PI3K/AKT and NF-kappaB/COX-2 signaling pathways. Onco Targets Ther 10:5471–5482. https://doi.org/10.2147/OTT.S149708

Zhu J-Y, Yang X, Chen Y et al (2017) Curcumin suppresses lung cancer stem cells via inhibiting Wnt/beta-catenin and Sonic Hedgehog pathways. Phytother Res 31:680–688. https://doi.org/10.1002/ptr.5791

Zou X, Liang J, Sun J et al (2016) Allicin sensitizes hepatocellular cancer cells to anti-tumor activity of 5-fluorouracil through ROS-mediated mitochondrial pathway. J Pharmacol Sci 131:233–240. https://doi.org/10.1016/j.jphs.2016.04.017

Zou J, Zhu L, Jiang X et al (2018) Curcumin increases breast cancer cell sensitivity to cisplatin by decreasing FEN1 expression. Oncotarget 9:11268–11278. https://doi.org/10.18632/oncotarget.24109

Integrated Palliative Cancer Care: From an Interdisciplinary Perspective

Amene Saghazadeh and Nima Rezaei

Abstract

The spread of cancer is, particularly, in the advanced stages, so wide that symptoms related to multiple systems are present, along with increasing the psychosocial distress, pain, and fatigue that demand for palliative care (PC). PC integration is crucial to both the general healthcare system and the specific oncologic care. Also, PC should take both patients' and their families' needs into account for integration. There have been efforts to apply integrated PC to cancer, with reports of improved life quality, symptoms management, and survival. However, findings are not consistent and vary across studies largely. Timing has been shown to crucially contribute to the impact of PC on cancer-related outcomes; early is superior over delayed PC. Challenges with integrated palliative and oncologic care are numerous, calling for an interdisciplinary approach. Interdisciplinary PC is necessary for cancer because advanced cancer

A. Saghazadeh
Integrated Science Association (ISA), Universal Scientific Education and Research Network (USERN), Tehran, Iran

Systematic Review and Meta-Analysis Expert Group (SRMEG), Universal Scientific Education and Research Network (USERN), Tehran, Iran

Research Center for Immunodeficiencies, Children's Medical Center, Tehran University of Medical Sciences, Tehran, Iran

N. Rezaei (✉)
Research Center for Immunodeficiencies, Children's Medical Center, Tehran University of Medical Sciences, Tehran, Iran

Department of Immunology, School of Medicine, Tehran University of Medical Sciences, Tehran, Iran

Cancer Immunology Project (CIP), Universal Scientific Education and Research Network (USERN), Stockholm, Sweden
e-mail: rezaei_nima@tums.ac.ir

Interdisciplinary Cancer Research, https://doi.org/10.1007/16833_2022_23
Published online: 28 October 2022

is a disease with multiple symptoms. Particularly, anorexia, pain, and psychosocial problems cause cancer to be a complicated to complex condition. Interdisciplinary PC offers hopes to provide a comprehensive and personalized care to improve well-being and reduce the clinical/economic burden of the end-of-life care. PC delivery through an interdisciplinary approach applies to both inpatient settings and outpatient clinics, both short-term (acute) and long-term (chronic) care facilities, both adults and children, and to both patients and their families/caregivers. Despite the importance of interdisciplinary PC for being integrated into standard cancer care, the status of interdisciplinary research on PC for cancer is not satisfactory, calling for an international effort to take integrated PC a step closer to the bright future-personalized PC for all patients living with cancer.

Keywords

Cancer · Integrated palliative cancer care · Interdisciplinary · Palliative care · Quality of life · Survival

1 Introduction

1.1 The Burden of Cancer

Cancer is a global issue associated with a high, growing burden in most countries during the past three decades, especially in developing countries (Smith and Mallath 2019). Prostate and breast cancer are the most common cancers seen in male and female subjects. Totally, tracheal, bronchus, and lung cancer account for the first cause of death from cancer. As the incidence of cancer increases, so does the cancer-associated burden. Importantly, in the advanced stage, the spread of cancer is so wide that symptoms related to multiple systems, including the gastrointestinal tract, pulmonary, neurologic, urologic, and hematologic systems, are present, along with increasing the psychosocial distress, spiritual demand, pain, and fatigue (Hung et al. 2013).

1.2 Definitions

1.2.1 Palliative Care

The definition of palliative care (PC) has changed over time to embrace more and more details. A PC patient was once considered by the World Health Organization (WHO) as a patient with a disease who does not respond to treatment for that given disease. Also, according to that organization's definition, PC was a practice aimed at bringing about life quality for a patient with a life-threatening disease and his/her family and caregiver(s). It is beyond the scope of this chapter to review the PC-related criteria/definitions and their ambiguities/limitations that have led to updates to them. According to the most recently published systematic reviews, the definition of a PC patient needs to include information related to the patients' disease, disease progression, patient's prognosis, and patient's setting (Van

Mechelen et al. 2013). However, to be more operational, it is suggested to integrate "disease trajectory, the type of disease and its progression, approach and outcome, and other elements" into the PC or terminal care patient definition (Van Mechelen et al. 2013). Also, PC is, per a 2020' consensus, referred to as "the active holistic care of individuals across all ages with serious health-related suffering due to severe illness and especially of those near the end of life" (Radbruch et al. 2020).

Team-working is crucial to PC (Crawford and Price 2003). A team that takes responsibility for the delivery of PC deals with the patients, their families and caregivers, and their care. It starts at the intake to the PC program and stands until the death in an effort to attenuate suffering and enhance life quality and well-being as much as possible (O'Connor et al. 2006).

1.2.2 Interdisciplinary and Multidisciplinary Palliative Care

Studies have used interdisciplinary and multidisciplinary PC in cancer patients and their caregivers, adults and children with cancer, and outpatient and inpatient settings. Under an interdisciplinary approach, the PC delivery is optimized. It is due to features interdisciplinary team members can meet, mainly including a common understanding of the role of norms, roles, and values, highly interdependent cooperation, and arriving at a cooperation-based decision that gives a higher value to the patient compared to a specific discipline-based decision. To emphasize, this final decision results from the interaction and cooperation between team members and the integration of their thoughts; so, no individual member could solely achieve it. To make such a patient-centered decision (Crawford and Price 2003), an interdisciplinary PC team is recommended to contain social workers, nurses, medical specialists, and psychologists (O'Connor et al. 2006). Noteworthy mentioning is that interdisciplinary PC-related benefits are not limited to the patients but extend to the team members who participated, i.e., practitioners and specialists, enabling them to develop the combination of skills (Crawford and Price 2003).

Like an interdisciplinary team, a multidisciplinary team comprises people from different disciplines to provide patients with PC. They differ in that, in general, integrated thoughts are the main product of interdisciplinary teamwork, while this integration does not occur in multidisciplinary teams (Bowen 2014). Multidisciplinary PC approaches for cancer mainly occurs in clinics and conferences (Shao et al. 2019). Multidisciplinary conferences are referred to as the collective of team meetings, case management meetings, and tumor boards. Multidisciplinary clinics comprise teams, rounds, a one-stop clinic, and a committee. Outcomes of multidisciplinary care are measured in relation to the patient, care provider, and system. Through a systematic literature review (Shao et al. 2019), studies concerning multidisciplinary PC for patients with breast cancer were included, leading to the identification of the following outcomes:

(i) Patient level: clinical outcomes and patient satisfaction
(ii) Provide level: provider satisfaction and clinical decision-making
(iii) System level: time to intervention, enrollment in clinical trials, and guideline adherence and implementation

As the main focus of this book is an interdisciplinary research, we do not discuss further multidisciplinary PC in this chapter.

1.3 Palliative Care for Cancer

The use of PC in the setting of oncology dates back to the 1950s (Clark 2007). In its earlier forms, the main objective of the PC was to relieve pain. In its current form, the PC comprises different domains: symptom management, life quality, patient and caregiver satisfaction, end-of-life care, survival, and care-related costs. Such applicability has led to the development of an integrated science that is integrated with PC and oncology that comprises oncology teams, psychosocial teams, and PC teams to provide the best possible mental health for patients with cancer who are incurable. The duration from the initiation of PC to death is between 15 and 18 days for patients with cancer, as estimated in a meta-analysis (Hung et al. 2013; Jordan et al. 2020). During this period, the care needs of patients are due to their cancer and comorbidities and their needs as a person. The latter range from acute and chronic issues to psychosocial, existential, and spiritual issues:

(i) Acute, physical symptoms: delirium and depression at risk of suicidality
(ii) Chronic, physical symptoms: anxiety, depression, and physical function
(iii) Psychosocial: advanced care planning, family structure, and caregiver care
(iv) Existential and spiritual: meaning, hopefulness, legacy and dignity, and religious and spiritual well-being

As in other integrated contexts, the integration of PC into oncology is faced with challenges and difficulties to achieve success (Hui and Bruera 2016). Successful integrated PC and oncology is indicated by items related to the clinical structure, clinical processes, education, research, and administration (Hui and Bruera 2016). A study of cancer institutes in the United States revealed that around 98% and 78% of national and non-national centers incorporated a PC program; however, there was great heterogeneity in resources and services (Hui et al. 2010). This warrants that there might be centers wherein the integration has not been properly implemented.

1.4 Objective

This chapter reviews the effect of integrated/interdisciplinary/multidisciplinary PC on cancer-related outcomes. To this end, we searched for systematic review and meta-analysis studies through PubMed using the combination of keywords: ("interdisciplinary," OR "multidisciplinary," OR "integrated," OR "integration") AND (palliative) AND (cancer) AND ("systematic review" OR "meta-analysis") on April 17, 2022. This part contains Sects. 2, 3, 4, 5, and 6 and discusses PC for cancer largely under an integrated framework. Then, an interdisciplinary-focused discussion is held in Sect. 7 to address the reasons, hopes, and requirements of an interdisciplinary approach to PC for cancer. Finally, the chapter concludes with a brief summary in Sect. 8.

2 Palliative Care for Cancer: Important Concepts

2.1 Supportive, Palliative, and Hospice Care

The origin of hospice dates back to the 1950s, when concerns emerged for patients dying from cancer–patients who have completed several interventions, including surgery, radiotherapy, chemotherapy, etc., but showing no effective response and therefore are expecting their death (Clark 2007). The concern is that these patients are still living, and so they are still our patients; however, their needs are different from those who are successfully cured; so there is a need for services that provide the patients beyond the conventional care, that is, diagnostics and therapeutics (Mor and Masterson-Allen 1990). The 1950s witnessed the research on understanding the psychosocial needs of patients came to physicians. During the 1960s, it evolved to embrace patients' caregivers as well, the importance of pain management, and communication with patients. Christopher's Hospice was built in 1967 to take a step toward modern hospice in practice through integrated clinical care, research, and education. Following Christopher's Hospice's success, other hospitals began to support the end-of-life or terminal, with more than 200 hospitals being active in hospice care by the end of 1996. In the 1980s, the efforts led to the development of palliative medicine, initially as a subspecialty and later as a specialty (Clark 2007).

In the literature, different terms apply when PC for cancer is under discussion, mainly the supportive care, PC, and hospice care. A range of definitions has been available for each with overlaps and differences, as reviewed in detail in Hui et al. (2013). To the purpose of this chapter, it needs to distinguish these concepts, so the implications of the following discussion which is totally on PC research become clear. "Hospice" is the oldest term, whereas "supportive" is the newest. Also, moving from the hospice care to the PC and supportive care, there is a less stigma associated with the term, the care has been based on hospital services rather than at-home care, more services have been working, and more stages of the disease have been captured–from the bereavement stage for the hospice care, the advanced and bereavement stages of disease for the PC, and early stages to the advanced and bereavement stages of disease for the supportive care (Fig. 1). During this positive movement, however, we see that the emergence of multiple definitions has caused ambiguities regarding the understanding of the terms and that the voluntary works have been diminishing.

2.2 Traditional Palliative Care and Early Palliative Care

PC was traditionally adopted as a strategy when life-prolonging or curative treatment is completed, but patients do not respond to the treatment (Kaasa et al. 2018). In

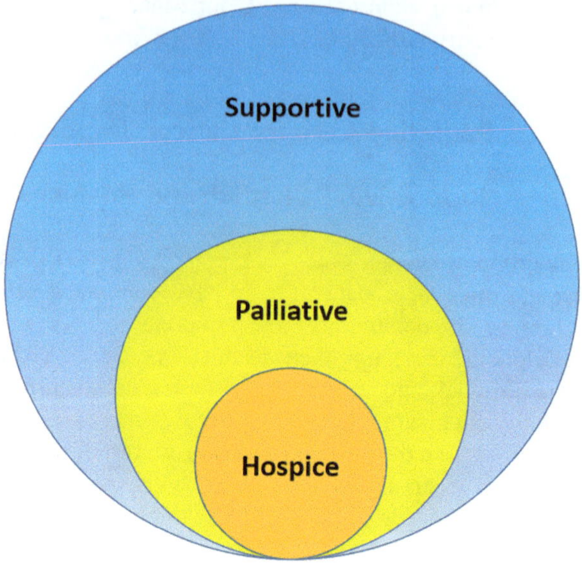

Fig. 1 The supportive, palliative, and hospice care

contrast, early PC is supposed to be administered early since diagnosis is made. Both forms are continued until the death of the patient. Both aim to enhance life quality and help with symptoms management.

3 Integration of Palliative Care for Cancer

3.1 Integration Levels

PC integration is crucial to both the general healthcare system and the specific oncologic care. Also, PC should take both patients' and their families' needs into account for integration. The main levels of integration are linkage, coordination, and full:

(i) In the linkage level, the patients' needs and the professions' skills are understood, and the components working occurs in parallel or in series, ensuring that an integrated system is provided for caring for patients;
(ii) In the coordination level, integration grows with a more structural approach. Different system structures start in an integrated manner, i.e., pathology, imaging, radiation, surgery, chemotherapy, etc. This integrated work has a regular plan for follow-up visits. A regular plan exists for evaluation and monitoring of the plan itself. These ensure the caring of patients in a structured and needs-based framework; and
(iii) Finally, all resources are unified at the full integration level, and silos are broken down, resulting in integrated products, such as multidisciplinary meetings (Kaasa et al. 2018).

3.2 Integration Components

Twelve components of integration broadly fall into the clinical structure and clinical processes (Hui et al. 2015a). As highlighted in a systematic review (Hui et al. 2015b), we can see the degree to which integration has been working in the seven included RCTs (Jordhøy et al. 2000; Temel et al. 2010, 2017; Zimmermann et al. 2014; Bakitas et al. 2015; Maltoni et al. 2016; Groenvold et al. 2017) as follows:

(i) Clinical structure
  - *Palliative care inpatient consultation team*, six studies met this item
  - *Palliative care outpatient clinic*, all studies met this item
  - *Community-based care or home palliative care*, two studies met this item

(ii) Clinical processes
  - *Multidisciplinary specialized palliative care team*, all studies met this item
  - *Routine symptom screening in the outpatient oncology clinic*, none of studies met this item
  - *Administration of systemic cancer therapy possible in patients admitted to palliative care service*, all studies met this item
  - *Follow prespecified palliative care guidelines*, five studies met this item
  - *Early referral to palliative care*, all studies met this item
  - *Availability of clinical care pathways (automatic triggers) for palliative care referral*, none of studies met this item
  - *Palliative care team routinely involved in multidisciplinary tumor conference for patient case discussions*, only one study met this item
  - *Communication, cooperation, and coordination between palliative and oncology service*, three studies met this item
  - *Routine discussion of prognosis, advance care planning with goals of care*, all studies met this item

Altogether, none of the studies could meet all items: two studies met nine out of 12 items, four studies met seven out of 12 items, and one study met six of 12 items. To arrive at an integrated PC for cancer in healthcare and cancer care is a long task, requiring policymakers' active contribution to spending proper funding to design and implement well-structured models at both national and international levels (Kaasa et al. 2018).

4 Palliative Care for Different Cancers

4.1 Breast Cancer

A systematic review (Drageset et al. 2021) identified six studies evaluating the effect of PC on life quality in patients with metastatic breast cancer. These studies supported that an interdisciplinary approach is required for the delivery of

PC. Patients receiving the integrated PC and standard oncologic care experienced a better quality of life and longer survival, felt less depressed, and were less likely to need chemotherapy than patients undergoing standard oncologic care alone. Other programs that have been used as a part of an interdisciplinary approach and could improve life quality include supervised exercise therapy (SET), art therapy, psychotherapy, and prayer. SET caused an increase in oxygen consumption and body composition, as well.

4.2 Hematological Cancer

Three studies investigating the PC in the interdisciplinary or multidisciplinary format for patients with hematological cancer were included in the review (Tanzi et al. 2020). Rodin et al. 2019 compared the effectiveness of integrated psychological care, PC, and standard care with that of standard care alone in patients with acute leukemia. For the integrated intervention, emotion and symptom-focused engagement (EASE) was used (Rodin et al. 2020). The integrated intervention was perceived as convenient and led to a significant reduction in stress symptoms, pain intensity, and pain interference. In the study by Hung et al. 2013, PC consultation was for the caring patients and their families delivered along with weekly phone interviews by an interdisciplinary team that comprised physicians, social workers, Buddhists, nurse specialists, and volunteer subjects (Hung et al. 2013). The third study by Selvaggi et al. 2014 held interdisciplinary meetings to provide PC consultation on the goals of care, including symptom control (Selvaggi et al. 2014), for patients with leukemia, lymphoma, multiple myeloma, and myelodysplastic syndrome. PC care could help pain management, with more than 60% of patients satisfied within only 2 days after PC consultation. Also, oncologists were happy with the care. The initiation of the program could noticeably increase hospice referrals by more than 30%. The systematic review found the lack of well-designed prospective studies on interdisciplinary/multidisciplinary PC in patients with hematological malignancies (Tanzi et al. 2020).

4.3 Pediatric Cancer

A systematic review of 32 studies of children with cancer and their parents investigated the effect of specialty pediatric palliative care (SPPC). Children undergoing SPPC showed symptom improvement, pain relief, and better life quality. They were also less likely to need intensive procedures and end-of-life care, while the likelihood of completing advanced care programs and dying at home increased. Children's families acknowledged the positive effect of SPPS; particularly, they felt they were better at communicating with their children (Kaye et al. 2021).

In the review (Piette et al. 2021), undergoing PC led to improve life quality and physical and psychological symptoms in children with cancer. In particular, as reported by the child or parent, life quality, amount of fun, events adding meaning to life, and communication were increased, whereas constipation, energy loss, pain, and dyspnea were decreased.

4.4 Thoracic Cancer

A systematic review (Brighton et al. 2019) aimed to investigate the impact of holistic services on patients suffering from chronic breathlessness. It included nine studies merely on patients with cancer, including lung cancer, intrathoracic malignancy, mesothelioma, etc. The services involved different disciplines, mainly including nursing, occupational therapy, social work, PC, oncology, physiotherapy, psychology, nutrition and dietetics, and complementary therapies. The duration of services ranged from one to 12 months. However, data synthesis was done for all 12 studies included, with more than 77% of patients having advanced cancer. In general, patients provided with holistic services showed an improvement in distress due to breathlessness and depression and anxiety scores; however, the life quality remained unchanged.

Eleven studies addressing the effectiveness of multidisciplinary PC were included in the review (Kochovska et al. 2020). Compared with those receiving the oncologic care alone, patients who underwent the combined specialized PC and oncologic care were less likely to experience lung cancer-related premature mortality and aggressive end-of-life care. Also, they had an improved life quality and were more satisfied with the PC and willing to share their thoughts about their death. However, a meta-analysis of two studies showed no significant difference between the two groups with regard to depressive symptoms, as assessed by the Patient Health Questionnaire 9 (PHQ-9). For caregivers, any improvement in overall life quality was absent with PC; however, depression, anxiety, and stress showed to improve somewhat.

The oncologic care alone was not different from a nutritional and physical exercise program and a nurse-directed face-to-face educational program in improving life quality in a mixed population of patients with cancer, including lung cancer. The same was true for multidisciplinary PC in patients with inoperable lung cancer. However, patients were satisfied with what a nurse-directed face-to-face educational program discussed. The caregivers of patients who underwent mindfulness-based stress reduction programs reported no improvement in life quality. Moreover, telephone symptom management (TSM) could not enable caregivers to control their own efficacy.

For patients with incurable lung cancer, early PC plus oncologic care was not different from usual care alone in improving personal competence. Even patients undergoing the usual care alone experienced an improvement in their social competence, whereas those receiving the integrated care did not do so. Moreover, health perceptions were deteriorating for both groups. These lines might imply that self-efficacy is an outcome that involves complex care, and current PC and oncologic care are not so to address it (Kochovska et al. 2020).

There were five studies of integrated early PC and anti-cancer treatment for patients with advanced lung cancer in the review (Ambroggi et al. 2018). However, no meta-analysis was done. The narrative synthesis concluded an improvement in life quality and survival with the intervention of interest.

4.5 Mixed

The study (Fulton et al. 2019) included ten randomized controlled trials (RCTs) of integrated PC for patients with advanced cancer. The authors appraised the level of integration for each study in terms of co-located care teams, routinely shared written or electronic information, bidirectional communication between care teams, information transmitted as a common and usual process, equal decision-making responsibilities for caregivers, standardized care for all patients, and a unified therapy strategy. Accordingly, the level of integration was rated low to moderate. Integrated PC led to improvement in life quality in the short-term but not at six to 12 months, physical symptoms but not psychological symptoms (i.e., depressive and anxiety symptoms), and survival at 12 months. For caregivers, it was associated with a better experience and improved depressive symptoms at month 3 of intervention. Such an effect could not be sustained after the patient died. Moreover, there was no improvement in caregivers' life quality. Worth mentioning is the lack of any association between integration levels and the influence of PC, both in general and particularly regarding life quality. This might imply that integration levels/elements might benefit from reform to represent changes in the intervention-related factors corresponding to changes to the outcomes of interest.

Another quantitative synthesis included eight RCTs providing high-quality and preliminary evidence, six of which were also included in the above study (Hoerger et al. 2019). However, the analyses are somewhat different, making them worth mentioning. Undergoing outpatient specialty PC led to a better survival associated with an absolute increase of about 6%, 11%, 14%, 10%, and 13% at six, nine, 12, 15, and 18 months compared to receiving usual care. However, such an effect was not observed at three, 21, and 24 months. According to the Kaplan–Meier curves, the median survival benefit for PC was about 4.6 months. The authors performed the analysis for life quality by including high-quality studies and could find a significant improvement in life quality with PC in all terms of physical, psychological, and global dimensions.

In the review (Kassianos et al. 2018), 11 studies on the effect of specialized PC on different types of cancer were included. Meta-analysis showed a significant effect of SPC on health-related life quality.

5 Timing: An Important Factor Contributing to the Impact of Palliative Care on Cancer-Related Outcomes

Timing is crucial to a PC's success. Despite this, a systematic review of 16 studies concerning PC for children with cancer shows that the issue is very vulnerable to neglect, with only around half of patients receiving PC before death (Cheng et al.

2019). Moreover, PC initiation was reported to take place late in relation to disease diagnosis, with a weighted mean of more than 500 days. As a result, PC duration is small, with a mean between about 56 and 70 days for patients in the pediatric oncology setting.

The two studies included in the review (Fadol et al. 2021) that compared early and delayed PC referral for patients with cancer are inconsistent with regard to results. One study by Temel et al. (2010) was conducted on patients with metastatic non-small-cell lung cancer. Compared with patients who received standard oncologic care alone, those undergoing integrated early PC and standard oncologic care alone showed better life quality, were less likely to develop depressive symptoms and need for the end-of-life aggressive care, and survived longer (median of around 12 vs. nine months). The other by Bakitas et al. (Bakitas et al. 2015) was run on patients with advanced cancer. Those with early PC were more likely to survive one year after enrollment in the study than those with delayed PC (delay of three months), but the two groups were not different with regard to patient-reported outcomes, e.g., mood, symptom impact, and life quality, as well as for hospitalization days, intensive care unit days, emergency room visits, chemotherapy over the past 2 weeks, and home death.

6 Challenges with Integrated Palliative Care and Oncologic Care

6.1 Limited Interaction with Palliative Care Services

As reported by patients, their interaction mainly occurs with healthcare professionals, and it is limited to general practitioners and PC services (Drageset et al. 2021)–being a cause of patients' dissatisfaction with their care.

6.2 Ambiguities with Regard to the Understanding of Palliative Care

As highlighted in Drageset et al. (2021), patients tend to misunderstand PC as a disease stage, treatment goal, and end-of-life care. For the latter, PC was not favorable for patients to follow. Moreover, patients did not consider complementary therapies/approaches as PC.

6.3 Delayed or Hindered Referral

Oncologists and hematologists believe making a referral is not cost-effective, and for this, they might decide to delay or cancel the referral-making task (Salins et al. 2020). Challenges with a delayed or hindered referral are, in turn, different, including the following:

- Role conflict, due to the therapeutic alliance rupture and a low degree of hope for treatment
- Diminished trust due to oncologists' and hematologists' desire to control the whole process themselves
- A daunting task, due to different factors, e.g., PC-related stigma, issues at the level of patients, families, and organizations
- Costs, mainly due to inconsistency of communication

For integrated care to address these challenges, it is essential to focus on the enhancement of PC resources (Salins et al. 2020).

In line with this, another systematic review (Dowling et al. 2020) highlighted that though hematologists acknowledge how integration is necessary for PC into cancer treatment, there are three major questions hematologists ask and repeat themselves, making them decide not properly about referrals:

- "Maybe we can pull another 'rabbit out of the hat'"
- "To tell or not to tell?"
- "Hospice, home or hospital?"

It seems the substitution of palliative with supportive would decrease the burden of concern hematologists feel with recommending a patient for PC referral (Dowling et al. 2020). However, by definition, PC is different from supportive care. So, to interchange terms, it is crucial for their definitions to be reformed in parallel.

6.4 Lack of Adequate Education

According to a systematic review, currently, about 70% of oncologists do agree that PC integration into standard care might help improve patients' life quality in China (Willemsen et al. 2021). Despite this, PC is not included in most undergraduate and postgraduate medical education programs. Efforts are required to design integrated medical education to offer to enhance understanding of the importance of PC.

6.5 Communication with Parents

For parents, it is often difficult to understand and accept that their children have a progressive condition that is cancer. Also, for pediatricians, it is challenging to keep parents updated on the most recent condition of their children and describe the outcomes they probably develop soon. Such difficulty lies mainly in a lack of trained physicians who are unable to communicate with parents truthfully while trying to care about their children hopefully. Indeed, what the parents of children with cancer really want is to speak about their children. This requires health professionals to make a conversation with the parents that is both open and empathetic (Wolfe et al. 2002). This, again, calls for a PC both being integrated into the standard care and working in an interdisciplinary manner to take into account both physical and psychological factors (Le Rouzic and Claudot 2020).

7 Interdisciplinary Palliative Care for Cancer

Looking at the results by time–obtained through our search mentioned earlier–it is realized that the topic has been under relative isolation, with less than ten studies published annually up to the year 2010 (Fig. 2). The number of publications per year has been between 15 and 44 since then; however, a point of concern again exists that it does not follow a regular increasing trend. Despite the importance of interdisciplinary PC for being integrated into standard cancer care, these facts about the status of interdisciplinary research on PC for cancer are not satisfactory, calling for an international effort to address the issue.

The major fields of interdisciplinary PC research on cancer include pain and symptoms control, access to PC services, translational research, education, and communication (Desa et al. 2008). Some important notes are provided further.

7.1 The Necessity of Interdisciplinary Palliative Care: The Reasons

PC is, in nature, an interdisciplinary specialty (Gelfman et al. 2008).

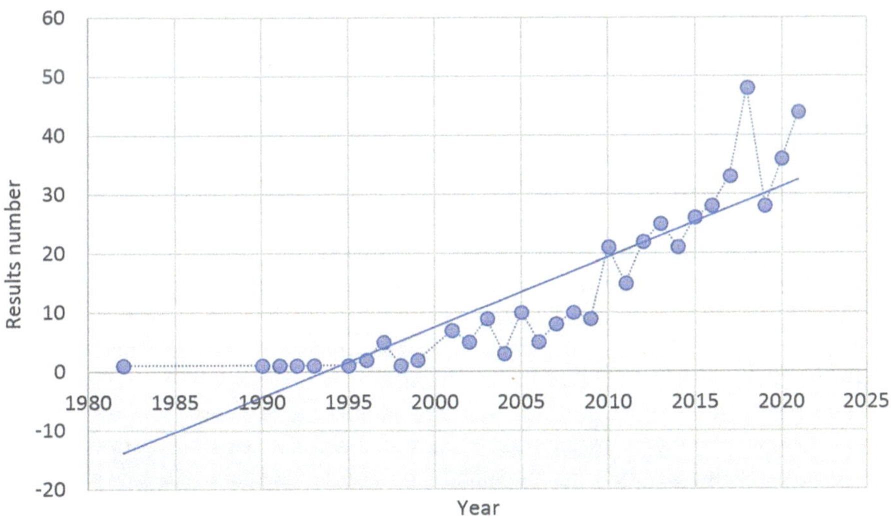

Fig. 2 The development of research on interdisciplinary palliative care for cancer

7.1.1 Advanced Cancer: A Disease with Multiple Symptoms

In the advanced stage of cancer, patients with cancer complain of a wide range of symptoms due to multiple systems affected and also as a consequence of anti-cancer therapy. In this stage, the disease is called incurable. According to evaluations by patients, nurses, and doctors, symptoms mainly include asthenia, pain, anorexia, and anxiety. However, these symptoms might vary by type of cancer; for example, patients with brain tumors might develop cognitive deficits as well (Ostgathe et al. 2010). Anyway, to deal with the problem of "advanced cancer," it means to treat different symptoms; so an interdisciplinary team including doctors, nurses, social workers, and psychologists is essential (Verger et al. 1992). There are hopes for the symptoms' management, providing the patients with opportunities to spend the remainder of their lives with quality and happiness.

7.1.2 Cancer Anorexia: Multiple Pathophysiological Mechanisms

Anorexia commonly happens to patients with cancer, with about half of patients reporting subjective anorexia. Anorexia is a major part of cancer anorexia-cachexia syndrome, characterized by appetite loss, weight loss, and nutritional deficiencies. About one-third of patients with cancer develop this condition, which affects physical functioning and, therefore, overall life quality. Anorexia-cachexia syndrome is thought to be the result of central and peripheral mechanisms. Central mechanisms are mediated by neurotransmitters, neuropeptides, and prostaglandins, affecting the patients' appetite. Peripheral mechanisms are numerous, including tumor-releasing substances, e.g., cytokines, lactate, and hormones that mediate harmful processes, such as inflammation and hypoxia or affect feeding, dysphagia due to cancer, and tumor-causing micronutrient deficiency (Ezeoke and Morley 2015). Such a condition, therefore, requires an approach to take multiple causes into consideration. Specialties crucial to the management of cancer anorexia-cachexia include doctors, nutritionists, and speech and swallowing specialties. They need to provide an individualized intervention suitable to treat the symptoms and improve the nutritional status and life quality of patients (Strasser and Bruera 2002; Granda-Cameron et al. 2010).

7.1.3 Cancer Pain: A Complicated Condition

Pain is common to patients with cancer, as experienced by up to 90% of terminally ill patients with cancer (Brennan 1993). Pain perception is under the influence of physical symptoms but also depends on a wide range of environmental, societal, and psychological factors (Scott 1982). For this, it is very expected that analgesics administration in a non-PC setting could not address the patients' pain adequately, but a PC unit working in an interdisciplinary manner is required to address all the issues collectively causing a cancer patient perceives severe pain. There is a need for a multidisciplinary team involving different specialties, e.g., consultative psychiatry, PC, supportive care, and rehabilitation (Brennan 1993), to act in place along with providing medical interventions and services.

7.1.4 Cancer Psychosocial Problems: A Complex Condition

Cancer-related stressors are numerous, causing the patients to feel a huge amount of psychosocial distress (Isikhan 2010). Consequently, psychosocial issues commonly happen to patients with cancer, observed from cancer diagnosis to advanced stages. They mainly include mood disorders and anxiety. Even psychosocial problems are more refractory to treatment than cancer pain. To exemplify, in one study (Verger et al. 1992), pain control was successful in more than 80% of patients with advanced cancer, standing in sharp contrast to the successful control of psychosocial distress, which was seen for less than 30% of patients. In particular, patients express existential suffering, which is the collective of anxiety due to uncertainty, guilt feelings, and meaninglessness due to dependency. To address this suffering, there have been developed numerous interventions, such as "supportive-expressive therapy," "providing comfortable environments," "meaning-centered approach," "being," "education and coping skills training," and "a religious approach" (Hirai et al. 2003). Importantly, these interventions need to be individualized by the patient's suffering; patients with anxiety might benefit from "providing comfortable environments" while those with meaningless from a "meaning-centered approach" and "being." It again calls for an integrated, interdisciplinary approach to identify the main causes of suffering and accordingly attenuate psychological distress while improving life quality.

7.1.5 Advanced Cancer: A Disease That Requires a Comprehensive Care

Once a cancer diagnosis is made, several disciplines are required to work jointly to manage the disease. For example, in the case of head and neck cancers, an interdisciplinary team of palliative specialists, otolaryngologists, oncologists, radiation oncologists, nutritionists, speech specialists, nutritionists, and occupational therapists is required. Moreover, in the advanced stage, the continuity of caring for cancer patients involves aggressive care, symptoms control, and interventions for life quality and comfort improvement. It includes palliative surgery for specific types of cancer as well, e.g., pancreatic cancer (Ferrell et al. 2003; Assfalg et al. 2011). This continuity is maintained when different specialties work together to ensure patients are well-cared in a comprehensive and personalized manner.

7.2 The Necessity of Interdisciplinary Palliative Care: The Hopes

7.2.1 To Improve Well-Being

Psycho-oncology is an interdisciplinary field addressing both PC and oncologic care. Examples of research projects in the field apply psychotherapy, music therapy, and attitude and spiritual care (Renz et al. 2005). They have shown positive effects on the complex suffering patients experience near-death, including a reduction in pain and anxiety and improvement of well-being. In particular, practicing spirituality in individual interviews and focused-group discussions enables patients to form the love in their souls but also to identify common values, inspiring them toward a collective soul (Sinclair et al. 2006). Music therapy can be used as a part of interdisciplinary PC for symptoms management and to help patients cope with the condition (Horne-Thompson et al. 2007). Also, interdisciplinary programs encouraging patients to do physical activity are recommended to restore physical functioning and thereby improve their life quality (Lowe 2011). It is, however, dependent upon whether the patient is able to do physical activity and, if so, how it is better to be scheduled. This calls for the inclusion of physical therapists in the interdisciplinary PC team.

7.2.2 To Reduce the Clinical/Economic Burden of End-of-Life Care

PC delivery through an interdisciplinary approach has a wide range of applications in both inpatient settings and outpatient clinics and in both short-term (acute) and long-term (chronic) care facilities (Ferris et al. 2009). Comprehensive, adaptable, life-affirming, longitudinal (CALL) intervention is another example. It has been shown to be effective in pain and symptoms control, with less than 30% of patients requiring hospitalization and less than 10% for admission to critical care (London et al. 2005). In line with this, the percentage of patients dying at home –that is, the desired outcome as it reflects the patient is satisfied with the end-of-life care – has been shown to be increased by interdisciplinary PC programs (Kurashima et al. 2005). For these reasons, interdisciplinary PC, especially home-based programs, is of interest to improve dying at home and thereby reducing resource utilization and cancer care-related costs as well (Enguidanos et al. 2005; Johnson et al. 2009). Indeed, interdisciplinary PC programs are helpful to reduce the burden of end-of-life cancer care in both clinical and economic terms (Hanson et al. 2008).

7.2.3 Interdisciplinary Palliative Care for Cancer

It applies to both adults and children and to both patients and their families/caregivers. For adults, an interdisciplinary program for patients with lung cancer often includes interviews with patients through which several life quality-related concerns can be highlighted, e.g., fatigue, dyspnea, pain, anxiety, family/psychological distress, isolation, cough, hemoptysis, depression, neuropathy, lack of energy, shortness of breath, sleep, weight loss, appetite, and daily functions. Based on patients' concerns, interviewers decide to provide patients with recommendations by, for example, referring to nutritionists, psychiatrists, psychologists, social workers, and rehabilitators. Such an interdisciplinary PC program has been shown to lead to improvement in the overall life quality, fatigue-related life quality, overall pain barriers score, overall fatigue barriers score, addiction danger, and Sensory–Piper fatigue scale (Borneman et al. 2008). The Pediatric Advanced Care Team (PACT) is an example project aimed to provide care for children with serious conditions like cancer and their families. A consult template of this program includes medical history, social history, physical examination, medications, and care-related discussion about the general goals of care, symptoms control, type of support required for the child and family, and how to deal with life-threatening events, such as death, communicating with the child to share his/her understanding of the current condition, fears and hopes, and preference for the location of death (Duncan et al. 2007). For caregivers, interdisciplinary PC consultation has proved to be more able to address family members' needs than standard care. Also, it could enhance caregivers' self-efficacy significantly (Gelfman et al. 2008).

7.3 The Necessity of Interdisciplinary Palliative Care: The Requirements

7.3.1 Tools for the Identification of Patients' Needs

Interdisciplinary tools are required to start with the screening of patients in need of PC. SPICT™ is such a tool that evaluates patients using two major classes of items that indicate the health status that is poor or worsening and the condition that limits life and functioning. Its evaluation ends with reviewing the current care and planning for future care (Bergenholtz et al. 2022).

7.3.2 Interdisciplinary Communication with Professions

Interdisciplinary teams for PC for cancer involve different professions. For an interdisciplinary team to act successfully, it is mandatory for team members to have consensus on the fundamental aspects of PC, i.e., how to communicate with patients and how to decide about them; otherwise, a program for arriving at consensus is indicated, so no significant interprofessional disagreement exists (Levorato et al. 2001). Particularly, nurses and physicians are the main actors of an interdisciplinary PC team, and their communication with patients is of utmost importance. They should take care mainly of what the patients perceive as their disease, what their needs are, and what they like to know.

7.3.3 Interdisciplinary Cooperation with Caregivers

Interdisciplinary at-home PC engages general practitioners and caregivers to work in cooperation with each other (Borgsteede et al. 2007). A Dutch national survey revealed cooperation between general practitioners and caregivers as the most common type of cooperation, followed by cooperation between general practitioners and cooperation between general practitioners and nurses.

7.3.4 Interdisciplinary Training

It is important for the training of health professionals to include interdisciplinary collaboration; however, multiple concerns exist mainly with regard to the goals, methods, and content of education and teaching emotional engagement (Papadatou 1997).

8 Conclusion

In summary, PC can help patients and their caregivers and physicians to better deal with the complicated condition of cancer. Also, the hospitals might benefit from PC. Studies show that PC can lead to a reduction in hospitalizations (Carmont et al.

2018). Supporting this, a meta-analysis of six cohort studies showed that early PC (initiated within the first 72 h of hospitalization) was associated with a significant decrease in total direct hospital costs (May et al. 2018). The first important factor is, therefore, to initiate PC as early as possible, and for early PC initiation, it is crucial to be integrated into the standard oncologic care. Then, this integration needs to continue its development so different dimensions of PC become a part of cancer care. Of note, there are various challenges with spiritual care programs, including, but not limited to, spaces suitable for spiritual care, professional issues, and academic considerations (Sinclair et al. 2009). Notably, spiritual care has been recently recommended to be incorporated into PC (Moosavi et al. 2020), ensuring that both patients and their caregivers are on spiritual support (Robert et al. 2019). More important is the implementation of cancer PC across the world in all settings. For this, resource-stratified guidelines have been developed, including recommendations for multiple domains (Osman et al. 2018) (Fig. 3), along with implementation strategies (Gilligan et al. 2017). Particularly, there is a need to develop PC programs for vulnerable populations with cancer who live in low- to middle-income countries and do not have access to PC services, crucially children (Delgado et al. 2010). For the future, a line of research is necessary to conduct quality studies addressing the

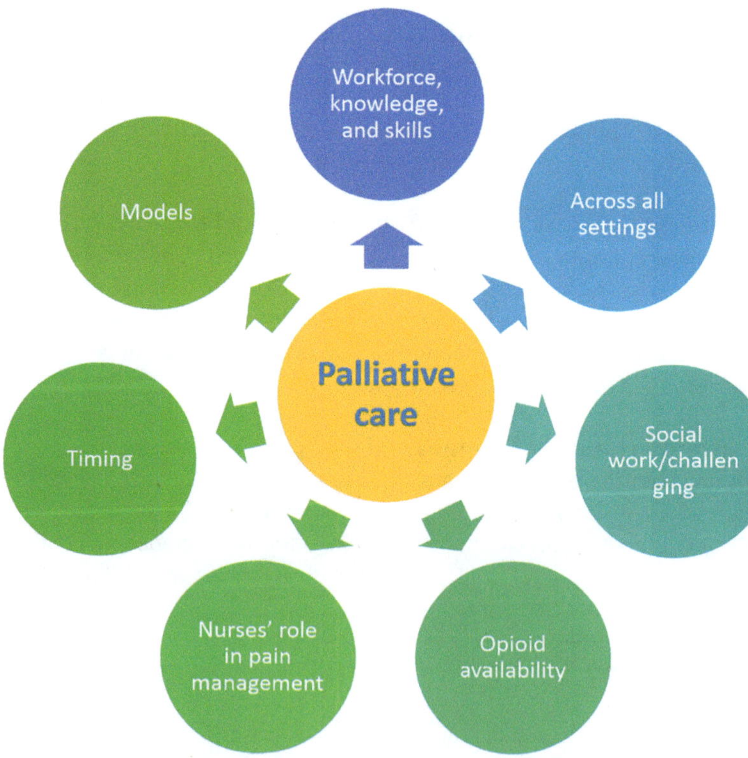

Fig. 3 Palliative care: recommendations

problems of the current literature that limit us in interpreting the results, most importantly methodological heterogeneity, publication bias, and potential sources of risk (Kassianos et al. 2018).

For PC to be integrated into cancer care, an interdisciplinary approach is not a catalyst but an essential to taking the multifactorial entity of cancer into the account of care. When all relevant sectors are available to contribute, then integrated palliative cancer care can set the goals and achieve outcomes that otherwise remain a dream. That is, we are looking forward to seeing each and every patient and all his/her family members and caregivers feel the power to cope effectively with cancer. That day, fears are not eliminated; of course, they exist; however, hopes are more than fears.

Acknowledgments None.

Compliance with Ethical Standards The authors declare that there is no conflict of interest.

References

Ambroggi M, Biasini C, Toscani I, Orlandi E, Berte R, Mazzari M, Cavanna L (2018) Can early palliative care with anti-cancer treatment improve overall survival and patient-related outcomes in advanced lung cancer patients? A review of the literature. Support Care Cancer 26: 2945–2953

Assfalg V, Hüser N, Michalski C, Gillen S, Kleeff J, Friess H (2011) Palliative interventional and surgical therapy for unresectable pancreatic cancer. Cancers (Basel) 3:652–661

Bakitas MA, Tosteson TD, Li Z, Lyons KD, Hull JG, Li Z, Dionne-Odom JN, Frost J, Dragnev KH, Hegel MT, Azuero A, Ahles TA (2015) Early versus delayed initiation of concurrent palliative oncology care: patient outcomes in the ENABLE III randomized controlled trial. J Clin Oncol 33:1438–1445

Bergenholtz H, Weibull A, Raunkiær M (2022) Supportive and palliative care indicators tool (SPICT™) in a Danish healthcare context: translation, cross-cultural adaptation, and content validation. BMC Palliat Care 21:41

Borgsteede SD, Deliens L, van der Wal G, Francke AL, Stalman WA, van Eijk JT (2007) Interdisciplinary cooperation of GPs in palliative care at home: a nationwide survey in The Netherlands. Scand J Prim Health Care 25:226–231

Borneman T, Koczywas M, Cristea M, Reckamp K, Sun V, Ferrell B (2008) An interdisciplinary care approach for integration of palliative care in lung cancer. Clin Lung Cancer 9:352–360

Bowen L (2014) The multidisciplinary team in palliative care: a case reflection. Indian J Palliat Care 20:142

Brennan MJ (1993) Overview of physiatric approaches to cancer pain. J Back Musculoskelet Rehabil 3:53–59

Brighton LJ, Miller S, Farquhar M, Booth S, Yi D, Gao W, Bajwah S, Man WD, Higginson IJ, Maddocks M (2019) Holistic services for people with advanced disease and chronic breathlessness: a systematic review and meta-analysis. Thorax 74:270–281

Carmont SA, Mitchell G, Senior H, Foster M (2018) Systematic review of the effectiveness, barriers and facilitators to general practitioner engagement with specialist secondary services in integrated palliative care. BMJ Support Palliat Care 8:385–399

Cheng BT, Rost M, De Clercq E, Arnold L, Elger BS, Wangmo T (2019) Palliative care initiation in pediatric oncology patients: a systematic review. Cancer Med 8:3–12

Clark D (2007) From margins to centre: a review of the history of palliative care in cancer. Lancet Oncol 8:430–438
Crawford GB, Price SD (2003) Team working: palliative care as a model of interdisciplinary practice. Med J Aust 179:S32
Delgado E, Barfield RC, Baker JN, Hinds PS, Yang J, Nambayan A, Quintana Y, Kane JR (2010) Availability of palliative care services for children with cancer in economically diverse regions of the world. Eur J Cancer 46:2260–2266
Desa V, Danjoux C, Matyas Y, Fitch M, Husain A, Horvath N, Myers J, Clemons M, Hux JE, Barnes EA (2008) An interdisciplinary and collaborative initiative in palliative care research. J Pain Res 2:1–3
Dowling M, Fahy P, Houghton C, Smalle M (2020) A qualitative evidence synthesis of healthcare professionals' experiences and views of palliative care for patients with a haematological malignancy. Eur J Cancer Care (Engl) 29. https://doi.org/10.1111/ecc.13316
Drageset S, Austrheim G, Ellingsen S (2021) Quality of life of women living with metastatic breast cancer and receiving palliative care: a systematic review. Health Care Women Int 42:1044–1065
Duncan J, Spengler E, Wolfe J (2007) Providing pediatric palliative care: PACT in action. MCN Am J Matern Child Nurs 32:279–287
Enguidanos SM, Cherin D, Brumley R (2005) Home-based palliative care study: site of death, and costs of medical care for patients with congestive heart failure, chronic obstructive pulmonary disease, and cancer. J Soc Work End Life Palliat Care 1:37–56
Ezeoke CC, Morley JE (2015) Pathophysiology of anorexia in the cancer cachexia syndrome. J Cachexia Sarcopenia Muscle 6:287–302
Fadol AP, Patel A, Shelton V, Krause KJ, Bruera E, Palaskas NL (2021) Palliative care referral criteria and outcomes in cancer and heart failure: a systematic review of literature. Cardiooncology 7:32
Ferrell BR, Chu DZ, Wagman L, Juarez G, Borneman T, Cullinane C, McCahill LE (2003) Online exclusive: patient and surgeon decision making regarding surgery for advanced cancer. Oncol Nurs Forum 30:E106–E114
Ferris FD, Bruera E, Cherny N, Cummings C, Currow D, Dudgeon D, Janjan N, Strasser F, von Gunten CF, Von Roenn JH (2009) Palliative cancer care a decade later: accomplishments, the need, next steps – from the American Society of Clinical Oncology. J Clin Oncol 27:3052–3058
Fulton JJ, LeBlanc TW, Cutson TM, Porter Starr KN, Kamal A, Ramos K, Freiermuth CE, McDuffie JR, Kosinski A, Adam S, Nagi A, Williams JW (2019) Integrated outpatient palliative care for patients with advanced cancer: a systematic review and meta-analysis. Palliat Med 33:123–134
Gelfman LP, Meier DE, Morrison RS (2008) Does palliative care improve quality? A survey of bereaved family members. J Pain Symptom Manag 36:22–28
Gilligan T, Coyle N, Frankel RM, Berry DL, Bohlke K, Epstein RM, Finlay E, Jackson VA, Lathan CS, Loprinzi CL, Nguyen LH, Seigel C, Baile WF (2017) Patient-clinician communication: American Society of Clinical Oncology consensus guideline. J Clin Oncol 35:3618–3632
Granda-Cameron C, DeMille D, Lynch MP, Huntzinger C, Alcorn T, Levicoff J, Roop C, Mintzer D (2010) An interdisciplinary approach to manage cancer cachexia. Clin J Oncol Nurs 14:72–80
Groenvold M, Petersen MA, Damkier A, Neergaard MA, Nielsen JB, Pedersen L, Sjøgren P, Strömgren AS, Vejlgaard TB, Gluud C (2017) Randomised clinical trial of early specialist palliative care plus standard care versus standard care alone in patients with advanced cancer: the Danish Palliative Care Trial. Palliat Med 31:814–824
Hanson LC, Usher B, Spragens L, Bernard S (2008) Clinical and economic impact of palliative care consultation. J Pain Symptom Manag 35:340–346
Hirai K, Morita T, Kashiwagi T (2003) Professionally perceived effectiveness of psychosocial interventions for existential suffering of terminally ill cancer patients. Palliat Med 17:688–694
Hoerger M, Wayser GR, Schwing G, Suzuki A, Perry LM (2019) Impact of interdisciplinary outpatient specialty palliative care on survival and quality of life in adults with advanced cancer: a meta-analysis of randomized controlled trials. Ann Behav Med 53:674–685

Horne-Thompson A, Daveson B, Hogan B (2007) A project investigating music therapy referral trends within palliative care: an Australian perspective. J Music Ther 44:139–155
Hui D, Bruera E (2016) Integrating palliative care into the trajectory of cancer care. Nat Rev Clin Oncol 13:159–171
Hui D, Elsayem A, De La Cruz M, Berger A, Zhukovsky DS, Palla S, Evans A, Fadul N, Palmer JL, Bruera E (2010) Availability and integration of palliative care at US cancer centers. JAMA 303: 1054–1061
Hui D, De La Cruz M, Mori M, Parsons HA, Kwon JH, Torres-Vigil I, Kim SH, Dev R, Hutchins R, Liem C (2013) Concepts and definitions for "supportive care," "best supportive care," "palliative care," and "hospice care" in the published literature, dictionaries, and textbooks. Support Care Cancer 21:659–685
Hui D, Bansal S, Strasser F, Morita T, Caraceni A, Davis M, Cherny N, Kaasa S, Currow D, Abernethy A (2015a) Indicators of integration of oncology and palliative care programs: an international consensus. Ann Oncol 26:1953–1959
Hui D, Kim YJ, Park JC, Zhang Y, Strasser F, Cherny N, Kaasa S, Davis MP, Bruera E (2015b) Integration of oncology and palliative care: a systematic review. Oncologist 20:77–83
Hung Y-S, Wu J-H, Chang H, Wang P-N, Kao C-Y, Wang H-M, Liau C-T, Chen J-S, Lin Y-C, Su P-J (2013) Characteristics of patients with hematologic malignancies who received palliative care consultation services in a medical center. Am J Hosp Palliat Med 30:773–780
Isikhan V (2010) Coping with stress in patients with advanced cancer. Asian Pac J Cancer Prev 11(Suppl 1):81–92
Johnson AP, Abernathy T, Howell D, Brazil K, Scott S (2009) Resource utilisation and costs of palliative cancer care in an interdisciplinary health care model. Palliat Med 23:448–459
Jordan RI, Allsop MJ, ElMokhallalati Y, Jackson CE, Edwards HL, Chapman EJ, Deliens L, Bennett MI (2020) Duration of palliative care before death in international routine practice: a systematic review and meta-analysis. BMC Med 18:368
Jordhøy MS, Fayers P, Saltnes T, Ahlner-Elmqvist M, Jannert M, Kaasa S (2000) A palliative-care intervention and death at home: a cluster randomised trial. Lancet 356:888–893
Kaasa S, Loge JH, Aapro M, Albreht T, Anderson R, Bruera E, Brunelli C, Caraceni A, Cervantes A, Currow DC (2018) Integration of oncology and palliative care: a Lancet Oncology Commission. Lancet Oncol 19:e588–e653
Kassianos AP, Ioannou M, Koutsantoni M, Charalambous H (2018) The impact of specialized palliative care on cancer patients' health-related quality of life: a systematic review and meta-analysis. Support Care Cancer 26:61–79
Kaye EC, Weaver MS, DeWitt LH, Byers E, Stevens SE, Lukowski J, Shih B, Zalud K, Applegarth J, Wong H-N, Baker JN, Ullrich CK (2021) The impact of specialty palliative care in pediatric oncology: a systematic review. J Pain Symptom Manag 61:1060–1079.e1062
Kochovska S, Ferreira DH, Luckett T, Phillips JL, Currow DC (2020) Earlier multidisciplinary palliative care intervention for people with lung cancer: a systematic review and meta-analysis. Transl Lung Cancer Res 9:1699–1709
Kurashima AY, Latorre Mdo R, Teixeira SA, De Camargo B (2005) Factors associated with location of death of children with cancer in palliative care. Palliat Support Care 3:115–119
Le Rouzic MA, Claudot F (2020) Characteristics of parental decision-making for children with advanced cancer who are offered enrollment in early-phase clinical trials: a systematic review. Pediatr Hematol Oncol 37:500–529
Levorato A, Stiefel F, Mazzocato C, Bruera E (2001) Communication with terminal cancer patients in palliative care: are there differences between nurses and physicians? Support Care Cancer 9:420–427
London MR, McSkimming S, Drew N, Quinn C, Carney B (2005) Evaluation of a comprehensive, adaptable, life- affirming, longitudinal (CALL) palliative care project. J Palliat Med 8: 1214–1225
Lowe SS (2011) Physical activity and palliative cancer care. Recent Results Cancer Res 186: 349–365

Maltoni M, Scarpi E, Dall'Agata M, Schiavon S, Biasini C, Codecà C, Broglia CM, Sansoni E, Bortolussi R, Garetto F (2016) Systematic versus on-demand early palliative care: a randomised clinical trial assessing quality of care and treatment aggressiveness near the end of life. Eur J Cancer 69:110–118

May P, Normand C, Cassel JB, Del Fabbro E, Fine RL, Menz R, Morrison CA, Penrod JD, Robinson C, Morrison RS (2018) Economics of palliative care for hospitalized adults with serious illness: a meta-analysis. JAMA Intern Med 178:820–829

Moosavi S, Borhani F, Akbari ME, Sanee N, Rohani C (2020) Recommendations for spiritual care in cancer patients: a clinical practice guideline for oncology nurses in Iran. Support Care Cancer 28:5381–5395

Mor V, Masterson-Allen S (1990) A comparison of hospice vs conventional care of the terminally ill cancer patient. Oncology (Williston Park) 4:85–91; discussion 94, 96

O'Connor M, Fisher C, Guilfoyle A (2006) Interdisciplinary teams in palliative care: a critical reflection. Int J Palliat Nurs 12:132–137

Osman H, Shrestha S, Temin S, Ali ZV, Corvera RA, Ddungu HD, De Lima L, Del Pilar Estevez-Diz M, Ferris FD, Gafer N, Gupta HK, Horton S, Jacob G, Jia R, Lu FL, Mosoiu D, Puchalski C, Seigel C, Soyannwo O, Cleary JF (2018) Palliative care in the global setting: ASCO resource-stratified practice guideline. J Glob Oncol 4:1–24

Ostgathe C, Gaertner J, Kotterba M, Klein S, Lindena G, Nauck F, Radbruch L, Voltz R (2010) Differential palliative care issues in patients with primary and secondary brain tumours. Support Care Cancer 18:1157–1163

Papadatou D (1997) Training health professionals in caring for dying children and grieving families. Death Stud 21:575–600

Piette V, Beernaert K, Cohen J, Pauwels NS, Scherrens AL, van der Werff Ten Bosch J, Deliens L (2021) Healthcare interventions improving and reducing quality of life in children at the end of life: a systematic review. Pediatr Res 89:1065–1077

Radbruch L, De Lima L, Knaul F, Wenk R, Ali Z, Bhatnaghar S, Blanchard C, Bruera E, Buitrago R, Burla C, Callaway M, Munyoro EC, Centeno C, Cleary J, Connor S, Davaasuren O, Downing J, Foley K, Goh C, Gomez-Garcia W, Harding R, Khan QT, Larkin P, Leng M, Luyirika E, Marston J, Moine S, Osman H, Pettus K, Puchalski C, Rajagopal MR, Spence D, Spruijt O, Venkateswaran C, Wee B, Woodruff R, Yong J, Pastrana T (2020) Redefining palliative care – a new consensus-based definition. J Pain Symptom Manag 60: 754–764

Renz M, Schütt Mao M, Cerny T (2005) Spirituality, psychotherapy and music in palliative cancer care: research projects in psycho-oncology at an oncology center in Switzerland. Support Care Cancer 13:961–966

Robert R, Stavinoha P, Jones BL, Robinson J, Larson K, Hicklen R, Smith B, Perko K, Koch K, Findley S, Weaver MS (2019) Spiritual assessment and spiritual care offerings as a standard of care in pediatric oncology: a recommendation informed by a systematic review of the literature. Pediatr Blood Cancer 66:e27764

Rodin G, Malfitano C, Rydall A, Schimmer A, Marmar CM, Mah K, Lo C, Nissim R, Zimmermann C (2020) Emotion And Symptom-focused Engagement (EASE): a randomized phase II trial of an integrated psychological and palliative care intervention for patients with acute leukemia. Support Care Cancer 28:163–176

Salins N, Ghoshal A, Hughes S, Preston N (2020) How views of oncologists and haematologists impacts palliative care referral: a systematic review. BMC Palliat Care 19:175

Scott JF (1982) Pain treatment in a palliative unit or team of a university hospital. Acta Anaesthesiol Scand Suppl 74:119–123

Selvaggi KJ, Vick JB, Jessell SA, Lister J, Abrahm JL, Bernacki R (2014) Bridging the gap: a palliative care consultation service in a hematological malignancy-bone marrow transplant unit. J Community Support Oncol 12:50–55

Shao J, Rodrigues M, Corter AL, Baxter NN (2019) Multidisciplinary care of breast cancer patients: a scoping review of multidisciplinary styles, processes, and outcomes. Curr Oncol 26:385–397

Sinclair S, Raffin S, Pereira J, Guebert N (2006) Collective soul: the spirituality of an interdisciplinary palliative care team. Palliat Support Care 4:13–24

Sinclair S, Mysak M, Hagen NA (2009) What are the core elements of oncology spiritual care programs? Palliat Support Care 7:415–422

Smith RD, Mallath MK (2019) History of the growing burden of cancer in India: from antiquity to the 21st century. J Glob Oncol 5:1–15

Strasser F, Bruera ED (2002) Update on anorexia and cachexia. Hematol Oncol Clin North Am 16:589–617

Tanzi S, Venturelli F, Luminari S, Merlo FD, Braglia L, Bassi C, Costantini M (2020) Early palliative care in haematological patients: a systematic literature review. BMJ Support Palliat Care 10:395–403

Temel JS, Greer JA, Muzikansky A, Gallagher ER, Admane S, Jackson VA, Dahlin CM, Blinderman CD, Jacobsen J, Pirl WF, Billings JA, Lynch TJ (2010) Early palliative care for patients with metastatic non-small-cell lung cancer. N Engl J Med 363:733–742

Temel JS, Greer JA, El-Jawahri A, Pirl WF, Park ER, Jackson VA, Back AL, Kamdar M, Jacobsen J, Chittenden EH (2017) Effects of early integrated palliative care in patients with lung and GI cancer: a randomized clinical trial. J Clin Oncol 35:834

Van Mechelen W, Aertgeerts B, De Ceulaer K, Thoonsen B, Vermandere M, Warmenhoven F, Van Rijswijk E, De Lepeleire J (2013) Defining the palliative care patient: a systematic review. Palliat Med 27:197–208

Verger E, Conill C, Pedro A, Chicote S, Salamero M, de Azpiazu P, Gil E, Biete A (1992) Palliative care in cancer patients. Frequency and priority of symptoms. Med Clin (Barc) 99:565–567

Willemsen AM, Mason S, Zhang S, Elsner F (2021) Status of palliative care education in Mainland China: a systematic review. Palliat Support Care 19:235–245

Wolfe J, Friebert S, Hilden J (2002) Caring for children with advanced cancer integrating palliative care. Pediatr Clin N Am 49:1043–1062

Zimmermann C, Swami N, Krzyzanowska M, Hannon B, Leighl N, Oza A, Moore M, Rydall A, Rodin G, Tannock I (2014) Early palliative care for patients with advanced cancer: a cluster-randomised controlled trial. Lancet 383:1721–1730

Correction to: Cancer: A Complex Problem Requiring Interdisciplinary Research

Niloufar Yazdanpanah, Filip Dochy, Gary L. Darmstadt, Godefridus J. Peters, Abraham Tsitlakidis, Elias C. Aifantis, Artemi Cerda, Elisabetta Comini, Serge Brand, Manoj Gupta, Bruce D. Cheson, Sabu Thomas, Michael Tanzer, Ralf Weiskirchen, Federico Bella, Seyed-Mohammad Fereshtehnejad, Konstantina Nikita, Imran Ali, Koichi Kato, Alessandro Poggi, Ernest Chua Kian Jon, Idupulapati M. Rao, Xiaoming Tao, Ji-Huan He, Lingamallu Jagan Mohan Rao, Alexander Leemans, Alessio Pomponio, Alfredo Martínez Hernandez, Hamid Ahmadieh, Mohammad Ali Sahraian, Roya Kelishadi, Visith Thongboonkerd, Seema Bahinipati, Masakazu Toi, Matthias von Herrath, Frank Sellke, Steven Sherwood, George Perry, Juan J. Nieto, Sudhir Gupta, Tommaso Dorigo, Bahram Mobasher, Hans D. Ochs, and Nima Rezaei

1 Correction to: Chapter "Cancer: A Complex Problem Requiring Interdisciplinary Research" in: N. Yazdanpanah et al., Interdisciplinary Cancer Research, https://doi.org/10.1007/16833_2022_116

In the published chapter, the affiliation "Universal Scientific Education and Research Network (USERN)" was incorrectly written as "Universal Scientific Education and Research Network (USERN); the World, Tehran, Iran". USERN is a network and does not belong to a specific country. This affiliation has now been corrected for all authors who were affiliated to it, to read as,

Universal Scientific Education and Research Network (USERN), https://usern.tums.ac.ir/

The updated original version of this chapter can be found at https://doi.org/10.1007/16833_2022_116

Interdisciplinary Cancer Research, https://doi.org/10.1007/16833_2023_173

Index

A
Ablation, 200, 344, 346–359, 362, 363, 367
Acute kidney injury (AKI), 159, 165–177, 179, 260
Acute tubulo-interstitial nephritis (ATIN), 159, 165–179
Antibody, 5, 21, 24, 30, 49–51, 53, 56, 57, 59, 60, 65–79, 118, 124, 132, 136, 139, 173, 191, 192, 200, 201, 203, 208, 253, 254, 258–260, 262, 271–274
Anticancer, vii, 9, 18, 20, 28, 56, 127, 158, 159, 189, 217–247, 385–388
Antitumor immunotherapy, 78, 251–263
Autoimmune disorders, 21, 268, 272–276

B
Biomarkers, 8, 28, 33, 54, 59–60, 92, 93, 99, 101–108, 110, 159, 173–175, 178, 179, 257
Biopsy, 59, 93, 95, 97, 101, 108, 110, 166, 172, 173, 344–346, 366, 367
Bone augmentation, 363

C
Cancer, 3, 47, 65, 92, 118, 158, 186, 217, 256, 268, 288, 324, 343, 384, 400
Cancer stem cells (CSCs), vii, 185–194, 384–385, 388
Cell therapy, vii, 21, 33, 55, 117–145, 261
Checkpoint blockade, 48, 260
Chimeric antigen receptor (CAR), vii, 5, 30, 33, 55, 56, 60, 65, 72–74, 76, 117–145, 192, 193
Combinational approaches, 385–387
Combination therapy, 16, 66, 69, 71, 73, 76, 77, 121–131, 139, 141, 142, 186, 192, 193
Complex problem, vii, 1–34
COVID-19, vii, 251–263
Cytotoxic T-lymphocyte-associated protein 4 (CTLA-4), 54, 55, 65, 67–69, 71, 72, 74, 77, 106, 110, 121, 124, 129, 138, 142, 144, 159, 160, 162, 164, 167, 193, 260, 268–273, 278, 279

D
Dendritic cells (DCs), 48, 50, 52, 58, 59, 66, 68, 70, 71, 73–77, 80, 95, 99, 104, 108, 122, 123, 125–127, 129, 190, 192, 200, 201, 205, 207, 254, 269, 271, 294
Design strategies, 33, 127
Diagnosis, 8, 12–15, 17, 18, 22–24, 26–29, 165, 168, 170–175, 344, 345, 404, 409, 413

E
Embolization, 344, 356–360
Enrichment, 200, 201, 203–204, 206–207

G
Graft manipulation, 200, 206
Graft-*versus*-host disease (GVHD), 132, 135, 200, 203–210

H
Hematopoietic stem cell transplantation (HSCT), 135, 200, 203–209, 261
Hyperbaric oxygen therapy (HBOT), vii, 323–337

Interdisciplinary Cancer Research, https://doi.org/10.1007/978-3-031-43983-4

I

Immune checkpoint, 54, 65–75, 106, 128, 129, 159, 161, 163, 169, 260, 262
Immune checkpoint inhibitor (ICIs), vii, 21, 30, 33, 54, 55, 59, 60, 65, 66, 69, 70, 72, 74, 76, 77, 79, 80, 106–108, 128–129, 157–179, 191, 259, 261–263, 268, 271–278, 280
Immune resistance, 65, 68, 77
Immunity, vii, 27, 48, 50, 51, 53–54, 79–80, 100, 123, 189, 204–208, 237, 253, 254, 256, 262, 270
Immuno-oncology, vii, 63–80
Immunotherapy, vii, 3, 5, 21, 23, 47–60, 65–67, 69, 72, 73, 76–78, 80, 93, 105–107, 110, 118, 122, 125, 127, 163, 171, 174, 176–178, 186, 190–194, 259–263, 267–280
Integrated palliative cancer care, vii, 399–417
Interdisciplinary, vii, 1–34, 343, 348, 399–417

K

Kidney biopsy, 165–167, 171–173, 179

L

Low-dose radiation (LDR), 290, 292, 298, 299, 309–312

M

Molecular docking, 222, 228–233, 236, 238

N

Nanoparticle, 13, 387
Nephrotoxicity, 158, 159, 165–167, 178

O

Onconephrology, 158

P

Palliative care (PC), 289, 362, 400–417
Phytochemicals, vii, 383–388
Prognostic biomarkers, 92, 93, 103–107, 351
Programmed cell death receptor 1, 106, 268, 271–272

Q

Quality of life, 5, 7, 23, 24, 26, 33, 293, 324, 362, 364, 406
Quinoline, vii, 217–247

R

Rejection, 164, 177, 178, 191, 200, 205, 209
Research, 7, 48, 65, 93, 122, 158, 258, 333, 350, 384, 402

S

Stem cell, vii, 57, 189, 200, 204, 206, 209, 259, 299, 310, 385, 387, 388
Survival, 16, 20, 24, 28, 54, 65, 76, 77, 92, 94, 98–108, 127, 129–131, 135, 139, 163, 178, 179, 192, 193, 206, 208, 209, 257, 299, 309, 310, 329–331, 333, 349–355, 359, 361, 362, 402, 406, 408

T

T-cell depletion (TCD), 71, 201–203, 205, 206, 208
T-cell response, 140, 190, 192, 205, 208, 254, 262
Tissue repair, 207
Transdisciplinary, 7, 26
Treatment, 3, 47, 66, 92, 118, 158, 186, 205, 218, 256, 268, 288, 324, 344, 384, 400
Tumor, 3, 48, 65, 92, 118, 158, 186, 208, 221, 256, 268, 289, 325, 344, 384, 401
Tumor-infiltrating lymphocytes (TILs), vii, 55, 60, 91–110, 118, 192
Tumor-initiating cells (TICs), 186
Tumor microenvironment (TME), 5, 17, 19, 25, 56–58, 60, 63–80, 92, 93, 96, 103, 119, 121, 123, 125, 127, 130, 131, 138, 141, 160, 189, 270, 331

W

Wound healing, vii, 287–313

SPRINGER NATURE

GPSR Compliance

The European Union's (EU) General Product Safety Regulation (GPSR) is a set of rules that requires consumer products to be safe and our obligations to ensure this.

If you have any concerns about our products, you can contact us on ProductSafety@springernature.com

In case Publisher is established outside the EU, the EU authorized representative is:

Springer Nature Customer Service Center GmbH
Europaplatz 3
69115 Heidelberg, Germany

MIX
Papier | Fördert gute Waldnutzung
FSC® C083411

Kolibri 360 GmbH
Ferdinand-Jühlke-Straße 7
99095 Erfurt, Deutschland
produktsicherheit@kolibri360.de